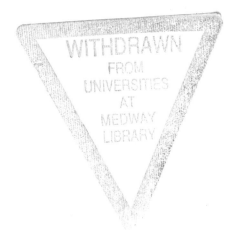

The Handbook of the Neuropsychology of Language

Volume 1
Language Processing in the Brain: Basic Science

Wiley-Blackwell Handbooks of Behavioral Neuroscience

The rapidly expanding field of behavioral neuroscience examines neurobiological aspects of behavior, utilizing techniques from molecular biology, neuropsychology, and psychology. This series of handbooks provides a cutting-edge overview of classic research, current scholarship, and future trends in behavioral neuroscience. The series provides a survey of representative topics in this field, suggesting implications for basic research and clinical applications.

Series editor: David Mostofsky, Boston University

The Handbook of Stress: Neuropsychological Effects on the Brain
Edited by Cheryl D. Conrad

The Handbook of Alzheimer's Disease and Other Dementias
Edited by Neil W. Kowall and Andrew E. Budson

The Handbook of the Neuropsychology of Language (2 Volumes)
Edited by Miriam Faust

The Handbook of the Neuropsychology of Language

Edited by Miriam Faust

Volume 1

Language Processing in the Brain: Basic Science

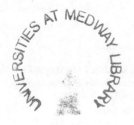

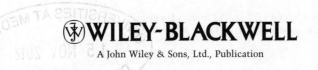

⊛WILEY-BLACKWELL

A John Wiley & Sons, Ltd., Publication

Library of Congress Cataloging-in-Publication Data

The handbook of the neuropsychology of language / edited by Miriam Faust.
    p. ; cm. – (Wiley-Blackwell handbooks of behavioral neuroscience)
  Includes bibliographical references and index.
  ISBN 978-1-4443-3040-3 (hardcover : alk. paper)
1. Neurolinguistics–Handbooks, manuals, etc.   I. Faust, Miriam.   II. Series: Wiley-Blackwell handbooks of behavioral neuroscience.
  [DNLM: 1. Language.   2. Neuropsychology–methods.   3. Brain–physiology.   4. Linguistics–methods.   WL 103.5]
  QP399.H365 2012
  612.8'2336–dc23

                          2011019728

A catalogue record for this book is available from the British Library.

This book is published in the following electronic formats: ePDFs 9781444345872; Wiley Online Library 9781444345902; ePub 9781444345889; mobi 9781444345896

Set in 10.5/13 pt Minion by Toppan Best-set Premedia Limited
Printed and bound in Singapore by Markono Print Media Pte Ltd

1   2012

I dedicate this book with love to the memory of my father, Professor Joseph Alexander Stein, who inspired me with a passion for knowledge, and to the memory of my mother, Yemima Gottesdiener-Stein, who provided me with the support and strength that enabled me to persist in my pursuit of this passion. A significant part of my accomplishments are theirs.

Contents

Volume 2   Language Processing in the Brain: Clinical Populations

Contributors

Jubin Abutalebi is a cognitive neurologist and an assistant professor of neuropsychology at the San Raffaele University in Milan. His main research activities focus on the cerebral architecture underlying bilingualism, which he studies by employing functional neuroimaging techniques.

Merav Ahissar works in the Department of Psychology, Center for Neural Computations and ELSC Center for Brain Research, The Hebrew University. Her research focuses on linking between behavioral patterns and neural mechanisms of perceptual and cognitive plasticity. She is interested in the relations between learning difficulties and perceptual and memory mechanisms.

Michael Andric is a graduate student in the Department of Psychology at the University of Chicago. He researches brain function in language processing and motor behaviors such as gesture.

Blair C. Armstrong is a graduate student in the PhD program of the Department of Psychology and the Center for the Neural Basis of Cognition at Carnegie Mellon University in Pittsburgh, Pennsylvania. His research involves using behavioral studies and computational modeling to examine the temporal dynamics of word comprehension and decision processes, and how these adapt in response to feedback.

Errol H. Baker, PhD, located at the VA Boston Healthcare System, is currently the biostatistician to the Research Office and to a VA Research Center of Excellence (Center for Organization, Leadership, and Management Research). He joined the Harold Goodglass Boston University Aphasia Research Center in 1971, and has collaborated with Dr Margaret Naeser since 1977. His research has focused on cognitive processes in patients with aphasia, and led to the development of a computer-based alternative communication system for severely impaired patients (C-ViC).

Juliana V. Baldo is a research neuropsychologist at Veterans Affairs Northern California Medical Center, where she is also the Associate Director of the Center for Aphasia and Related Disorders. Her work focuses on the neural basis of memory and language. She has worked primarily with brain-injured patients and has used a variety of structural neuroimaging techniques to better characterize brain regions critical for mediating specific cognitive processes. Dr Baldo's work has also addressed how those cognitive processes interact with each other, such as the critical role that language plays in higher reasoning.

Karen Banai, PhD, works at the Department of Communication Sciences and Disorders, University of Haifa. Her research focuses on the interaction between perceptual and cognitive skills in typical and atypical populations and on whether the perception of linguistic and nonlinguistic attributes can be explained by shared mechanisms. She is also interested in perceptual learning and development.

Kathleen Baynes is Professor of Neurology in the Center for Mind and Brain at the University of California, Davis. She studies language processing with a particular focus on understanding language changes after neurological damage. She researches how language is lateralized in the brain by studying healthy young adults, left and right hemisphere focal lesioned patients, and split-brain patients. In recent research, she has been developing intervention programs to support the recovery of naming disorders.

Mark Beeman is an associate professor in the Psychology Department at Northwestern University.

Jeffrey R. Binder is Director of the Language Imaging Laboratory at the Medical College of Wisconsin. His research examines the neural basis of normal language processes and applications of language mapping in neurological patients.

Jesse Bledsoe, MA, is a doctoral candidate in clinical psychology at Michigan State University. Currently, he is a psychology resident at the University of Washington School of Medicine and Seattle Children's Hospital. His master's thesis examined neuropsychological aspects of ADHD and his doctoral dissertation will examine cortical thickness in children with ADHD on and off medication. He has presented this work at several national and international conferences.

Katy Borodkin, PhD, is a research associate in the Department of Psychology, Bar Ilan University. Her research focuses on individual differences in second-language acquisition.

Hiram Brownell received his PhD in psychology from the Johns Hopkins University. His research interests include language, language disorders, and treatment approaches, with a focus on the role of the right hemisphere.

Deborah M. Burke is the W. M. Keck Distinguished Service Professor at Pomona College, Claremont, CA. Her research focuses on cognitive aging, especially aging-related change in language production and the neural substrate.

Cristina Cacciari is full Professor of Psychology at the Department of Biomedical Sciences at the University of Modena. Her research interests concern language comprehension from behavioral and brain-based perspectives.

Christine Chiarello is Professor of Psychology at the University of California, Riverside. She received her PhD from the University of California, Berkeley. Her research explores the unique role of the right hemisphere in language comprehension, specifically processes of meaning access and retrieval, and visual word recognition. More recent interests include individual differences in brain organization for language, and biologically informed models of human variation.

Joanna A. Christodoulou, EdD, conducts research at the intersection of education and cognitive neuroscience, with a focus on reading development and difficulties, and works clinically with struggling students. She has an EdD in human development and psychology from the Harvard Graduate School of Education (HGSE), an EdM in mind, brain, and education from HGSE, and an MA in child development from Tufts University. She is a postdoctoral associate in the Gabrieli Laboratory in the Department of Brain and Cognitive Sciences at Massachusetts Institute of Technology.

Dorothee Chwilla is a cognitive neuroscientist in the field of language at the Donders Institute for Brain, Cognition, and Behavior. She investigates semantic, syntactic, and prosodic processes in language comprehension across contexts (single words, sentences, and discourse). Recent research areas are the processing of semantics in a second language and the interactions of language and attention and of language and emotion.

Henri Cohen is editor of the *Journal of Neurolinguistics* and associate editor of *Brain and Cognition*. He holds appointments in the departments of psychology at Université du Québec, Montreal, and at Université Paris Descartes where he served as Director of Laboratoire de Psychologie et Neurosciences Cognitives (UMR8189 – CNRS). His research interests are wide and include language and speech production in normal and brain-damaged populations, cognition and emotion in movement disorders, the role of complexity in learning and consolidation, among others. He is the organizer or co-organizer of several international conferences, including the 2011 IASCL conference in Montreal. He is fortunate in his collaborations with exciting colleagues in many parts of the world. When he has time, he loves to scuba dive, travel to exotic places, and practice photography.

Max Coltheart is Emeritus Professor of Cognitive Science at Macquarie University in Sydney, having held previous positions elsewhere in Australia and also in Canada and England. He works on normal and impaired processes of reading and spelling (including computational modeling), and also on delusional beliefs.

Lisa Tabor Connor, PhD, is Assistant Professor of Occupational Therapy, Radiology, and Neurology at Washington University School of Medicine. She received her PhD in experimental psychology from Washington University and completed postdoctoral fellowships at the Georgia Institute of Technology in cognitive aging and Boston University School of Medicine in adult communicative disorders. Her research focuses on language and cognitive rehabilitation, and reintegration of people with aphasia into the community after stroke.

Seana Coulson is Associate Professor in the Cognitive Science Department at the University of California, San Diego, where she heads the Brain and Cognition Laboratory. She is the author of *Semantic Leaps* (2001).

Tristan S. Davenport is a graduate student in the Cognitive Science Department at the University of California, San Diego. Advised by Seana Coulson, his primary research interest is the neural basis of semantic processing.

Annette M. B. de Groot is Professor of Experimental Psycholinguistics at the University of Amsterdam. She completed a master's degree in general linguistics and a doctorate in psycholinguistics at the University of Nijmegen, the Netherlands. Her present research focuses on bilingualism, with a special interest in bilingual word processing, foreign language vocabulary learning, and simultaneous interpreting.

Pasquale Anthony Della Rosa, PhD, is a post-doc at the Psychology Faculty of the University San Raffaele. His research activities are mainly based on functional neuroimaging studies of cognitive functions.

Rutvik H. Desai is Assistant Professor of Neurology at the Medical College of Wisconsin. His research investigates the neural basis of language and speech processing, with emphasis on the relationship between conceptual processing and sensori-motor systems.

Ton Dijkstra holds a Chair in Psycholinguistics and Multilingualism and is head of the Division of Psycholinguistics in the Donders Centre for Cognition, part of the Donders Institute for Brain, Cognition, and Behavior at Radboud University Nijmegen, the Netherlands.

Nina F. Dronkers is Director of the Center for Aphasia and Related Disorders at the Department of Veterans Affairs Northern California Health Care System and professor of neurology at the University of California, Davis. She specializes in the study of aphasia and other language and communication disorders that can occur with neurological disease. Her research, concerning the localization of language functions in the brain, uses lesion–symptom mapping to assess the relationship between patients' specific behavioral deficits and the areas of the brain that were injured.

Andrew W. Ellis is Professor of Psychology at the University of York, UK. He is interested in the psychology of word recognition and production in both healthy speakers/listeners and people with neuropsychological conditions such as aphasia and dementia. He also has an interest in object and face recognition. His current research combines cognitive, neuropsychological, and neuroimaging approaches, including the use of magnetoencephalography to explore the time course of processing within the brain.

Zohar Eviatar is Associate Professor in the Psychology Department and a member of the Institute for Information Processing and Decision Making, at the University of Haifa, Israel.

Franco Fabbro is full Professor of Developmental Neuropsychiatry at the University of Udine (Italy) and scientific director at the Research Institute E. Medea in San Vito al Tagliamento, Italy. He is author of a number of books and articles in peer-reviewed journals.

Miriam Faust, PhD, is Professor of Psychology in the Department of Psychology and the director of the Brain and Language Laboratory in the Gonda Center for Brain Research at Bar-Ilan University. She studies language processing, focusing mainly on semantic processing by the two cerebral hemispheres, word retrieval, and phonological processing. Two of her recent research projects focus on the neural bases of verbal creativity and on individual differences in foreign language attainment.

Kara D. Federmeier received her PhD in cognitive science from the University of California, San Diego. She is currently an associate professor in the Department of Psychology and the Program in Neuroscience at the University of Illinois and head of the Cognition and Brain Laboratory, located in the Beckman Institute for Advanced Science and Technology.

Patricia Marinaro Fitzpatrick, PhD, CCC-SLP, is a research speech/language pathologist at the Harold Goodglass Aphasia Research Center affiliated with the Department of Neurology at the Boston University School of Medicine and the Boston VA Healthcare System. She received her MSc from the University of Pittsburgh and her PhD from Emerson College. Her research focuses on treatment of aphasia, quality of life issues, and long-term recovery from aphasia.

John D. E. Gabrieli, PhD, is Professor of Health Sciences and Technology and Cognitive Neuroscience at the Massachusetts Institute of Technology (MIT). He has a dual appointment in the Harvard-MIT Division of Health Sciences and Technology and in the Department of Brain and Cognitive Sciences. He is Director of the Imaging Center at the McGovern Institute for Brain Research and co-director of the MIT Clinical Research Center. He has a BA in English from Yale and a PhD in behavioral neuroscience from MIT, and was a postdoctoral fellow in the Psychology Department at Harvard. His area of research is human cognitive neuroscience, in which he studies the brain basis of memory, language, and thought.

Morton Ann Gernsbacher is Vilas Research Professor and Sir Frederic Bartlett Professor at the University of Wisconsin–Madison, USA.

Matthew Goldrick is Associate Professor of Linguistics at Northwestern University, Evanston, Illinois, where he is affiliated with the Northwestern Cognitive Science Program and Northwestern Institute on Complex Systems. He received his undergraduate and postgraduate degrees in cognitive science from Johns Hopkins University.

Mira Goral, PhD, CCC-SLP, is Associate Professor of Speech-Language-Hearing Sciences at Lehman College, The City University of New York. Her research focuses on multilingualism, aphasia, language attrition, and language and cognition in aging.

Elizabeth R. Graham is currently completing her PhD in applied cognitive psychology at Claremont Graduate University.

William W. Graves is a cognitive neuroscientist in the Language Imaging Laboratory, Department of Neurology, at the Medical College of Wisconsin. He received his PhD in neuroscience from the University of Iowa in 2006. His research into the neural basis of language production and understanding draws on a variety of techniques, including functional magnetic resonance imaging, computational modeling, and, most recently, magnetoencephalography.

Taomei Guo is Associate Research Professor for Cognitive Neuroscience at Beijing Normal University. Her research mainly focuses on the cognitive and neural mechanisms of bilingual language processing and has been supported by the National Science Foundation of China.

Prahlad Gupta graduated from Carnegie Mellon University in Pittsburgh, Pennsylvania, with an MS in computational linguistics and a PhD in cognitive psychology. He is currently a faculty member in the Psychology Department at the University of Iowa, where his research focuses on the relationship between language processing/learning, working memory, implicit memory, explicit memory, and the neural and computational bases of these processes.

Michael Ho, PhD, is a postdoctoral fellow at Boston University School of Medicine, working in the Neuroimaging/Aphasia Research Lab of Dr Margaret Naeser, VA Boston Healthcare System and the Harold Goodglass Boston University Aphasia Research Center. He is interested in functional neuroimaging of language, and has studied language recovery after stroke using functional magnetic resonance imaging (fMRI) and language processing using fMRI and magnetoencephalography.

Ken J. Hoyte received his PhD in neuroscience from Brandeis University. His research applies behavioral and imaging paradigms to topics such as speech prosody and understanding why the ability to use language to communicate effectively in social contexts is impaired in children and adolescents who have been diagnosed with autism or an autistic spectrum disorder.

Peter Indefrey holds PhDs in linguistics and medicine. Until 2009 he was head of the research group Dynamics of Multilingual Processing at the Max Planck Institute for Psycholinguistics (together with Marianne Gullberg) and principal investigator at the Donders Centre for Cognitive Neuroimaging (Nijmegen, the Netherlands).

The focus of his research is on the neurocognition of monolingual and bilingual sentence processing and word production. He is Professor for Psycholinguistics and Neurolinguistics at Heinrich Heine University Düsseldorf, Germany.

Clinton L. Johns, PhD, is a postdoctoral scholar at Haskins Laboratories, a research institute for the study of speech, language, and reading. He studies language comprehension in mature readers with a particular focus on the processes that are involved in understanding pronouns and other referring expressions.

Eunike Jonathan is a graduate student in the Department of Psychology at the University of California, Davis. She is the recipient of a National Science Foundation graduate research fellowship. She studies the role of controlled attention in reading by investigating reading processes during episodes of mind wandering.

Elina Kaplan, BS, is a doctoral student in the Neuroscience and Behavior Program at the University of Massachusetts, Amherst. Her area of interest is audiovisual integration in speech processing, and which sensory and cognitive factors predict young and older adults' ability to benefit in comprehension from seeing a speaker talk. She is also interested in visual search and auditory selective attention.

Kristina A. Kellett is a doctoral student in the Cognitive and Cognitive Neuroscience Program at the University of Wisconsin–Madison, USA.

Michael Kiang is Assistant Professor in the Department of Psychiatry and Behavioral Neurosciences at McMaster University in Hamilton, Ontario, Canada.

Saskia Kohnen is a postdoctoral research fellow at Macquarie University in Sydney. She is interested in subtypes of developmental reading and spelling disorders and their remediation.

Sonja A. Kotz is a linguist and cognitive neuroscientist who investigates speech, language, emotion, rhythm, and timing in healthy, clinical (aphasic, neurodegenerative), and bilingual populations using neuroimaging methods such as event-related potentials, magnetoencephalography, functional magnetic resonance imaging, and transcranial magnetic stimulation. She recently received a five-year award from the Max Planck Society's "W 2 Special Programme for the Advancement of Outstanding Female Scientists at the Max Planck Society" that supports her independent research group: Neurocognition of Rhythm in Communication, at the Max Planck Institute for Human Cognitive and Brain Sciences in Leipzig, Germany.

Ioulia Kovelman, PhD, is Assistant Professor at the Department of Psychology, University of Michigan. She has a BA in psychology from Queen's University (Canada) and a PhD from Dartmouth College. She was a postdoctoral associate at the Department of Brain and Cognitive Sciences at Massachusetts Institute of Technology. She is a developmental cognitive neuroscientist interested in bilingual and monolingual language and literacy acquisition.

Judith F. Kroll is Distinguished Professor of Psychology, Linguistics, and Women's Studies and Director of the Center for Language Science (http://www.cls.psu.edu) at Pennsylvania State University. The research that she and her students conduct concerns the acquisition, comprehension, and production of two languages during second-language learning and in proficient bilingual performance.

Marta Kutas is a Distinguished Professor in the Departments of Cognitive Science and Neuroscience and Director of the Center for Research in Language at the University of California, San Diego.

Michal Lavidor is Associate Professor in the Department of Psychology in Bar Ilan University, Israel, and a Reader at the Department of Psychology, University of Hull, UK. While studying for her PhD at Bar Ilan University, she specialized in visual word recognition, in particular hemispheric differences in processing written words. She moved to the University of York as a Marie Curie Research Fellow and developed further her research interests to investigate brain structures involved in ortho-graphic processing of words and letters. She now has her own transcranial magnetic stimulation laboratory with the aim of investigating the neural pathways of word processing, prosody, and gestures comprehension.

Chia-lin Lee received an MA in linguistics from the National Taiwan Normal University and a PhD in psychology from the University of Illinois. She is currently a post doctoral research fellow at the Moss Rehabilitation Research Institute.

Christiana M. Leonard is Professor Emeritus of Neuroscience at the University of Florida, where she has been since 1976. She was educated at Radcliffe College and Massachusetts Institute of Technology. In her early career, she investigated the neural substrate of taste, olfaction, and birdsong in rodents and canaries. She now uses magnetic resonance imaging to study the cognitive correlates of individual variation in brain structure in children and adults.

Laurence B. Leonard is Rachel E. Stark Distinguished Professor at Purdue University. His research is concerned with the proper characterization of the lin-guistic and cognitive difficulties experienced by children with specific language impairment. Along with his work with English-speaking children, Leonard and his collaborators have studied children with specific language impairment acquiring such languages as Italian, Hebrew, Swedish, Cantonese, Spanish, Hungarian, and Finnish.

Debra L. Long, PhD, is Professor of Psychology at the University of California, Davis, and International Research Professor at the University of Central Lancashire in England. She studies language comprehension in healthy, young adults and in patients with focal lesions in the brain. She focuses primarily on understanding how variation in language-specific processes (e.g., word recognition, syntactic analysis) and general cognitive abilities (e.g., working-memory capacity, reasoning) give rise to individual differences in language comprehension.

Nira Mashal received her PhD in brain science (The Leslie and Susan Gonda Multidisciplinary Brain Research Center) at Bar-Ilan University and currently she is a senior lecturer at the School of Education at Bar-Ilan University. She studies the cognitive and the brain mechanisms of nonliteral language processing in healthy individuals and in special populations including schizophrenia, attention deficit hyperactive disorder, and learning disability.

Andrea Marini is Assistant Professor in Cognitive Psychology at the University of Udine, Italy. He is responsible for research projects about the neuropsychology of language in the research institutes E. Medea in San Vito al Tagliamento and Santa Lucia in Rome. He is author of a number of books and articles in peer-reviewed journals.

Paula I. Martin, BS, is a graduate student in the Behavioral Neuroscience PhD program at Boston University School of Medicine. Since 1999, she has worked in the Neuroimaging/Aphasia Research laboratory of Dr Margaret Naeser at the VA Boston Healthcare System, and the Harold Goodglass Boston University Aphasia Research Center. Her projects include functional neuroimaging of speech output in aphasia patients and transcranial magnetic stimulation to improve naming in aphasia. Her interests include language processing, language recovery after stroke, and language and aging.

Heather J. Mirous is a graduate student in the Cognitive Psychology Program at Northwestern University, under the direction of Mark Beeman.

Maya Misra is a cognitive neuroscientist who received her PhD from Tufts University. Her research uses event-related potentials and functional magnetic resonance imaging to investigate the cognitive and neural mechanisms underlying language processing, with specific emphasis on lexical processing in bilinguals and on the development of component skills in reading.

Margaret A. Naeser, PhD, located at the VA Boston Healthcare System, is Research Professor of Neurology, Boston University School of Medicine. She joined the Harold Goodglass Boston University Aphasia Research Center in 1977. Her earlier aphasia research focused on lesion localization on structural CT scan or magnetic resonance imaging scan, and potential for recovery in aphasia. Her current aphasia research investigates transcranial magnetic stimulation to improve naming and speech, in chronic aphasia patients. She also conducts research on transcranial, red, and near-infrared light-emitting diode (LED) therapy to improve cognitive function in chronic, mild traumatic brain injury.

Loraine K. Obler, PhD, is Distinguished Professor of Speech-Language-Hearing Sciences at the CUNY Graduate Center, and affiliated with the Linguistics Program there, and the Language in the Aging Brain Laboratory at Boston University School of Medicine and the Boston VA Healthcare System. Her books include *Language and the Brain*, with K. Gjerlow, *The Bilingual Brain: Neuropsychological and Neurolinguistics Aspects of Bilingualism*, with M. L. Albert, *Agrammatic Aphasia: A*

Cross-Language Narrative Sourcebook, edited with L. Menn, and *The Exceptional Brain: Neuropsychology of Talents and Special Abilities,* edited with D. Fein.

Costanza Papagno, MD, PhD, neurologist, is full Professor of Physiological Psychology at the Department of Psychology at the University of Milano-Bicocca. Her research interests concern language and memory processes in brain-damaged patients.

Alvaro Pascual-Leone, MD, PhD, is Professor of Neurology at Harvard Medical School, Director of the Berenson-Allen Center for Noninvasive Brain Stimulation, and the program director of the Harvard-Thorndike Clinical Research Center at Beth Israel Deaconess Medical Center, Boston, MA. Dr Pascual-Leone is internationally recognized as one of the pioneers in the field of transcranial magnetic stimulation (TMS). His work has been fundamental in establishing TMS as a valuable tool in cognitive neurology, increasing knowledge about its mechanisms of action, critically improving the technology and its integration with several brain imaging methodologies, and helping to create the field of therapeutic noninvasive brain stimulation. His primary interest is to understand neural plasticity at the system's level. This includes learning enough about the mechanisms of plasticity in order to manipulate them, suppressing some changes and enhancing others, to gain a clinical benefit and behavioral advantage for a given individual.

Seija Pekkala, PhD, is a University Lecturer in Logopedics and a speech and language pathologist working at the Institute of Behavioral Sciences of the University of Helsinki, Finland. Her research interests focus on language and communication in normal aging and dementia.

Orna Peleg, PhD, is a lecturer at the program of Cognitive Studies of Language Use at Tel-Aviv University. Her research focuses on the processes and mechanisms underlying real-time language comprehension, specifically focusing on how readers access the meaning of written words.

Daniela Perani, MD (Vita-Salute San Raffaele University, Milan Italy; Nuclear Medicine Department and Division of Neuroscience, San Raffaele Scientific Institute, Milan, Italy), is a neurologist and neuropsychologist with long-standing experience in neuroimaging research. Her research activities concern language and bilingualism, dyslexia, dementia, and other neurological and psychiatric diseases.

Tepring Piquado received her PhD in Neuroscience from Brandeis University. She currently is a postdoctoral fellow in the Department of Cognitive Sciences, University of California, Irvine. Her research interests include auditory perception and language processing.

David C. Plaut is Professor in the Department of Psychology and the Center for the Neural Basis of Cognition at Carnegie Mellon University in Pittsburgh, Pennsylvania. His research involves using computational modeling, complemented by empirical studies, to investigate the nature of normal and disordered cognitive processing in the domains of reading, language, and semantics.

Alexander Michael Rapp, MD, is a senior psychiatrist and researcher at the Department of Psychiatry at the University of Tuebingen, Germany. His research interests include the functional neuroanatomy of nonliteral language in healthy subjects and patients with psychiatric diseases.

Kathrin Rothermich is a linguist and educational scientist who is currently a PhD candidate in cognitive neuroscience in the independent research group Neurocognition of Rhythm in Communication at the Max Planck Institute for Human Cognitive and Brain Sciences in Leipzig, Germany. Her research focuses on semantics, syntax, and the interface of semantics and prosody utilizing event-related potentials, magnetoencephalography, and functional magnetic resonance imaging.

Maren Schmidt-Kassow received training in linguistics, phonetics, psychology, and cognitive neuroscience. She obtained a PhD in cognitive science from the University of Potsdam in Germany, and is currently working as a postdoctoral fellow at the Institute of Medical Psychology in Frankfurt, Germany. She is investigating the interface of prosody and syntax in second-language acquisition as well as the role of rhythmic patterns in poetry with event-related potentials and functional magnetic resonance imaging.

Richard G. Schwartz, PhD, is Presidential Professor in the PhD Program in Speech-Language-Hearing Sciences, The Graduate Center, City University of New York. He has served as an editor of the *Journal of Speech, Language, and Hearing Research*. He has published widely on children's language development and disorders, most recently focusing on language processing for production and comprehension.

Mark S. Seidenberg is Hilldale and Donald O. Hebb Professor of Psychology and Cognitive Neuroscience at the University of Wisconsin-Madison. He studies normal and disordered reading and language, with an emphasis on the role of statistical learning mechanisms in acquisition and skilled performance.

Margaret Semrud-Clikeman, PhD, is Professor of Pediatrics and Division Head of Behavioral Neuroscience at the University of Minnesota Medical School in Minneapolis. She is the author of numerous articles, chapters, and books. Her research areas are in neuroimaging of developmental disorders as well as the neuropsychology of attention deficit hyperactivity disorder and autistic spectrum disorders.

Valerie L. Shafer, PhD, is Professor in the PhD Program in Speech-Language-Hearing Sciences, The Graduate Center, City University of New York. She has published widely on neurophysiological indices of speech and language processing in child language development and disorders and on cross-linguistic and bilingual speech perception.

John J. Sidtis is Director of the Brain and Behavior Laboratory in the Geriatrics Division of the Nathan Kline Institute and a research professor in the Department of Psychiatry at the New York University School of Medicine. He was an original member of the first Cognitive Neuroscience Program at Cornell University Medical School and Rockefeller University. He has used functional imaging in his research for 30 years and has been a licensed neuropsychologist over that same period. He is currently studying the effects of deep brain stimulation on speech and brain function in Parkinson's disease.

Steven Small, PhD, MD, is Stanley van den Noort Professor and Chair of Neurology at the University of California, Irvine, and Professor Emeritus of Neurology and Psychology at the University of Chicago. He is editor-in-chief of the international journal *Brain and Language,* and founder of the Society for the Neurobiology of Language. His work focuses on the human brain organization for language, both in the healthy state and in the face of neurological injury, particularly stroke. The basic work emphasizes distributed neural processing of language comprehension, with focus on network models of context- and task-dependent disambiguation processes. The stroke work brings the distributed network approach to the study of both natural recovery and the systems neurobiology of treatment interventions. Most of this work involves functional magnetic resonance imaging, but this is often coupled with computer modeling, and sometimes also coupled with electrophysiological and electromagnetic approaches.

Avron Spiro III, PhD, is a Research Career Scientist at VA Boston Healthcare System, and Research Professor of Epidemiology at Boston University School of Public Health. He is co-editor of *Handbook of Health Psychology and Aging* (with Carolyn Aldwin and Crystal Park), and has written widely on cognition, health, personality, and aging. He has been affiliated with the Aphasia Research Center and the Language in the Aging Brain laboratory at Boston University for nearly 15 years.

John Stein is Emeritus Professor of Neuroscience and Fellow in Medicine at Magdalen College, University of Oxford. His research focuses on the specialized system of "magnocellular" nerve cells that mediate temporal processing, and their role in movement disorders and dyslexia. He doesn't cook fish and his younger brother, British TV fish chef, Rick Stein, doesn't do neuroscience!

Jennifer L. Stevenson is Assistant Professor in the Psychology Department at Ursinus College, USA.

Kim Sweeney is a doctoral candidate in the Department of Cognitive Science at the University of California, San Diego.

Marco Tettamanti, PhD (Nuclear Medicine Department and Division of Neuroscience, San Raffaele Scientific Institute, Milan, Italy), studied neurobiology in Basel and then took a doctoral training in neurosciences at the University of Zurich. His main interests focus on neuroimaging research on the neural bases of language acquisition and aphasia.

Ethan Treglia, MS, CCC-SLP, is a speech-language pathologist working in the Neuroimaging/Aphasia Research laboratory of Dr Margaret Naeser, VA Boston Healthcare System, and the Harold Goodglass Boston University Aphasia Research Center. He screens potential participants, and provides evaluations and treatments to patients with aphasia. His interests include novel treatments for aphasia, language processing, and language recovery after stroke.

Cosimo Urgesi is Assistant Professor in Cognitive Neuroscience at the University of Udine, Italy. He is responsible for research projects concerning the neurocognitive substrates of body representation in the Research Institute E. Medea in San Vito al Tagliamento, Italy. He is author of a number of articles in peer-reviewed journals.

Walter J. B. Van Heuven is a lecturer in the School of Psychology at the University of Nottingham, UK. His research interests include bilingual word processing, language processing in the bilingual brain, orthographic processing, and computational modeling.

Diana Van Lancker Sidtis, PhD, CCC-SLP, is Professor of Communicative Sciences and Disorders at New York University and a research scientist in the Geriatrics Division at the Nathan Kline Institute for Psychiatric Research in New York. Licensed and certified as a speech pathologist, she teaches and performs speech science and neurolinguistic research.

Christine E. Watson is a postdoctoral research fellow in the Department of Neurology and the Center for Cognitive Neuroscience at the University of Pennsylvania in Philadelphia. She uses behavioral studies of normal and brain-damaged individuals, in conjunction with computational modeling, to elucidate the relationship between action and event comprehension and verb knowledge, as well as the neural bases of solving verbal and nonverbal analogies.

Christine Weber-Fox is Professor in the Department of Speech, Language, and Hearing Sciences at Purdue University. She studies the development of neural functions for language processing in children with typical speech and language abilities and in children with communication disorders, such as specific language impairment and stuttering.

Stephen R. Welbourne graduated from the University of Oxford in 1989 with a physics degree. For the next 12 years he worked in the IT industry. In 2000 he made a major career change and started training in psychology. He did his PhD with Professor Matthew Lambon Ralph at Manchester University, where he now works as a lecturer in cognitive neuroscience.

Suzanne E. Welcome received her PhD from the University of California, Riverside, exploring relationships between brain anatomy and reading ability. She is currently working on functional magnetic resonance imaging studies of reading ability and disability in children and adults as a postdoctoral fellow at the University of Western Ontario.

Stephen M. Wilson is Assistant Professor in the Department of Speech, Language and Hearing Sciences at the University of Arizona. His research combines structural and functional neuroimaging techniques with linguistic analysis to study the neural basis of language processing, and how it breaks down in patients with different kinds of aphasia.

Arthur Wingfield received his DPhil in experimental psychology from the University of Oxford. His research interests include cognitive aging with special focus on hearing acuity, language comprehension, and memory.

Preface

The capacity for language is generally acknowledged as one of the characteristics of what it is to be human. Onkelos, a second-century CE translator of the Old Testament into Aramaic, the then common language of the Middle East, makes this point vividly. In Genesis chapter 2, verse 7, the Bible concisely describes the creation of man in the following manner: "The LORD GOD formed man of the dust of the ground, and breathed into his nostrils the breath of life and man became a living soul." Back translating from Onkelos' Aramaic to modern English, the expression "man became a living soul" becomes "and it became in Adam a discoursing spirit." Thus, according to Onkelos, language, the innate desire and ability to discourse with others, breathed into Adam by the LORD GOD, constitutes the essence of the human spirit – what many today would prefer to term the human mind.

This two-volume book consists of 46 chapters that present the most current state-of-the-art understanding of how the above innate capacity for language and discourse is embodied in the brain. These chapters were authored by scientists from a variety of disciplines concerned with the theoretical and clinical implications of the brain–language relationship. Specifically, these chapters are concerned with the bidirectional nature of these implications and this relationship. Accordingly, they explicate what the brain can teach us about language as well as how advances in our understanding of language require that we expand our comprehension of the brain. In addition, the chapters of Volume 1 describe basic research into the brain–language relationship and attempt to show how theories describing this relationship can contribute to our ability to cope with problems associated with the use of language. The chapters of Volume 2 describe how various clinical phenomena can motivate the theoretical work described in Volume 1. The book thus relates to some of the modern hot debates concerning brain–language relationship, including nature versus nurture, basic versus applied clinical research, and the interactions between genetics, early experiences, and later events such as multilingualism and brain injury.

The two volumes could have been divided into parts and chapters in many different ways. Thus, the way they are organized and presented here is just one of several plausible options. Volume 1 includes 25 chapters divided into five parts. Part I focuses on the differences between the two brain hemispheres in language processing. This issue has raised much interest since the discoveries of language areas in the human brain in the mid-nineteenth century. Part I opens with a chapter by Chiarello, Welcome, and Leonard on individual differences in brain organization for language. The chapter documents the range of variation in brain anatomy and behavior within a large, normally functioning group of young adults. The authors consider variation in brain structure, in behavior, and in the relation between structure and behavior.

The second chapter, by Cohen, deals with a major theoretical issue related to hemispheric involvement in language processing, i.e., whether hemispheric involvement is absolute or relative. The chapter presents a new technique to examine the above issue and to properly assess the relative contribution of each hemisphere to the presentation of speech sounds. In the third chapter, by Lavidor, the author reviews transcranial magnetic stimulation (TMS) and language studies. This chapter highlights the evolution of TMS-language studies and shows how the initial concept of "virtual lesion" (or, in other words, TMS-induced inhibition) has evolved to encompass hemispheric connectivity and facilitation.

Peleg and Eviatar present in Chapter 4 a model which is a general account of how the integration between phonological, orthographic, and semantic representations occurs in the two cerebral hemispheres. They propose the three representations are related to each other differently in each hemisphere. Chapter 5, by Long, Johns, Jonathan, and Baynes, describes a method, called item priming in recognition, for examining the nature of discourse representation and the use of this method to understand how discourse concepts are stored and organized in the two cerebral hemispheres.

The central theme of parts II and III of Volume 1 is language comprehension and language production. Part II approaches this issue from a computational perspective whereas the Part III offers an empirical perspective. Chapter 6, by Watson, Armstrong, and Plaut, illustrates how connectionist modeling has furthered our understanding of normal and impaired processing in semantic memory, knowledge of grammatical class, and word reading and how the connectionist approach has provided for theoretical advancement that would not have occurred using the double-dissociation rubric of traditional cognitive neuropsychology.

Chapter 7, by Goldrick, focuses on three core principles of connectionist theories of speech production, and the impact of each of these principles on psycholinguistic theories of speech production is reviewed. The author examines how learning-based modification of spreading activation may (or may not) lead to novel theories of cognitive processes. In the last chapter of Part II, Gupta reviews evidence for the proposal that the processing and learning of words can usefully be understood as lying at the intersection of a variety of memory mechanisms. He offers a framework that integrates functional and computational considerations in word processing and word learning.

Part III, on empirical studies of the neural correlates of language production and comprehension, opens with Chapter 9, by Graves, Binder, Seidenberg, and Desai. They present behavioral and hemodynamic neuroimaging studies on three variables thought to influence the degree of semantic processing in reading aloud: imageability, spelling–sound consistency, and word frequency. They attempt to clarify the different contributions of neural systems supporting semantic processing in reading aloud.

In Chapter 10, Lee and Federmeier review behavioral and eye-tracking studies on lexical frequency, word class, linguistic concreteness, and lexical semantic ambiguity and relate the findings to event-related potential (ERP) studies. Taken together, these studies suggest that word recognition is a flexible and dynamic process that is sensitive to features within the lexical item itself as well as to information in the surrounding linguistic context. In Chapter 11, Indefrey reviews research that used hemodynamic techniques for studying syntactic processing. Based on meta-analysis of the relevant studies he concludes that there is good and largely consistent evidence for Broca's area and the left posterior temporal lobe as neural substrates of syntactic processing in sentence comprehension and production. It is suggested that Broca's area may be involved in the bidirectional mapping of thematic and syntactic structures.

Chapter 12, by Tettamanti and Perani, presents evidence from a wide host of empirical studies showing that the same anatomical brain structures, and notably the pars opercularis of Broca's area, play a crucial role in the processing and in the acquisition of hierarchical syntactic dependencies in adult subjects. The authors suggest that this computational capacity may be at the core of what makes us a linguistic species. The central topic of Chapter 13, by Chwilla, is how the mind/brain creates meaning. The author presents recent ERP results revealing that familiar meanings, and, crucially, novel meanings too, are immediately accessed/integrated into the ongoing context and argues that the electrophysiological findings support embodied views of language and challenge abstract symbol theories of meaning.

Mashal, Andric, and Small discuss in Chapter 14 motor regions of the cerebral cortex and their participation in a number of functions related to human language, i.e., producing and perceiving speech and language and representing the meaning of words and sentences. The authors elaborate on motor system involvement in articulate speech, continue to characterize its involvement in manual gesture, and, lastly, discuss its more general role in interpreting a message's content. In the final chapter of this part, Chapter 15, Kellett, Stevenson, and Gernsbacher examine the role of the cerebellum in language processing by reviewing brain imaging studies of healthy adults performing phonological, lexical, semantic, syntactic, and discourse-level processes. Their review includes experiments that employed a high-level baseline that controls for motor processes and reports cerebellar lobular regions across studies to identify similar areas of activations for language tasks.

Part IV of Volume 1 focuses on the representation of higher-level language processes in the brain, emphasizing figurative language and linguistic creativity. This part opens with Chapter 16 by Mirous and Beeman, describing some of the cognitive processes and neural substrates that underlie a few categories of creative language use, highlighting similarities and a few differences. The chapter discusses how each hemisphere contributes to processing jokes, drawing inferences, and creatively solving problems and outlines a theoretical mechanism for these hemispheric differences. Van Lancker Sidtis presents in Chapter 17 a historical and critical survey of phraseology, the study of formulaic language, in the context of analytic, experimental, and biological approaches, culminating in current views of formulaic language as an integral component of speech performance and language competence. The author concludes that the empirical evidence supports a dual-process model of language, whereby novel expressions and formulaic expressions differ essentially in how they are learned or acquired, stored, and processed.

Chapter 18, by Cacciari and Papagno, reviews literature concerning the neural architecture underlying idiom comprehension in language-unimpaired and language-impaired participants. The review includes neuropsychological, brain imaging (fMRI), and TMS data and the authors draw some conclusions about possible answers to the basic question that motivated this chapter, i.e., hemispheric involvement in idiom comprehension. Coulson and Davenport focus in Chapter 19 on two well-defined examples of creative language that utilize frames and mappings: jokes and metaphors. The authors review cognitive neuroscience research used to test and develop models of the comprehension of these phenomena and evidence for the importance of the right hemisphere in each. They conclude with some speculations about the potential relevance of such research to general issues relevant to meaning in language.

In Chapter 20, Rapp postulates that nonliteral expressions constitute a challenge for comprehension as they go beyond the literal meaning of the words and require the ability to process more than the literal meaning of an utterance in order to grasp the speaker's intention in a given context. This chapter reviews the current functional brain imaging evidence on the comprehension of metaphors, idioms, proverbs, and ironic expressions. In the concluding chapter of this part, Chapter 21, Faust presents research on the processing of novel metaphoric expressions and discusses the relation to linguistic creativity. The chapter presents converging evidence from studies using behavioral, brain imaging (fMRI, magnetoencephalography), electrophysiological (ERP), and TMS techniques suggesting that the right hemisphere plays a major role in processing novel metaphoric word combinations.

In our increasingly globalizing modern society, learning and mastering foreign languages has become a basic requirement. Consequently, in Part V of Volume 1, the linguistic processes discussed in the previous parts are reassessed from the perspective of the multilingual brain. Part V begins with Chapter 22, by Dijkstra and van Heuven, describing a number of assumptions shared or discussed by researchers in bilingual word recognition, and assesses to what extent the findings of neuroimaging and electrophysiological studies with bilinguals agree with these. The authors conclude that, overall, the neuroscientific data support many of the architecture and processing assumptions shared by behavioral models. In Chapter 23, de Groot discusses aspects of the acquisition of vocabulary in two very different populations of learners, monolingual and bilingual infant first-language (L1) learners and late second-language (L2) learners. The chapter highlights the fact that L1 vocabulary learning involves the learning of both word form and word meaning, whereas in L2 vocabulary learning the targeted L2 meanings are already largely in place in the form of lexical concepts in the learners' L1.

Chapter 24, by Kroll, Guo, and Misra, considers a set of research questions on bilingualism comparing behavioral and electrophysiological research. The chapter reviews the empirical evidence from behavioral and ERP studies demonstrating the presence of cross-language activity. The implications of these results for claims about the neural basis for a bilingual advantage in executive function tasks that require the resolution of competition are discussed. The closing chapter of this part, Chapter 25 by Abutalebi and Della Rosa, reviews and analyzes functional neuroimaging research showing how the brain acquires, processes, and controls an L2. The authors conclude that the reviewed works support a dynamic view concerning language acquisition. "Dynamic" because there may be proficiency-related changes in the brain, i.e., once an L2 learner has gained sufficient proficiency, she will engage exactly the same brain areas as she would for her native language.

Volume 2 of the book focuses on neuropsychological research and on the connections between basic science and clinical research. The research described in this volume shows how clinical work drives research in basic neuroscience. Thus, for example, existing brain–language theories may have to be re-examined and adjusted to account for new clinical findings. This process may generate new hypotheses and stimulate basic neuroscientific research on brain–language relations.

Volume 2 includes 21 chapters divided into three parts. Part I emphasizes methods and paradigms used in neuropsychological research and opens with Chapter 26, by Kutas, Kiang, and Sweeney, on event-related brain potentials and neuropsychology. This chapter describes how the use of this technique has impacted our understanding of normal cognitive processes, including language, and thus has great potential for investigating their disruption by disease states. The authors claim that ERP components are one of the few available tools for demarcating and dissecting the human language architecture in all human brains – young or old, intact or compromised, compliant, defiant, or simply incapable.

Chapter 27, by Sidtis, invites serious reflection on the assumptions, methods, and meaning of functional imaging studies. The author argues that the long and often insightful history of clinical observations of brains that cannot speak, brains that speak nonsense, or brains that speak poorly should not be ignored in the age of functional imaging and that listening to these accounts may lead to a better understanding of what functional imaging is trying to tell us. Baldo, Wilson, and Dronkers present in Chapter 28 a new lesion analysis technique, called voxel-based lesion–symptom mapping (VLSM), that has been applied to a number of questions regarding the brain basis of language. This approach has produced a number of unique findings and has shown that many regions of the left hemisphere outside Broca's and Wernicke's classical language areas play a critical role in linguistic functions.

Chapter 29, by Brownell, Hoyte, Piquado, and Wingfield, uses the investigation of naming deficits to illustrate some current methodological issues and options associated with patient-based research. The authors discuss a study of naming in several mildly impaired aphasic patients, explore the distinction between group studies and case studies, and bring to bear a variety of analytic techniques that are straightforward, already in the literature, and accessible. Chapter 30, by Pekkala, shows how the use and analysis of performance on verbal fluency tasks can not only reveal the cognitive processes underlying the tasks but also lead to a successful differentiation between normal and impaired word retrieval. Pekkala suggests that verbal fluency tasks can be used as a reliable method when assessing word retrieval skills of individuals with different cultural and language backgrounds.

Chapter 31 by Ellis opens Part II, on language loss, and deals with the acquisition, retention, and loss of vocabulary in aphasia, dementia, and other neuropsychological conditions. The author concludes that age of acquisition is clearly a powerful determinant of processing speed and retention or loss of knowledge, although it is by no means the only determinant. In Chapter 32, Welbourne traces the evolving relationship between cognitive neuropsychology and computational models of language focusing on language processing and its breakdown in aphasia. The author discusses the use of computational neuropsychological techniques and shows how they can significantly enhance our understanding of the underlying brain disorders and the mechanisms that allow recovery. Chapter 33, by Naeser, Martin, Ho, Treglia, Kaplan, Baker, and Pascual-Leone, reviews functional brain imaging studies related to recovery of language in aphasia, and presents the rationale for the use of repetitive TMS (rTMS) in treating aphasia patients. The authors describe their current rTMS treatment protocol used with aphasia patients and a diffusion tensor imaging (DTI) study that examined possible white matter connections between specific brain areas. Finally, they address the potential role of mirror neurons in relationship to improved naming post-TMS with nonfluent aphasia patients.

The main aim of Chapter 34, by Fitzpatrick, Obler, Spiro, and Connor, was to address the question of long-term recovery in aphasia using confrontation naming and word-finding measures. Their results indicate that single-word naming continues to show significant improvement at least as long as 15 years post-onset. This finding supports the observations of Geschwind and other clinicians that it is possible for patients to continue to recover long after 1 year. Chapter 35, by Goral, focuses on multilingualism. The author reviews two types of neurolinguistic studies, namely, neuroimaging of multilinguals and multilingual aphasia in order to answer questions about the representation and processing of multiple languages in the brain. In the last part of the chapter current data concerning cognitive abilities and multilingualism are briefly presented. Marini, Urgesi, and Fabbro conclude in Chapter 36 that bilingual patients with different etiologies and ages may present differential patterns of impairment and/or recovery of their languages. This applies to adult aphasia, childhood aphasia, specific language impairment, neuropsychiatric disorders, and neurodegenerative disorders. The authors thus assume that the cerebral representation of different languages must be implemented in different cerebral circuits.

In Chapter 37, Kotz, Rothermich, and Schmidt-Kassow discuss the temporal and neural correlates of language subprocesses by providing ERP and fMRI evidence from healthy and brain-damaged populations. The chapter ends with an overview of the possible interfaces between language subprocesses, including syntax, prosody, and semantics, in sentence processing. Their review suggests that investigations of dependencies between language subprocesses are necessary to understand the dynamics of sentence comprehension. In the last chapter of the part on language loss, Chapter 38, Burke and Graham discuss the neural basis for aging effects on language. The authors review evidence for the behavioral dissociation in aging effects on semantic and phonological retrieval processes and then consider research that might link this dissociation to an asymmetry in how the brain ages. They note that language provides a promising approach for examining the neurobiological substrates that are associated with functional cognitive decline and cognitive preservation, as occurs in phonological and semantic processing, respectively.

The final part of the book focuses on developmental language disorders. The goal of the first chapter in this part, Chapter 39, by Semrud-Clikeman and Bledsoe, was to provide insight into developmental language disorders as well as into the underlying brain function in language development. The authors emphasize intervention and conclude that fruitful research that continues to tease apart the similarities and differences in these diagnoses will be helpful not only for understanding the disorders but also for developing appropriate remediation programs. In Chapter 40, Leonard and Weber-Fox describe processing deficits in linguistic, cognitive, and sensory domains in specific language impairment (SLI). They point to weaknesses in the detection, perception, storage, and integration of information and conclude that one of the next steps toward understanding SLI will come from attempts to relate the particular weaknesses in processing that are seen in SLI to the specific language symptoms that individuals with this disorder exhibit. The neurobiology of SLI is discussed in Chapter 41 by Schwartz and Shafer. The authors review MRI, fMRI, and ERP studies and emphasize the use of these methods to provide early identification of children at risk for SLI, as well as their use to measure changes following intervention. They argue that the great challenges remaining in the study of the neurobiology of SLI include the continuing establishment of relations between neurological findings and behavior, determining the specific cognitive and linguistic implications of anatomical and functional differences between children with SLI and their typically developing peers.

Chapters 42–45 focus on developmental reading disabilities. In Chapter 42, Kovelman, Christodoulou, and Gabrieli postulate that there are multiple pathways to dyslexia and that individuals with dyslexia vary with regard to their strengths and weaknesses. They review neuroimaging research showing that children undergo functional and anatomical reorganization as a result of reading experience, but that there are important differences between typical and dyslexic readers. These differences may be related to the learning and perceptual differences in the processing patterns of individuals with dyslexia. Chapter, 43 by Coltheart and Kohnen, describes the features of eight subtypes of acquired dyslexia and considers how each might be interpreted as arising via specific selective impairments of a general information-processing model of visual word recognition and reading aloud. The authors argue that developmental dyslexia is very similar to acquired dyslexia in that seven of the eight acquired dyslexias they describe can also be seen in developmental form.

In Chapter 44, Banai and Ahissar present evidence that normal anchoring mechanisms, i.e., the implicit formation of internal representations, which allow most individuals to benefit from the statistics that characterize each episode or context, are malfunctioning in dyslexia and that this malfunction can account for dyslexics' difficulties in discriminating both simple tones and speech elements. The authors list evidence for interrelations across cognitive domains that are typically studied in isolation and present anchoring as a putative mechanism that could account for these interrelations and provide evidence for its failure in dyslexia. In Chapter 45, Stein argues that all the manifestations of developmental dyslexia could be explained by a single underlying cause, namely impaired development of a discrete system of nerve cells throughout the brain, magnocellular neurones, that are specialized for timing functions. The final chapter of the volume and book, Chapter 46 by Borodkin and Faust, is similar to the first chapter of this part in that it relates to developmental language impairments including both SLI and dyslexia. However it adds a third, subclinical group of persons who have marked difficulties in learning foreign languages. The chapter reviews research on word retrieval difficulties in developmental language disorders, focusing on the application of the tip-of-the-tongue experimental paradigm for studying impaired phonological processes in these populations.

I would like to conclude the preface by making the point that the 46 chapters of the two volumes were not intended to cover all relevant issues related to brain–language research in a systematic manner. Instead we aimed to provide a comprehensive overview of current trends and recent advances in neuroscientific and neuropsychological research, emphasizing state-of-the-art methodologies and paradigms and their application to the central questions in brain–language relationship. I hope this goal was achieved.

Miriam Faust

Acknowledgments

This project could not have been completed without the help and encouragement of many people. I'm extremely grateful to them. I would like to thank all authors who have contributed to this two-volume book for their highly interesting contributions, their enthusiasm, and their full cooperation throughout this long process. I would also like to thank Christine Cardone, Constance Adler, Matt Bennett, and Nicole Benevenia from Wiley-Blackwell for being so patient, supportive, and unintrusive. I'm particularly grateful to Shlomo Kravetz from the Psychology Department at Bar-Ilan University for his thought-provoking comments. The preparation of this book was greatly aided by the excellent editorial assistance of Katy Borodkin; I'm deeply indebted to her.

Last, but definitely not least, I gratefully acknowledge the endless love and support of my husband, Raphael, and my children, Achinoam, Tirtsa, Abigail, and Joseph.

Part I

Language and Hemispheres: From Single-Word Recognition to Discourse

1

Individual Differences in Brain Organization for Language

Christine Chiarello, Suzanne E. Welcome,
and Christiana M. Leonard

Variation is a defining characteristic of biological entities. Complex gene-environment interactions within each organism endow all species with a rich assortment of unique individuals. Humans are no different. Look around – people come in all shapes and sizes, with varying talents and limitations across a range of motor, personality, linguistic, and cognitive domains. Our memory and perceptual systems have evolved to enable us to recognize a nearly endless number of individuals from seeing their faces or hearing their voices. Clearly, there are strong pressures on the evolution of neural systems to permit us to respond to conspecifics as individuals. Indeed, every parent, clinician, and teacher knows that an approach that succeeds with one person may fail miserably with another.

Yet although both biology and "folk wisdom" acknowledge the importance of understanding individual variation, until very recently the fields of cognitive science and cognitive neuroscience have been largely silent on this issue. Here the primary emphasis has been on understanding the cognitive architecture that underlies acts of thinking, speaking, perceiving, and remembering, and the neural instantiation of this architecture, as it applies to all persons regardless of variation in skill or strategy.[1] Once the "master plan" has been identified, then perhaps individual differences can be explored by tweaking parameters within a generalized model. In the meantime, individual differences are often treated as noise to be managed statistically.

We have been exploring a more biologically oriented approach in which individual variation is a primary phenomenon to be explained. We consider it plausible that the human brain can support cognitive and linguistic functions in a variety of ways, and that individual differences in brain structure may have functional significance. In this chapter we report initial findings from the Biological Substrates for

The Handbook of the Neuropsychology of Language, First Edition. Edited by Miriam Faust.

Language Project, which was designed to examine the range of variation in cortical morphology, reading skill, and visual field (VF) lateralization in a sample of 200 college students. One goal of the project was purely descriptive: to document the range of variation in brain anatomy and behavior within a large, normally functioning group of young adults. It is often the case that such individuals are included as an undifferentiated control group in neuropsychological studies of impairment (such as dyslexia) or special talent. However, this approach often conceals the range of variation that exists within the normal population, and the frequency of unusual features (such as reversed planum temporale asymmetry) within this typically functioning group is not reported. Another goal was to examine the amount of this individual variation that can be attributed to easily measured subject variables such as sex and handedness, and then to explore other more novel dimensions of individual difference. In each case we considered variation in brain structure, in behavior, and in the relation between structure and behavior.

Our project was informed by a view of individual variation that was prompted by current work in developmental biology (Siegal & Bergman, 2002; Rice, 2008). Research in that field suggests that development is regulated by a complex genetic network that acts to buffer the developing organism from random influences. One outcome of this buffering is to quiet random genetic and environmental variation, thereby promoting regression toward the population mean, similar to the "canalization" idea originally proposed by Waddington (1957). We hypothesized that individuals differ in the extent to which their neural development is buffered from random genetic and environmental influences. Those with well-buffered development should demonstrate cortical and behavioral features that approximate the population mean, while those with less buffered development should evidence more extreme values and a greater extent of inter- and intra-individual variation. At the conclusion of this chapter we propose a framework that acknowledges the very high dimensionality of the individual difference "space."

Project Methods

Two hundred native English-speaking college students (100 female) from the University of California, Riverside, volunteered to participate. There was no selection criterion for hand preference in order to obtain a sample representative of the population as a whole. Each individual received the Wechsler Abbreviated Scale of Intelligence (WASI), three subtests (word identification, word attack, passage comprehension) from the Woodcock Reading Mastery Test – Revised (WRMT-R), a hand preference inventory, and Annett's pegboard moving test of hand skill. Additional demographic data was obtained to assess familial sinistrality, socioeconomic status, college major, and a self-report measure of reading history. In addition, each student participated in eight divided VF experiments. Due to the anatomy of the visual system, the divided VF method allows us to directly transmit visual information to a single hemisphere. Thus words or letter strings briefly presented to the right visual field (RVF) are received in the left hemisphere, and vice versa. An advantage for stimuli presented in one VF allows us to infer a processing advantage for the opposite hemisphere. The divided VF tasks were selected to assess basic word recognition processes (word naming – 2 administrations, nonword naming, masked word recognition, lexical decision) and meaning access and retrieval (semantic decision, verb and category generation). Details about stimuli and experimental procedure have been described in previous publications (Chiarello, Welcome, Halderman, & Leonard, 2009a; Chiarello et al., 2009b; Chiarello, Welcome, & Leonard, in press; Welcome et al., 2009).

Following the five behavioral test sessions, all participants received a structural MRI scan. Imaging procedure and measurement techniques are described elsewhere (Chiarello et al., 2009b, submitted; Leonard et al., 2008; Leonard, Towler, Welcome, & Chiarello, 2009). Hemispheric volumes of gray and white matter were estimated, and measurements of total corpus callosum area and seven callosal subdivisions were calculated. Left–right asymmetries were measured for seven cortical regions that show reliable asymmetries at the population level: pars opercularis and pars triangularis (Broca's area), Heschl's gyrus (primary auditory cortex), planum temporale (overlaps Wernicke's area), midparacingulate sulcus (all typically larger in left hemisphere), and planum parietale (supramarginal gyrus) and anterior cingulate sulcus (typically larger in right hemisphere) – see Figure 1.1. For a smaller,

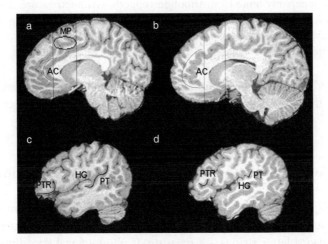

Figure 1.1   Sagittal MRI images depicting asymmetric structures in medial (top) and perisylvian (bottom) cortex. (a) Left hemisphere: Vertical lines through the genu of the corpus callosum and the anterior commissure separate anterior cingulate (AC) from midcingulate cortex. The paracingulate in midcingulate cortex (MP) is generally larger in the left hemisphere while the anterior cingulate cortex is larger in the right. (b) Right hemisphere: The paracingulate sulcus is absent in this example. (c) Left hemisphere: Thick lines outline the pars triangularis (PTR) and planum temporale (PT), while a thinner line outlines Heschl's gyrus (HG). These structures are typically larger in the left hemisphere. (d) Right hemisphere.

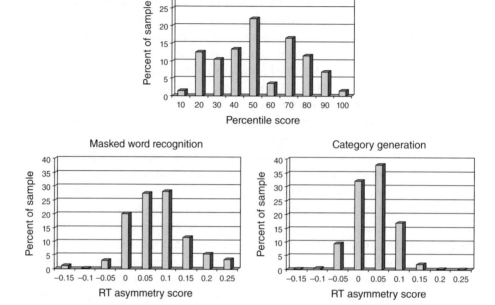

Figure 1.2   Variability in selected behavioral measures. Percentile scores for word attack have a broad, apparently bimodal distribution (upper). Asymmetry scores (response time – RT) for masked word recognition (lower left) and category generation (lower right) indicate both individual and task variation in asymmetry. Positive asymmetry scores represent a RVF/left hemisphere advantage.

partially overlapping sample stratified by reading subskills, local brain size and gray matter thickness were calculated (Welcome, Chiarello, Thompson, & Sowell, in press).

Normal Variation in Brain Anatomy and Behavior

Figure 1.2 displays the range of variation in some of our behavioral measures. The word attack subtest of the WRMT-R requires participants to pronounce increasingly difficult nonword letter strings – a measure of phonological decoding. As can be seen, even in a group of typical college students there is extensive variation in this reading skill, with an apparent bimodal distribution – some individuals can perform this task with relative ease while others have great difficulty. Figure 1.2 also indicates the variation in VF asymmetries for two representative tasks, one involving word recognition (masked word recognition) and one requiring semantic retrieval (category generation). Reaction time asymmetries were calculated using a standard asymmetry index (LVF − RVF/LVF + RVF) such that a positive score indicates a RVF/left hemisphere (LH) processing advantage. Although reliable RVF advantages

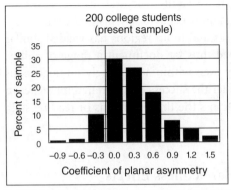
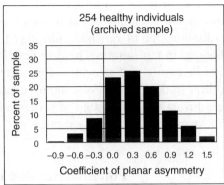
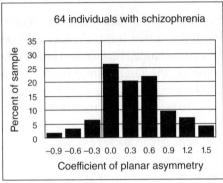
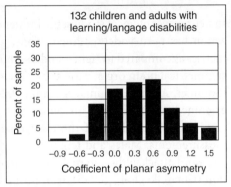

Figure 1.3 Variability in asymmetry of the planum temporale in the present sample (upper left), another control sample (upper right), and two samples with clinical diagnoses: schizophrenia (lower left), and language/learning disabilities (lower right). Coefficient of asymmetry is calculated by subtracting the left measure from the right and dividing by the average, so that leftward asymmetries yielded positive coefficients.

were obtained in our tasks at the group level, there is considerable individual variation in the degree and direction of asymmetry, with some individuals demonstrating reversed or exaggerated asymmetries.

In Figure 1.3, we plot the distribution of asymmetry for the planum temporale for the current sample (upper left), a heterogeneous sample of healthy adults and children (N = 258; upper right), a sample of 64 schizophrenics (lower left), and a group of individuals with dyslexia and/or specific learning impairment (N = 132; lower right). The latter three samples were obtained from numerous studies imaged at various sites but analyzed at the University of Florida using the same methods. It is striking that the mean and range of planar asymmetry is nearly identical across all samples, with approximately two thirds of each sample demonstrating leftward asymmetry. Although measurement error is likely a source for some of the observed variation, the consistency of the mean and range of variation across samples points to powerful underlying biological mechanisms. It also suggests that the probability of reversed asymmetry is similar within normal "control" samples and large clinically diagnosed samples.[2] These findings belie simplistic attempts to associate complex behavioral disorders with a single aberrant structural feature. However, this should not imply that structural variation is behaviorally insignificant.

Examination of variability for other tasks and brain regions has yielded similar findings in our sample. The data described thus far document a range of ability, and behavioral and structural asymmetry even within a seemingly homogeneous college student sample. We can now consider the success of different approaches in identifying the relationship of variation across the three domains of reading skill, VF asymmetry, and brain structure.

Potential Sex and Handedness Effects

In neuropsychological studies, the influence of sex and handedness on brain organization has been widely studied. Non-right-handers often display reduced asymmetries as compared to right-handers, and it is often claimed that women have more symmetrical brain organization than men, although the latter claim is controversial (Sommer, Aleman, Bouma, & Kahn, 2004; Wallentin, 2009). We have thoroughly examined sex differences in our sample, and have concluded that this variable accounts for very little of the individual variation in behavioral and anatomical measurements. Males and females performed similarly in passage comprehension and word attack, although males had somewhat greater accuracy in word identification (Chiarello et al., 2009b). Composite measures of VF asymmetry across all our tasks also obtained no evidence of sex differences. We also considered whether men and women might differ in the variability of their VF asymmetries. However, there were no sex differences in the variability of visual lexical asymmetry across different tasks, within any given task, or within a task across two different administrations (Chiarello et al., 2009b). Women did demonstrate reduced asymmetry for two of our eight VF tasks (nonword naming, category generation), but only for the accuracy measure. Furthermore, this sex difference only accounted for 2% of the variance in asymmetry, and follow-up analyses were unable to replicate the sex difference using a split-sample technique.

Asymmetry of the planum temporale, planum parietale, Heschl's gyrus, pars triangularis, pars opercularis, and the anterior cingulate sulcus did not differ by sex (Chiarello et al., 2009b; Leonard et al., 2009). The size of the total corpus callosum, and all seven callosal subregions was also similar for males and females, when the effects of brain volume were partialled out (Welcome et al., 2009b). As expected, males had significantly greater brain volume, but most previously reported sex differences in regional brain size (e.g., Harasty, Seldon, Chan, Halliday, & Harding, 2003) were not observed when the effects of overall brain volume were removed (Leonard et al., 2008). We recently found evidence for one sex difference in structural asymmetry that could not be attributed to brain volume confounds (Leonard et al., 2009). Leftward asymmetry of the midparacingulate sulcus was significantly *greater* for female, than for male, participants. In general, however, very little of the readily observable variation in cortical morphology could be attributed to sex, and there was no evidence for reduced structural asymmetry in women. These findings comport with other large-scale investigations of behavioral and neuroanatomical asymmetry (e.g., Boles, 2005; Sommer et al., 2004).

Our sample contained the expected number of left-handers (N = 32), and thus far we have not observed any significant differences between left- and right-handers for any of our measurements (and all reported effects remain significant when left-handers' data are removed). However, a much larger number of left-handed participants would be needed to draw any strong conclusions from this result. We have obtained some handedness-related effects when contrasting consistent handers (those strongly preferring one hand for all activities, N = 103) to mixed handers (N = 97). Using standard VF asymmetry indices no differences between these groups were observed (Chiarello et al., 2009a). However, when we examined the degree of VF asymmetry, independent of direction (i.e., absolute value of asymmetry index), then consistent handers had marginally greater asymmetries than mixed handers, due to somewhat greater frequency of extreme rightward and extreme leftward asymmetries for consistent handers. Structural asymmetries generally did not distinguish between these handedness groups. However, consistent handers had greater leftward asymmetry of the pars opercularis than did mixed handers, $p = .05$. Consistent and mixed handers did not differ in callosal area (Welcome et al., 2009).

One is left with the impression that only a small degree of the individual variation in reading skill, VF lateralization, or brain structure can be attributed to easily measured subject variables such as sex and handedness. However, it is also important to investigate the relationships between the domains of skill, behavioral laterality, and brain structure for groups differentiated by sex and/or handedness. Similar behavioral or neuroanatomical features across groups need not imply that the mapping between these domains is comparable. We have obtained some evidence for differences in these associations for sex/handedness groups.

First, we observed positive associations between reading skill and VF lateralization for consistent handers, but not for mixed handers. For consistent handers, larger VF asymmetries were associated with better reading performance (accounting for approximately 6% of the variance; Chiarello et al., 2009a). This effect was not moderated by sex. Second, planum temporale asymmetry was positively correlated (albeit weakly) with VF response-time asymmetry for men, but not for women (Chiarello et al., 2009b). Third, although there were minimal differences in either VF asymmetry or callosal area for sex X handedness groups, these groups did differ in the *relationship between* callosal area and VF asymmetry (Welcome et al., 2009). Among consistent handed males a negative association was observed – larger callosal area was associated with smaller RVF advantages, accounting for 12.4% of the variance. This relationship held for total callosal area, but was most robust for the splenium (no relationship was observed for any anterior subregion). In contrast, mixed handed females demonstrated a positive correlation – larger callosa were associated with larger RVF/LH advantages, accounting for 21.4% of the variance. For this group, the relationship was demonstrated for total callosal area, and nearly all callosal subregions, with an especially robust relationship for the genu. For the remaining groups (mixed handed males, consistent handed females) no association was observed.

These data imply a rather different role for the corpus callosum in mediating interaction between lateralized processors for males with consistent handedness and females with mixed handedness. For male consistent handers, larger callosa appear to support a greater degree of bilateral processing, while smaller callosa support more highly lateralized processing. The splenium locus implies that, for this group, hemispheric interaction for reading processes may depend on the rapid transfer of visual sensory information, since large fast-conducting fibers predominate in the splenium. In contrast, for mixed handed females a very different functional organization is implied, as those with larger callosa had the most asymmetrical processing. This implies that the callosum in this group may function to inhibit information transfer between lateralized processors. There has been great debate in the literature as to whether the corpus callosum serves a primarily facilitatory or inhibitory function for interhemispheric interaction (Bloom & Hynd, 2005; Innocenti, 2009). Our data raise the intriguing possibility that there are subpopulations that differ in the balance between facilitatory and inhibitory callosal mediation. The fact that mixed handed males and consistent handed females display no net correlation of VF asymmetry and callosal size might indicate a combination of facilitatory and inhibitory influences (perhaps some reading subprocesses involve hemispheric interaction, while others require isolation between lateralized processors).

Findings such as these hint that individual differences, at least those related to subject characteristics such as sex and handedness, may be more evident when second-order relationships are examined. In our sample, group differences were difficult to observe for various measures of reading skill, VF lateralization, or neuroanatomy, when each domain was investigated separately. However, as described above, relationships across these domains revealed some interesting contrasts, suggesting that individual differences can become evident in cross-domain mappings. This implies that structure–function relationships can differ even for individuals with similar levels of skill, functional lateralization, or neurostructural features.

Subtypes of College Student Readers

We have also considered whether variations in reading subskills are associated with alternate forms of brain organization. Although phonological encoding skill (the ability to make print-to-sound associations) is widely viewed as essential for reading acquisition, among college student readers text comprehension can be dissociated from this lower-level skill. Resilient readers are those with poor phonological encoding (word attack scores below 35th percentile), but normal-to-excellent passage comprehension (scores above 45th percentile). This group was compared to proficient readers (word attack and passage comprehension above 45th percentile) and poor readers (below 35th percentile on both subtests) – see Table 1.1. Behavioral

Table 1.1   Mean scores for proficient, resilient, and poor readers.

	Proficient (N = 22)	*Resilient (N = 21)*	*Poor (N = 12)*
Word attack percentile	62.3	20.2	20.8
Passage comprehension percentile	69.5	66.0	28.8
Semantic priming (ms)	+33	+74	+34
Planum temporale asymmetry (sd)	.152 (.169)	.143 (.307)	.210 (.286)

investigations of these groups indicated that both resilient and poor readers were equally impaired at phonological coding, even when the task did not require decoding print (auditory phoneme deletion; Welcome, Leonard, & Chiarello, 2011). Both groups also were less accurate than proficient readers in an orthographic choice task, implying that resilient readers are not relying on enhanced orthographic analysis as a compensatory strategy. However, we obtained evidence that resilient readers made greater use of word meaning relationships than either proficient or poor readers – resilient readers had significantly greater semantic priming than either of the other groups (see Table 1.1). Hence, resilient readers may achieve good reading comprehension, despite poor phonological decoding, by increased reliance on semantic context.

Manual measurements of planum temporale asymmetry and automated measurements of regional differences in cortical thickness were examined in the three reading subgroups (Welcome et al., 2010; in press). Although these groups did not differ in mean asymmetry of planum temporale surface area, the resilient readers had significantly greater variability in planar asymmetry as compared to proficient readers (see Table 1.1), and poor readers showed a similar (albeit nonsignificant) trend. Follow-up analyses verified a greater percentage of resilient (23.8%) and poor readers (33.3%) having extreme planar surface area asymmetries (greater than two standard deviations from the mean) than proficient readers (4.5%), due mainly to increased variability in the right planum. Increased variability may suggest that buffering mechanisms that normally maintain an optimal trajectory of neural development are less efficient, permitting more extreme asymmetries to emerge.

In contrast to the manual measures, the automated measures suggested that, relative to proficient readers, both resilient and poor readers had reduced asymmetry of temporoparietal gray matter thickness (Welcome et al., in press). It remains for future research to determine whether the reduced or more variable asymmetry is the more robust finding. The automated and manual procedures are measuring different aspects of cortical asymmetry (cortical thickness vs. planar length, respectively). One possibility is that the groups have sulci of equivalent length, but differing depth, within this temporoparietal region. Because reading comprehension was normal for the resilient group, the reduced gray matter asymmetry appears to be associated with deficient phonological decoding, rather than poor overall reading skill. In contrast, poor, but not proficient or resilient, readers had reduced volume of the right lateral inferior frontal region that was not associated with a reduction of gray matter. A reduction in either gyrification or white matter in the right frontal area could account for this result, which may be associated with poor text comprehension.

Taken together the data imply a dysregulation of asymmetry in the temporoparietal region for adult readers with poor phonological decoding skills. When poor decoding co-occurs with diminished reading comprehension, additional atypical features in the right inferior frontal area were observed. These data suggest that some fairly subtle differences in reading skills among college students can be associated with differences in brain morphology, particularly within the right hemisphere. Greater research emphasis on the neuroanatomical correlates of variations in specific dimensions of reading skill could reveal behavioral–anatomical associations that are obscured when more global comparisons between "normal" and a heterogeneous collection of dyslexic readers are made.

Reading-Lateralization Profiles Revealed by Cluster Analysis

A paradox arises when we attempt to understand *individual* differences by contrasting the behavior or neural functioning of *groups* of individuals, be they groups defined by subject characteristics such as sex or handedness, or behavioral traits such as reading subskills. On the one hand, the study of individual differences is motivated by a desire to understand what makes each of us unique, but on the other hand, we try to investigate this by grouping individuals in order to permit statistical assessments. Furthermore, the groups are formed based on investigators' a priori notions about what should be relevant dimensions of individual difference for brain organization (e.g., sex, intelligence, imagery ability, etc.). We have no way of knowing whether nature has deemed these to be the relevant dimensions for the organization of psychological functions in the brain, as opposed to a myriad of other possibilities (e.g, fertility, swimming ability, degree of extroversion, etc.). And because individual differences are inherently multidimensional, it may be that investigating specific combinations of traits holds the key to understanding variations in brain organization, rather than grouping individuals along single dimensions.

We have recently explored an alternate approach (cluster analysis) in which subject groups are discovered by identifying similarities in patterns across a set of behavioral measures (Chiarello et al., in press). We can then examine whether the resulting "bottom-up" subject classifications are associated with distinct neurostructural characteristics. A subset of our behavioral variables was used in the cluster analysis to identify subgroups (clusters) with similar performance: word attack from the WRMT-R, and asymmetry scores for masked word recognition (RT [response time] and accuracy), verb generation (RT and accuracy), lexical decision (RT and accuracy), and nonword naming RT. All but 17 of our 200 participants were successfully classified into one of four clusters (described below). The remaining 17 individuals were identified as multivariate "outliers"; these participants had behavioral profiles that did not resemble any of the clusters, and were not similar enough to each other to form their own cluster. After describing the four cluster groups, we will examine the behavioral and neuroanatomical findings from the outliers. Because these individuals have idiosyncratic behavioral features we suspect that they may have a less buffered type of neurodevelopment, resulting in atypical neuroanatomical characteristics.

The cluster analysis identified four distinct reading/VF lateralization profiles, and these differences across clusters generalized to reading and VF measures that were not included in the cluster analysis (Chiarello et al., in press). Therefore we present the findings across all our measures to provide a more complete portrait of these groups (see Table 1.2) – note that the data are reported as z-scores. Because we obtain RVF/LH advantages for all the divided VF tasks (Chiarello et al., 2009b), a z-score of 0 for the VF measures indicates the typical RVF/LH advantage for that task; small negative z-scores indicate a reduced RVF/LH advantage and large negative z-scores a reversed asymmetry. The composite asymmetry score is the average of the z-scored asymmetries obtained in each task.

Cluster 1 (N = 61) consisted of individuals with the poorest reading skill, for our sample. Their VF asymmetries across all tasks were somewhat smaller than average. Cluster 2 individuals (N = 26) had superior reading skill and reduced or reversed asymmetry in our lexical tasks. Cluster 3 (N = 63) comprised persons with average reading skill and quite large LH advantages for the VF tasks. Finally, Cluster 4 represented a second group with very good reading skill, but their VF asymmetries

Table 1.2   Mean Z-scores, by cluster, for reading subtests and composite visual field asymmetry. F-tests indicate that there were significant differences across clusters for all behavioral indices.

	Cluster 1 (N = 61)	Cluster 2 (N = 26)	Cluster 3 (N = 63)	Cluster 4 (N = 33)	F(3,179)
Reading skill	Poorer	Good	Average	Good	
VF asymmetry	Low-to-average	Low	Large	Varies by task	
Reading subtests					
Word identification	−.535	.434	.037	.528	12.7***
Passage comprehension	−.382	.376	−.117	.362	6.3**
Word attack	−.748	.851	−.032	.600	34.9***
Composite VF asymmetry					
Accuracy	−.036	−.522	.275	−.111	18.4***
Response time	−.204	−.449	.217	.189	28.1***

**p < .001, ***p > .0001.

varied depending on the task. For example, individuals in this cluster had the highest asymmetries in masked word recognition, average asymmetries in lexical decision, and reduced asymmetries for nonword naming, and for verb generation accuracy. It is notable that the clusters did not vary significantly in sex or handedness, indicating that there is identifiable variance in reading and lateralization that is not captured by typical subject variables. Although the cluster analysis identified associations between reading skill and VF lateralization, the data do not support the view that weaker lateralization is associated with poor reading: the group with the least evidence for LH lateralization had very good reading ability, while the group with the largest LH advantages had average reading ability. The poorest readers in our sample did not demonstrate extreme asymmetries in either direction.

Somewhat to our surprise, cortical asymmetries for both anterior (pars triangularis, pars opercularis, anterior cingulate and midparacingulate sulci) and posterior (planum temporale, planum parietale, Heschl's gyrus) regions did not differ significantly by cluster. However, we did observe some differences for the callosal area measurements. First, the posterior body (and to a lesser extent the midbody) of the corpus callosum was larger for Cluster 1 (poor readers, low/average VF asymmetries) than for Cluster 4 (good readers, task-dependent VF asymmetries). Second, Cluster 2 individuals (good reading, reduced/reversed VF asymmetry) had much larger splenia than individuals from any other cluster (Chiarello et al., in press).

The techniques we used did not provide any evidence for an association between VF/reading profiles and cortical asymmetry. Additional techniques such as voxel based morphometry or diffusion tensor imaging and/or alternate behavioral measures may be needed to identify correlates of variation in cortical asymmetry. However, the data indicate an association between the size of posterior callosal regions and VF asymmetry for the skilled-reader clusters: reduced VF asymmetry associated with enlarged splenia (Cluster 2) and larger, although variable, VF asymmetry associated with reduced callosal posterior body (Cluster 4). The corpus callosum, and especially the splenium, has a protracted period of maturation extending well into adulthood (Giedd et al., 1999; Muetzel et al., 2008). We suggest that the most proficient readers will have accumulated greater reading experience during this extended maturation period, increasing the probability of experience-dependent sculpting of callosal organization relevant to reading processes. If this is the case, then skilled readers could continue to "fine tune" the relationship between hemispheric specialization for reading and interhemispheric channels, resulting in associations between lateralization and callosal area that are not found in less skilled readers.

To summarize, distinct behavioral/lateralization profiles were revealed by the cluster analysis, and a few neuroanatomical correlates were noted. The findings become more interesting when we consider the data for the outliers, those individuals whose behavioral data (for measures used to identify clusters) was dissimilar to any of the identified clusters. In what way was their data unusual, and are any atypical neuroanatomical features observed for these individuals? Although the outliers, by definition, do not resemble each other on the variables used in the cluster analysis, a consideration of their behavior across all our measures revealed some intriguing observations.

Statistical analyses consisted of comparisons between the outliers and the remainder of the sample considered as one group (see Chiarello et al., in press, for details). Although the outliers' performance on the WRMT-R word level tests (word identification, word attack) was unremarkable, they had extremely high scores on passage comprehension ($z = .526$) relative to the rest of the sample ($z = -.049$). In other words, in contrast to any of the clusters (see Table 1.2), their reading comprehension dissociated from lower-level reading skills. The outliers also had higher IQs than the rest of the sample. With respect to our VF tasks, analysis of the composite task asymmetries revealed that the outliers had greater RVF/LH advantages ($z = .249$ vs. $.024$), at least for reaction time. Most remarkable, however, was the finding that the outliers had much more extreme variations in asymmetry across tasks, relative to the individuals with more normative behavioral profiles. This was indicated by a standard deviation measure of the consistency of their asymmetries across tasks (for previous use of this measure see Chiarello, Kacinik, Manowitz, Otto, & Leonard, 2004; Chiarello et al., 2009b): outliers $z = 1.43$ vs. clusters $z = .851$, $p < .0001$, indicating much more extreme variations in asymmetry scores across tasks for the outliers.

The outliers were also less likely to have leftward asymmetry of the planum temporale, and their mean asymmetry did not differ from zero (Chiarello et al., in press). In contrast, the clustered individuals as a group, and every individual cluster, had leftward planar asymmetries that significantly differed from zero. The absence of asymmetry for the outliers was due to significantly larger right plana for the outliers, relative to the rest of the sample; left planum size did not differ. The outliers also differed significantly from the rest of the sample in that they were less likely to have the typical rightward asymmetry of the anterior cingulate sulcus. In this case, the absence of asymmetry was due to larger left anterior cingulate for the outliers; the right cingulate did not differ from the rest of the sample. Thus, the reduced asymmetry for these two cortical areas among outliers was due to increased size of the typically smaller hemisphere (RH for the planum temporale, LH for the anterior cingulate), resulting in greater symmetry for these typically asymmetrical structures. However, there were no differences in any of our corpus callosum measurements when we compared the outliers to the clustered individuals.

We note, in the behavioral data obtained from the outliers, some dissociations between measures that co-vary for the remainder of the sample: between word-level and text-level reading skill, and between VF asymmetries across various tasks. This may be why these individuals were statistically identified as outliers. This may suggest a less well-regulated type developmental trajectory with less buffering from random influences, which could result in unusual (although not necessarily harmful[3]) behavioral features. It is interesting that the atypical behavioral profiles found for the outliers co-occurred with some atypical neuroanatomical features, specifically reduced asymmetry in the planum temporale and anterior cingulate sulcus. Because the reduced asymmetry was due to increased size of the (normally smaller) right planum and left anterior cingulate, we cannot localize the unusual neuroanatomical findings to a single hemisphere or brain region. Rather, it appears that the unusual behavioral profiles were associated with alterations across multiple regions of the cortex, which is consistent with the dysregulation view.

To summarize, the cluster analysis revealed several distinct profiles of reading skill and visual lateralization that would not have been evident from more standard ways of grouping individuals a priori. The clusters were not differentiated on the basis of sex or handedness, nor on any particular behavioral trait. Rather, they represent behavioral subtypes differentiated by their within-group similarity across multiple behavioral measures. But some individuals in our sample did not "fit" into any cluster, indicating more idiosyncratic profiles of reading and visual lateralization. Some neuroanatomical differences were associated with individual clusters and with the outliers. This suggests that some anatomical–behavioral correlations may be obscured when we rely on a priori ideas about how to categorize individuals.

Conclusions and an Alternate View of Individual Differences

The study of the neural correlates of individual differences is still at a very early stage of development. Nevertheless, although our project is ongoing, we can offer some preliminary conclusions. First, easily measured grouping variables such as sex and handedness at best only account for a very small amount of the variance in brain lateralization and reading ability. Second, even when subject groups are similar behaviorally and anatomically, the association between behavior and brain can differ. That is, neural and behavioral variation can map onto each other in different ways within different subgroups of persons. This suggests that there is more than one way in which the human brain can support cognitive functions such as reading. Third, novel multivariate statistical approaches can reveal profiles of individual variation that may not be observable when the investigator determines a priori what the appropriate subgroups should be. Finally, it is just as important to investigate those individuals who cannot be classified into definable subtypes, as those who can. Such outliers can potentially inform us about the costs and benefits of atypical developmental outcomes.

Our findings on anatomical and behavioral variability in healthy young adults have implications for the search for neurological substrates of disorders such as autism, dyslexia, and schizophrenia. Given the variability that is characteristic of such healthy "control" populations, simple comparisons of control and clinically identified groups that rely on group averaging may not yield the sort of insights we seek. Greater attention to the relation of individual behavioral and anatomical profiles is essential if we are to understand the ways in which various disorders depart from the normal range.

Because individuals can differ from each other in a multitude of ways, no single approach to the study of human variation can explain even a fraction of this diversity. For example, although the cluster analysis described above identified some interesting differences between subgroups, no doubt a different grouping of the same individuals would have resulted had we examined a different set of measures. We make no claim that our analysis is any more valid than other ways to carve up the individual difference "space." If we think of each individual as a single point in a multidimensional space, where each dimension represents one facet of variation, then there can be a nearly infinite number of empirically valid subgroups within this space. Hence it may be a fruitless quest to attempt to understand the mapping between behavioral and neural variation by identifying a small number of relevant dimensions, be they subject characteristics such as sex or handedness, or information processing differences such as Phoenician versus Chinese reading styles (e.g., Bowey, 2008).

We propose a kaleidoscope metaphor as an appropriate approach to the study of individual differences and their neural correlates. A kaleidoscope consists of a tube containing a set of colored beads and internal mirrors. When looking through a kaleidoscope a range of different patterns can be seen by rotating the tube that adjusts the mirrors. Although the patterns change, the elements (beads) out of which the patterns are formed do not. Similarly, different subgroups (patterns) can be revealed when the same individuals are examined in different ways. This implies that even small adjustments in our analytical lens (i.e., variations in variables and statistical methods) can reveal a succession of patterns latent in the population under study, each of which is a "true" reflection of the associations underlying individual variation. As investigators, then, it will behoove us to continually vary our analytical lenses in order to better understand the many ways in which individuals are similar and different.

Notes

This research was supported by NIH grant DC006957. We thank Dr Ronald Otto for facilitating this research, and Laura K. Halderman, Janelle Julagay, Travellia Tjokro, and Stephen Towler for assistance with data collection and analysis.

1   Variations due to sex or handedness are often considered, but this can only go so far in understanding *individual* differences. Subdividing groups by sex or handedness does not generally have a substantial effect on the range of individual variation. A large range of variation is still evident when examining groups such as right-handed females.

2   Note that although there appears to be slightly more learning disabled individuals with reversed asymmetry, this is actually due to a less peaked distribution overall.

3   In general, greater "openness" to random genetic and environmental influences should have both positive and negative outcomes, since random factors are not biased in any direction (see Belsky & Pluess, 2009, for a similar hypothesis). Yet in our sample, the "outliers" seemed to have somewhat superior intellectual skill. We hypothesize that unregulated individuals with net negative outcomes would be unlikely to attend college, and hence not represented in our sample. A larger, community-based sample would be needed to confirm this conjecture.

References

Belsky, J., & Pluess, M. (2009). The nature (and nurture?) of plasticity in early human development. *Perspectives on Psychological Science, 4*, 345–351.

Bloom, J. S., & Hynd, G. W. (2005). The role of the corpus callosum in interhemispheric transfer of information: Excitation or inhibition? *Neuropsychology Review, 15*, 59–71.

Boles, D. B. (2005). A large-sample study of sex differences in functional cerebral lateralization. *Journal of Clinical and Experimental Neuropsychology, 27*, 759–768.

Bowey, J. A. (2008). Is a "Phoenician" reading style superior to a "Chinese" reading style? Evidence from fourth graders. *Journal of Experimental Child Psychology, 100*, 186–214.

Chiarello, C., Kacinik, N., Manowitz, B., Otto, R., & Leonard, C. (2004). Cerebral asymmetries for language: Evidence for structural–behavioral correlations. *Neuropsychology, 18*, 219–231.

Chiarello, C., Welcome, S. E., Halderman, L. K., & Leonard, C. M. (2009a). Does degree of asymmetry relate to performance? An investigation of word recognition and reading in consistent and mixed handers. *Brain and Cognition, 69*, 521–530.

Chiarello, C., Welcome, S. E., Halderman, L. K., Towler, S., Julagay, J., Otto, R., et al. (2009b). A large-scale investigation of lateralization in cortical anatomy and word reading: Are there sex differences? *Neuropsychology, 23*, 210–222.

Chiarello, C., Welcome, S. E., & Leonard, C. M. (in press). Individual differences in reading skill and language lateralization: A cluster analysis. *Laterality*.

Giedd, J. N., Blumenthal, J., Jeffries, N. O., Rajapakse, J. C., Vaituzis, A. C., Liu, H., et al. (1999). Development of the human corpus callosum during childhood and adolescence: A longitudinal MRI study. *Progress in Neuro-Psychopharmacology and Biological Psychiatry, 23*, 571–588.

Harasty, J., Seldon, H. L., Chan, P., Halliday, G., & Harding, A. (2003). The left human speech-processing cortex is thinner but longer than the right. *Laterality, 8*, 247–260.

Innocenti, G. M. (2009). Dynamic interactions between the cerebral hemispheres. *Experimental Brain Research, 192*, 417–423.

Leonard, C. M., Towler, S. D., Welcome, S., & Chiarello, C. (2009). Paracingulate asymmetry in anterior and midcingulate cortex: Sex differences and the effect of measurement technique. *Brain Structure and Function, 213*, 553–569.

Leonard, C. M., Towler, S., Welcome, S., Halderman, L. K., Otto, R., Eckert, M. A., et al. (2008). Size matters: Cerebral volume influences sex differences in neuroanatomy. *Cerebral Cortex, 18*, 2920–2931.

Muetzel, R. L., Collins, P. F., Mueller, B. A., Schissel, A. M., Lim, K. O., & Luciana, M. (2008). The development of the corpus callosum microstructure and associations with bimanual task performance. *NeuroImage, 39*, 1918–1925.

Rice, S. H. (2008). Theoretical approaches to the evolution of development and genetic architecture. *Annals of the New York Academy of Sciences, 1133*, 67–86.

Siegal, M. L., & Bergman, A. (2002). Waddington's canalization revisited: Developmental stability and evolution. *Proceedings of the National Academy of Sciences, USA, 99*, 10528–10532.

Sommer, I. E. C., Aleman, A., Bouma, A., & Kahn, R. S. (2004). Do women really have more bilateral language representation than men? A meta-analysis of functional imaging studies. *Brain, 127*, 1845–1852.

Waddington, C. H. (1957). *The strategy of genes.* London: George Allen & Unwin.

Wallentin, M. (2009). Putative sex differences in verbal abilities and language cortex: A critical review. *Brain and Language, 108,* 175–183.

Welcome, S. E., Chiarello, C., Thompson, P. M., & Sowell, E. R. (in press). Reading skill is related to individual differences in brain structure in college students. *Human Brain Mapping.*

Welcome, S. E., Chiarello, C., Towler, S., Halderman, L. K., Otto, R., & Leonard, C. M. (2009). Behavioral correlates of corpus callosum size: Anatomical/behavioral relationships vary across sex/handedness groups. *Neuropsychologia, 47,* 2427–2435.

Welcome, S. E., Leonard, C. M., & Chiarello, C. (2010). Alternate reading strategies and variable asymmetry of the planum temporale in adult resilient readers. *Brain and Language, 113,* 73–83.

2

The Perceptual Representation of Speech in the Cerebral Hemispheres

Henri Cohen

Introduction

Results from a large number of experiments have demonstrated a right ear advantage (REA) in the perception of speech sounds. One widely accepted interpretation of these results holds that the REA reflects the specialization of the left cerebral hemisphere for the treatment of speech information whereas the perception of nonspeech sounds is either not lateralized or is better with left ear presentations (e.g., Benson et al., 2001; Whalen, Richardson, Swainson, et al., 2001). However, the neural substrates underlying speech perception are still not well understood.

Task demand is also a modulating effect of cerebral hemispheric involvement in the processing of information, showing the complex interaction between type of information and hemispheric specialization. In a classic study by Veroff (1976), the performance of patients with severe right hemisphere (RH) lesions was compared to those with severe left hemisphere (LH) lesions on a task of arranging three pictures (place set and category set) in their correct sequence. The groups showed a complete dissociation on these tasks: the LH-lesioned group was both slower and less accurate on the change-of-category sets, while the RH-lesioned group was both slower and less accurate on the change-of-place sets. What would appear to be a similar task, ordering three pictures in a correct sequence, seems to involve different kinds of cognitive processing specificity that would engage both hemispheres to different degrees. Results such as these suggest that subjects can process various stimuli in different ways depending on their psychological set. Thus an individual's processing strategy may dictate to a certain extent how information is dealt with in the brain.

The Handbook of the Neuropsychology of Language, First Edition. Edited by Miriam Faust.
© 2012 Blackwell Publishing Ltd. Published 2012 by Blackwell Publishing Ltd.

Although processing strategies seem to contribute greatly to the effects observed in laterality research, it should be noted that there are examples where certain properties of the stimulus happen to be crucial. Using synthetic fricative-vowel syllables, Darwin (1971) found that fricatives with rapid formant transitions showed a REA while those without such transitions failed to reveal any asymmetry. A possible interpretation of these results is that the LH is specialized for the extraction of rapid frequency changes, and that stimuli lacking such transitions may engage either hemisphere. In this conception, the phonetic properties of the stimuli would be more important than the acoustic properties. One would predict from this model a LH involvement even for phonetically impossible stimuli as long as they contain formant transitions. Cutting (1974) has reported precisely that, leading to the suggestion that there may be two LH mechanisms operating on incoming auditory information, one primarily acoustic and the other primarily phonetic (see also Hertich, Mathiak, Lutzenberger, & Ackermann, 2002). In the first, the analysis of the speech signal results in a corresponding set of nonlinguistic parameters such as the frequency of the signal, its amplitude, and changes in parameters over time. In the second, the listener presumably focuses on certain aspects of these parameters, or combination of cues, and processes them further in order to reach an organized linguistic description.

However, there is no need to postulate a specialized LH processor to deal with the processing of the speech signal. According to motor theory (e.g., Fridriksson, Moss, Davis, Baylis, et al., 2008), speech perception is mediated by mechanisms of speech production. Whether operating by mechanisms involving feature analysis or motor synthesis, the LH has traditionally been thought to be endowed with specialized segmentation processors that decipher the continuous speech stream into phonetic elements, track the rapid formant transitions (important cues in the identification of complex speech sounds such as consonants) and adjust for differences in vocal tract.

However, at a more general level, a serious argument against postulating a specialized speech processor has emerged from studies demonstrating that phonetic-like processing can occur for natural events, outside of speech, throughout the auditory domain. Rise time, for example, is a musical dimension that is categorically perceived (Cutting, 1977; Vatakis & Spence, 2006). Notes perceived from musical instruments are identified as either plucked (rapid rising times – 0 through 30 ms) or bowed (more slowly rising times – 50 through 80 ms). The perception of the plucked–bowed distinction meets all the criteria for categorical perception and has been shown to be categorically perceived by 2-month old infants (Jusczyk, Rosner, Cutting, Foard, & Smith, 1977). This parallels the infant's categorical perception of consonants.

Results from electrophysiological correlates of speech perception suggest an alternative viewpoint on how the brain may process speech sounds. For example, early work by Molfese (1978a, 1978b), using average evoked responses to bilabial stops varying in voice onset time (VOT), a distinctive feature of speech, showed among other things, RH components that categorically differentiated voiced from voiceless stimuli but a different pattern of differentiation in the LH. Using a nonspeech tone-onset analogue of VOT, Molfese (1980) again found a RH component. Segalowitz and Cohen (1989) replicated Molfese's general results with natural speech and also concluded to an active participation of RH mechanisms, as revealed by principal components analysis of evoked responses. In a study where lateralization for non-familiar speech (Mandarin Chinese) categories was investigated, Cohen and Segalowitz (1990) also observed a differential involvement of the cerebral hemi-spheres. Their results showed that the RH "acquired" the voicing distinction faster than the left and that only the LH distinguished between aspirated and nonaspirated speech exemplars (aspiration is not a phonemic feature in English). One possible interpretation of this result is that voicing may be cued by auditory features that lie within the competence of the RH (see also Simos, Molfese, & Brenden, 1997).

This interpretation has found support with researchers studying speech percep-tion in brain-damaged patients. Early studies by Miceli, Caltagirone, Gainotti, and Payer-Rigo (1978) presented pairs of phonemes distinguished by voicing or place of articulation to normal controls, aphasic, and nonaphasic brain-damaged patients. They found discrimination of voice contrasts less difficult than place contrasts in the aphasic (that is, LH-damaged) patients. Perecman and Kellar (1981) similarly reported that left-damaged patients relied significantly more on voice features than place in sorting stop consonants, and were more severely impaired in making place-of-articulation distinctions compared to normal and RH-damaged subjects (but see Ravizza, 2002). Oscar-Berman, Zurif and Blumstein (1975) also found such results with their patients and suggested that the feature voice is more easily recovered from the acoustic signal and hence can be processed by both hemispheres. Also, in a study with speech-impaired children (Cohen, Gélinas, Lassonde, & Geoffroy, 1991), the general pattern of errors indicated that these children had more difficulty than controls in discriminating place-of-articulation contrasts only when they were pre-sented to the right ear, as well as a difficulty in discriminating voice contrasts selec-tive to the left ear. Together, such early studies raise the possibility that both hemispheres are involved in the processing of speech information, but that they may differ with respect to the particular features they best handle. It thus appears that tasks that might superficially be labeled linguistic are comprised of processing stages that individually engage one hemisphere or the other.

The studies just cited present evidence from very different sources: neurophysi-ological recordings with normal subjects and behavioral evidence, using dichotic listening, from normal and brain-damaged patients. While dichotic listening studies have contributed much to our current ideas about the nature of hemispheric asym-metries in normal subjects, the meaning of results obtained from these studies is not always clear. One concern is that repeated testing of the same subjects does not always produce the same results, and that the reliability of dichotic (and tachisto-scopic) tests is lower than one might expect (e.g., Bethmann, Tempelmann, De Bleser, Scheich, & Brechmann, 2007).

In spite of these shortcomings, dichotic listening techniques have helped raise interesting theoretical issues. One of these is whether hemispheric involvement is absolute or relative. Does a difference in performance between ears reflect the fact that only one hemisphere is capable of performing the task? Or does it simply mean that one is better at the task than the other? The typical study does not allow teasing these alternatives out because better performance may result either from more efficient processing by a specialized hemisphere or from processing by a specialized hemisphere after transfer of information across the cerebral commissures. The results would be presumably the same in either case: a difference in performance between the two sides. To examine this issue and properly assess the relative contribution of each hemisphere to the presentation of speech sounds, a new technique is proposed and used in experiments described later.

In this listening technique, subjects are presented with pairs of speech sounds given in random order to the left, right, or both ears. White noise in the opposite ear accompanies the occurrences of the speech stimuli only when they are presented to the left or right ear. Thus, each subject is asked to judge each stimulus pair under three conditions: with white noise in the left ear, with white noise in the right ear, and without noise. White noise was chosen because its broad spectral band covers the frequency range of the stimuli used in the experiments, and to serve, at a low signal-to-noise ratio, as an inhibitor of ipsilateral and cross-callosal transfer of speech information. Subjects are asked to judge the degree of dissimilarity between the stimuli within each pair.

Presumably, differences in the perceptual configurations derived from multidimensional scaling analyses would reflect differences in perception and information processing. A structural analysis of each configuration can thus yield both qualitative and quantitative information about hemispheric functional asymmetry with respect to speech perception. The manner in which these structural analyses of the configurations help us probe the processes involved in speech perception is taken up below.

Perceptual Representation of Information

Much of the work on the representation of complex stimuli, whether auditory or visual, supports the notion that perception is based on an analysis of stimulus patterns along a number of psychological dimensions or features. This process of feature extraction is thought to reflect a selective reduction of information whereby perceptually salient features are extracted from the pattern while other information is not retained.

One may conceive of these dimensions as forming a multidimensional space in which each stimulus is represented as a point. This space, of course, is not directly observable and both the set of dimensions comprising the space and the loci of the stimuli within the space must be inferred or derived by indirect methods. Multidimensional scaling (MDS) is an important method for deriving a representation of the perceptual space (Graef & Spence, 1979). MDS techniques are designed to decompose a matrix of pairwise similarity or dissimilarity judgments on a set of complex stimuli into a metric space of some (investigator-specified) number of orthogonal dimensions. Each stimulus is defined as a point in space such that, ideally, the distances between pairs of stimuli in the space are monotonically related to the degrees of judged dissimilarity of the pairs. MDS methods are thus designed to find the dimensions given the dissimilarities. The typical input data consists of an $N \times N$ (or $(N \times (N - 1)/2)$) matrix whose cell values indicate the dissimilarity of pairs of the N stimuli. Dissimilarities are generally assumed to measure the psychological distance between the stimuli (e.g., Nishimura, Maurer, & Gao, 2009).

The central assumption underlying MDS techniques for perception is that the stimuli are "coded" internally in terms of continuously varying parameters or dimensions. The aim of MDS is to discover the number of dimensions relevant to the perception of the stimuli under consideration and to determine the stimulus coordinates on each dimension, i.e., to determine the dimensionality and the configuration of stimuli in multidimensional space.

The set of abstracted dimensions and the relative loci of the stimuli within the space may be interpreted to reflect the structure of psychological space. Having thus obtained an abstracted multidimensional solution, an investigator may attempt to relate the derived psychological dimensions to the known physical structure of the stimuli. Success in identifying the psychophysical functions relating psychological to physical dimensions is typically measured by a high correlation between values on a psychological dimension and values on the candidate physical measure across stimuli.

A few studies have used MDS techniques with success to identify psychological dimensions underlying the perception of speech sounds (e.g., Shepard, 1972; Hebben, 1986), but none used the techniques to derive perceptual spaces reflecting the extent to which each cerebral hemisphere is involved in the representation of specific aspects, or features, of speech sounds.

The purpose of the studies presented in this chapter was thus to determine the extent to which each cerebral hemisphere is involved in the process of speech perception, and, given that it is, to determine the nature of this participation. The first experiment addressed the problem of hemispheric involvement in the perception of English consonants. The second explored each hemisphere's contribution to two important defining features of consonants, voicing and place of articulation. The third experiment investigated vowel perception in an effort to determine whether traditional classification systems of vowel sounds, in terms of tongue height and advancement, could account for the perceptual representations derived from presentations to each ear. Lastly, individual differences in the perceptual representations of speech sounds were highlighted.

Experiment 1

Several investigators have already reported differences in performance in consonant identification as a function of ear of presentation. In general, significant REAs are found for initial and final stop consonants, and for the features of voicing and place of articulation. Because left ear input is usually correctly perceived above chance, it is often concluded that the RH shares with the LH a general capability to extract the auditory parameters of a speech signal, while the LH is additionally specialized for the extraction of linguistic features from those parameters.

In the present experiment a somewhat different approach was taken to the study of hemisphere involvement in speech perception. Instead of being required to provide some form of identification or recognition of a speech stimulus, subjects were asked to rate the extent to which two consonant–vowel stimuli differed when presented one after the other to a single ear. In the listening paradigm used, as mentioned above, stimulus pairs were presented either to left ear or the right ear with white noise in the opposite ear, or to both ears without noise. Subjects were asked to judge the degree of dissimilarity between the stimuli within each pair. The judgment task allowed subjects to develop their own strategies and imposed no constraint on the manner in which the stimuli were to be judged. The dissimilarity ratings obtained for these exemplars were subjected to MDS analysis to obtain perceptual representations for each of the three ear conditions.

The following listening technique was used in the other two experiments as well. Subjects were presented with two successive target speech sounds in one ear with white noise presented simultaneously in the other ear. They were required to perform a dissimilarity rating task with the pair of target sounds. Thus, for example, on a given trial subjects might hear/bi/followed by/ti/ in the left ear and white noise in the right ear and they would have to rate the dissimilarity of the two consonants on a rating scale sheet. Such ratings were obtained for target sounds presented in the right ear opposed by white noise in the left, for sounds presented in the left ear opposed by white noise in the right, and for sounds presented in both ears (binaurally) without noise. The dissimilarity ratings obtained in each of the ear conditions were subsequently submitted to MDS analysis. From these analyses perceptual spaces were generated for each of the ear conditions. Differences in the perceptual configurations derived from MDS analyses were presumed to reflect hemispheric differences in the perception of the speech sounds used. In particular, analyses of these perceptual spaces permitted not only observation of global similarities and differences between ear conditions in the perception of particular sounds, but also comparison of the relative importance of the features underlying each of the sounds in each ear condition.

The subjects were four men and four women right-handed university students, native speakers of English, with no reported hearing deficits. The stimuli used in this experiment consisted of 16 consonant–vowel (CV) syllables: /ba, da, fa, ga, ka, ma, na, pa, sa, ta, va, za, a, a, a, a/, spoken by a male phonetician. A tape was made consisting of three randomized sets of the 136 possible random paired combinations of the stimuli, excluding permutations. Interstimulus interval was 1 second and interpair interval was 5 seconds.

The subjects listened through headphones to the presentation of the stimulus pairs (see Figure 2.1). Pairs were presented in blocks of 16, each block randomly

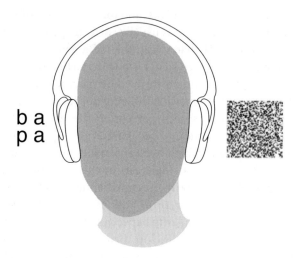

Figure 2.1 In the left and right ear stimulus presentations, subjects listened to pairs of stimuli presented to one ear with white noise presented in the other ear. There is no white noise in bilateral presentations of stimulus pairs.

assigned to the left, right, or both ears with no two consecutive blocks to the same ear. White noise simultaneously accompanied right and left ear presentations of speech stimuli. The signal to noise ratio was measured with a Bruel and Kjoer Impulse Precision Sound Level Meter and noise was about 6 dB louder than speech. Sound level was the same for all subjects. The subjects' task was to indicate, by marking a stroke on a 100 mm continuous line, the extent to which the two stimuli in each pair were dissimilar. The scale was labeled "very similar" at one end and "very dissimilar" at the other. Subjects were not given any description of the stimuli. The session lasted about 1 hour.

Results of Experiment 1

Each subject contributed 136 observations per ear condition. Inspection of the diagonal entries (data from trials not included in the analysis when a stimulus was paired with itself) revealed that all subjects assigned zero or near-zero values to all 16 pairs of identical stimuli. The remaining 120 observations per subject were submitted to MDS analysis using the MULTISCALE for group data (Ramsay, 1978, 2003) program. All subjects produced acceptable data, that is, the within-subject statistics provided by MULTISCALE indicated no unacceptably high standard error estimates (>1.3) or unacceptably low exponents (<.3) that would suggest ratings which were at either end of the scale or exactly in the middle. The stopping rule of dimensionality indicated that 4-dimensional solutions were superior to 3-dimensional solutions in each listening condition ($p.<.05$). Figures 2.2, 2.3, and 2.4 show the projections of CVs onto dimensions 1 and 2 in the left, right, and both ears' perceptual spaces, respectively.

In the left ear (RH; see Figure 2.2a) condition there does not appear to be any meaningful interpretation in addition to manner of articulation to the way sounds are arrayed along Dimension 1. Dimension 2 appears to reflect voicing, with perhaps a sharper distinction among the fricatives than among the stops. These results suggest that in the RH voicing information figures predominantly. No interpretation could be assigned to Dimensions 3 and 4.

In the right ear condition (LH; see Figure 2.2b), ordering by place of articulation (bilabial to velar) is also evident among stop consonants along Dimension 1. In fricatives, except for the placement of /z/, there is, as in the both ears condition, a contrast between those sounds produced with frontal articulators and those produced with articulators further back in the articulatory apparatus, i.e., labiodental and dental versus alveolar and palato-alveolar. These results confirm the findings of others regarding LH involvement in the processing of place of articulation information. Dimension 2 here also appears to reflect voicing. Again, dimensions 3 and 4 could not be interpreted.

The first dimension extracted in the MDS analysis when stimuli are presented to both ears (see Figure 2.2c) clearly refers to manner of articulation. The location of the consonant stimuli along Dimension 1, however, reveals more than manner of articulation information. The fricatives appear to be further divided into sibilants and nonsibilants, and, among these, the labiodentals /f, v/ and the dentals /ð, θ/ are distinguished from the alveolars /s, z/ and the palato-alveolars /ʃ, ʒ/. This distinction contrasts fricatives produced at frontal places of articulation from those produced further back. This result is similar to that obtained by Shepard (1972) in his MDS analysis of Miller and Nicely's (1958) consonant confusion data. Dimension 2 appears to reflect voicing, with the distinction strongest among fricatives. Dimensions 3 and 4 could not be readily interpreted.

In summary, these results suggest that the features of manner, voicing, and place of articulation underlie the perceptual representations obtained for each of the ear conditions. Manner of articulation was found to be the most salient dimension in all ear conditions. Differences were, however, observed between the two single ear conditions with respect to voicing and place of articulation. In the right ear condition, Dimension 1 reflected place of articulation more clearly than it did in the left ear condition. Also, in the right ear condition Dimension 2 appeared to reflect both voicing and place contrasts, but in the left ear condition it appeared to reflect voicing only.

These results may be taken, tentatively, to suggest that consonants presented to each hemisphere may be perceived in terms of the features manner, place of articulation, and voicing; in each hemisphere the various properties of the stimulus are differentially reflected. In the case of oral stops in particular, the LH representations appear to reflect place information more strongly than voicing information while the RH representations appear to strongly reflect voicing information. These differences are explored further in the next experiment.

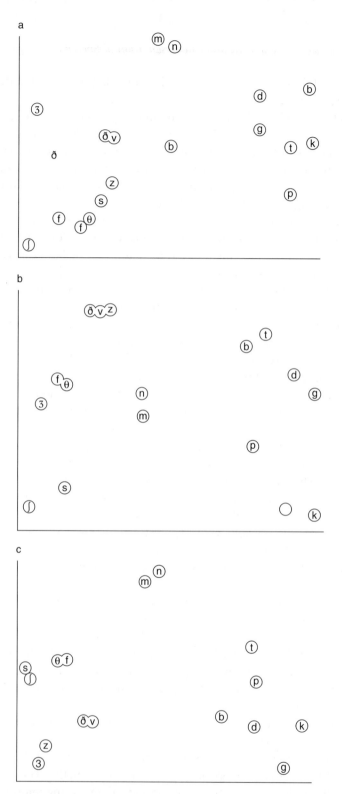

Figure 2.2 a Plot of Dimension 1 (horizontal axis) against Dimension 2 for the configuration of consonants derived from presentations to the left ear. b Plot of Dimension 1 (horizontal axis) against Dimension 2 for the configuration of consonants derived from presentations to the right ear. c Plot of Dimension 1 (horizontal axis) against Dimension 2 for the configuration of consonants derived from presentations to both ears (without white noise).

Experiment 2

The second experiment addressed the more specific question of hemispheric rep-resentation of natural speech English stop consonants contrasted on voicing (voiced /b, d, g/ vs voiceless /p, t, k/) and on place of articulation (bilabial /b, p/; alveolar /d, t/; velar /g, k/). Stimuli were embedded in three vocalic contexts (_/i/; /i/_/u/; /a/_) to provide different exemplars of each consonant. Native speakers of English listened to pairings of these 18 speech stimuli. Trials were presented in blocks either to the left, right, or both ears. Thus, as in Experiment 1, each subject judged each stimulus pair under three different conditions: presented to the right ear with white noise in the left ear; presented to the left ear with white noise in the right ear; and presented to both ears without noise. As before, the dissimilarity ratings obtained for these exemplars were subjected to MDS analysis to obtain perceptual representa-tions for each of the three ear conditions.

The subjects were 12 right-handed native speakers of English, six men and six women, with no reported hearing deficits. These subjects participated only in this experiment. Three exemplars of six consonants contrasted on voicing and place of articulation, spoken by a male phonetician, were used as stimuli. The voiced con-sonants /b, d, g/ and their voiceless cognates /p, t, k/ contrasted also on place of articulation: the bilabials /b, t/, the labiodentals /d, t/, and the velars /g, k/. These sounds were embedded in three different vowel environments: prevocalic /_ i/, intervocalic /i_u/, and postvocalic /a_ / to yield 18 different monosyllabic and disyl-labic exemplars. A tape was made consisting of three sets of all possible combina-tions of pairs of stimuli excepting permutations. Each set thus contained 170 pairs. Stimulus pairs were randomly presented in blocks of 16, with blocks randomly assigned to the left, right, or both ear conditions. The procedure was the same as in Experiment 1.

Data Analysis for Experiment 2

After submitting the data to MDS, the differentiation of these consonant categories was assessed in a manner proposed elsewhere for the study of visual (Homa, Rhoads, & Chambliss, 1979), tactile (Cohen & Levy, 1986, 1988), and auditory (Cohen & Segalowitz, 1990) concept category formation. Briefly, the interpoint distances between the exemplars in the perceptual configurations derived from MDS analysis were calculated to obtain a measure of category differentiation as follows. The degree to which categories are differentiated from each other is reflected both in how small the interpoint distances are for items within the same category – since small distances in perceptual space are assumed to reflect similarity – and in how large the interpoint distances are between items taken from different categories. The ratio of these within-category to between-category distances provides an index of category structure. This structure index reflects the degree to which the perceptual

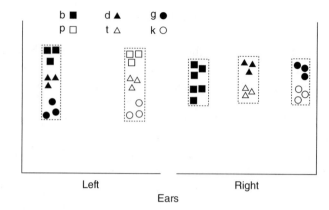

Figure 2.3 Schematized perceptual representation of consonant categories derived from presentations of stimulus pairs presented to the left and right ears. Dimension 1 (horizontal axis) is the first extracted dimension and accounts for the larger proportion of explained variance. It is hypothesized that the left ear (RH) is preferentially involved in the processing of voicing information, and the right ear (LH) in place-of-articulation information.

space is structured along category lines. The lower the structure index, the more the elements in perceptual space are differentiated along category lines. Figure 2.3 shows a schematized, hypothesized representation of the perceptual spaces derived from the presentation of stimulus pairs.

Structure indices were computed for each category, for each listening condition, and for each subject in the following manner. To obtain an evaluation of the voicing contrast, category structure indices were first obtained for categories differentiated on voice but sharing the same place value (e.g., /b/ vs. /p/; /d/ vs. /t/; /g/ vs. /k/). This permitted an assessment of how well differentiated the voiced exemplars were from the voiceless exemplars. The same operation was then performed on the voiceless categories (e.g., /p/ vs. /b/; etc.). Structure indices were thus obtained for voiced versus voiceless consonants as well as for voiceless versus voiced consonants, across all three places of articulation, then summed and finally averaged over the number of comparisons to yield an index of category structure for voicing (holding place of articulation constant).

To evaluate the place of articulation contrast, category structure indices were similarly computed for differentiating the exemplars of different places of articulation but of the same voice (e.g., /b/ vs. /d/ and /g/). This was repeated for each of the six consonants and the structure indices were then averaged over the number of comparisons to yield an index of category structure for place of articulation. These indices were therefore computed for each category, for each ear condition, and for each subject.

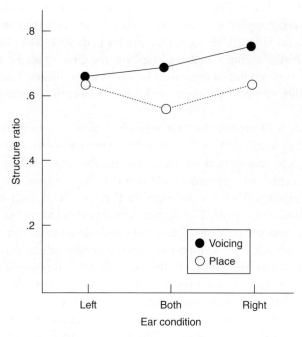

Figure 2.4 Ear differences (mean structure ratios) in the perception of the features of place of articulation and voicing.

Results of Experiment 2

Each subject contributed 170 observations per condition. All subjects in the experiment produced acceptable data. With the application of the stopping rules, the dimensionality retained for the final configurations derived for each condition was three in some cases and two in others. The projections for each of the 18 stimuli on the axes defining the final dimensional space accepted for each subject were further analyzed to compute the structure indices described earlier which reflect the degree to which the space is differentiated along category lines.

Derived structure indices were then subjected to a two-way analysis of variance with two levels of feature (voicing, place of articulation) and three levels of ear of presentation (left, right, both ears) with repeated measures on both factors. The analysis yielded a main effect of ear of presentation ($F(2,22) = 4.14$, $MSe = 0.044$, $p < .05$) indicating overall ear differences (see Figure 2.4). There was also a significant feature by ear interaction ($F(2,22) = 3.65$, $MSe = .0012$, $p < .05$). Subsequent post hoc Neuman-Keuls tests indicated there was greater place differentiation than voice differentiation with right ear (LH) presentations (mean structure indices of 0.380 and 0.422 respectively, $p < .05$) whereas there were no differences in the left ear (RH; 0.303 vs. 0.314) and both ears conditions (0.245 vs. 0.249). Moreover, category structure was better in the Left than in the right ear condition both for voice (0.303 vs. 0.422) and for place (.314 vs. .308) ($p < .05$; see Figure 2.4). Finally, a group analysis based on the data of all 12 subjects using MULTISCALE was conducted separately for each ear condition. The stopping rule of dimensionality yielded a 4-dimensional solution in each of the three ear conditions ($p < .05$).

Figure 2.5 a, b illustrates the first two dimensions of the perceptual spaces derived from the group's data for the left and right presentations of stop consonants, respectively. These representations are similar in the sense that both perceptual spaces can be explained in terms of the two defining features under study, that is, place and voicing. They are different in the sense that each representation emphasizes a different feature. The first dimension extracted by the MDS analysis accounts for the larger portion of the explained variance. It can be seen from projections of stimuli onto Dimension 1 in the configuration derived from the left ear presentations (Figure 2.5a) that stimuli were discriminated according to their voicing value on Dimension 1 with the voiced consonants /b, d, g/ at one extreme and the voiceless consonants /p, t, k/ at the other. It is also evident from projections of these stimuli onto Dimension 2 that subjects took into consideration place of articulation when rating speech sounds presented to the left ear since the labials, alveolars, and velars appear to be systematically differentiated along this dimension. The dispersion of elements in Figure 2.5a thus shows that voicing (Dimension 1) was emphasized to a greater extent than place of articulation (Dimension 2) for the left ear representation. The configuration derived from presentations to the right ear (LH; Figure 2.5b) indicates that subjects emphasized in this case place of articulation (Dimension 1) over voicing (Dimension 2).

There exists a further distinction between the two configurations described. In the case of the right ear representation, the projection of the consonants onto the place of articulation dimension are ordered in a manner similar to their relative place of production in the vocal tract (labials, alveolars, then velars). Such a relationship is absent in the left ear representation and is perhaps indicative of the particular specialization of the LH for place perception. Place and voicing also account for the interpretation of the dimensions defining the perceptual space derived from stimulus presentations to both ears, with place corresponding to Dimension 1, although not as clearly as in the right ear representation.

Finally, relative differentiation of contrasts was examined more closely by considering the category structure indices described earlier. These structure indices indicated better category differentiation for both voicing and place for stimuli presented to the left ear (RH) than for those presented to the right ear (LH). The results also showed a difference for the right ear condition, but not the left, favoring differentiation by place over differentiation by voice.

These data suggest both place and voicing information are represented in each hemisphere but they are represented differently. They confirm the

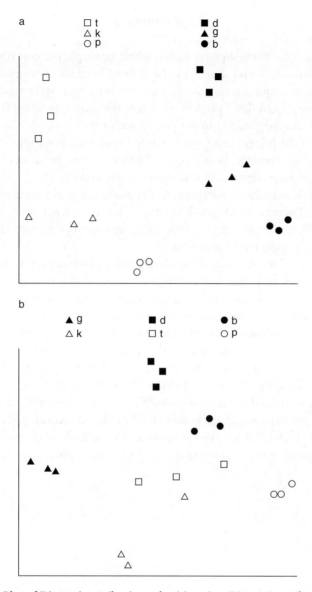

Figure 2.5   a Plot of Dimension 1 (horizontal axis) against Dimension 2 for the configuration of consonant categories derived from stimulus presentations to the left ear. b Plot of Dimension 1 (horizontal axis) against Dimension 2 for the configuration of consonant categories derived from stimulus presentations to the right ear.

results of Experiment 1 in showing stronger reflection of place than voice information in the LH representations and stronger reflection of voice in the RH than in the LH. Unexpectedly however, the present results also indicated better overall differentiation in the left ear condition than in the right (RH better than LH).

Experiment 3

The third experiment investigated each cerebral hemisphere's contribution to the perception of vowels. Vowel sounds can be defined in terms of acoustic parameters such as formant frequencies F_1, F_2, F_3 and duration, and MDS studies of vowel perception have shown that F_1 and F_2 constitute the most important characteristics taken into account by subjects in the perception of these sounds (Shepard, 1972). The purpose of the present experiment was to explore the possibility that, as in the previous two experiments, hemispheric differences may be associated with the analysis of particular component features of vowel sounds.

The eight subjects who participated in Experiment 1 also served in this study a few days later. Twelve natural speech vowels (/i, I, e, ɛ, æ, a, ʌ, o, U, u, ə, ɔ/) embedded in /h/ _ /d/, spoken by a male phonetician, were used as stimuli. The procedure was exactly the same as in Experiment 1.

MDS analysis of the subjects' dissimilarity ratings (105 observations per subject per condition after exclusion of identity pairs) revealed that two subjects produced unacceptable data (exponents < .3). As these data suggested inconsistency in the use of the scale, they were eliminated from further analysis. The group data based on the remaining six subjects were subjected to analysis by MULTISCALE. Applying the stopping rule, four dimensions provided a significantly better fit to the data than three for vowels presented to both ears and to the left ear (p < .05). Three dimensions were accepted for stimuli presented to the right ear (p < .05).

MDS analysis yielded for each ear condition a perceptual space that resembled the auditory space into which the vowels could be placed according to their acoustic properties (see Figure 2.6 for presentations to the left ear). To obtain a measure of the extent to which acoustic features of the stimuli corresponded to the dimensions

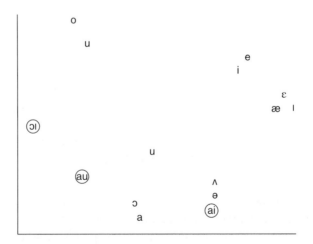

Figure 2.6   Plot of Dimension 2 (vertical axis) against Dimension 1 for the configuration of vowels presented to the left ear. Circled symbols refer to diphthongs.

Table 2.1 Summary table of canonical correlation analyses for each ear of presentation condition.

	Left ear		Both ears		Right ear	
	CANVAR 1	CANVAR 2	CANVAR 1	CANVAR 2	CANVAR 1	CANVAR 2
1st set	.975 (F2)	.759 (F1)	−1.087 (F2)	.976 (F3)	.884 (F1)	.868 (F2)
2nd set	.789 (D1)	−.794 (D2)	.94 (D1)	1.106 (D2)	−.68 (D3)	.802 (D1)
CANCOR	.993	.979	.998	.915	.989	.969
X^2	56.739	26.707	59.326	21.2	52.18	23.35
df	16	9	16	9	12	6
p	.0001	.002	.0001	.012	.0001	.001

CANVAR 1: First canonical variate
CANVAR 2: Second canonical variate
CANCOR: Canonical correlation coefficient

of perceptual spaces, canonical correlations were computed between the physical parameters defining the vowel sounds used (F_1, F_2, F_3 and duration) and the projections of the points on the axes defining the perceptual space for the vowels as determined by MDS (see Table 2.1).

The first observation of interest is that the intercorrelation matrix showed excellent correspondence between F_2 and Dimension 1 for all ear conditions (0.944, 0.950 and 0.956, $p < .001$, $df = 11$ for left, both, and right ear conditions respectively), F_1 and Dimension 2 (−0.821, 0.654 and −0.650, $p < .01$, $df = 11$), and F_1 and Dimension 3 (0.691, and −0.710 in the both and right ear conditions, $p < .005$, $df = 11$).

The canonical correlation extracted two significant canonical variates in each of the ear conditions, with the first variate accounting for at least 97% of the explained variance in each condition and the second variate accounting for at least 84% of the remaining variance. The observation of interest here is that the ear conditions differed with respect to which variables contributed to the formation of these variates (see Table 2.1).

In the right ear condition (LH) F_1 and Dimension 3 had the largest weights in the first canonical variate while F_2 and Dimension 1 had the largest weight in the second canonical variate. In the left ear condition (RH) the pattern was reversed, with F_2 and Dimension 1 contributing most to the first canonical variate. This suggests that the LH places more emphasis on the analysis of F_1 than F_2 while the RH does the reverse in the perception of vowel sounds. The results of canonical correlation analysis for the both ears data yielded a pattern of results similar to that for the RH.

Thus, as was the case with consonants, each hemisphere appears to be involved in the perception of these two physical characteristics. However, the hemispheres differ with respect to the relative importance given to each feature. This suggests that, in vowel perception, there is a coordinate combination of these two sources of information with the RH probably playing a larger role, given the similarity of the pattern obtained with stimuli presented to both ears (without noise) and to the left ear.

Individual Differences in the Perceptual Representations of Speech Sounds

Individual differences characterize neurolinguistic research just as much as any other field involving live organisms. Such differences may be due to individual variations in task performance, differences in brain morphology, as well as to differences in developmental experiences that may affect the way language comes to be organized in the brain. It can readily be accepted that no two individuals will perceive a set of stimuli in exactly the same way. Moreover, no two individuals will use the response medium in exactly the same way.

This is especially true with MDS analyses. For example, MDS results obtained from group data may reveal a higher dimensionality than individual data because different individuals use different dimensions or properties in making the judgments. Dimensionality for grouped data should thus be interpreted partly as a consequence of intersubject variation in dimensions used as well as the dimensionality of any subject's perceptions. The MDS program used here assumes that the subjects share a common perspective on the speech stimuli but that they nonetheless vary with respect to their relative use of the dimensions underlying the group's perceptual representations. A glance at Figure 2.7 reveals the extent of individual variation in the left and right ear conditions. The figure shows that subjects appear to use each dimension differently (as reflected by the weight estimates, an index of the subjects' consideration of a particular dimension) from other subjects and to a different extent from one condition to the next. Furthermore, there are important differences in the number of dimensions underlying the spaces derived from presentations to the left or right ear as well as in the salience each ear "gives" to each dimension. In Experiment 3, for example, four dimensions account for a better fit of the data for presentations to the left ear while only three do so for the right ear. The extraction of a larger number of dimensions may be indicative of a more complex perceptual skill in that more features or properties of the stimuli are taken into account.

These variations suggest different degrees of involvement on the part of each hemisphere in the perception of different classes of speech sounds. These data argue for the notion that the two hemispheres do not give equal consideration to the defining features or properties of a set of stimuli, and that listeners vary with respect to the relative significance accorded to each dimension

Conclusion

The results of the first two experiments indicated that the consonant features voice and place of articulation are reflected in the perceptual representations correspond-

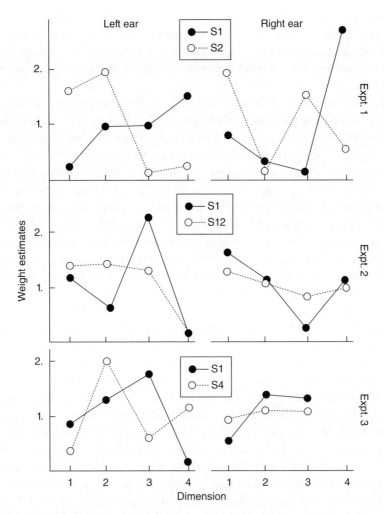

Figure 2.7   Final weight estimates of the dimensions derived for two subjects in Experiments 1, 2, and 3.

ing to both left and right ear presentation conditions, and hence by inference in the RH and LH. These features are not, however, reflected to the same degree in each condition. In Experiments 1 and 2 differentiation of stop consonants by voice appeared stronger in the left than in the right ear condition (stronger in RH than in LH); in the right ear condition (LH) differentiation by place was stronger than differentiation by voice. These results are in agreement both with the early neurophysiological data obtained with normal subjects (Molfese, 1978, 1980) and with the brain-damaged patients (Miceli et al., 1978; Perecman & Kellar, 1981). The present data provide behavioral confirmation of these effects with normal subjects.

The results of the third experiment showed ear differences in the perception of the most important acoustic parameters of vowels, F_1 and F_2. In the LH (right ear condition) canonical correlation indicated greater representation of this F_2 information while in the RH (left ear result) the pattern was reversed. Thus while these two physical characteristics of vowels were clearly represented in each hemisphere, they nevertheless differed with respect to their relative importance in each hemisphere.

These interpretations of the results depend on the assumption that both hemispheres processed the speech stimuli as speech. This is likely given the overall similarities in the left and right ear representations in terms of the clustering of exemplars and in terms of the dimensions that emerged to define the perceptual spaces.

In a sense, however, this issue is part of the larger difficult problem of whether speech perception in general involves a special speech mode of processing and whether aspects of speech production intervene in speech perception. Important evidence on the question of speech mode versus auditory mode of perceptual processing may come from the study of trading relations between features underlying phonetic distinctions (that is, trade-offs between very different types of acoustic features that maintain constant phonetic percepts). In light of the present results indicating bilateral but differential representation of feature information, it would seem useful to explore such trading relations in each cerebral hemisphere.

The studies introduced a novel approach to the study of hemispheric functional involvement that can be used to test for the psychological reality of the processes assumed to be involved. This approach can also be applied to the study of the specificity and plasticity of brain functions underlying speech during normal and atypical language development, and in the dissolution and recovery of speech or language after cerebral lesions. At one level, differences in the recovered perceptual configurations, for example, would argue for the existence of specific differences between age groups in the processing of speech or language. At another level, we can advance our knowledge of the organization and reorganization of linguistic or other cognitive functions in the brain by investigating differences between clinical populations and reference groups. Finally, the experiments reported here have shown, with different classes of speech sounds, the active role played by both hemispheres in speech perception. More importantly, the results also suggest that this participation to the process of speech analysis occurred along divisions defined by the features of the stimulus rather than by the class of the stimulus.

References

Agnew, J. A., Zeffiro, T. A., & Eden, G. F. (2004). Left hemisphere specialization for the control of voluntary movement rate. *NeuroImage, 22*, 289–303.

Benson, R. R., Whalen, D. H., Richardson, M., Swainson, B., Clark, V. P., Lai, S., et al. (2001). Parametrically dissociating speech and nonspeech perception in the brain using fMRI. *Brain and Language, 78*, 364–396.

Bethmann, A., Tempelmann, C., De Bleser, R., Scheich, R., & Brechmann, A. (2007). Determining language laterality by fMRI and dichotic listening. *Brain research, 1133*, 145–157.

Cohen, H., Gélinas, C., Lassonde, M., & Geoffroy, G. (1991). Auditory lateralization for speech in language-impaired children. *Brain and Language, 41*, 395–401.

Cohen, H., & Levy, J. (1988). Hemispheric specialization for tactile perception opposed by contralateral noise. *Cortex, 24*, 425–431.

Cohen, H., & Segalowitz, N. (1990). Cerebral hemispheric involvement in the acquisition of new phonetic categories. *Brain and Language, 38*, 398–409.

Cutting, J. (1974). The left hemisphere mechanism in speech perception. *Perception and Psychophysics, 16*, 601–612.

Darwin, C. J. (1971). Ear differences in the recall of fricatives and vowels. *Quarterly Journal of Experimental Psychology, 23*, 46–62.

Fridriksson, J., Moss, J., Davis, B., Baylis, G. C., Bonilha, L., & Rorden, C. (2008). Motor speech perception modulates the cortical language areas. *NeuroImage, 41*, 605–613.

Graef, J., & Spence, I. (1979). Using distance information in the design of large multidimensional scaling experiments. *Psychological Bulletin, 86*, 60–66.

Hebben, N. (1986). The role of the frontal and temporal lobes in the phonetic organization of speech stimuli: A multidimensional scaling analysis. *Brain and Language, 29*, 342–357.

Hertich, I., Mathiak, K., Lutzenberger, W., & Ackermann, H. (2002). Hemispheric lateralization of the processing of consonant–vowel syllables (formant transitions): Effects of stimulus characteristics and attentional demands on evoked magnetic fields. *Neuropsychologia, 40*, 1902–1917.

Homa, D., Rhoads, D., & Chambliss, D. (1979). Evolution of conceptual structure. *Journal of Experimental Psychology: Human Learning and Memory, 5*, 11–23.

Iacoboni, M. (2008). The role of the premotor cortex in speech perception: Evidence from fMRI and rTMS. *Journal of Physiology-Paris, 102*, 222–236.

Jusczyk, P. W., Rosner, B. S., Cutting, J. E., Foard, C. F., & Smith, L. (1977). Categorical perception of nonlinguistic sounds by two-months old infants. *Perception and Psychophysics, 21*, 50–54.

Miceli, G., Caltagirone, C., Gainotti, G., & Payer-Rigo, P. (1978). Discrimination of voice versus place contrasts in aphasia. *Brain Language, 6*, 47–51.

Miller, G., & Nicely, P. E. (1955). An analysis of perceptual confusions among some English consonants. *Journal of the Acoustical Society of America, 27*, 338–352.

Molfese, D. L. (1978a). Left and right hemisphere involvement in speech: Electrophysiological correlates. *Perception and Psychophysics, 23*, 237–243.

Molfese, D. L. (1978b). Neuroelectrical correlates of categorical speech perception in adults. *Brain and Language, 5*, 25–35.

Molfese, D. L. (1980). Hemispheric specialization for temporal information: Implication for the perception of voicing cues during speech perception. *Brain and Language, 11*, 285–299.

Nishimura, M., Maurer, D., & Gao, X. (2009). Exploring children's face-space: A multidimensional scaling analysis of the mental representation of facial identity. *Journal of Experimental Child Psychology, 103*, 355–375.

Oscar-Berman, M., Zurif, E., & Blumstein, S. (1975). Effects of unilateral brain damage on the processing of speech sounds. *Brain and Language, 2*, 345–355.

Perecman, E., & Kellar, L. (1981). The effect of voice and place among aphasic, nonaphasic right-damaged, and normal subjects on a metalinguistic task. *Brain and Language, 12*, 213–223.

Ramsay, J. O. (1978). *Multiscale*. National Educational Resources: Chicago.

Ravizza, S. M. (2002). Relating selective brain damage to impairments with voicing contrasts. *Brain and Language, 77*, 95–118.

Segalowitz, S., & Cohen, H. (1989). Right hemisphere EEG sensitivity to speech. *Brain and Language, 37*, 220–231.

Shepard, R. N. (1972). Psychological representation of speech sounds. In E. David & P. Denes (Eds), *Human communication: A unified view* (pp. 67–113). New York: McGraw Hill.

Simos, P. G., Molfese, D. L., & Brenden, R. A. (1997). Behavioral and electrophysiological indices of voicing-cue discrimination: Laterality patterns and development. *Brain and Language, 57*, 122–150.

Vatakis, A., & Spence, C. (2006). Audiovisual synchrony perception for speech and music assessed using a temporal judgment task. *Neuroscience Letters, 393*, 40–44.

Veroff, A. E. (1978). A structural determinant of hemispheric processing of pictorial material. *Brain and Language, 5*, 139–148.

3

Mechanisms of Hemispheric Specialization: Insights From Transcranial Magnetic Stimulation (TMS) Studies

Michal Lavidor

Introduction

Studies of patients with brain lesions provided the foundations for our knowledge of the cortical organization of human cognitive abilities. Lesions produced dramatic deficits that provide clues about which brain regions are necessary for which cognitive processes – and their influence on language research has been as deep and perennial as in any field: Broca (1865) suggested that the language areas are located in the left hemisphere (LH); Wernicke (1874) revealed the language functions of the area in and around the Sylvian fissure, and Dejerine (1892) associated damage to the left angular gyrus with specific reading difficulties.

Early neuropsychological findings thus established the dominant role of the LH in language processing. However, although the language deficits following right hemisphere (RH) damage may be subtler than those following LH insult, they nonetheless affect language and communication and thus impact daily functions, social interactions, and quality of life. Joanette and Goulet (1994) found that over 50% of patients with RH damage presented with verbal communication problems. Despite the fact that the LH is crucially responsible for the programming of motor commands required for speech production, the RH supplements the LH by controlling the prosodic and nonpropositional components of expressive language. Not surprisingly, Larsen, Skinhøj, and Lassen (1979) concluded that during verbal recitation both hemispheres are highly active in the normal brain.

Lesion studies continue to provide new and insightful evidence for brain functions, but are known to have fundamental limitations. The behavior of patients with brain lesions may not delineate what process is subserved by the injured tissue, but

The Handbook of the Neuropsychology of Language, First Edition. Edited by Miriam Faust.
© 2012 Blackwell Publishing Ltd. Published 2012 by Blackwell Publishing Ltd.

rather reflect what the uninjured brain regions can accomplish after the lesion. Lomber (1999) termed this analytical problem "the specter of neural compensations." Further, naturally occurring lesions often impair multiple brain systems, making it difficult to determine which deficit is the consequence of which part of a lesion. In addition, in recent years, brain imaging studies have fostered the development of cognitive models, but these are constrained by anatomical considerations (e.g., Price, 2000). Functional neuroimaging studies using positron emission tomography (PET) or functional magnetic resonance imaging (fMRI) now permit the visualization of cognitive processes in the healthy brain. Functional neuroimaging studies make feasible the design of psychological experiments targeted at specific cognitive processes such as language. However, these imaging techniques are limited conceptually by the fact that they only measure correlations between brain activity and behavior, leaving it open to speculation whether activations reported are epiphenomenal rather than representative of processing the task at hand. Other technical restrictions make only limited manipulations of linguistic variables possible (Joseph, 2001), and subtle effects such as word frequency, age of acquisition, word length, and the like (which are often used in psycholinguistics studies) are difficult to obtain in imaging studies.

Other neuroscience tools that enable observation of the brain during language tasks are based on electrical activity recordings such as event-related potential (ERP), electroencephalography (EEG), and magnetoencephalography (MEG). Although these methods offer excellent temporal resolution, as do brain imaging techniques, they can demonstrate correlational links between brain regions and cognitive tasks rather than account for causality or connectivity. An alternative way of probing cognitive variables is to use transcranial magnetic stimulation (TMS), now a standard lab tool for investigating perceptual and cognitive functions (Walsh & Pascual-Leone, 2003). TMS has the ability to interfere with brain processes at well-defined spatial locations at a temporal precision of single milliseconds. This combination of reasonable spatial resolution and excellent temporal resolution is unique to TMS.

This chapter reviews TMS and language studies. It highlights the evolution of TMS language studies and shows how the initial concept of "virtual lesion" (or, in other words, TMS-induced inhibition) has evolved to encompass connectivity and facilitation. The evolution of TMS studies provides a timeline for research on the segregated and integrated hemispheric processes of language.

TMS Principles

During TMS a focal electric current is induced in the cortex by a magnetic pulse which undergoes minimal attenuation by the intervening soft tissue and bone. The magnetic pulse is generated after a brief current is discharged from a capacitor into a circular or figure-of-eight-shaped coil, which is held above the subject's scalp. The induced electric field is strongest near the coil and typically stimulates a cortical area of a few centimeters in diameter. TMS pulses cause coherent firing of neurons in the stimulated area as well as changes in firing due to synaptic input. At the microscopic level, the electric field affects the neurons' transmembrane voltage and thereby the voltage-sensitive ion channels. Brain imaging tools can be used to detect the associated electrical currents and changes in blood flow of metabolism. In motor cortex stimulation, peripheral effects can be observed as muscle activity with surface electromyography (EMG, Rothwell et al., 1994). Moreover, there may be behavioral changes; for instance, stuttering when TMS is applied over Broca's area of healthy subjects (Stewart, Walsh, Frith, & Rothwell, 2001).

TMS Modes and Stimulation Protocols

When TMS was first developed (Barker, Jalinous, & Freeston, 1985), it served to stimulate the motor cortex. Later developments led to its applications in language studies. Amassian et al. (1989) were the first to demonstrate suppression of visual perception with TMS; participants were unable to identify visually presented letters when a TMS pulse was given over the occipital pole between 80 ms and 100 ms after the letters were briefly presented. This experiment might arguably be considered the first TMS language experiment. Another landmark was introduced about 18 years ago when Pascual-Leone and colleagues used TMS to investigate speech production in pre-surgical epilepsy patients (1991).

The ability to impair performance such as inducing (temporary and reversible) stuttering in healthy subjects with TMS was termed the "virtual lesion" mode (Cowey & Walsh, 2000; Walsh & Cowey, 1998) and was employed to map cognitive functions of cortical areas. The term "virtual lesion" refers to the temporal inhibition effects generated by TMS, which either slow down response times (RT) (for example, slower lexical decision times to mixed-case words following TMS over the right parietal cortex, see Braet & Humphreys, 2006) or decrease accuracy (for example, a drop of 60% in accuracy in identifying letter triplets subsequent to TMS over the occipital pole, Ammassian et al., 1989, 1993). Following magnetic stimulation, a healthy subject's performance is impaired for a short period of time, from milliseconds to minutes (depending on stimulation protocols – see details below). Since performance under TMS can be compared to a control condition which could be sham, placebo, a different site and/or a different timing stimulation, a within-subjects experimental design overcomes the known problems of real lesion studies. The concept of the "virtual lesion" mode therefore captures the unique nature of inhibition-induced TMS studies which make it possible to establish (heuristically sound and replicable) causal relationships between brain regions and cognitive functions.

More recent technological developments resulted in another TMS mode designed to explore connectivity between cortical networks. The combination of TMS with brain imaging techniques (e.g., PET, fMRI) allows researchers to examine functional connections between neural processes (Paus, 2005; Paus, Castro-Alamancos, &

Petrides, 2001; Paus et al., 1997). For example, TMS effects have been shown to induce changes in brain activity locally (in the cortex beneath the TMS coil) and in distant cortical areas interconnected to the stimulated site (Barrett, Della-Maggiore, Chouinard, & Paus, 2004; Bohning, George, & Epstein, 2001; Munchau, Bloem, Irlbacher, Trimble, & Rothwell, 2002; Rounis et al., 2005). Research combining TMS with functional neuroimaging techniques has shown that TMS can also have effects in distant brain regions that are neuroanatomically connected to the area targeted by stimulation (Paus, 2005; Paus et al., 1997). For instance, a PET study showed that 1 Hz-TMS over the left dorsolateral frontal cortex (DLPFC) induced neurophysiological changes in the DLPFC but also in the anterior cingulate cortex (Barrett et al., 2004). In addition, Rounis et al. (2005) showed that repetitive TMS over the primary motor cortex induced changes in the motor cortex and also in the cerebellum. It is clear now that the effects induced by TMS are not restricted to the stimulated site but also induce different functional changes in remote interconnected sites (Barrett et al., 2004; Munchau et al., 2002; Paus et al., 1997; Rounis et al., 2005).

An exciting possibility which has been studied recently in neuropsychological settings is the generation of facilitative, rather than inhibitory TMS effects. However, before examining these three TMS modes in language research, the common stimulation protocols will be summarized (Figure 3.1). In fact, the TMS effect on

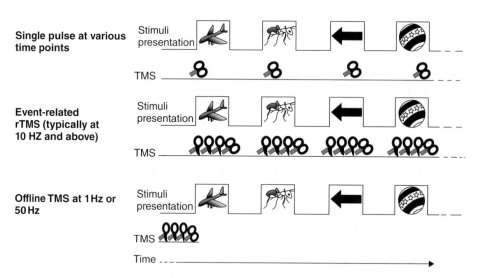

Figure 3.1   Three schematic TMS protocols in a picture naming task. The magnetic stimulation is given at various points during the visual presentation. In a single pulse protocol and repetitive online protocols, the pulse or train of pulses is given when the visual stimuli are presented. During offline protocols the train of magnetic pulses is given before the naming task. A control condition is required in all protocols so that the TMS effect can be calculated as the difference in behavior when TMS is applied compared to the control condition.

cognitive behavior is dictated by many parameters including stimulation intensity, frequency, duration, cortical location, coil type, and type of task, to mention only some. This chapter focuses primarily on stimulus frequency and timing, and will touch on other aspects when interpreting the main findings in TMS language research.

The single pulse protocol (upper panel, Figure 3.1) has the best temporal resolution and can reveal critical processing times of cognitive stimuli. In this protocol, a single pulse is applied at different predefined points in time when subjects are engaged in their task (picture naming in the plotted example). The prototype of this protocol is the seminal work by Amassian et al. (1989) that induced errors in identifying letters only when the TMS pulse was applied over the primary visual cortex at around 80 ms following the letters. Using the same stimulation at other time points (for example 120 ms following letter presentation) did not affect letter identification accuracy. Topper, Mottaghy, Brugmann, Noth, and Huber (1998) induced longer response latencies to picture naming when the single pulse TMS was applied over Wernicke's region 80 ms following the to-be-named picture, but not when applied at other time points.

Event-related online protocols (middle panel, Figure 3.1) apply a train of pulses synchronized with stimuli presentation. The number of pulses given depends on frequency and duration; for example, a common protocol of 10 HZ for 500 ms translates that subjects receive a train of 5 pulses for 500 ms. Pobric, Mashal, Faust, and Lavidor (2008), for example, applied such a protocol coupled with word pair presentation in a semantic decision task. Any protocol that applies trains of magnetic pulses is called repetitive TMS (rTMS), and can be interwoven with stimuli presentation in an online protocol, or applied before or after stimuli presentation in an offline protocol.

Offline protocols (lower panel, Figure 3.1) are a train of pulses applied before stimuli presentation, so that subjects' pre-TMS and post-TMS responses can be compared. There are two typical frequencies that are used in offline rTMS protocols: one that uses 1 Hz frequency for 5–20 minutes, at a rate of one pulse per second. The newer offline rTMS protocol is set at 50 Hz, where 300 pulses are applied within 20 seconds (Huang, Edwards, Rounis, Bhatia, & Rothwell, 2005). Many previous studies have established the 1 Hz protocol as inhibitory; for example, Oliveri, Romero, and Papagno (2004) reported slower reaction times and poorer accuracy in idiom comprehension following 5-minute 1 Hz rTMS over Wernicke's area. Knecht, Ellger, Breitenstein, Ringelstein, and Henningsen (2003) showed that the inhibitory effect of the 1 Hz protocol lasts about half the stimulation time; i.e., 10-minute stimulation will affect behavior for about 5 minutes.

There are fewer cognitive studies using the 50 Hz protocol (also known as Theta burst, Huang et al., 2005) compared to the 1 Hz, though the few published studies report consistent inhibition effects that last about an hour. Vallesi, Shallice, and Walsh (2007), for example, showed how 50 Hz rTMS over the right dorsolateral prefrontal cortex (rDLPFC) impaired temporal processing.

Stimulation Areas in Language Studies

The majority of TMS studies of language have stimulated Wernicke's and Broca's areas and their homologues. Linguistic processing may emerge from the activation of a network of several ensembles in the superior temporal gyrus, each interconnected to Wernicke's and Broca's areas by the arcuate fasciculus. Wernicke's area occupies the phonological/lexical/semantic pole of the network but also participates in articulation and syntax, whereas Broca's area occupies the articulatory/syntactic pole of the network but is also involved in phonological discrimination and lexical generation.

TMS language studies do not really differentiate the main stimulation areas; however, the localization of target brain areas to be stimulated relies on a variety of methods. Sparing et al. (2001) used cranial coordinates in the international 10–20 electrode system to localize Wernicke's area (i.e., CP5). A more precise method is to use MRI images of the subjects and co-register the TMS coil with the specific scanned brain (Pobric et al., 2008). An interesting alternative that has the best functional resolution was applied by Devlin, Matthews, and Rushworth (2003) who located a particular region in Broca's area based on performance in a pilot naming task.

Although TMS studies on language processing have mainly focused on stimulation of a limited number of brain areas (i.e., language-related areas), differing (inconsistent) effects have been obtained. The overview below attempts to pinpoint the sources of these discrepancies and draws conclusions for future studies.

Facilitation and Inhibition Processes

Various TMS protocols have been used in healthy subjects to explore causal relationships between brain regions and language functions (Andoh et al., 2006, 2008; Devlin et al., 2003; Nixon, Lazarova, Hodinott-Hill, Gough, & Passingham, 2004; Sakai, Noguchi, Takeuchi, & Watanabe, 2002). Various effects have been found that are not only reflective of the functional differences but are also sensitive to stimulation parameters. For example, Andoh et al. (2006, 2008) applied rTMS over Wernicke's area and reported a facilitation effect on auditory language processing. They interpreted the observed effects as a change in activity in brain regions engaged during the language task (e.g., bilateral middle temporal gyrus, left superior temporal gyrus, and inferior frontal gyrus). Moreover, they also showed that rTMS could have differential effects on language processing depending on the stimulation frequency used, namely 1 Hz rTMS facilitated detection of the native language, whereas 50 Hz bursts of rTMS facilitated detection of foreign languages (Andoh et al., 2008). These results suggest that rTMS could induce changes in cortical excitability and connectivity depending on the *intensity* of the "virtual lesion" induced in the stimulated area.

Repetitive TMS of the same area, e.g., Broca's area, can induce opposite effects depending on the information processes tapped by the task (see Table 3.1). For instance, high-frequency rTMS (5–10 Hz) over Broca's area has been associated with the facilitation of phonological and syntactic performance on the one hand, and impaired semantic performance on the other (Devlin et al., 2003; Nixon et al., 2004; Sakai et al., 2002; Thiel et al., 2005). Similarly, low-frequency rTMS (1 Hz) over Wernicke's area has been documented to have no effect during a picture naming task (Sparing et al., 2001), but to induce facilitative effects when performing a speech fragment detection task in the native language (Andoh et al., 2006).

Another factor that might account for the different TMS effects but is often ignored is subject's handedness, or rather their brain organization. Knecht et al. (2002) showed that 1 Hz rTMS over the LH slowed down language processing in subjects with left-side language dominance, but not in subjects with right-side language dominance, demonstrating that the susceptibility of TMS effects was strongly correlated to the degree of language lateralization.

In addition to these factors, an obvious important factor accounting for the differences in the effects of TMS is the anatomical location of the stimulated areas. Dräger, Breitenstein, Helmke, Kamping, and Knecht (2004) tested healthy volunteers with left language lateralization on a picture–word verification task prior to and after rTMS (1 Hz for 10 minutes at 110% of subjects' resting motor thresholds). Compared to the control conditions, there were opposite effects on picture–word verification for stimulation of Wernicke's area and Broca's area; namely, a relative inhibition in the case of Wernicke's area and a relative facilitation in the case of Broca's area. These results may indicate that low-frequency rTMS has both general arousing effects and domain-specific effects.

Despite the various factors that modulate TMS effects in language studies, the summary of the main TMS language studies in Table 3.1 reveals some consistent patterns. When low frequency rTMS (1–4 Hz) is applied over language areas for several minutes in an offline protocol, subjects' RT typically increase (Drager et al., 2004; Knecht et al., 2002; Oliveri et al., 2004; Thiel et al., 2005). The only exception was found by Andoh (Andoh et al., 2006, 2008) in a study that reported faster RT following the offline 1 Hz rTMS protocol rather than the expected inhibition, perhaps due to the auditory nature of the task. When high-frequency rTMS (10–40 Hz) is applied over language areas, there is no consistent pattern: whereas some studies have reported a decrease in RT (Mottaghy et al. 1999; Nixon et al., 2004; Sparing et al., 2001), newer studies with more complex semantic tasks have found inhibition effects (Devlin et al., 2003; Gough, Nobre, & Devlin, 2005; Pobric et al., 2008; Schuhmann, Schiller, Goebel, & Sack, 2009). In fact, the various and sometimes contrasting TMS effects on language tasks have helped to develop contemporary ideas on the way the two hemispheres collaborate when processing language, a view which differs significantly from the older concept of LH dominance for language. The last section of this chapter presents these collaboration models and outlines a way to generate facilitative TMS effects via interhemispheric collaboration.

Table 3.1 A summary of TMS studies of language areas using language tasks. While TMS-induced inhibition is usually achieved with low-frequency TMS, higher-frequency TMS has yielded mixed results in terms of enhancing or inhibiting linguistic task performance.

	LH	RH	Control	Frequency & Duration	Intensity	Task	Results
Facilitation							
Topper et al. 98	CP5	CP6	M1	Single pulse	35%, 55%, 75% and 95% MO	Picture naming	Decrease of RT (80 ms) at 35% and 55% MO;
Mottaghy et al. 99	CP5, F3		V1, vertex	20 Hz, 2 s	55% MO	Picture naming	TMS over CP5 decreased RT (40 ms)
Sparing et al. 01	CP5, F3	–	sham	1 Hz, 40 s and 20 Hz, 2 s	35%, 45%, 55% MO	Picture naming	TMS CP5 decreased RT (21 ms) at by 20 Hz 55% MO
Sakai et al. 02	F3	F2	sham	Double pulse	55% and 98% MT	Semantic and phonological	TMS over F3 decreased RT (20 ms)
Nixon et al. 04	F3	–	sham	13.3 Hz, 375 ms and 10 Hz, 500 ms	55% and 75% MO	phonological	TMS over F3 decreased RT (100 ms)
Andoh et al. 06	CP5, F3	–	sham	1 Hz, 600 s	110% MT	Auditory fragment-detection	Decrease of RT (199 ms) by CP5 stimulation
Andoh et al. 08	CP5	–	sham	1 Hz, 600 s and 50 Hz-burst of rTMS	110% MT and 90% MT	Semantic	1 Hz decreased RT (64 ms); 50 Hz-bursts of rTMS decreased RT (95 ms)
Inhibition							
Knecht et al. 02	CP5	CP6	vertex	1 Hz, 600 s	110% MT	Picture–word verification	For right handers, CP5 increased RT (12 ms); for left handers, TMS over CP6 increased RT (18 ms)

	LH	RH	Control	Frequency & Duration	Intensity	Task	Results
Devlin et al. 03	LIPC	–	No-TMS	10 Hz, 300 ms and single pulse	110% MT	Semantic and phonological	Increase of RT (72 ms)
Drager et al., 04	CP5, F3	CP6, F2	V1	1 Hz 600 s	110% MT	Picture–word verification	inhibition in CP5 (10 ms), facilitation in F3 (12 ms)
Oliveri et al., 04	CP5, F3	CP6, F2	No-TMS	1 Hz 300 s	110% MT	Semantic (idioms)	TMS over CP5 increased RT (60 ms)
Thiel et al. 05	F3	F2	Vertex,	4 Hz, 10 s	55% and 65% MO	Semantic	Increase of RT (40 ms)
Gough et al., 05	IFG	–	No-TMS	10 Hz 300 ms	60% MO	Semantic and phonological	Increased RT (52 ms)
Pobric et al. 08	CP5, F3	CP6, F2	Vertex	10 Hz 500 ms	110% MT	Semantic (metaphors)	CP5: increased RT (80 ms) CP6: increased RT for novel metaphors (120 ms)
Schuhmann et al. 08	F2	–	Sham	Triple Pulse 40 Hz	120% MT	Picture naming	RT increased (50 ms) when the pulse was given 300 ms after the picture

LH, RH: left and right hemispheres stimulation sites. rTMS: repetitive transcranial magnetic stimulation. CP5: Wernicke's area in the international 10–20 electrode system. CP6: right hemispheric homologue of Wernicke's area. F3: pars opercularis/pars triangularis of Broca's area. F2: right hemispheric homologue of Broca's area. MT: motor threshold. MO: maximal stimulator output (around 2.2 tesla).

Hemispheric Collaboration During Language Processing

Jung-Beeman (2005) put forward a conceptual framework that highlights the complementary roles of the left and right hemispheres in processing language tasks. The model suggests that at least three distinct but highly interactive components of semantic processing, supported by three distinct brain areas, are crucial for natural language comprehension: *semantic activation, semantic integration,* and *semantic selection.* The three components are claimed to have counterparts in both hemispheres (i.e., a RH and a LH version of each process), and to interact across processes and across hemispheres. Although each type of semantic processing occurs bilaterally, the hemispheres compute information differently, such that the RH performs relatively *coarser semantic coding.* LH semantic coding is relatively fine compared with that of the RH. Numerous previous studies have documented the preference of the LH to process routine (Goldberg & Costa, 1981), frequent (Sergent, 1982), and salient meanings of words (Giora, 2007). Correlatively, the RH has an advantage in processing a Gestalt mode (Levy-Agresti & Sperry, 1968), novel (Goldberg & Costa, 1981), infrequent (Sergent, 1982), and nonsalient meanings (Giora, 2007). These differences are elegantly conceptualized in the coarse and fine coding lateralization proposed in Jung-Beeman's model (2005; see also Mirous & Beeman, Volume 1, Chapter 16). These qualitative differences allow for a two-pronged approach to natural language comprehension: rapid interpretation and tight links in the LH, and maintenance of broader meaning activation and recognition of distant relations in the RH. Jung-Beeman's (2005) framework can successfully account for the contrasting inhibition and facilitation effects induced by TMS in language studies (see Table 3.1) as detailed below.

Recently, TMS applied over motor or cognitive functions has highlighted a mechanism that may underlie performance changes by providing experimental support for the hypothesis that some brain functions operate in a state of inter-hemispheric compensation; i.e., TMS may reflect use of adaptive plasticity in the nondominant hemisphere for function recovery (Fries, Danek, Scheidtmann, & Hamburger, 1993). These plastic, adaptive changes of the intact hemisphere could intervene rapidly and be specific to functions that are normally mediated by the perturbed area (Johansen-Berg et al., 2002; O'Shea, Johansen-Berg, Trief, Gobel, & Rushworth, 2007). For example, Kobayashi, Hutchinson, Theoret, Schlaug, and Pascual-Leone (2004) observed that rTMS applied over the left motor cortex during a motor task facilitated performance with the ipsilateral hand (decreased RT in the left hand). According to these authors, given that the LH controls the right hand, low-frequency rTMS over the left motor cortex could lead to the disinhibition of the contralateral right motor cortex (Kobayashi et al., 2004) – presumably through the suppression of transcallosal inhibition (Gerloff et al., 1998; Theoret, Kobayashi, Valero-Cabre, & Pascual-Leone, 2003) – and thus to subsequent better performance with the ipsilateral left hand.

More recently, O'Shea et al. (2007) provided direct evidence for interhemispheric compensation by showing that if the pattern of reorganization causes recovered behavior, then recovery performance should break down when activity is disrupted in the compensatory hemisphere. The authors applied 1 Hz rTMS over the left dorsal premotor cortex (PMd) and fMRI was used to investigate short-term reorganization in the right PMd. The results indicated a compensatory increase in activity in the right PMd and connected medial premotor areas. In addition, subsequent TMS of the reorganized right PMd disrupted performance, confirming that the pattern of functional reorganization of the right PMd made a causal contribution in preserving behavior after neuronal interference. Interhemispheric compensation has also been observed in higher-order cognitive functions. Hilgetag, Theoret, and Pascual-Leone (2001) reported that right hemispheric parietal stimulation improved the ipsilateral detection of visual stimuli. They suggested that the inhibition induced at the site of stimulation was matched by increased excitability in the contralateral hemisphere, resulting in measurable behavioral enhancement.

The idea of interhemispheric compensation might explain some of the contrasting TMS effects found in TMS studies and thus elucidate mechanisms of interhemispheric collaboration during language processing. The basic assumption here is a competitive race model where both hemispheres are not just busy processing stimuli but at the same time inhibit each other via transcallosal connections. The idea that TMS of one region may disinhibit the homologous regions in the contralateral hemisphere (Seyal, Ro, & Rafal, 1995) suggests, for instance, that the stimulation of the Wernicke's area in the LH decreases the inhibitory effect of this region on the homologous right area, resulting in faster processing of some semantic tasks (for example, Pobric et al, 2008; see Table 3.1). This hypothesis is supported by Oliveri et al. (2004) who reported that stimulation over the right temporal lobe improved performance via disinhibition of the LH in a semantic task of processing idioms. According to this explanation, both hemispheres activate transcallosal inhibition during semantic processing as they operate in a competitive mode. Since the LH is dominant for semantic processing in typical brain organization, in accordance it activates a larger transcallosal inhibition over the RH homologous semantic areas as part of normal LH semantic processing mechanisms. This inhibition may interfere with the ability of the RH to carry out semantic processing to a larger degree than the RH is interfering with LH processing. Indeed transcallosal disinhibition was directly demonstrated in healthy subjects by applying rTMS at a frequency of 4 Hz over the left inferior frontal gyrus (IFG), while simultaneously measuring language activity with PET (Thiel et al., 2006). Repetitive TMS decreased left IFG activity and increased right IFG activity, showing a rightward shift of language activity caused by a "virtual brain lesion," thus further supporting the hypothesis that right homologous activations may be linked to a disinhibition phenomenon (Voets et al., 2006).

A different interpretation of interhemispheric TMS effects that might be useful as well in applying disinhibition principles was introduced recently by Sandrini,

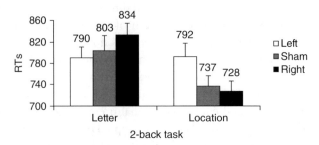

Figure 3.2 An example of indirect TMS effects. The effects are compared to the sham condition (grey bars). Recall of letter identities was impaired due to TMS over the right dorsolateral prefrontal cortex (DLPFC) but not with TMS over the left DLPFC. This seems surprising since memory processes for letters are known to be related to the left and not the right DLPFC. The interpretation suggested by Sandrini et al. (2008) is that the TMS affects inhibition of the irrelevant information (letter location in the case where letter identities are the target). Such results pave the way to using TMS to explore the inhibitory intercorrelations between homologous brain areas whose contribution to behavior is as important as, if not greater than, direct feed-forward brain processes. Taken from Sandrini et al. (2008), with permission.

Rossini, and Miniussi (2008). In a working memory task, the researchers applied rTMS over the left and right DLPFC. Sandrini et al. (2008) discovered a double dissociation between TMS location and task: during the letter condition, when applied to the right DLPFC, rTMS significantly delayed task performance, whereas the same result was observed during the location condition, but only when rTMS was applied to the left DLPFC (see Figure 3.2). This pattern seems counterintuitive at first glance, because if one assumes a direct "virtual lesion" TMS effect, it would be expected that TMS over the left site would impair letter processing, while spatial processing would be impaired by RH-TMS. Sandrini et al. (2008) proposed a novel interpretation which opens up new possibilities in TMS research. They argued that the functional dichotomy of the hemispheres may be due to mechanisms of cognitive control over interference, which resolve conflict through the inhibition of task-irrelevant information. In other words, part of normal processing of one hemisphere is to inhibit competing irrelevant information that activates the homologue hemisphere, for example, the left DLPFC, while processing letter identities, needs to inhibit spatial information regarding the letter location which is processed by the homologue right region. Sandrini et al. (2008) generated TMS interference that affected lateralized inhibition processes.

Future Directions – Rehabilitation

TMS studies may play an explanatory role in the framework of intrahemispheric or interhemispheric compensation in language processing in clinical populations.

Meister et al. (2006) investigated the functional relationship between linguistic and hand movement processing in patients who were recovering from post-stroke aphasia. In patients, reading aloud enhanced the excitability of the right hemispheric hand motor cortex, whereas in the control group, an increased excitability of the left hemispheric hand motor system was found during reading aloud. This may indicate that the RH participates in language processing in patients recovering from aphasia. Further, Meister et al. (2006) suggested that the coactivation between cerebral representations of hand movements and language may be used therapeutically for aphasia rehabilitation. Such a proposal is consistent with the notion of interhemispheric compensation and reinforces the value of TMS as an ideal tool to apply it.

One hypothesis being explored in this author's laboratory is that during interference with a local brain area, rTMS could induce a functional reorganization in remote areas homologous to the "virtual lesion" to compensate the stimulated and disturbed area. More specifically, the reported therapeutic effects of rTMS could be attributed to an inhibition of the stimulated area, and its compensation by the homologue area in the contralateral hemisphere.

How can performance enhancement in clinical populations be achieved via remote stimulation? There are some examples of TMS studies of aphasia that have led to behavioral improvement. For example, in a preliminary study on patients with nonfluent aphasia, Naeser et al. (2005) observed significant and persistent improvement in naming pictures after rTMS application over the right IFG, the homologue to Broca's area (see also Naeser et al., Volume 2, Chapter 33). The authors postulated that rTMS decreased excitation in the right IFG, which in turn modulated activity in the distributed, bi-hemispheric language network. This result suggests a contralateral facilitation attributable to transcallosal disinhibition and supports the application of rTMS as a promising tool for aphasia rehabilitation.

These improvements are thought to be due to selective disinhibition in structures connected to the lesion site. In fact, lesions may form new sets of excitatory and inhibitory interactions, and facilitation could be related to the reduction or suppression of interference effects (Kapur, 1996). In line with this hypothesis, authors of PET studies of patients with focal cerebral lesions have noted that mechanisms underlying functional facilitation have been related to paradoxical increases in blood flow in structures distal but connected to the lesion site (Weiller, Chollet, Friston, Wise, & Frackowiak, 1992). This increase in cerebral blood flow has been interpreted as a functional disinhibition of structures that are connected by interhemispheric or intrahemispheric pathways to the critical lesion site.

Similarly, Musso et al. (1999) used PET to investigate short-term changes in the cortical network involved in language comprehension during recovery from Wernicke's aphasia. The results showed a correlation between blood flow in the right homologue of Wernicke's area and performance during a verbal comprehension task, supporting the mechanism of interhemispheric compensation to improve performance in some patients with Wernicke's aphasia.

Future applications following the "paradoxical" disinhibition effect are relevant as well for treatment of language disorders in schizophrenia. Aleman, Sommer, and Kahn (2007) demonstrated that rTMS in Wernicke's area induced inhibition, which in turn led to activation changes in the right hemispheric homologue of Wernicke's area. Since atypical patterns of language lateralization are often found in schizophrenia (Mitchel & Crow, 2005), this hypothesis raises the issue of the role of homologue areas in the contralateral hemisphere for the recovery of psychiatric disorders related to dysfunctions of language processing, such as schizophrenia.

In summary, this chapter reviewed the various TMS protocols that can modulate language-related behavior either directly in a "virtual lesion" mode (for example, all the inhibition studies in Table 3.1) or via cortico-cortical spreading (Paus et al., 1997). The latter protocol is the most intriguing, because TMS can be used to actually enhance recovery (Naeser et al., 2005). These enhancement effects illustrate a very long-lasting effect of TMS, far beyond transient first-order effects of stimulation. Presumably, TMS modulates activity throughout the language system via cortico-cortical spreading, and this activity is sufficient to promote plastic changes (i.e., reorganization) that improve performance. If these findings can be independently replicated and shown to rely on a controlled regimen of TMS "treatments," rTMS might become an important part of rehabilitative therapy to enhance recovery, at least in some aphasic patients. Currently TMS, together with direct current stimulation, are the only research tools that can reveal the causal roles of language functions in the left and right regions in healthy brains.

Note

Michal Lavidor is supported by an ERC starting grant (INSPIRE 200512).

References

Aleman, I. Sommer E., & Kahn, R. S. (2007). Efficacy of slow repetitive transcranial magnetic stimulation in the treatment of resistant auditory hallucinations in schizophrenia: A meta-analysis. *Journal of Clinical Psychiatry, 68*, 416–421.

Amassian, V. E., Cracco, R. Q., Maccabee, P. J., Cracco, J. B., Rudell, A., & Eberle, L. (1989). Suppression of visual perception by magnetic coil stimulation of human occipital cortex. *Electroencephalography and Clinical. Neurophysiology, 74*, 458–462.

Amassian, V. E., Maccabee, P. J., Cracco, R. Q., Cracco, J. B., Rudell, A. P., & Eberle, L. (1993). Measurement of information processing delays in human visual cortex with repetitive magnetic coil stimulation. *Brain Research, 605*, 317–321.

Andoh, J., Artiges, E., Pallier, C., Riviere, D., Mangin, J. F., Cachia, A., et al. (2006). Modulation of language areas with functional MR image-guided magnetic stimulation, *Neuroimage, 29*, 619–627.

Andoh, J., Artiges, E., Pallier, C., Riviere, D., Mangin, J. F., Paillere-Martinot, M. L., et al. (2008). Priming frequencies of transcranial magnetic stimulation over Wernicke's area modulate word detection. *Cerebral Cortex, 18*, 210–216.

Barker, A. T., Jalinous, R., & Freeston, I. L. (1985). Non-invasive magnetic stimulation of human motor cortex. *Lancet*, *1*, 1106–1107.

Barrett, J., Della-Maggiore, V., Chouinard, P. A., & Paus, T. (2004). Mechanisms of action underlying the effect of repetitive transcranial magnetic stimulation on mood: Behavioral and brain imaging studies. *Neuropsychopharmacology*, *29*, 1172–1189.

Bohning, D. E., He, L., George, M. S., & Epstein, C. M. (2001). Deconvolution of transcranial magnetic stimulation (TMS) maps. *Journal of Neural Transmission*, *108*, 35–52.

Bohning, D. E., Shastri, A., McConnell, K. A., Nahas, Z., Lorberbaum, J. P., Roberts D. R., et al. (1999). A combined TMS/fMRI study of intensity-dependent TMS over motor cortex. *Biological Psychiatry*, *45*, 385–394.

Braet, W., & Humphreys, G. W. (2006). The "Special Effect" of case mixing on word identification: Neuropsychological and transcranial magnetic stimulation studies dissociating case mixing from contrast reduction. *Journal of Cognitive Neuroscience*, *18*, 1666–1675.

Broca P. (1865). Sur le siège de la faculté du language articule. *Bulletin de la Société Anatomique de Paris*, *6*, 337–393.

Cowey, A., & Walsh, V. (2000). Magnetically induced phosphenes in sighted, blind and blind-sighted observers. *NeuroReport*, *11*, 3269–3273.

Dejerine J. (1892). Contribution à l'étude anatomo-pathologique et clinique des différentes variétés de cécité verbale. *Mémoires de la Société de Biologie*, *4*, 61–90.

Devlin, J. T., Matthews, P. M., & Rushworth, M. F. (2003). Semantic processing in the left inferior prefrontal cortex: A combined functional magnetic resonance imaging and transcranial magnetic stimulation study. *Journal of Cognitive Neuroscience*, *15*, 71–84.

Dräger, B., Breitenstein, C., Helmke, U., Kamping, S., & Knecht, S. (2004). Specific and non-specific effects of transcranial magnetic stimulation on picture–word verification. *European Journal of Neuroscience*, *20*, 1681–1687.

Fries, W., Danek, A., Scheidtmann, K., & Hamburger, C. (1993). Motor recovery following capsular stroke. Role of descending pathways from multiple motor areas. *Brain*, *116*, 369–382.

Gerloff, C., Cohen, L. G., Floeter, M. K., Chen, R., Corwell, B., & Hallett, M. (1998). Inhibitory influence of the ipsilateral motor cortex on responses to stimulation of the human cortex and pyramidal tract. *Journal of Physiology*, *510*, 249–259.

Giora, R. (2007). Is metaphor special? *Brain and Language*, *100*, 111–114.

Goldberg, E., & Costa, D. L. (1981). Hemisphere differences in the acquisition and use of descriptive systems. *Brain and Language*, *14*, 144–173.

Gough, P. M., Nobre, A. C., & Devlin, J. T. (2005). Dissociating linguistic processes in the left inferior frontal cortex with transcranial magnetic stimulation. *Journal of Neuroscience*, *25*, 8010–8016.

Hilgetag, C. C., Theoret, H., & Pascual-Leone, A. (2001). Enhanced visual spatial attention ipsilateral to rTMS induced "virtual lesions" of human parietal cortex. *Nature*, *4*, 953–957.

Huang, Y., Edwards, M., Rounis, E., Bhatia, K., & Rothwell, J. (2005). Theta burst stimulation of the human motor cortex. *Neuron*, *45*, 201–206.

Joanette, Y., & Goulet, C. (1994). Right hemisphere and verbal communication: Conceptual, methodological and clinical issues. *Clinical Aphasiology*, *22*, 1–23.

Johansen-Berg, H., Rushworth, M. F., Bogdanovic, M. D., Kischka, U., Wimalaratna, S., & Matthews, P. M. (2002). The role of ipsilateral premotor cortex in hand movement after stroke. *Proceedings of the National Academy of Sciences of the United States of America,* *99,* 14518–14523.

Joseph, J. E. (2001). Functional neuroimaging studies of category specificity in object recognition: A critical review and meta-analysis. *Cognitive, Affective and Behavioral Neuroscience, 1,* 119–136.

Jung-Beeman, M. (2005). Bilateral brain processes for comprehending natural language. *Trends in Cognitive Sciences, 9,* 512–518.

Kapur, N. (1996). Paradoxical functional facilitation in brain-behaviour research. A critical review. *Brain, 119,* 1775–1790.

Knecht, S., Ellger, T., Breitenstein, C., Ringelstein, E. B., & Henningsen, H. (2003). Changing cortical excitability with low-frequency transcranial magnetic stimulation can induce sustained disruption of tactile perception. *Biological Psychiatry, 53,* 175–179.

Knecht, S., Floel, A., Drager, B., Breitenstein, C., Sommer, J., Henningsen H., et al. (2002). Degree of language lateralization determines susceptibility to unilateral brain lesions. *Nature Neuroscience, 5,* 695–699.

Kobayashi, M., Hutchinson, S., Theoret, H., Schlaug, G., & Pascual-Leone, A. (2004). Repetitive TMS of the motor cortex improves ipsilateral sequential simple finger movements. *Neurology, 62,* 91–98.

Larsen, B., Skinhøj, E., & Lassen, N. (1979). Cortical activity in the left and right hemisphere provoked by reading and visual naming. *Acta Neurologica Scandinavia, 72,* 6–7.

Levy-Agresti, J., & Sperry, R. W. (1968). Differential perceptual capacities in major and minor hemispheres. *Proceedings of the National Academy of Science, 61,* 1.

Lomber, S. (1999). The advantages and limitations of permanent or reversible deactivation techniques in the assessment of neural function. *Journal of Neuroscience Methods, 86,* 109–118.

Meister, I. G., Sparing, R., Foltys, H., Gebert, D., Huber, W., Topper, R., et al. (2006). Functional connectivity between cortical hand motor and language areas during recovery from aphasia. *Journal of the Neurological Sciences, 247,* 165–168.

Mitchell, R. L. C., & Crow, T. J. (2005). Right hemisphere language functions and schizophrenia: The forgotten hemisphere? *Brain, 128,* 963–978.

Mottaghy, F. M., Hungs, M., Brügmann, M., Sparing, R., Boroojerdi, B., Foltys, H., et al. (1999). Facilitation of picture naming after repetitive transcranial magnetic stimulation. *Neurology, 53,* 1806–1812.

Munchau, A., Bloem, B. R., Irlbacher, K., Trimble, M. R., & Rothwell, J. C. (2002). Functional connectivity of human premotor and motor cortex explored with repetitive transcranial magnetic stimulation. *Journal of Neuroscience, 22,* 554–561.

Musso, M., Weiller, C., Kiebel, S., Muller, S. P., Bulau, P., & Rijntjes, M. (1999). Training-induced brain plasticity in aphasia. *Brain, 122,* 1781–1790.

Naeser, M. A., Martin, P. I., Nicholas, M., Baker, E. H., Seekins, H., Kobayashi, M., et al. (2005). Improved picture naming in chronic aphasia after TMS to part of right Broca's area: An open-protocol study. *Brain and Language, 93,* 95–105.

Nixon, P., Lazarova, J., Hodinott-Hill, I., Gough, P., & Passingham, R. (2004). The inferior frontal gyrus and phonological processing: An investigation using rTMS. *Journal of Cognitive Neuroscience, 16,* 289–300.

Oliveri, M., Romero, L., & Papagno, C. (2004). Left but not right temporal involvement in opaque idiom comprehension: A repetitive transcranial magnetic stimulation study. *Journal of Cognitive Neuroscience, 16,* 848–855.

O'Shea, J., Johansen-Berg, H., Trief, D., Gobel, S., & Rushworth, M. F. (2007). Functionally specific reorganization in human premotor cortex. *Neuron, 54,* 479–490.

Pascual-Leone, A., Gates, J. R., & Dhuna, A. (1991). Induction of speech arrest and counting errors with rapid-rate transcranial magnetic stimulation. *Neurology, 41,* 697–702.

Paus, T. (2005). Inferring causality in brain images: A perturbation approach. *Philosophical Transactions of the Royal Society of London. Series B, Biological sciences, 360,* 1109–1114.

Paus, T., Castro-Alamancos, M. A., & Petrides, M. (2001). Cortico-cortical connectivity of the human mid-dorsolateral frontal cortex and its modulation by repetitive transcranial magnetic stimulation. *European Journal of Neuroscience, 14,* 1405–1411.

Paus, T., Jech, R., Thompson, C. J., Comeau, R., Peters, T., & Evans, A. C. (1997). Transcranial magnetic stimulation during positron emission tomography: A new method for studying connectivity of the human cerebral cortex. *Journal of Neuroscience, 17,* 3178–3184.

Pobric, G., Mashal, N., Faust, M., & Lavidor, M. (2008). The role of the right cerebral hemisphere in processing novel metaphoric expressions: A TMS study. *Journal of Cognitive Neuroscience, 20,* 170–181.

Price, C. J. (2000). Functional-imaging studies of the nineteenth-century neurological model of language. *Revue Neurologique, 157,* 833–836.

Rothwell, J., Burke, D. T., Hicks, R., Stephen, J., Woodforth, I., & Crawford, M. (1994). Transcranial electrical stimulation of the motor cortex in man: Further evidence for the site of activation. *Journal of Physiology, 481*(1), 243–250.

Rounis, E., Lee, L., Siebner, H. R., Rowe, J. B., Friston K. J., Rothwell J. C., et al. (2005). Frequency specific changes in regional cerebral blood flow and motor system connectivity following rTMS to the primary motor cortex. *Neuroimage, 26,* 164–176.

Sakai, K. L., Noguchi, Y., Takeuchi, T., & Watanabe, E. (2002). Selective priming of syntactic processing by event-related transcranial magnetic stimulation of Broca's area, *Neuron, 35,* 1177–1182.

Sandrini, M., Rossini, P. M., & Miniussi, C. (2008). Lateralized contribution of prefrontal cortex in controlling task-irrelevant information during verbal and spatial working memory tasks: rTMS evidence. *Neuropsychologia, 46,* 2056–2063.

Schuhmann, T., Schiller, N. O., Goebel, R., & Sack, A. T. (2009). The temporal characteristics of functional activation in Broca's area during overt picture naming. *Cortex, 45,* 1111–1116.

Sergent, J. (1982). The cerebral balance of power: Confrontation or cooperation? *Journal of Experimental Psychology: Human Perception and Performance, 8,* 253–72.

Seyal, M., Ro, T., & Rafal, R. (1995). Increased sensitivity to ipsilateral cutaneous stimuli following transcranial magnetic stimulation of the parietal lobe. *Annals of Neurology, 38,* 264–267.

Sparing, R., Mottaghy, F. M., Hungs, M., Brugmann, M., Foltys H., Huber W., et al. (2001). Repetitive transcranial magnetic stimulation effects on language function depend on the stimulation parameters. *Journal of Clinical Neurophysiology, 18,* 326–330.

Stewart, L., Walsh, V., Frith, U., & Rothwell, J. (2001). TMS produces two dissociable types of speech disruption. *Neuroimage, 13,* 472–478.

Theoret, H., Kobayashi, M., Valero-Cabre, A., & Pascual-Leone, A. (2003). Exploring paradoxical functional facilitation with TMS. *Supplements to Clinical Neurophysiology, 56,* 211–219.

Thiel, A., Habedank, B., Herholz, K., Kessler, J., Winhuisen, L., Haupt, W. F., et al. (2006). From the left to the right: How the brain compensates progressive loss of language function. *Brain and Language, 98,* 57–65.

Thiel, A., Haupt, W. F., Habedank, B., Winhuisen, L., Herholz, K., Kessler, J., et al. (2005). Neuroimaging-guided rTMS of the left inferior frontal gyrus interferes with repetition priming. *Neuroimage, 25,* 815–823.

Topper, R., Mottaghy, F. M., Brugmann, M., Noth, J., & Huber, W. (1998). Facilitation of picture naming by focal transcranial magnetic stimulation of Wernicke's area. *Experimental Brain Research, 121,* 371–378.

Vallesi, A., Shallice, T., & Walsh, V. (2007). Role of the prefrontal cortex in the foreperiod effect: TMS evidence for dual mechanisms in temporal preparation. *Cerebral Cortex, 17,* 466–474.

Voets, N. L., Adcock, J. E., Flitney, D. E., Behrens, T. E., Hart, Y., Stacey, R., et al. (2006). Distinct right frontal lobe activation in language processing following left hemisphere injury. *Brain, 129,* 754–766.

Walsh, V., & Cowey, A. (1998). Magnetic stimulation studies of visual cognition. *Trends in Cognitive Sciences, 2,* 103–110.

Walsh, V., & Pascual-Leone, A. (2003). *Transcranial magnetic stimulation: A neurochronometrics of mind.* Harvard: MIT press.

Weiller, C., Chollet, F., Friston, K. J., Wise R. J. S., & Frackowiak, R. S. J. (1992). Functional reorganization of the brain in recovery from striatocapsular infarction in man. *Annals of Neurology, 31,* 463–472.

Wernicke, C. (1874). *Das aphasische symptomencomplex.* Breslau: Cohn & Weigert.

4

Understanding Written Words: Phonological, Lexical, and Contextual Effects in the Cerebral Hemispheres

Orna Peleg and Zohar Eviatar

In this chapter we present a model of the functional architecture of the way in which meaning is accessed during reading. The model is based on well-established general models of reading, and is applied to what we know about the division of labor in the cerebral hemispheres in the process of visual word recognition and meaning activation.

It is an arresting fact that all of the major models of language use in general, and of reading in particular, have been triangular, from Lichtheim Wernicke's and model of the relations between the centers for motor images, sound images, and concepts, to Seidenberg and McClelland's (1989) well-known connectionist model with orthographic, phonological, and semantic units. This triangular structure is based on the fact that the processing of written words requires readers to rapidly access and integrate knowledge about spelling, pronunciation, and meaning

The model we present is a general account of how this integration occurs in the two cerebral hemispheres. We propose that phonological, orthographic, and semantic representations are related to each other differently in each hemisphere. Specifically, we propose that there are no direct connections between orthographic and phonological representations in the right hemisphere (RH), whereas all three processes are completely interactive in the left hemisphere (LH) (see Figure 4.1).

The model is parsimonious, in that this single difference in architecture can account for many hemispheric asymmetries in reading reported in the literature. The model is general, because it is tested on a language that is very different from English, allowing for more precise generalizations about how the modal brain works. The model is timely, reflecting our growing realization of the dynamism and complexity of hemispheric abilities and relations, as it is clear that these

The Handbook of the Neuropsychology of Language, First Edition. Edited by Miriam Faust.
© 2012 Blackwell Publishing Ltd. Published 2012 by Blackwell Publishing Ltd.

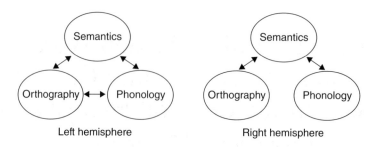

Figure 4.1 The functional architecture of reading in the two hemispheres.

underlie our experience of unity and diversity of consciousness, and higher cognitive functions.

Introduction

Phonological and orthographic asymmetries in visual word recognition

Although visual word recognition is normally conceptualized as being driven primarily by the analysis of orthography, it is now commonly accepted that the processing of a printed word is also influenced by information concerning its pronunciation. For example, behavioral studies using the masked-priming paradigm (e.g., Ferrand & Grainger, 1992, 1993) show that target recognition is speeded by the prior brief presentation of a masked pseudo-homophone prime (e.g., koat – COAT) relative to an orthographic control (poat – COAT). This literature has led a number of researchers (e.g., Frost, 1998) to suggest that phonological recoding is a mandatory, automatic phase of print processing.

Research on commissurotomy patients, however, suggests that this automatic phonological process proposed by Frost (1998) may be an accurate description of reading processes supported by the LH, but may not be applicable to the RH (e.g., Baynes & Eliassen, 1998; Zaidel, 1985; Zaidel & Peters, 1981). The basic finding, reported by Zaidel and Peters (1981), revealed that while the disconnected RH is able to connect the "sound image of a word" (i.e., its phonological representation) with a picture (i.e., its semantic representation) and to access the meaning of a word from its written form (i.e., its orthographic representation), it is unable to access the phonological form of a word from its written form. The disconnected LH, of course, can access all the representations of the word from its written form.

The majority of the studies examining hemispheric differences during reading in healthy participants use the divided visual field (DVF) paradigm. This technique takes advantage of the fact that stimuli presented in the left side of the visual field are initially processed exclusively by the RH and vice versa. Although information presented that way can be later transmitted to both hemispheres, the interpretation of DVF studies rests on the assumption that responses to stimuli presented briefly to one visual field reflect mainly the processing of that stimulus by the contralateral hemisphere, so that responses to targets in the right visual field (RVF) reflect LH processes and responses to targets in the LVF reflect RH processes. (For theoretical and electrophysiological support for this assumption, see Banich, 2003; Berardi & Fiorentini, 1997; Coulson, Federmeier, van Petten, & Kutas, 2005).

Similar to the split-brain results, DVF studies with intact participants demonstrate that the LH is more influenced by the phonological aspects of written words, whereas word recognition processes in the RH are more influenced by orthography (e.g., Lavidor & Ellis, 2003; Marsollek, Kosslyn, & Squire, 1992; Marsolek, Schacter, & Nicholas, 1996; Smolka & Eviatar, 2006). For example, Halderman and Chiarello (2005) utilized a backward masking paradigm in conjunction with a DVF display. In that experiment, target words (e.g., *bowl*) were presented and backward masked by nonwords that differed in the degree to which they shared orthographic and phonological information with the target. Three types of nonwords were used: pseudo-homophone (e.g., *bowl* – BOAL), orthographically similar, but phonologically less similar (e.g., *bowl* – BOOL), or unrelated controls (e.g., *bowl* – MANT). Stimuli were briefly presented to the LVF or to the RVF. The results indicated that responses to targets presented to the RVF/LH were facilitated in the phonological, pseudo-homophone condition relative to the orthographically similar condition. In contrast, responses to targets presented to the LVF/RH showed a greater degree of facilitation for the orthographically similar condition relative to the unrelated condition. Overall, these observations are consistent with the view that both hemispheres can recognize words visually via orthographic–semantic connections, but orthographic–phonological connections are available only to the LH.

Asymmetries in meaning activation

Lexical and contextual effects on ambiguity resolution   Understanding written words during sentence comprehension requires readers to rapidly access and integrate not only lexical knowledge related to the word itself (e.g., its spelling, pronunciation, and meaning), but also contextual knowledge related to the sentential context in which the word is embedded. This process is further complicated by the fact that many words have more than one distinct meaning and thus part of the comprehension process entails a selection of one of those meanings. Ample evidence from behavioral research indicates that this selection process is governed by lexical factors (for example, relative meaning frequency) and by contextual factors (for example, prior semantic information). However, despite decades of intensive research, the processes underlying ambiguity resolution are still controversial and not fully fleshed out.

On the one hand, serial models argue that all meanings of an ambiguous word are immediately activated regardless of either frequency or contextual bias. According to this view, contextually inappropriate meanings are discarded only at a later, postlexical selection stage (e.g., Onifer & Swinney 1981; Swinney, 1979). On the other hand, direct access models suggest that a strong biasing context can selectively activate the contextually appropriate meaning of an ambiguous word, regardless of relative meaning frequency (e.g., Martin, Vu, Kellas, & Metcalf, 1999; Vu, Kellas, & Paul, 1998). Between these two extremes, hybrid models such as the Reordered Model (Duffy, Morris, & Rayner, 1988) or the Graded Salience Hypothesis (Giora, 1997, 1991, 2003; Peleg, Giora, & Fein, 2001, 2004) suggest that both contextual and lexical factors influence meaning activation immediately and independently of each other. According to these models, context can facilitate the activation of the contextually appropriate meaning, but it cannot override relative meaning frequency. Thus, salient (frequent) meanings would be activated, even when contexts favor the less salient meaning of an ambiguous word.

Importantly, recent neuropsychological studies show that ambiguity resolution requires the intact functioning of both hemispheres. For example, not just unilateral LH damage, but also unilateral RH damage leads to deficits in ambiguity resolution (e.g., Grindrod & Baum, 2003). Similarly, imaging studies reveal bilateral activation during ambiguity resolution (e.g., Mason & Just, 2007). However, the unique contribution of each hemisphere to reading in general and to the resolution of homographs in particular remains to be elucidated.

Hemispheric asymmetries in lexical ambiguity resolution – The received view   Research using the DVF technique has led to the conclusion that the hemispheres differ significantly in the way they deal with lexical and contextual factors during ambiguity resolution (e.g., Burgess & Simpson, 1988; Faust & Chiarello, 1998; Faust & Gernsbacher, 1996). According to the received view, in the LH all meanings are immediately activated and shortly afterwards one meaning is selected on the basis of frequency and/or contextual information. The RH, on the other hand, activates all meanings more slowly and maintains these meanings irrespective of context or frequency.

Within this "standard model," the functioning of the LH is maximized: it has the ability to immediately activate both salient and less salient meanings and then to use both lexical and contextual information in order to select a single appropriate meaning. As a result, in the absence of contextual bias, it quickly selects the salient, more frequent meaning (e.g., Burgess & Simpson, 1988), while in the presence of a biasing prior context, it quickly selects the contextually appropriate meaning (e.g., Faust & Chiarello, 1998; Faust & Gernsbacher, 1996). The RH abilities, however, are minimized: first, activation of the less salient meaning is slower (e.g., Burgess & Simpson, 1988). In addition, it is viewed as less able to use lexical and/or contextual information for selection. As a result, it maintains alternate meanings regardless of their salience or contextual appropriateness (e.g., Burgess & Simpson, 1988; Faust & Chiarello, 1998; Faust & Gernsbacher, 1996).

A number of attempts have been made to account for this pattern of asymmetries. The fine/coarse coding hypothesis postulates that the cerebral hemispheres differ in their breadth of semantic activation, with the LH activating a narrow, focused semantic field and the RH weakly activating a broader semantic field (e.g., Beeman,

1998; Jung-Beeman, 2005; Mirous & Beeman, Volume 1, Chapter 16). As a result, meaning activation in the RH is relatively sustained and nonspecific, whereas meaning activation in the LH is faster and restricted to more frequent or closely associated meanings. According to the "message-blind RH" model (e.g., Faust, 1998), the LH is sensitive to sentence-level context, while the RH primarily processes word-level meaning and is therefore less able to use sentential information for selection. Finally, it was proposed that the RH is simply slower (e.g., Burgess & Lund, 1998). Because activation processes are slower, selection processes start later. As a result, alternative meanings are maintained for a longer period of time in the RH than in the LH. Taken together, current models of hemispheric differences in ambiguity resolution converge on a proposal that LH language processing is relatively more focused and faster than RH language processing, and takes place at higher (e.g., the sentence message) levels of analysis.

However, the idea that the RH is insensitive to higher-level, contextual processes seems at odds with neuropsychological studies reporting discourse-level deficits after RH damage (e.g., Brownell, Potter, Birhle, & Gardner, 1986), as well as the findings that patients with damage to either hemisphere display deficits in their ability to exploit sentence-level information to determine the appropriate meaning of homographs (e.g., Grindrod & Baum, 2003). Further, in contrast to the message-blind model, recent behavioral and neurological studies suggest that context sensitivity characterizes *both* hemispheres (e.g., Coulson et al., 2005; Federmeier & Kutas, 1999; Gouldthorp & Coney, 2009). We therefore suggest an alternative explanation for asymmetries in meaning activation from written words. Our explanation relates to the different ways in which orthographic, phonological, and semantic processes interact in the two hemispheres. Thus, rather than assuming asymmetries at higher (e.g., semantic) levels of analysis, we propose asymmetries at lower (e.g., phonological) levels of analysis.

Alternative Proposal

The dual hemispheric reading model

Generally speaking, there are two ways to access meaning from print: visually (from orthography directly to meaning) and phonologically (from orthography to phonology to meaning). As mentioned earlier, previous studies suggest that orthographic–semantic connections exist in both hemispheres, whereas orthographic–phonological direct associations are available only to the LH (e.g., Lavidor & Ellis, 2003; Smolka & Eviatar, 2006; Zaidel & Peters, 1981). On the basis of these findings, we propose a simple model in which both hemispheres exploit orthographic, phonological, and semantic information in the processing of written words. However, in the LH, orthographic, phonological, and semantic representations are fully interconnected, while there are no direct connections between phonological and orthographic units in the RH. The model is illustrated in Figure 4.1. We make no other assumptions about the nature of these representations in the two hemispheres. Indeed, we claim that this single difference in hemispheric functional architecture results in hemisphere asymmetries, in the disambiguation of homographs in particular, and, more broadly, in the processing of written words.

Processing implications – Homophonic versus heterophonic homographs

Because an orthographic representation of an English word (as well as other Latin orthographies) is usually associated with one phonological representation, most studies of lexical ambiguity used *homophonic homographs* – multiple meanings associated with a single orthographic and phonological representation (e.g., *bank*). As a result, models of hemispheric differences in lexical processing focus mainly on semantic organization (e.g., Jung-Beeman, 2005). We suggest that this reliance on homonyms has limited our understanding of hemispheric involvement in meaning activation, neglecting the contribution of phonological and orthographic asymmetries to hemispheric differences in semantic activation.

The unvoweled Hebrew orthography offers an opportunity to examine other types of homographs as well. In Hebrew, letters represent mostly consonants, and vowels can optionally be superimposed on consonants as diacritical marks. Since the vowel marks are usually omitted, Hebrew readers frequently encounter not only homophonic homographs (*bank*), but also *heterophonic homographs* – a single orthographic representation associated with multiple phonological codes each associated with a different meaning (e.g., *tear*). Both types of homographs have one orthographic representation associated with multiple meanings. They are different however, in terms of the relationship between orthography and phonology.

According to our proposed model (Figure 4.1), when orthographic and phonological representations are unambiguously related (as in the case of homophonic homographs like *bank*), meaning activation is faster in the LH than in the RH, because all related meanings are *immediately* boosted by both orthographic and phonological sources of information. However, when a single orthographic representation is associated with multiple phonological representations, (as in the case of heterophonic homographs like *tear*) meanings may be activated more slowly in LH than in the RH, due to the competition between the different phonological alternatives.

In order to contrast the received view with our proposal, we examined the disambiguation of homophonic versus heterophonic homographs in the two hemispheres: if hemispheric differences in processing homophonic homographs are due to differences in scope of semantic activation or in the ability to select a single meaning, then a similar pattern should be observed with heterophonic homographs. If, however, hemispheric differences in processing homophonic homographs are due to phonological asymmetries, then opposite asymmetries should be observed in the case of heterophonic homographs.

Table 4.1 Translated examples of stimuli.

Homograph type	Sentence context	Homograph	Pronunciation	Target words
Homophonic homograph	Unbiased: They looked at the	חזה	/XOZE/	Dominant – document
	Dominant: The buyers signed the	contract		Subordinate – prophet
	Subordinate: The Children of Israel listened to the	seer		
Heterophonic homograph	Unbiased: The young man looked for the	ספר	/SEFER/ /SAPAR/	Dominant – reading
	Dominant: The students were asked to buy the	book		Subordinate – hair
	Subordinate: The bride made an appointment with the	barber		

Experiments Demonstrating That Semantic Asymmetries are Modulated by Phonological Asymmetries

In our studies (Peleg & Eviatar, 2008, 2009, in preparation), a DVF technique was employed in conjunction with the lexical-priming paradigm. Participants were asked to silently read sentences that ended with either homophonic or heterophonic homographs and to perform a lexical decision task on targets presented laterally (to the LVF or to the RVF), 150 ms, 250 ms, or 1000 ms after the onset of the final homograph. Sentential contexts were either biased towards one interpretation of the final homograph, or unbiased. Targets were either related to one of the meanings of the ambiguous prime, or unrelated. Magnitude of priming was calculated by subtracting reaction time (RT) to related targets from RT to unrelated targets. Translated examples of the stimuli in the different conditions are presented in Table 4.1.

Predictions – Phonological, lexical, and contextual effects

Although the model does not assume any architectural asymmetries in sensitivity to contextual (e.g., prior semantic information) or experiential (e.g., frequency of occurrence) factors, it does make a number of predictions with regard to the way phonological asymmetries (direct orthographic–phonological connections in the LH vs. indirect connections in the RH) interact with lexical and contextual processes.

Effects of phonology   First, the model predicts that phonological effects will occur earlier in the reading process in the LH than in the RH. As a result, at early sites of activation (SOAs), differences between heterophonic and homophonic homographs will be more pronounced in the LH than in the RH. Specifically, it predicts that direct connections between orthographic and phonological representations in the LH should speed up lexical (bottom-up, stimulus driven) processes in the case of homophonic homographs, but should slow down lexical processes in the case of heterophonic homographs. Thus, in the case of homophonic homographs, multiple meanings may be activated faster in the LH than in the RH. Importantly, however, in the case of heterophonic homographs, multiple meanings may be activated more slowly in the LH than in the RH.

Effects of context   When a sentential context is biased, meanings can be activated via two separate routes: the contextual predictive route, and the lexical bottom-up route (e.g., Peleg et al., 2001, 2004). When contexts favor the salient meaning, activation of this meaning is facilitated by both contextual and lexical processes. However, when contexts favor the less salient meaning, contextually appropriate meanings would be activated via the contextual predictive route, whereas salient, more frequent meanings would be activated via lexical bottom-up processes. Importantly, when lexical bottom-up processes are fast, contextually inappropriate meanings are more likely to be immediately activated, resulting in simultaneous activation of multiple meanings. In contrast, when lexical bottom-up processes are slowed down, contextually inappropriate meanings are less likely to be immediately activated, resulting in a more ordered meaning activation, where the contextually appropriate meaning is activated before the more frequent but contextually inappropriate meaning. Thus, in the case of homophonic homographs, where lexical processes are faster in the LH, contextually inappropriate meanings may be activated more slowly in the RH than in the LH. However, in the case of heterophonic homographs, where lexical processes are slowed down in the LH, contextually inappropriate meanings may be activated more slowly in the LH than in the RH.

Effects of lexical frequency (salience)   The direct connections between orthography and phonology in the LH have implications for frequency effects as well. In principle, when homographs are polarized (one meaning is more frequent or salient than the other), we expect salient meanings to be activated before less salient meanings (Giora, 1997, 2003; Peleg et al., 2001, 2004). Given that heterophonic homographs are both phonologically and semantically ambiguous, whereas homophonic homographs are only semantically ambiguous, we expect larger effects of frequency for heterophones than for homophones. Frequency effects are found in both semantic and phonological representations of words. For homophonic homographs, frequency differences reflect relative exposure to different meanings. For heterophonic homographs, frequency differences reflect not only relative exposures to different meanings, but also relative exposures to different pronunciations. As a result, polarization (difference between the dominant and the subordinate meanings) should be larger for heterophonic homographs than for homophonic homographs. Thus, in the case of heterophonic homographs, frequent meanings may be more activated in the LH, whereas less frequent meanings may be more activated in the RH.

Effects of time   While our model predicts differences at earlier stages of the reading process, we assume that these differences affect later stages as well. First, given our assumption that both hemispheres are sensitive to lexical and contextual constraints, we expect salient and/or contextually appropriate meanings to be retained for a longer period of time in both hemispheres. In addition, we assume that when meanings are activated later in one hemisphere relative to the other hemisphere, decay processes may start later as well. As a result, in the case of homophonic homographs, meanings are more likely to be retained in the RH, whereas in the case of heterophonic homographs, meanings are more likely to be retained in the LH.

Results

As predicted by our model, different patterns of priming were found between homophonic and heterophonic homographs, indicating that hemispheric contributions to ambiguity resolution are modulated by the phonological status of the homograph. Overall, we show that in the case of homophonic homographs, meanings are activated and decay faster in the LH than in the RH. In contrast, the opposite pattern was found with heterophonic homographs: both activation and decay processes are faster in the RH than in the LH. In the following we report the timeline of ambiguity resolution for each context condition separately.

When contexts are kept neutral   In a neutral, non-biasing context, we see a different pattern of results in the two visual fields and for the two types of homographs. These are illustrated in Figure 4.2. In the RVF/LH (see Figure 4.2b), both meanings of homophonic homographs were available at 150 SOA. However, 100 ms later, only the dominant, more frequent meaning remained active. At 1000 SOA, none of the meanings were retained. In the LVF/RH (see Figure 4.2a), the less salient meaning was activated more slowly, so that 150 ms after the onset of the ambiguous prime, only salient meanings were significantly activated. Shortly afterwards (at 250 SOA), the less salient meaning was activated alongside the salient one. At 1000 SOA, only the dominant meaning remained active. Overall, these results indicate that in the case of homophonic homographs, multiple activation and decay processes are faster in the LH.

Heterophonic homographs, however, revealed a different pattern of results. In the RVF/LH (see Figure 4.2d), salient meanings were activated exclusively, regardless of SOA. Alternatively, in the LVF/RH (see Figure 4.2c), 150 ms after homograph presentation, only salient meanings were significantly activated. However, shortly afterwards (at 250 SOA), the less salient meaning was activated alongside the salient one. At 1000 SOA none of the meanings were retained. Overall, these results indicate

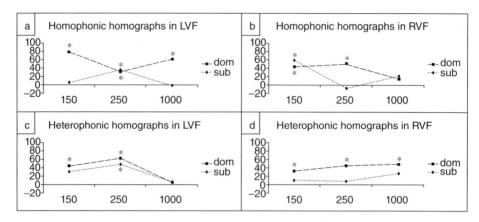

Figure 4.2 Magnitude of priming effects (in ms) for targets related to the dominant/ frequent, more salient meaning of homographs (dashed lines), and to targets related to the less salient meaning (dotted lines), as a function of SOA (150 ms, 250 ms, or 1000 ms), when contexts are kept neutral. Note: *Significant, $p < 0.5$.

that in the case of heterophonic homographs, multiple activation and decay processes are faster in the RH.

When contexts favor the salient meaning In a context biasing towards the salient, more frequent meaning, this meaning is activated exclusively, regardless of SOA, location of target (LVF or RVF), or type of homograph. This indicates that *both* hemispheres are able to selectively access the contextually appropriate meaning, when this meaning is both salient and supported by contextual information.

When contexts favor the subordinate meaning In a context biasing towards the less salient meaning, we see a different pattern of results in the two visual fields and for the two types of homographs. These are illustrated in Figure 4.3. For homophonic homographs, both meanings (the contextually compatible less salient meaning as well as the contextually inappropriate salient meaning) were activated at 150 SOA and remained active at 250 SOA, regardless of target location (RVF or LVF). However, at 1000 SOA, only the compatible subordinate meaning remained active and only in the LVF/RH (see Figure 4.3a,b). Overall, these results indicate that in the case of homophonic homographs, meanings are retained for a longer period of time in the RH.

Heterophonic homographs, however, were processed differently: in the RVF/LH (see Figure 4.3d), at 150 SOA, the contextually subordinate meaning was activated exclusively. Shortly afterwards, however, at 250 SOA, the salient inappropriate meaning was also activated. Both meanings remained active at 1000 SOA. In contrast, in the LVF/RH (see Figure 4.3c), both meanings were immediately activated (150 SOA) and remained active at 250 SOA. However, at 1000 SOA, the contextually appropriate subordinate meaning was activated exclusively. Overall, these results

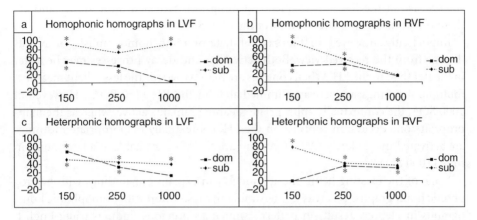

Figure 4.3   Magnitude of priming effects (in ms) for targets related to the dominant/ frequent, more salient meaning of homographs (dashed lines), and to targets related to the less salient meaning (dotted lines), as a function of SOA (150 ms, 250 ms, or 1000 ms), when contexts favor the less salient, subordinate meaning. Note: *Significant, $p < 0.5$.

indicate that in the case of heterophonic homographs, salient but contextually inappropriate meanings are available earlier in the RH, but are retained for a longer period of time in the LH.

Conclusions

According to the received view, when readers encounter an ambiguous word, multiple meanings are available immediately in the LH, but shortly afterwards one meaning is selected on the basis of relative frequency and/or contextual information. The RH, on the other hand, activates all meanings more slowly and maintains these meanings irrespective of context or frequency. On the basis of such findings, current hemispheric models of ambiguity resolution have converged on the proposal that LH language processing is relatively more focused, faster, and takes place at higher levels of analysis than RH language processing. The work we have described here and in Peleg and Eviatar (2008, 2009, in preparation) suggests a different, more complex picture of hemispheric abilities. Our use of heterophonic homographs in a language in which these are frequent, reveals complementary hemispheric contributions which are much more dynamic than previously assumed.

   As predicted by our model, our findings show that hemispheric differences in the time course of meaning activation and meaning decay are modulated by the phonological status of the homograph. In the case of homophonic homographs, our results converge with the received view. Both activation and decay processes are faster in the LH than in the RH. In neutral contexts, both meanings are activated immediately in the LH (150 SOA). However, shortly afterwards (250 SOA), the salient, more frequent meaning remains active, while the less frequent one decays.

In contrast, in the RH, less frequent meanings are activated more slowly and are therefore available at a later point in time (250 SOA).

Importantly, however, in the case of heterophonic homographs, our results diverge from the received view. Both activation and decay processes may be faster in the RH than in the LH. When contexts are biased towards the less salient meaning, multiple meanings are activated immediately in the RH (150 SOA). However, at 1000 SOA, the contextually appropriate meaning remains active, whereas the inappropriate one decays. In contrast, in the LH, contextually inappropriate meanings are activated more slowly (250 SOA) and are therefore available at a later point in time (1000 SOA).

None of the existing hemispheric models can explain our findings with heterophonic homographs. Whereas testing ambiguity resolution with homophonic homographs in Hebrew results in patterns similar to previous findings using English (e.g. Burgess & Simpson, 1988), testing heterophonic homographs, which are quite common in Hebrew but quite rare in English, results in patterns of activation and decay quite different from those found in previous studies. In fact, as shown above, the RH seems to be able to immediately activate multiple meanings, and also to quickly choose the contextually appropriate meaning. In contrast, when dealing with these heterophonic homographs, the LH activates meanings more slowly and retains them for a longer period of time. Recall that this pattern is reversed relative to the pattern described by the received view.

Our model is highly parsimonious: rather than assuming differences in the scope of meaning activation (e.g., Beeman et al., 1994; Jung-Beeman, 2005; Mirous & Beeman, Volume 1, Chapter 16), or in the processes involved in meaning selection (e.g., Faust & Chiarello, 1998; Copland, Chenery, & Murdoch, 2002), we propose that all these asymmetries can be accounted for by one difference in the functional architecture in the two hemispheres. Specifically, our model postulates no direct connections between orthographic and phonological representations in the RH. However, in the LH, phonological, orthographic, and semantic representations are entirely interactive (see Figure 4.1). Importantly, as mentioned above, this model not only explains existing data based on homophonic homographs, but also accounts for reverse asymmetries in the disambiguation of heterophonic homographs.

We assume that meaning activation depends on both contextual processes (e.g., prior semantic information) and lexical processes sensitive to experiential familiarity (e.g., frequency of occurrence, or salience; see Giora, 1997). Both processes occur in both hemispheres. As a result, contextually appropriate and/or salient meanings are more likely to be activated earlier and to remain active for longer periods of time, while inappropriate and/or less salient meanings may be activated more slowly and are more likely to decay faster. However, as a result of the two functional architectures (see Figure 4.1), contextual and lexical processes may occur at different temporal stages in the two cerebral hemispheres and may have differential effects for the two types of homographs.

First, in the case of polarized heterophonic homographs, frequency effects may be more pronounced in the LH than in the RH, because in the LH they immediately affect not only semantic processes but also phonological processes. In contrast, in the RH phonological effects are delayed. As a result, when a biasing context is not provided and meaning activation is guided only by frequency, frequent meanings are more likely to be activated and retained in the LH, whereas less frequent meanings are more likely to be activated in the RH. Second, when lexical processes are fast, frequent meanings are more likely to be immediately activated, regardless of context. However, when lexical information is activated more slowly, as in the case of heterophonic homographs in the LH, context (predictive) effects may precede relative frequency effects. As a result, when contexts favor the less frequent meaning, inappropriate frequent meanings are activated more slowly in the LH than in the RH.

Thus, in agreement with other studies examining homophonic homographs (e.g., Burgess & Simpson, 1988), our findings demonstrate that, when contexts are kept neutral or favor the less salient meaning, multiple meanings are immediately activated in the LH. Under similar circumstances (when contexts are kept neutral), a more ordered activation is observed in the RH. In contrast, in the case of heterophonic homographs, our findings demonstrate that, when contexts favor the less salient meaning, immediate activation of multiple meanings is observed in the RH, whereas a more ordered activation is observed in the LH.

While our model mainly explains differences at earlier stages of the reading process, these differences also affect later processing stages. First, recall that in accordance with our assumption that both hemispheres are sensitive to lexical and contextual constraints, we show that in both hemispheres, salient and/or contextually appropriate meanings are retained for a longer period of time, whereas less frequent and/or contextually inappropriate meanings are more likely to decay earlier. In addition, our results indicate that when meanings are activated later in one hemisphere compared to the other hemisphere, decay processes may start later as well. As a result, in the case of homophonic homographs, meanings are more likely to be retained in the RH, whereas in the case of heterophonic homographs, meanings are more likely to be retained in the LH. These reverse asymmetries in the time course of meaning activation and decay can only be explained by taking into account phonological asymmetries.

Beyond hemispheric differences, our results have implications for general models of reading and ambiguity resolution. Contrary to the predictions of the direct-access (context-sensitive) model (e.g., Vu et al., 1998), suggesting that a strong context can selectively activate the contextually appropriate meaning, regardless of salience, we show that *both* context and salience influence the retrieval of word meanings. Importantly, in agreement with hybrid models such as the Graded Salience Hypothesis (e.g., Giora, 1997, 2003; Peleg et al., 2001, 2004, 2008), our results show that context can enhance activation of the contextually appropriate meaning, but it cannot inhibit salient meanings even when these are contextually inappropriate.

Thus, even when contexts favor the less salient meaning, salient, more frequent meanings are still activated: in the case of homophonic homographs, both meanings were activated immediately (150 SOA) and remained active 100 ms later, regardless of visual field. Interestingly, even when contextual processes preceded lexical processes, as in the case of heterophonic homographs, in which the contextually appropriate meaning was activated exclusively in the LH (150 SOA), 100 ms later (250 SOA) the salient but contextually inappropriate meaning also became available, regardless of context.

In addition, our results shed light on one of the main controversies in the reading literature; namely, the role phonology plays in silent reading. One class of models suggests that printed words activate orthographic codes that are directly related to meanings in semantic memory. An alternative class of models asserts that access to meaning is always mediated by phonology. (For a review, see Frost, 1998; van Orden & Kloos, 2005.) Current models of reading incorporate both phonological and orthographic processes. Dual route models (e.g., Coltheart & Kohnen, Volume 2, Chapter 43; Coltheart, Rastle, Perry, Langdon, & Ziegler, 2001) assume that meanings can be accessed either via the direct, orthographic/visual route, or via orthography–phonology decoding. Connectionist models (e.g., Harm & Seidenberg, 2004) propose an interactive system that always uses both orthography and phonology to access the meaning of words.

By looking at differential hemispheric involvement in orthographic and phonological processes, we may be able to resolve these differences. Recall that our model assumes that in the LH orthographic units are directly related to both phonological and semantic units. It therefore predicts that meaning activation in the LH will be instantly influenced by phonology. As expected, our results indeed show that when a short SOA (150 ms) was used, homophonic and heterophonic homographs, which diverge on how their meanings are related to phonology, were processed differently in the LH. Recall further that our model assumes that in the RH, phonological codes are not directly related to orthographic codes and are activated indirectly, via semantic codes. This organization, in the RH, should result in a different timing of activation: the phonological computation of orthographic representations should begin later than the semantic computation of the same representations. As a result, lexical access in the RH should initially be affected to a greater extent by orthography than by phonology. As expected, our results demonstrate that, in the RH, at a short SOA (150 ms) similar patterns (in terms of significant priming effects) were obtained for both types of homographs. These results converge with previous studies showing that the LH is more influenced by the phonological aspects of a written word (e.g., Halderman & Chiarello, 2005; Lavidor & Ellis, 2003; Zaidel, 1982; Zaidel & Peters, 1981), whereas lexical processing in the RH is more sensitive to the visual form of a written word (e.g., Halderman & Chiarello 2005; Lavidor & Ellis, 2003; Marsollek et al., 1992; Marsolek et al., 1996; Smolka & Eviatar, 2006).

The overall picture that emerges from the present results is that hemispheric processes may be more similar than assumed earlier. It seems that both hemispheres have access to the same sources of information (orthographic, phonological, lexical, and contextual); however, as a result of the two functional architectures (see Figure 4.1) these may be used differently, and at different temporal stages. We thus propose that RH processing reflects a different pattern of interaction between orthographic, phonological, and semantic information, rather than, as suggested by other models, lower sensitivity to lexical and contextual constraints. This view of RH abilities converges with many neuropsychological studies, both behavioral and imaging studies, showing RH involvement in comprehending the full meaning of words, phrases, and texts (e.g., Coulson & Williams, 2005; Eviatar & Just, 2006; Federmeier & Kutas, 1999; Giora, Zaidel, Soroker, Batori, & Kasher, 2000; Mashal, Faust, & Hendler, 2005; McDonald, 1996, 1999).

It is clear that during normal reading, both hemispheres are involved in accessing the meaning of print stimuli. In real life, multiplicity of meaning is very common, and skilled readers are able to access and manipulate these multiple meanings easily and flexibly. We have begun to specify how the hemispheres may cooperate in this very complex task, and suggest complementary hemispheric contributions during the disambiguation processes of homographs, which are much more dynamic than previously assumed. By exploiting the distinction between homophonic and heterophonic homographs in Hebrew, we show that a single architectural difference (namely, direct vs. indirect orthographic–phonological connections) can explain existing data based on homophonic homographs (in Hebrew and English), as well as reverse asymmetries in the disambiguation of heterophonic homographs. In this way, our model provides a more comprehensive, coherent, and general framework for understanding the hemispheres' separable abilities and tendencies during normal reading comprehension.

References

Banich, M. T. (2003). Interaction between the hemispheres and its implications for the processing capacity of the brain. In R. Davidson & K. Hughdahl (Eds.), *Brain asymmetry* (2nd ed., pp. 261–302). Cambridge, MA: MIT Press.

Baynes, K., & Eliassen, J. (1998). The visual lexicon: Its access and organization in commissurotomy patients. In M. Beeman & C. Chiarello (Eds.), *Right hemisphere language comprehension* (pp. 79–104). Mahwah, NJ: Erlbaum.

Beeman, M. (1998). Coarse semantic coding and discourse comprehension. In M. Beeman & C. Chiarello (Eds.), *Right hemisphere language comprehension: Perspectives from cognitive neuroscience* (pp. 255–284). Mahwah, NJ: Erlbaum.

Beeman, M., Friedman, R., Grafman, J., Perez, E., Diamond, S., & Lindsay, M. (1994). Summation priming and coarse coding in the right hemisphere. *Journal of Cognitive Neuroscience, 6*, 26–45.

Berardi, N., & Fiorentini, A. (1997). Interhemispheric transfer of spatial and temporal frequency information. In S. Christman (Ed.), *Cerebral asymmetries in sensory and perceptual processing* (pp. 55–79). New York: Elsevier Science.

Brownell, H. H., Potter, H. H., Birhle, A. M., & Gardner, H. (1986). Inference deficits in right brain-damaged patients. *Brain and Language, 27*, 310–321.

Burgess, C., & Lund, K. (1998). Modeling cerebral asymmetries of semantic memory using high-dimensional semantic space. In M. Beeman & C. Chiarello (Eds.), *Right hemisphere language comprehension: Perspectives from cognitive neuroscience.* Hillsdale, NJ: Erlbaum.

Burgess, C., & Simpson, G. B. (1988). Cerebral hemispheric mechanisms in the retrieval of ambiguous word meanings. *Brain and Language, 33,* 86–103.

Coltheart, M., Rastle, K., Perry, C., Langdon, R., & Ziegler, J. (2001). Drc: A dual route cascaded model of visual word recognition and reading aloud. *Psychological Review, 108*(1), 204–256.

Copland, D. A., Chenery, H. J., & Murdoch, B. E. (2002). Hemispheric contributions to lexical ambiguity resolution: Evidence from individuals with complex language impairment following left hemisphere lesions. *Brain and Language, 81,* 131–143.

Coulson, S., Federmeier, K., van Petten, C., & Kutas, M. (2005). Right hemisphere sensitivity to word and sentence level context: Evidence from event-related brain potentials. *Journal of Experimental Psychology: Learning, Memory, and Cognition, 31,* 129–147.

Coulson, S., & Williams, R. W. (2005). Hemispheric asymmetries and joke comprehension. *Neuropsychologia, 43,* 128–141.

Duffy, S. A., Morris, R. K., & Rayner, K. (1988). Lexical ambiguity and fixation times in reading. *Journal of Memory and Language, 27,* 429–446.

Eviatar, Z., & Just, M. A. (2006). Brain correlates of discourse processing: An fMRI investigation of irony and metaphor comprehension. *Neuropsychologia, 44,* 2348–2359.

Faust, M. (1998). Obtaining evidence of language comprehension from sentence priming. In M. Beeman & C. Chiarello (Eds.), *Right hemisphere language comprehension: perspectives from cognitive neuroscience* (pp. 161–186). Hillsdale, NJ: Erlbaum.

Faust, M., & Chiarello, C. (1998). Sentence context and lexical ambiguity resolution by the two hemispheres. *Neuropsychologia, 36,* 827–835.

Faust, M., & Gernsbacher, M. A. (1996). Cerebral mechanisms for suppression of inappropriate information during sentence comprehension. *Brain and Language, 53,* 234–259.

Federmeier, K. D., & Kutas, M. (1999). Right words and left words: Electrophysiological evidence for hemispheric differences in meaning processing. *Cognitive Brain Research, 8,* 373–392.

Ferrand, L., & Grainger, J. (1992). Phonology and orthography in visual word recognition: Evidence from masked nonword priming. *Quarterly Journal of Experimental Psychology, 45A,* 353–372.

Ferrand, L., & Grainger, J. (1993). The time-course of phonological and orthographic code activation in the early phases of visual word recognition. *Bulletin of the Psychonomic Society, 31,* 119–122.

Frost, R. (1998). Toward a strong phonological theory of visual word recognition: True issues and false trails. *Psychological Bulletin, 123,* 71–99.

Giora, R. (1991). A probabilistic view of language. *Poetics Today, 12*(1), 165–179.

Giora, R. (1997). Understanding figurative and literal language: The graded salience hypothesis. *Cognitive Linguistics, 7*(1), 183–206.

Giora, R. (1999). On the priority of salient meanings: Studies of literal and figurative language. *Journal of Pragmatics, 31,* 919–929.

Giora, R. (2003). *On our mind: Salience, context, and figurative language.* New York: Oxford University Press.

Giora, R., Zaidel, E., Soroker, N., Batori, G., & Kasher, A. (2000). Differential effect of right and left hemispheric damage on understanding sarcasm and metaphor. *Metaphor and Symbol, 15,* 63–83.

Gouldthorp, B., & Coney, J. (2009). The sensitivity of the right hemisphere to contextual information in sentences. *Brain and Language, 110*, 95–100.

Grindrod, C. M., & Baum, S. R. (2003). Sensitivity to local sentence context information in lexical ambiguity resolution: Evidence from left- and right-hemisphere-damaged individuals. *Brain and Language, 85*, 503–523.

Halderman L, K., & Chiarello, C. (2005). Cerebral asymmetries in early orthographic and phonological reading processes: Evidence from backward masking. *Brain and language 95*(2), 342–52.

Harm, M. W., & Seidenberg, M. S. (2004). Computing the meanings of words in reading: Cooperative division of labor between visual and phonological processes. *Psychological Review, 111*, 662–720.

Jung-Beeman, M. (2005). Bilateral brain processes for comprehending natural language. *Trends in Cognitive Sciences, 9*, 512–518.

Lavidor, M., & Ellis, A. W. (2003). Orthographic and phonological priming in the two cerebral hemispheres. *Laterality, 8*, 201–223.

Marsolek, C. J., Kosslyn, S. M., & Squire, L. R. (1992). Form-specific visual priming in the right cerebral hemisphere. *Journal of Experimental Psychology: Learning, Memory, and Cognition, 18*, 492–508.

Marsolek, C. J., Schacter, D. L., & Nicholas, C. D. (1996). Form-specific visual priming for new associations in the right cerebral hemisphere. *Memory and Cognition, 24*, 539–556.

Martin, C., Vu, H., Kellas, G., & Metcalf, K. (1999). Strength of discourse context as a determinant of the subordinate bias effect. *Quarterly Journal of Experimental Psychology, 52A*, 813–839.

Mashal, N., Faust, M., & Hendler, T. (2005). The role of the right hemisphere in processing nonsalient metaphorical meanings: Application of principal components analysis to fMRI data. *Neuropsychologia, 43*(14), 2084–2100.

Mason, R. A., & Just, M. A. (2007). Lexical ambiguity in sentence comprehension. *Brain Research, 1146*, 115–127.

McDonald, S. (1996). Clinical insights into pragmatic theory: Frontal lobe deficits and sarcasm. *Brain and Language, 68*, 486–506.

McDonald, S. (1999). Exploring the process of inference generation in sarcasm: A review of normal and clinical studies. *Brain and Language, 68*, 486–506.

McDonald, S., & Pearce, S. (1996). Clinical insights into pragmatic theory: Frontal lobe deficit and sarcasm. *Brain and Language, 53*, 81–104.

Onifer, W., & Swinney, D. A. (1981). Accessing lexical ambiguities during sentence comprehension: Effects of frequency of meaning and contextual bias. *Memory and Cognition, 9*(3), 225–236.

Peleg, O., & Eviatar, Z. (2008). Hemispheric sensitivities to lexical and contextual constraints: Evidence from ambiguity resolution. *Brain and Language, 105*(2), 71–82.

Peleg, O., & Eviatar, Z. (2009). Semantic asymmetries are modulated by phonological asymmetries: Evidence from the disambiguation of heterophonic versus homophonic homographs. *Brain and Cognition 70*, 154–162.

Peleg, O., & Eviatar, Z. (in preparation). Meaning selection in the two cerebral hemispheres: Evidence from the disambiguation of heterophonic versus homophonic homographs.

Peleg, O., Giora, R., & Fein, O. (2001). Salience and context effects: Two are better than one. *Metaphor and Symbol, 16*, 173–192.

Peleg, O., Giora, R., & Fein, O. (2004). Contextual strength: The whens and hows of context effects. In I. Noveck & D. Sperber (Eds.), *Experimental pragmatics* (pp. 172–186). Palgrave: Basingstoke.

Peleg, O., Giora, R., & Fein, O. (2008). Resisting contextual information: You can't put a salient meaning down. *Lodz Papers in Pragmatics 4*(1), 13–44.

Seidenberg, M. S., & McClelland, J. L. (1989). A distributed, developmental model of word recognition and naming. *Psychology Review, 96*, 523–568.

Smolka, E., & Eviatar, Z. (2006). Phonological and orthographic visual word recognition in the two cerebral hemispheres: Evidence from Hebrew. *Cognitive Neuropsychology, 23*(6), 972–989.

Swinney, D. (1979). Lexical access during sentence comprehension: Reconsideration of context effects. *Journal of Verbal Learning and Verbal Behavior, 18*, 645–660.

Van Orden, G. C., & Kloos, H. (2005). The question of phonology and reading. In M. S. Snowling & C. Hulme (Eds.), *The science of reading: A handbook* (pp. 61–78). Oxford: Blackwell.

Vu, H., Kellas, G., & Paul, S. (1998). Sources of sentence constraint on lexical ambiguity resolution. *Memory and Cognition, 26*(5), 979–1001.

Zaidel, E. (1982). Reading in the disconnected right hemisphere: An aphasiological perspective. *Dyslexia: Neuronal, cognitive and linguistic aspects* (vol. 35, pp. 67–91). Oxford: Pergamon Press.

Zaidel, E. (1985). Language in the right hemisphere. In D. F. Benson & E. Zaidel (Eds.), *The dual brain: Hemispheric specialization in humans* (pp. 205–231). New York: The Guilford Press.

Zaidel, E., & Peters, A. M. (1981). Phonological encoding and ideographic reading by the disconnected right hemisphere: Two case Studies. *Brain and Language, 14*, 205–234.

5

The Organization of Discourse in the Brain: Results From the Item-Priming-in-Recognition Paradigm

Debra L. Long, Clinton L. Johns, Eunike Jonathan,
and Kathleen Baynes

Two important aims of language comprehension research are to understand how mental representations of discourse are constructed from linguistic input and to understand how these representations are stored and organized in long-term memory. In the last two decades, most comprehension research has focused on the first of these aims, understanding language processing in real time ("online"), as words and sentences are processed. This focus has both theoretical and methodological origins. An important theoretical impetus was Fodor's (1983) modularity hypothesis. He argued that language comprehension involves processes much like those in visual perception. They operate in an autonomous bottom-up manner, in the sense that linguistic processes (e.g., word recognition, syntactic analysis) are isolated from the influence of world knowledge and context. The modularity hypothesis can only be tested by examining the time course of language comprehension to determine when contextual information is used. Methodological developments also contributed to the real-time focus in studies of language comprehension. Researchers have developed sophisticated eye-tracking and electrophysiological techniques, allowing them to track the activation of information during comprehension with millisecond accuracy.

We have made substantial gains in our knowledge about the time course of online language processing; however, these gains have been achieved at the expense of research aimed at specifying the nature of discourse in long-term memory. The lack of attention to this issue is unfortunate because understanding the nature of discourse representation is important for several reasons. First, online methods alone cannot discriminate the temporary activation of concepts during comprehension

The Handbook of the Neuropsychology of Language, First Edition. Edited by Miriam Faust.
© 2012 Blackwell Publishing Ltd. Published 2012 by Blackwell Publishing Ltd.

from the integration of those concepts into a stable and permanent representation. Many concepts are activated by the individual words in a sentence; however, only a few of these are incorporated into a long-term memory representation (Graesser, Singer, & Trabasso, 1994; McKoon & Ratcliff, 1992, 1998). Second, discourse representations in natural language contexts are constructed over extended periods of time. New linguistic input is understood in light of representations that were constructed previously and stored in memory (Gernsbacher, 1989, 1990; Kintsch, 1988). Understanding how discourse is organized in memory is important in understanding how new input is integrated into the developing discourse representation. Finally, and most relevant to the topic of this chapter, understanding how discourse is represented can constrain theories of comprehension and yield new hypotheses about real-time language comprehension, including theories of language organization in the brain.

Our goal in this chapter is to describe a method for examining the nature of discourse representation and our use of this method to understand how discourse concepts are stored and organized in the two cerebral hemispheres. In the first section, we describe theories of discourse representation. Next, we describe a method, called item-priming-in-recognition, for investigating memory for discourse concepts. We then describe how we have used this method to examine discourse representation in both neurologically healthy young adults and brain-damaged patients. We conclude by discussing how our findings inform theories of discourse comprehension in the brain.

The Nature of Discourse Representation

Most theories of discourse representation claim that comprehenders construct at least two interrelated representations during language understanding (Gernsbacher, 1990; Graesser et al., 1994; Greene, McKoon, & Ratcliff, 1992; Kintsch, 1988; Kintsch & van Dijk, 1978; McKoon & Ratcliff, 1990, 1992, 1998). One representation consists of the concepts that are explicit in discourse and the relations among them. This is often called a propositional network or a textbase. Word-level and sentence-level processes are essential in constructing this network. Idea units are derived from sentences by assigning thematic roles to predicates. These units are connected to one another by means of syntactic, referential, and semantic relations. Thus, the network is structured such that some concepts and ideas are more closely related than are other concepts and ideas.

A second representation, called a discourse model or situation model, consists of the comprehenders' understanding of the real or fictional situation that discourse describes (Kintsch, 1988; Sanford & Garrod, 1998; Zwaan & Radvansky, 1998). This involves mapping concepts and ideas in the propositional network to relevant world knowledge. The discourse model contains information about people and their goals, causes and consequences, and temporal/spatial relations among people and objects.

A classic example from Bransford and Johnson (1972) illustrates the distinction between a propositional network and a discourse model. Consider the following sentence:

1   The haystack was important because the cloth ripped.

The execution of word-level and sentence-level processes will result in a propositional network consisting of three ideas: (1) there was an important haystack; (2) there was a cloth that ripped; and (3) the important haystack and the ripped cloth have a causal connection such that former was important because of the latter. The successful construction of a propositional network, however, is not sufficient for understanding what the sentence is about. The sentence is presented in the absence of context and the particular words in this sentence do not evoke relevant world knowledge (e.g., a schema) that can be used to construct the discourse model. This can be remedied by telling the reader that the sentence is about skydiving. With this knowledge, the reader can map the concept *cloth* to a sensible referent (i.e., parachute) and can make appropriate inferences such as "a ripped parachute caused the skydiver to fall" and "the haystack was important because it cushioned the skydiver's landing."

We have conducted a series of experiments to examine how the propositional network and discourse model are represented in the two hemispheres (Baynes, Long, Gillette, Dronkers, & Davis, 2002; Long & Baynes, 2002; Long, Baynes, & Prat, 2005, 2007; Prat, Long, & Baynes, 2007). We have investigated two hypotheses. First, the propositional network and discourse model may be represented similarly across the hemispheres. This might occur if the two hemispheres have similar roles in constructing the representations or if the hemispheres have somewhat different roles, but the outcome of processing is shared. Second, the hemispheres may store different information about discourse. This might occur if the hemispheres have different roles in constructing the propositional network and discourse model and if these different roles have consequences for how discourse information is represented in memory. In the next section, we describe our method for investigating these hypotheses.

Item-Priming-in-Recognition

The item-priming-in-recognition paradigm was developed by McKoon and Ratcliff (1980) to study the nature of discourse representation. The logic of the paradigm relies on the assumption that comprehension results in a network of concepts and that the retrieval of one concept can facilitate the retrieval of other concepts as a function of their connection strength. If two concepts are "close" in the network, that is, strongly connected, then one concept will act as a prime or cue for the other.

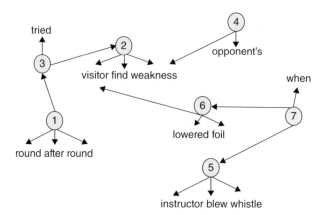

Figure 5.1 Graphic depiction of the explicit concepts and their relations in the passage "Round after round, the visitor tried to find his opponent's weakness. When the instructor blew his whistle, the visitor lowered his foil."

Consider the following short passage from Long and Baynes (2002):

2   Round after round, the visitor tried to find his opponent's weakness. When the instructor blew his whistle, the visitor lowered his foil.

Figure 5.1 depicts the concepts that are explicit in the passage and some of the relations among them. Note that some concepts in the network are more closely (strongly) connected than others. For example, *instructor* and *whistle* are more closely connected than are *visitor* and *whistle* even though *whistle* is as close to *visitor* in the surface structure of the passage as *instructor* is to *whistle*. This is because *instructor* and *whistle* are part of the same idea unit; that is, they are related to the same predicate (*blew*), whereas *whistle* and *visitor* belong to different idea units, that is, they are associated with different predicates.

Previous research has shown that connections among concepts in a propositional network have implications for memory retrieval (Baynes et al., 2002; Long & Baynes, 2002; Long et al., 2005, 2007; Prat et al., 2007; Ratcliff & McKoon, 1980). When readers are asked to recognize words from a passage, their speed and accuracy is influenced by cues that precede the target words. For example, a reader's ability to recognize *whistle* as a word from the passage will be faster and more accurate if it is preceded by the word *instructor* than by the word *visitor*. This is because *whistle* and *instructor* are more closely connected in the network than are *whistle* and *visitor*; thus, *whistle* will be a better retrieval cue than *visitor*.

The item-priming-in-recognition paradigm can also be used to examine the representation of semantic information that is associated with the passage, but is not explicit in it (Baynes, Gillette, et al., 2002; Long & Baynes, 2002; Long et al., 2005). For example, passage (2) should evoke a "fencing" schema. Readers who have constructed a discourse model of the passage should have fencing-related concepts as part of their discourse model, including a representation of the word *foil* as referring to a sword even though the word has another meaning (i.e., aluminum foil). Imagine that readers are asked if the words *sword* or *fencing* appeared in the passage. Readers may false alarm to these words, or be slow to reject them, because the concepts will match information that readers have included in their discourse model.

We have used the item-priming-in-recognition paradigm to investigate the representation of discourse in the two hemispheres in divided visual field (DVF) and patient experiments (Baynes, Gillette, Mostofian, Long, & Dronkers, 2002; Baynes, Gillette, et al., 2002; Long & Baynes, 2002; Long et al., 2005, 2007; Prat et al., 2007). In DVF experiments, test words are flashed to the left or right of a fixation point for a brief period of time. The time is sufficient to permit recognition, but is too fast to allow eye movement. Using this methodology, the retinal locus at which the word appears in the right and left eyes is controlled, routing the retinal input selectively to either the right or the left hemisphere (Barton, Goodglass, & Shai, 1965). We examine responses to a target as a function of the relation between the prime and target and the visual field of presentation. In our patient experiments, test words are presented centrally to groups with various neurological impairments. The data are analyzed to reveal differences in priming patterns as a function of the locus of damage.

All of our experiments involve a series of study-test trials. Participants read a set of four short passages like the one above. They then receive a simple recognition test. The test words are presented one at a time. Participants are asked to make simple recognition judgments, responding "yes" if the word was presented in the passage and "no" if it was not explicitly presented. Embedded in the list, but unbeknownst to participants, are sets of prime–target pairs. Some of the targets are words that were explicitly presented in the passages. The correct answer to these items is "yes." These targets are preceded by prime words (words that were also explicit in one of the passages). The prime words vary in their relation to the targets. Some are closer in the propositional network than are others. We examine the speed and accuracy of responses to the targets as a function of their relation to the primes.

We also include targets that were not presented in the passages, but are relevant to a reader's discourse model. Some targets are words that are thematically related to the passage; others are context-appropriate senses of ambiguous words. These targets are preceded by a content word from the passage. The correct answer to these items is "no." We examine the speed and accuracy with which readers can reject these items relative to test words that were not presented in the passages and were not semantically related to them.

The item-priming-in-recognition paradigm has some methodological advantages over other priming tasks that can be used to investigate language comprehension in the two hemispheres. In tasks such as lexical decision and word naming, baseline response times often differ across the two hemispheres. Lexical-decision latencies are usually faster when words are presented to the right visual field/left hemisphere (RVF/LH) than when they are presented to the left visual field/right hemisphere (LVF/RH) because phonological and orthographic abilities tend to be LH dominant. Naming latencies are also faster to words presented in the RVF/LH than in the LVF/RH because the RH has limited word production abilities. The difference in baseline rates can complicate the interpretation of priming differences. The item-priming-in-recognition paradigm does not involve discriminating words from nonwords nor does it involve word production; it requires only a simple recognition judgment of a previously presented stimulus; thus, the stimulus can be processed as an object rather than a word. Object recognition ability is strong in the RH and can compensate for limited word recognition abilities. In all of our studies, we have found priming differences across the two hemispheres, but similar baseline response latencies.

We have also found that the item-priming-in-recognition paradigm works well in patient studies. The paradigm has low production demands and does not require that patients reflect on their understanding of the passages. They make simple recognition judgments to lists of test words. We have found that patients with aphasia can perform the task with considerable accuracy, even when they have very low scores on standardized tests such as the Boston Naming Test and the Nelson-Denny Reading Comprehension Test. In the following section, we describe some of our experiments and our conclusions about discourse representation in the two hemispheres.

Discourse Representation in the Hemispheres

We have used the item-priming-in-recognition paradigm to compare the representation of discourse in the two hemispheres. Our strongest prediction is that the LH is likely to have a representation of discourse concepts that is more structured than the one in the RH. This hypothesis has its foundation in research showing that the LH has much better syntactic processing abilities than does the RH (Baynes & Gazzaniga, 1988; Zaidel, 1978, 1990). Syntactic analysis is critical in identifying and representing propositions because propositions are defined by predicate and argument relations among the words in a sentence. Syntactic information is necessary in determining these relations. Moreover, propositions are often connected to one another by means of referential relations. These relations rely on the readers' understanding of "who did what to whom" in a sentence.

If the propositional network is more strongly represented in the LH than the RH, is there an asymmetrical representation of the discourse model as well? We have considered two possibilities. First, the RH may represent a broader range of semantic information that is relevant to the discourse model than does the LH. Considerable evidence suggests that the RH plays an important role in integrating ideas among sentences and in making inferences; these processes are essential in constructing a discourse model (Beeman, 1993; Brownell, Gardner, Prather, & Martino, 1995; Brownell, Potter, Bihrle, & Gardner, 1986; Delis, Wapner, Gardner, & Moses, 1983; Hough, 1990; Joanette, Goulet, & Hannequin, 1990; Myers, 1994; Rehak, Kaplan, &

Gardner, 1992; Robertson et al., 2000; Tompkins, 1995; Tompkins, Baumgaertner, Lehman, & Fassbinder, 2000). Some researchers have suggested that the RH has diffuse, overlapping semantic representations of words and that this is important in the activation of world knowledge (e.g., Beeman, 1993). If so, then the RH may represent more diverse (but, possibly underspecified) information about the situation described in a text or conversation than does the LH.

A second possibility is that the discourse model is distributed across the two hemispheres. Theories of discourse representation claim that the propositional network and the discourse model are interrelated representations (Kintsch, 1988; Kintsch & van Dijk, 1978; McKoon & Ratcliff, 1990, 1992, 1998). The RH may be involved in activating concepts from world knowledge that are relevant to the discourse model, but these concepts may then be represented in both hemispheres, that is, represented in the RH because the RH played a role in activating them, and represented in the LH because the concepts are strongly connected to the propositional representation.

We have investigated the hemispheric distribution of the propositional network and the discourse model across the two hemispheres using the item-priming-in-recognition paradigm in combination with a DVF procedure (Long & Baynes, 2002). In one experiment, young adults received a series of study-test trials; each trial consisted of four passages presented one at a time for study. Sample passages appear in Table 5.1. Each passage consisted of two sentences and contained a homograph (e.g., *mint*) at the end of the first or second sentence. Each block of passages was followed by a recognition test. The test items were words; some had appeared in the passages and some items were new. The recognition items were presented one at a time. Participants made yes/no recognition judgments to each item. Embedded in the recognition list were sets of prime–target pairs. Three types of priming pairs were interleaved among true and false filler items. *Propositional priming* pairs consisted of a target (e.g., *structure*) that was preceded by a prime from the same proposition (e.g., *disaster*) or by a prime from a different proposition in the same sentence (e.g., *danger*). *Associate priming* pairs consisted of a target that was either the context-appropriate associate of the homograph in the sentence (e.g., *money*) or the inappropriate associate (e.g., *candy*). These test items were preceded by a prime from the sentence containing the homograph (e.g., *townspeople*). Finally, *topic priming* pairs consisted of a target that was either the topic of a passage (e.g., *earthquake*) or was an unrelated word (e.g., *breath*). These items were preceded by a prime from the final sentence of the passage (e.g., *architect*). Note that the correct response to the associate and topic words was "no." These items did not appear in the sentences. Primes were presented in the center of a computer screen; targets were briefly presented in either the LVF/RH or the RVF/LH.

We asked three questions in this study. First, do both hemispheres represent structural (i.e., propositional) relations among concepts in passages? If so, then propositional priming effects should be found in both the RVF/LH and the LVF/RH such that we should find faster responses to targets in the same-proposition condition than in the different-proposition condition. Second, do both hemispheres

Table 5.1 Sample passages and example prime–target pairs from Long and Baynes (2002, Experiment 1).

Priming Relation	Prime	Target
The townspeople were amazed to find that all the buildings had collapsed except the <u>mint</u>. Obviously, the architect had foreseen the danger because the structure withstood the natural disaster.		
Propositional priming pairs		
Same proposition	disaster	structure
Different proposition	danger	structure
Associate priming pairs		
Appropriate associate	townspeople	money
Inappropriate associate	townspeople	candy
Topic priming pairs		
Appropriate topic	architect	earthquake
Inappropriate topic	architect	breath
The guest ate garlic in his dinner, so the waiter brought a <u>mint</u>. The worried guest soon felt comfortable socializing with his friends.		
Propositional priming pairs		
Same proposition	guest	garlic
Different proposition	waiter	garlic
Associate priming pairs		
Appropriate associate	dinner	candy
Inappropriate associate	dinner	money
Topic priming pairs		
Appropriate topic	friends	breath
Inappropriate topic	friends	earthquake

represent semantic information related to the context-appropriate senses of ambiguous words? If so, then we should find associate-priming effects in both hemispheres, that is, slower latencies to reject targets in the context-appropriate than context-inappropriate condition. Third, do both hemispheres represent thematically related information about the passages? If so, then we should find thematic priming in both hemispheres, that is, slower latencies to reject targets in the thematically related than thematically unrelated condition.

The reaction-time results from Long and Baynes (2002, Experiment 1) appear in Figure 5.2. The priming patterns show both differences and similarities in how discourse was represented in the two hemispheres. Propositional priming was found only in the LH. No propositional priming was found for targets presented in the LVF/RH. The priming patterns in the two hemispheres were similar, however, with respect to the representation of context-appropriate senses of ambiguous words and thematically related information. Participants had difficulty rejecting both appropriate associates and related topic words irrespective of visual field presentation.

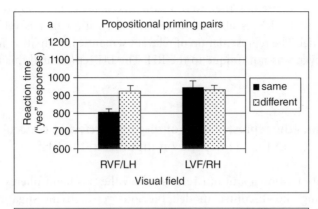

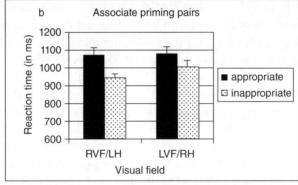

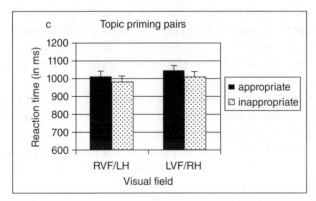

Figure 5.2 Mean reaction time and standard errors from Long and Baynes (2002, Experiment 1). Panel (a) depicts time to respond "yes" to targets in propositional priming pairs. Panels (b) and (c) depict time to respond "no" to targets in associate and topic priming pairs, respectively.

Presumably, the semantically relevant targets resonated with information stored in memory making it difficult for participants to reject the items.

These results confirmed our prediction that the LH has a representation of explicit text concepts that is structured according to predicate–argument relations. In contrast, the RH had access to the stored concepts, but the concepts did not appear to be structured as they were in the LH. The results also confirmed our prediction that the RH is able to represent information that is relevant to the discourse model. The representation of relevant semantic information in our experiments, however, was not unique to the RH. The LH represented this information as well.

Does the representation of discourse-relevant concepts in the LH depend on input from the RH?

An important question about our results is how the two hemispheres participated in constructing the discourse model. Previous research investigating language comprehension in the RH has suggested that it plays an important role in understanding the gist of a text. Patients with RH damage exhibit a range of comprehension difficulties. In particular, they have difficulty making many of the inferences that are necessary to understand discourse as a connected whole (Beeman, 1993; Brownell et al., 1986; Delis et al., 1983; Myers, 1994). If the RH plays a unique role in supporting semantic information that is relevant to the discourse model, then the associate and topic priming that we found in Long and Baynes (2002) may have resulted from activities that occurred in the RH. For example, the RH may have activated the relevant concepts and then activation spread to the other hemisphere, leading to similar representations across the hemispheres. Alternatively, the hemispheres may have constructed the discourse representations redundantly and independently. Both hemispheres have semantic networks and these may support the representation of discourse-relevant concepts by means of semantic priming. We investigated these possibilities by replicating the Long and Baynes study (2002, Experiment 1) in a group of callosotomy patients (Long & Baynes, 2002, Experiment 2).

Participants were three patients who had undergone surgery to sever the corpus callosum as treatment for intractable epilepsy (for details see Long & Baynes, 2002, Experiment 2). The materials and procedures were the same as those used in Long and Baynes (2002, Experiment 1) except that all test items were presented centrally on the computer screen and remained there until participants made a response. All responses were made with the patients' right hands.

The patients showed a propositional priming effect in both their reaction time and accuracy data. Although the patients responded more slowly than did the normal, young adults in Long and Baynes (2002, Experiment 1), the pattern of reaction times was the same as that depicted in Figure 5.2: responses were faster in the same-proposition than different-proposition condition. Patients also showed the expected priming effects in the associate and the topic conditions, making more errors in the context-appropriate conditions than the context-inappropriate conditions.

These results suggest that the LH represents discourse-relevant concepts in the absence of substantial RH input. One caveat to this conclusion is that our interpretation of these results is based on the assumption that right-handed responses in callosotomy patients result from cognitive activities that occur in the LH alone. Both hemispheres had access to similar input in our task; thus, we cannot completely exclude the possibility of some RH contribution to the priming results.

How do LH-damaged and RH-damaged patients represent discourse in memory?

We mentioned previously that the item-priming-in-recognition paradigm can be used with aphasic patients who have language processing problems that can impair their ability to understand complex sentences or to produce fluent utterances. Because the paradigm involves simple recognition judgments, patients can perform the task even if they do not completely understand the sentences in which the test items are presented.

We have examined propositional, associate, and topic priming in heterogeneous groups of left-hemisphere damaged (LHD) and right-hemisphere damaged (RHD) patients, all of whom suffered a single unilateral stroke. The LHD patients were of mixed aphasia types, but all had a reading score on the Western Aphasia Battery of at least 6. Twenty-two LHD and ten RHD patients participated. We also included a group of age and education matched controls.

The materials were the same as those used in Long and Baynes (2002). Participants received a set of study-test trials. Each trial consisted of four passages and then a test list of single words. Each test item was presented in the center of the screen and remained until the participant responded. Embedded in the test list were the prime–target pairs described above. We collected both accuracy and latency data. Participants made relatively few errors to propositional priming targets (old items); thus, we had very little missing data. This was not true for the associate and topic targets. Patients made many false alarms; thus, we examined only the accuracy data.

Our analyses revealed that control participants showed the same patterns of priming as we saw in both young adults and callosotomy patients. They responded faster to targets that were preceded by a word from the same proposition relative to one from a different proposition. In contrast, neither patient group showed propositional priming. With respect to priming in the associate and topic conditions, all groups showed reliable priming. Participants were more likely to falsely recognize a contextually appropriate associate or an appropriate topic word than they were to falsely recognize unrelated items.

The propositional priming results in this experiment differed from the pattern that we observed in the callosotomy patients (Long & Baynes, 2002, Experiment 2). The callosotomy patients all showed robust propositional priming in the LH, suggesting that input from the RH was not necessary for the representation of discourse structure. In contrast, neither brain-damaged group in this experiment showed propositional priming. It is no surprise that the LH group showed no representation of propositional structure. A structured representation is strongly dependent on syntactic abilities. These abilities are often impaired after LH damage. It is surprising, however, that the RHD patients showed no propositional priming. If the LH alone is responsible for constructing a structural representation of discourse, then the RHD patients, who have intact LHs should have shown propositional priming. Further research will be necessary to determine why the callosotomy patients, but not the RHD patients, showed propositional priming; however, two possibilities seem likely. First, priming in our callosotomy patients may have been influenced by some RH input even though the patients responded with their right hands. The second (and, in our opinion, the more likely) possibility is that damage to either hemisphere affects memory, such that patients have difficulty maintaining structural relations in memory or have difficulty retrieving them at test.

Does the RH represent intersentential relations?

In all of the experiments described above, propositional priming, when it was found, occurred only in the LH. Our results, however, tell us little about how discourse concepts are organized in the RH. The results tell us only that the RH does not represent structural relations among concepts that appeared in the same sentence. It is possible, however, that the RH represents structural relations at a more coarse-grained level than does the LH. The RH may be insensitive to connections within a sentence, but may represent connections across sentences. This might occur because connections within a sentence are often based on syntactic relations among words. The RH may be more sensitive to semantic relations than syntactic ones and cluster sentence concepts accordingly. Thus, we conducted a study to examine connections among concepts both within and across sentence boundaries.

We used the item-priming-in-recognition paradigm with a new set of materials (Long et al., 2005). Participants read sets of passages and then received recognition tests consisting of single words. Four types of prime–target pairs were embedded in the test list. Table 5.2 contains sample passages and test items. In the *same-proposition* condition, a target from one of the sentences (e.g., *hunter*) was preceded by a prime from the same proposition (e.g., *pheasant*). In the *different*-proposition condition, the target was preceded by a prime from a different proposition in the same sentence (e.g., *deer*). In the different-*sentence* condition, the target was preceded by a prime from a different sentence in the same passage (e.g., *birds*). Finally, in the different-*passage* condition, the target was preceded by a prime from a different passage in the same block of passages (e.g., *apples*). Primes were presented centrally and targets were presented to the LVF/RH or to the RVF/LH. It is important to note that the primes and targets in all of the within-passage conditions (same-proposition, different-proposition, and different-sentence conditions) are all semantically related, whereas the primes and targets in the different-passage condition were unrelated.

Our priming results appear in Figure 5.3. We found that the LH was sensitive to the distance between the prime and target in the propositional structure of the

Table 5.2 Sample passages and example prime–target pairs from Long, Baynes, and Prat (2005, Experiment 1).

Priming Relation	Prime	Target
While the hunter (who was wearing an orange vest) stalked the pheasant, the deer ate leaves in the meadow. The birds sang as they roosted in the trees and watched the creatures below.		
Same proposition	pheasant	hunter
Different proposition	deer	hunter
Different sentence	birds	hunter
Different passage	apples	hunter
The children laughed at the silly sight. The elephant (that was large and gray) pulled the cart, while the monkey juggled the apples.		
Same proposition	elephant	cart
Different proposition	monkey	cart
Different sentence	sight	cart
Different passage	creatures	cart

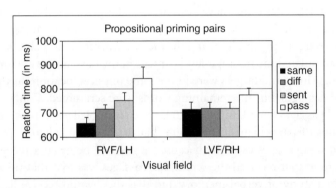

Figure 5.3 Mean reaction time and standard errors from Long, Baynes, and Prat (2005, Experiment 1) as a function of distance in the propositional network.

passages, as expected. We observed the greatest priming in the same-proposition condition and the least priming in the between-passage condition. We found no within-passage priming in the LVF/RH; however, responses to targets that followed within-passage primes (i.e., same-proposition, different-proposition, and different-sentence conditions) were faster than those that followed different-passage primes. Thus, the RH appeared to represent concepts within a passage as distinct from those in other passages.

Why did the RH show priming across passages, but not within passages? One possibility is that the concepts within a passage were represented according to their semantic relations. That is, concepts in the same passage (e.g., *hunter, pheasant, deer, birds)* were associated in the RH because they were thematically related. We were concerned, however, that the semantic relations among these concepts were pre-existing and did not reflect connections that were made when the passages were comprehended. We investigated this possibility in two ways. First, we examined association norms for connections among the primes and targets. We found no difference in association across priming pairs. Second, we conducted a lexical-decision priming test in which the primes and targets were embedded in a list of words and nonwords. The test words were presented in the absence of the passages. We found no priming differences across the prime–target conditions. Thus, the propositional priming that we observed in our study did not appear to result from pre-existing semantic relations.

Does the RH represent message-level content?

The results of our previous studies show that the RH represents discourse concepts even though it does not represent the structural relations among them. The absence of a structured representation in the RH raises a question about its representation of message-level content. Does the RH represent words in a passage as a set of semantically related items that have been presented together or does it represent the meaning of discourse? We addressed this question in a DVF study using the item-priming-in-recognition paradigm and the materials from Long et al (2005; see Table 5.2). We manipulated the message-level content in the passages by creating versions in which the primes and targets were in the same physical locations as they were in the original passages, but the remaining words were scrambled. Coherent versions (the original passages from Long et al., 2005) and scrambled versions were presented to two groups of participants. The group that received the coherent passages was told to read the passages carefully because they would be given a recognition test later. The group that received the scrambled passages was told that they were participating in a study of verbal memory and that they would receive lists of words to study. These lists would be followed by tests in which they would be asked to judge whether test items had been presented in the lists that they had studied or if the items were new.

The pattern of priming in the coherent-passage condition replicated the results that we observed in Long et al. (2005; see Figure 5.3). Participants showed a propositional distance effect when targets were presented in the RVF/LH, whereas priming in the LVF/RH was found only when the within-passage conditions were compared to the between-passage condition. Our primary interest was the pattern of priming in the scrambled condition. We found that the scrambling manipulation had no influence on priming in the RH. Reaction times were slower in the passage condition relative to all other conditions. The LH, however, showed the pattern that is usually associated with the RH: participants responded faster to targets that were preceded by primes from the same passage relative to primes from different passages.

These results suggest that the RH did not store the message-level content of the passages. The same pattern of priming in the RH occurred when concepts were presented as a coherent message and when they were presented as a scrambled list. Only the LH showed an effect of presentation condition: we found a propositional priming effect when passages had a coherent message and we found the RH pattern when concepts were presented in list format.

It is important to note that our claim concerns the representation of message-level content in *long-term* memory. Research on RH sensitivity to message-level content "online" during the comprehension process has produced inconsistent findings; some studies have found that the RH is unable to integrate syntactic and semantic information to construct a message-level representation (Faust, 1998; Faust, Babkoff, & Kravets, 1995; Faust & Gernsbacher, 1996; Faust, Kravetz, & Babkoff, 1993), whereas other studies have found that the RH does represent message-level content and is involved in the integration of content across sentences (Chiarello, Liu, & Faust, 2001; Coulson, Federmeier, van Petter, & Kutas, 2005; Faust, Bar-lev, & Chiarello, 2003; Federmeier, Mai, & Kutas, 2005). Even if the RH is sensitive to message-level content during the comprehension process, our research suggests that this representation is not maintained for an extended period of time.

Does the RH represent spatial/temporal relations among concepts?

Our previous experiment showed that the RH does not represent structural or message-level relations among concepts, but it provides no information about the types of relations that the RH does represent. We think it is very likely that the RH represents semantic relations among concepts based on substantial research showing semantic priming in the RH. In this experiment, we asked whether the RH also represents spatial/temporal relations among concepts.

In all of our experiments, the two sentences in each passage were presented on the same screen and different passages were presented on different screens. Thus, spatial and temporal proximity was confounded with our manipulation of propositional distance. That is, explicit concepts that were later used as primes and targets in the within-passage conditions were presented simultaneously, whereas explicit concepts that were later used as primes and targets in the different-passage condition were presented at different times. Our goal in the current experiment was to examine the extent to which the temporal and spatial proximity of the primes and targets in the within-passage conditions influenced the pattern of priming.

Considerable research has shown that the RH has spatial/temporal abilities that are greater than those in the LH. This has been found in behavioral, neuroimaging, and lesion studies (Kosslyn, Maljkovic, Hamilton, Horwitz, & Thompson, 1995; Kounios & Holcomb, 1994; Laeng, Zarrinpar, & Kosslyn, 2003). We hypothesized that the organization of discourse concepts in the RH may be influenced by the spatial/temporal properties of the stimuli. We investigated this hypothesis by manipulating the presentation of the passages in a between-subjects design. In the

Debra L. Long et al.

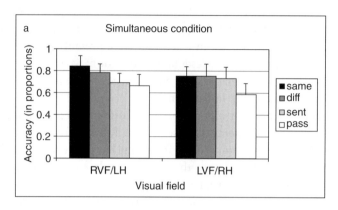

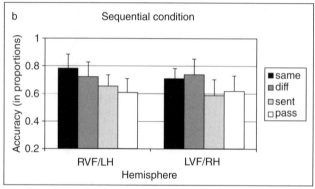

Figure 5.4 Percentage accuracy and standard errors to targets as a function of distance in the propositional network. Panel (a) depicts results from the simultaneous condition and Panel (b) depicts results from the sequential condition.

simultaneous condition, the two-sentence passages were presented simultaneously (as in our previous experiments). In the separate condition, the two sentences were presented sequentially on separate screens. We signaled the beginning and end of each passage so that participants understood that the two sentences were part of the same passage. Each passage was preceded by a set of asterisks and instructions to press the space bar to read the next passage. In both conditions, a block of four passages was presented followed by a recognition test with the embedded prime–target pairs.

Our priming results appear in Figure 5.4. The results for targets presented in the RVF/LH replicate the pattern that we have found in previous experiments. Priming was a function of distance in the propositional structure of the passage. This was true in both the simultaneous and sequential conditions. Thus, the LH represented the passages as a coherent message even when the two sentences of a passage were presented on separate screens.

We found a different pattern of results in the RH. Responses to targets in the simultaneous condition replicated our previous findings: faster responses in the within-passage conditions than in the different-passage condition. In the sequential condition, however, responses to targets in the same-proposition and different-proposition conditions were faster than responses to targets in the between-sentence and between-passage conditions. Critically, we found no difference in response times in the latter two conditions. Thus, the RH stored stronger connections among concepts when they were presented simultaneously than when they were presented sequentially. This was the case even though concepts in the between-sentence condition were thematically related to concepts in the same-sentence conditions (same proposition and different proposition) by virtue of the passage content.

Our priming results in the RH are consistent with our hypothesis that the spatial/temporal abilities of the RH affect its representation of discourse concepts. We do not claim, however, that the RH is insensitive to semantic relatedness even though we did not find greater priming in the between-sentence than between-passage condition when the passages were presented sequentially. Although primes and targets in the between-sentence condition were related, they were not strong associates. Moreover, the primes and targets were not members of the same semantic category; they were related by virtue of a schema or scenario that was relevant to the situation described in the passage (e.g., birds are a target of hunters). We discuss the relevance of our findings for theories of discourse processing in the next section.

Implications for Understanding RH Discourse Comprehension

The studies that we have described have implications for understanding how the RH participates in constructing a coherent representation of discourse. In particular, theories of discourse comprehension will be constrained by five findings about how discourse is represented in the RH. First, the RH stores explicit concepts from discourse, but these concepts are not organized according to predicate–argument relations. That is, the RH has no permanent representation of "who did what to whom" in a sentence. Second, the RH represents semantic information that is relevant to the message conveyed in a sentence, including the context-appropriate senses of ambiguous words and topic-related concepts. Although the RH stores contextually relevant information, it does not appear to do so uniquely; we found similar patterns in the LH. Third, the RH does not appear to *store* message-level information that is conveyed by a sentence. We found no difference between the representation of concepts in discourse and the representation of the same concepts in a list format. Fourth, the RH stores temporal/spatial information about concepts in discourse. It clusters concepts more closely when they are presented simultaneously than when they are presented sequentially. We found that this occurred even when sequentially presented information was semantically related. Finally, brain damage seems to impair the representation of structural

information, but not the representation of contextually relevant semantic information. Moreover, we found that the representation of structural relations was impaired
after both LH and RH damage.

Our examination of memory representations in the RH may help clarify some
of the many inconsistencies that are found in the literature on RH language comprehension. In the neuroimaging literature, some studies have reported greater RH
than LH activation for high-level comprehension processes, such as the establishment of coherence relations, inference generation, and the processing of figurative
language (Bottini, Corcoran, Sterzi, Paulesu, 1994; Mashal, Faust, Hendler, & Jung-
Beeman, 2008; Mason & Just, 2004; St George, Kutas, Martinez, & Sereno, 1999),
whereas other studies have found either bilateral activation or greater LH than RH
activation (Ferstl, 2007; Ferstl, Neumann, Bogler, & von Cramon, 2008; Rapp, Leube,
Erb, Grodd, & Kircher, 2004).

Similar inconsistencies have been found in lesion studies. Some studies have
found that RHD patients are impaired in using thematic information to organize
sentence ideas into a coherent discourse model (Delis et al., 1983; Schneiderman,
Murasagi, & Saddy, 1992). Other research has found that RHD patients comprehend
main ideas as accurately as do LHD patients (Brookshire & Nicholas, 1984; Hough,
1990; Wegner, Brookshire, & Nicholas, 1984). Consider, also, the literature on inference generation after RHD. Numerous studies have shown that RHD patients are
impaired in generating inferences to construct a coherent discourse representation
(Beeman, 1993; Brownell et al., 1986; Harden, Cannito, & Dagenais, 1995; Myers &
Brookshire, 1996), whereas other studies have found no such deficits (Lehman-
Blake & Lesniewicz, 2005; Leonard & Baum, 1998; Leonard, Waters, & Caplan,
1997a, 1997b; McDonald & Wales, 1986; Tompkins, Fassbinder, Lehman-Blake,
Baumgaertner, & Jayaram, 2004).

Two issues may be important in reconciling inconsistencies in the literature
on RH language comprehension. The first issue concerns the distinction between
inferences that are based on activation of concepts in a semantic network and
inferences that require knowledge about predicate–argument relations. We have
argued that both hemispheres represent inferences that are thematically related
by virtue of the semantic overlap among explicit concepts in a sentence and related
concepts stored in semantic memory. Indeed, the RH may have some advantage in
activating certain types of inferences based on semantic overlap. Jung-Beeman
(2005) has argued that both hemispheres contribute to semantic processing, but
do so somewhat differently. The LH has a finely coded network that supports the
strong activation of the dominant features of words, whereas the RH has a coarsely
coded network that supports the weak, diffuse activation of distantly related or
subordinate semantic features. These distantly related concepts can provide information that is essential for elaborating a discourse representation with inferences
or for reinterpreting a word or phrase when the LH has selected an inappropriate
meaning.

Not all inferences, however, can be generated solely on the basis of semantic
overlap. Some inferences require access to knowledge about predicate–argument

relations. Consider, for example, inferences that are necessary to establish referential relations as in the following:

3   John saw Paul fall down the stairs. He ran to get help.

Some of the information that is relevant to understanding this short passage can be activated by means of priming in a semantic network. For example, the concept *fall* is semantically related to the concept *hurt*. It is also necessary, however, to represent exactly *who* fell in order to understand who ran to get help. This involves the representation of *Paul* as the agent of fall; thus, Paul is the one who needs help. This information is important for the inference that *John* is the agent of the verb *ran*. If the RH is limited in its representation of predicate–argument relations then its ability to generate inferences of this type will be limited even though it may have some advantage in generating inferences that are supported by lexical–semantic relations.

A second issue that may be important in reconciling inconsistent findings in the literature on RH language comprehension is the distinction between temporary activation of concepts and their more permanent representation in memory. Consider a recent study by Tompkins and her colleagues. Tompkins, Sharp, Meigh, and Fassbinder (2008) found that RHD patients were impaired in maintaining the peripheral features of words, but not in activating them. Similarly, Lehman-Blake and Lesniewicz (2005) found that RHD patients generated inferences during comprehension, but did not maintain these inferences over time unless the inferences were supported by strong semantic associates in the context. These findings are consistent with our claim that early activation of concepts does not necessarily lead to the integration of these concepts into a long-term memory representation of discourse.

Finally, our finding that the RH represents temporal/spatial properties of discourse may be relevant to understanding the RH's role in repair processes in comprehension. Studies have found that the RH is involved in the reinterpretation of discourse when initial interpretations are inconsistent with previously processed information (Rehak et al., 1992; Schneiderman & Saddy, 1988), including syntactic revision after misanalysis (Meyer, Friederici, & von Cramon, 2000). The RH representation of temporal/spatial information about concepts in sentences may offer a mechanism by which repair can occur. Memory for the temporal order of information would be very helpful in revising an interpretation when an initial analysis is inappropriate.

Concluding Remarks

Our goal in this chapter was to describe a method for examining how discourse is represented in the two hemispheres of the brain. The results that we have found using this method suggest both similarities and differences in the representations that are stored after readers have comprehended a text. Both hemispheres maintain representations of explicit text concepts and semantic information relevant to understanding the situation to which a text refers. The LH maintains structural relations among explicit text concepts, whereas the RH maintains some spatial/temporal information about their presentation. Our findings have the potential to resolve some inconsistencies in the literature on RH language comprehension and suggest interesting questions for future research.

References

Barton, M. I., Goodglass, H., & Shai, A. (1965). Differential recognition of tachistoscopically presented English and Hebrew words in the right and left visual fields. *Perceptual and Motor Skills, 21,* 431–437.

Baynes, K., & Gazzaniga, M. (1988). Right hemisphere language: Insights into normal language mechanisms? In F. Plum (Ed.), *Language, communication, and the brain* (pp. 117–126). New York: Raven.

Baynes, K., Gillette, E., Mostofian, E., Long, D., & Dronkers, N. (2002). Modes of processing in the right and left hemispheres of aphasic patients. *Journal of the International Neuropsychological Society, 8,* 280.

Baynes, K., Long, D. L., Gillette, J., Dronkers, N. F., & Davis, C. (2002). Priming of discourse relations in left-hemisphere injured patients. *Cognitive Neuroscience Abstracts, 9,* 81.

Beeman, M. (1993). Semantic processing in the right hemisphere may contribute to drawing inferences from discourse. *Brain and Language, 44,* 80–120.

Bottini, G., Corcoran, R., Sterzi, R., & Paulesu, E. (1994). The role of the right hemisphere in the interpretation of figurative aspects of language: A positron emission tomography activation study. *Brain: A Journal of Neurology, 117,* 1241–1253.

Bransford, J. D., & Johnson, M. K. (1972). Contextual prerequisites for understanding: Some investigations of comprehension and recall. *Journal of Verbal Learning and Verbal Behavior, 11,* 717–726.

Brookshire, R. H., & Nicholas, L. E. (1984). Comprehension of directly and indirectly stated main ideas and details in discourse by brain-damaged and non-brain-damaged listeners. *Brain and Language, 21,* 21–36.

Brownell, H., Gardner, H., Prather, P., & Martino, G. (1995). Language, communication, and the right hemisphere. In H. S. Kirshner (Ed.), *Handbook of neurological speech and language disorders* (pp. 325–349). New York: Marcel Dekker.

Brownell, H. H., Potter, H. H., Bihrle, A. M., & Gardner, H. (1986). Inference deficits in right brain-damaged patients. *Brain and Language, 27,* 310–321.

Chiarello, C., Liu, S., & Faust, M. (2001). Bihemispheric sensitivity to sentence anomaly. *Neuropsychologia, 39,* 1451–1463.

Coulson, S., Federmeier, K. D., van Petter, C., & Kutas, M. (2005). Right hemisphere sensitivity to word- and sentence-level context: Evidence from event-related brain potentials. (2005). *Journal of Experimental Psychology: Learning, Memory, and Cognition, 31,* 129–147.

Delis, D., Wapner, W., Gardner, H., & Moses, J. (1983). The contribution of the right hemisphere to the organization of paragraphs. *Cortex, 19,* 43–50.

Faust, M. (1998). Obtaining evidence of language comprehension from sentence priming. In M. Beeman & C. Chiarello (Eds.), *Right hemisphere language comprehension: Perspectives from cognitive neuroscience* (pp. 161–185). Mahwah, NJ: Erlbaum.

Faust, M., Babkoff, H., & Kravetz, S. (1995). Linguistic processes in the two cerebral hemispheres: Implications for modularity and interactionism. *Journal of Clinical and Experimental Neuropsychology, 17*, 171–192.

Faust, M., Bar-lev, A., & Chiarello, C. (2003). Sentence priming effects in the two cerebral hemispheres: Influences of lexical relatedness, word order, and sentence anomaly. *Neuropsychologia, 41*, 480–492.

Faust, M., & Gernsbacher, M. A. (1996). Cerebral mechanisms for suppression of inappropriate information during sentence comprehension. *Brain and Language, 53*, 234–259.

Faust, M., Kravetz, S., & Babkoff, H. (1993). Hemisphericity and top-down processing of language. *Brain and Language, 44*, 1–18.

Federmeier, K. D., Mai, H., & Kutas, M. (2005). Both sides get the point: Hemispheric sensitivities to sentential constraint. *Memory and Cognition, 33*, 871–886.

Ferstl, E. C. (2007). The functional neuroanatomy of text comprehension: What's the story so far? In F. Schmalhofer & C. A. Perfetti (Eds.) *Higher level language processes in the brain: Inference and comprehension processes* (pp. 53–102). Mahwah, NJ: Erlbaum.

Ferstl, E. C., Neumann, J., Bogler, C., & von Cramon, D. Y. (2008). The extended language network: A meta-analysis of neuroimaging studies on text comprehension. *Human Brain Mapping, 29*, 581–593.

Fodor, J. (1983). *Modularity of Mind*. Cambridge, MA: MIT Press

Gernsbacher, M. A. (1989). Mechanisms that improve referential access. *Cognition, 32*, 99–156.

Gernsbacher, M. A. (1990). *Language comprehension as structure building*. Hillsdale, NJ: Erlbaum.

Graesser, A. C., Singer, M., & Trabasso, T. (1994). Constructing inferences during narrative text comprehension. *Psychological Review, 101*, 371–395.

Greene, S. B., McKoon, G., & Ratcliff, R. (1992). Pronoun resolution and discourse models. *Journal of Experimental Psychology: Learning, Memory, and Cognition, 18*, 266–283.

Harden, W. D., Cannito, M. P., & Dagenais, P. A. (1995). Inferential abilities of normal and right hemisphere damaged adults. *Journal of Communication Disorders, 28*, 247–259.

Hough, M. S. (1990). Narrative comprehension in adults with right and left hemisphere brain-damage: Theme organization. *Brain and Language, 38*, 253–277.

Joannete, Y., Goulet, P., & Hannequin, D. (1990). *Right hemisphere and verbal communication*. New York: Springer-Verlag.

Jung-Beeman, M. (2005). Bilateral brain processes for comprehending natural language. *Trends in Cognitive Sciences, 9*, 512–518.

Kintsch, W. (1988). The role of knowledge in discourse comprehension: A construction-integration model. *Psychological Review, 95*, 163–182.

Kintsch, W., & van Dijk, T. A. (1978). Toward a model of text comprehension and production. *Psychological Review, 85*, 363–394.

Kosslyn, S. M., Maljkovic, V., Hamilton, S. E., Horwitz, G., & Thompson, W. L. (1995). Two types of image generation: Evidence for left and right hemisphere processes. *Neuropsychologia, 33*, 1485–1510.

Kounios, J., & Holcomb, P. J. (1994). Concreteness effects in semantic processing: ERP evidence supporting dual-coding theory. *Journal of Experimental Psychology: Learning, Memory, and Cognition, 20*, 804–823.

Laeng, B., Zarrinpar, A., & Kosslyn, S. M. (2003). Do separate processes identify objects as exemplars versus members of basic-level categories? Evidence from hemispheric specialization. *Brain and Cognition, 53*, 15–27.

Lehman-Blake, M., & Lesniewicz, K. S. (2005). Contextual bias and predictive inferencing in adults with and without right hemisphere brain damage. *Aphasiology, 19*, 423–434.

Leonard, C. L., & Baum, S. R. (1998). On-line evidence for context use by right-brain-damaged patients. *Journal of Cognitive Neuroscience, 10*, 499–508.

Leonard, C. L., Waters, G. S., & Caplan, D. (1997a). The use of contextual information by right brain-damaged individuals in the resolution of ambiguous pronouns. *Brain and Language, 57*, 309–342.

Leonard, C. L., Waters, G. S., & Caplan, D. (1997b). The use of contextual information related to general world knowledge by right brain-damaged individuals in pronoun resolution. *Brain and Language, 57*, 343–359.

Long, D. L., & Baynes, K. (2002). Discourse representation in the two cerebral hemispheres. *Journal of Cognitive Neuroscience, 14*, 228–242.

Long, D. L., Baynes, K., & Prat, C. S. (2005). The propositional structure of discourse in the two cerebral hemispheres. *Brain and Language, 95*, 383–394.

Long, D. L., Baynes, K., & Prat, C. S. (2007). Sentence and discourse representation in the two cerebral hemispheres. In C. Perfetti & F. Schmalhofer (Eds.), *Higher-level language processes in the brain* (pp. 329–353). Mahwah, NJ: Erlbaum.

Mashal, N., Faust, M., Hendler, T., & Jung-Beeman, M. (2008). Hemispheric differences in processing the literal interpretation of idioms: Converging evidence from behavioral and fMRI studies. *Cortex, 44*, 848–860.

Mason, R., & Just, M. A. (2004). How the brain processes causal inferences in text: A theoretical account of generation and integration component processes utilizing both cerebral hemispheres. *Psychological Science, 15*, 1–7.

McDonald, S., & Wales, R. (1986). An investigation of the ability to process inferences in language following right hemisphere brain damage. *Brain and Language, 29*, 68–80.

McKoon, G., & Ratcliff, R. (1980). Priming in item recognition: The organization of propositions in memory for text. *Journal of Verbal Learning and Verbal Behavior, 19*, 369–386.

McKoon, G., & Ratcliff, R. (1990). Textual inferences: Models and measures. In D. A. Balota, G. B. Flores d'Arcais, & K. Rayner (Eds.), *Comprehension processes in reading* (pp. 403–421). Hillsdale, NJ: Erlbaum.

McKoon, G., & Ratcliff, R. (1992). Inference during reading. *Psychological Review, 99*, 440–466.

McKoon, G., & Ratcliff, R. (1998). Memory based language processing: Psycholinguistic research in the 1990s. *Annual Review of Psychology, 49*, 25–42.

Meyer, M., Friederici, A. D., von Cramon, D. Y. (2000). Neurocognition of auditory sentence comprehension: Event related fMRI reveals sensitivity to syntactic violations and task demands. *Cognitive Brain Research, 9*, 19–33.

Myers, P. S. (1994). Communication disorders associated with right hemisphere brain damage. In R. Chapey (Ed.), *Language intervention strategies in adult aphasia* (pp. 514–534). Baltimore: Williams & Wilkins.

Myers, P., & Brookshire, R. H. (1996). Effect of visual and inferential variables on scene description by right-hemisphere-damaged and non-brain-damaged adults. *Journal of Speech and Hearing Research, 39*, 870–880.

Prat, C. S., Long, D. L., & Baynes, K. (2007). Individual differences in the hemispheric representation of discourse. *Brain and Language, 100*, 283–294.

Rapp, A. M., Leube, D. T., Erb, M., Grodd, W., & Kircher, T. J. (2004). Neural correlates of metaphor processing. *Cognitive Brain Research, 20*, 395–402.

Rehak, A., Kaplan, J. A., & Gardner, H. (1992). Sensitivity to conversational deviance in right-hemisphere-damaged patients. *Brain and Language, 42*, 203–217.

Rehak, A., Kaplan, J. A., Weylman, S. T., Kelly, B., Brownell, H. H., & Gardner, H. (1992). Story processing in right-hemisphere brain-damaged patients. *Brain and Language, 42*, 320–336.

Robertson, D. A., Gernsbacher, M. A., Guidotti, S. J., Robertson, R. R. W., Irwin, W., Mock, B. J., et al. (2000). Functional neuroanatomy of the cognitive process of mapping during discourse comprehension. *Psychological Science, 11*, 255–260.

Sanford, A. J., & Garrod, S. C. (1998). The role of scenario mapping in comprehension. *Discourse Processes, 26*, 159–1990.

Schneiderman, E. I., Murasagi, K. G., & Saddy, J. D. (1992). Story arrangement ability in right brain-damaged patients. *Brain and Language, 43*, 107–120.

Schneiderman, E. I., & Saddy, J. D. (1988). A linguistic deficit resulting from right-hemisphere damage. *Brain and Language, 34*, 38–53.

St George, M., Kutas, M., Martinez, A., & Sereno, M. I. (1999). Semantic integration in reading: Engagement of the right hemisphere during discourse processing. *Brain: A Journal of Neurology, 122*, 1317–1325.

Tompkins, C. A. (1995). *Right hemisphere communication disorders: Theory and management.* San Diego, CA: Singular Publishing.

Tompkins, C. A., Baumgaertner, A., Lehman, M. T., & Fassbinder, W. (2000). Mechanisms of discourse comprehension impairment after right hemisphere brain damage: Suppression in lexical ambiguity resolution. *Journal of Speech, Language, and Hearing Research, 43*, 62–78.

Tompkins, C. A., Fassbiner, W., Lehman-Blake, M., Baumgaertner, A., & Jayaram, N. (2004). Inference generation during text comprehension by adults with right hemisphere brain damage: Activation failure versus multiple activation. *Journal of Speech, Language and Hearing Research, 47*, 1380–1395.

Tompkins, C. A., Scharp, V. L., Fassbinder, W., Meigh, K. M., & Armstrong, E. M. (2008). A different story on "theory of mind" deficits in adults with right hemisphere brain damage. *Aphasiology, 22*, 42–61.

Wegner, M. L., Brookshire, R., & Nicholas, L. (1984). Comprehension of main ideas and details in coherent and noncoherent discourse by aphasic and nonaphasic listeners. *Brain and Language, 21*, 37–51.

Zaidel, E. (1978). Lexical organization in the right hemisphere. In P. Buser & A. Gougeul-Buser (Eds.), *Cerebral correlates of conscious experience* (pp. 177–197). Amsterdam: Elsevier.

Zaidel, E. (1990). Language functions in the two hemispheres following complete cerebral commissurotomy and hemispherectomy. In F. Boller & G. Grafman (Eds.), *Handbook of neuropsychology* (Vol. 4, pp. 115–150). Amsterdam: Elsevier.

Zwaan, R. A., & Radvansky, G. A. (1998). Situation models in language comprehension and memory. *Psychological Bulletin, 123*, 162–185.

Part II

Computational Modeling
of Language

6

Connectionist Modeling of Neuropsychological Deficits in Semantics, Language, and Reading

Christine E. Watson, Blair C. Armstrong, and David C. Plaut

Introduction

Representations of linguistic information and the neural substrates that underlie them are incredibly complex. This chapter illustrates how connectionist modeling has furthered our understanding of normal and impaired processing in three related domains – semantic memory, knowledge of grammatical class, and word reading – and how the development of these models engenders a reciprocal relationship between theoretical and empirical research. In particular, we highlight the value of employing domain-general learning and information-processing principles to derive explicit accounts of the ways in which factors which make contact with, or are central to, linguistic abilities can interact to give rise to a range of behaviors. We also detail how the connectionist approach has provided for theoretical advancement that would not have occurred using the double-dissociation rubric of traditional cognitive neuropsychology and how it has allowed the exploration and development of ideas that would have been difficult, if not impossible, to formulate verbally.

Semantic Memory Impairments

Developing a theory of how semantic memory is represented and processed is central to understanding key aspects of human cognition, as this knowledge is required for a variety of language-related tasks and beyond. A key source of empirical data for theory development is derived from the study of patients with various neurological impairments (e.g., cerebral infarction, viral infection, dementia) who

The Handbook of the Neuropsychology of Language, First Edition. Edited by Miriam Faust.
© 2012 Blackwell Publishing Ltd. Published 2012 by Blackwell Publishing Ltd.

exhibit consistent and specific patterns of semantic memory impairment. The present section focuses on two contrasting types of "pure" semantic memory deficits – that is, impairments to semantic memory in which other cognitive functions such as lower-level perception and short-term memory have (in some cases, at least) been documented as being relatively intact – in which there is either selective loss of knowledge for particular semantic categories or a more uniform loss of knowledge which spans all semantic categories. These data have been particularly challenging for and central to the development of recent theories. (Note that we use the term "category" to refer to both broad superordinate-level categories, such as *living things*, as well as narrower basic-level semantic categories, such as *birds*.)

The first type of impairment consists of so-called category-specific semantic deficits (CSDs), in which knowledge for one category is substantially impaired while other categories are relatively preserved, albeit with some important exceptions. These impairments tend to manifest themselves as increased commission or category coordinate errors, wherein the incorrect responses patients produce to items from the impaired category are also members of the impaired category (e.g., in a picture naming task, participants with impaired knowledge of living things might respond "dog" to an image of a sheep; Lambon Ralph, Lowe, & Rogers, 2007). Two key patterns of selective impairment have emerged in the literature (see Capitani, Laiacona, Mahon, & Caramazza, 2003, for a review of over 100 case studies of these impairments). The most frequently reported pattern consists of a selective loss of living thing knowledge while knowledge of nonliving things is preserved (e.g., Warrington & Shallice, 1984). Associated with this general loss of living thing knowledge are several exception categories. Knowledge of musical instruments, for example, tends to be lost along with living things, whereas knowledge of exception categories such as body parts and manufactured foods is preserved. The opposite pattern of impairment – selective loss of nonliving thing knowledge, which is accompanied by loss of knowledge for exception categories such as foods and body parts – has also been reported (Caramazza & Shelton, 1998; Warrington & McCarthy, 1983, 1987), though far less frequently. Note that of these cases, though there have been a number of "pure" selective impairments without any apparent additional impairments to particular sensorimotor modalities (e.g., Caramazza & Shelton, 1998), a large number of cases have also been reported in which knowledge for particular sensorimotor modalities and semantic categories have both been impaired (e.g., Magnié, Ferreira, Giusiano, & Poncet, 1999; McCarthy & Warrington, 1988).

CSDs have been linked to a variety of etiologies, with approximately half of the known cases being associated with damage from herpes simplex virus encephalitis (HSVE) and the remaining cases being mainly associated with various forms of dementia and cerebrovascular accident. Cases of selective loss of living thing knowledge are primarily associated with HSVE and damage to the left temporal lobe; there is less specificity and consistency in impaired brain regions associated with the less frequently observed loss of nonliving thing knowledge (Capitani et al., 2003).

In contrast to the CSD cases, there have also been many documented cases of general semantic impairments in which all categories of knowledge have been documented as being equally affected, with the impairment usually taking the form of errors of omission (that is, patients are unable to make any response to a probe stimulus; Lambon Ralph et al., 2007). These general semantic impairments are primarily associated with *semantic dementia*, a disease which selectively affects the anterior and inferolateral temporal cortex. This region largely overlaps with the regions associated with HSVE and living thing deficits, though semantic dementia may uniquely involve more lateral regions and the HSVE more medial regions of the temporal lobe (Noppeney et al., 2007).

Traditional accounts of semantic impairments

Employing double-dissociation logic, Caramazza and Shelton (1998; see also Santos & Caramazza, 2002; Sartori & Job, 1988) argued that the separate cases of category-specific semantic impairments for living things and nonliving things suggest that these categories are subserved by anatomically distinct neural substrates; they further provide a post hoc evolutionary basis for this view. Their perspective is known as the *domain-specific* hypothesis. Accounting for category-specific deficits is trivial under this framework – selective lesions to brain regions subserving each category would leave the other categories intact. Though Caramazza and Shelton did not attempt to explain uniform deficits in semantic knowledge, their likely account for this phenomenon is straightforward, as well: uniform semantic deficits would result from equal damage to each semantic module.

The domain-specific hypothesis has obvious intuitive and theoretical appeal. This theory is also the only one to date that is able to account for the extreme selective impairment of particular categories while leaving the others completely intact (patient E. W. being a highly controlled example of these effects; Caramazza & Shelton, 1998). Nevertheless, despite these high-level successes, we find the domain-specific hypothesis to be lacking in several key respects. First, the theory is in essence nothing more than a recapitulation of the data. As a result, though it may be able to *explain* some phenomena, it is not a very useful tool for making new *predictions* with which to expand our understanding of semantic memory. Second, though the domain-specific hypothesis succeeds in accounting for some extreme cases not currently captured by reductionist accounts and their supporting connectionist models, the theory also shows no promise of parsimonious incorporation of the broader semantic deficit literature and cognitive neuroscience research which suggests that knowledge is partially organized by modality (Martin & Chao, 2001). In particular, cases in which the impaired category is also associated with a differential impairment of knowledge from a particular sensorimotor modality (e.g., McCarthy & Warrington, 1988; Lambon Ralph, Howard, Nightingale, & Ellis, 1998), or in which knowledge of particular *grammatical* categories is impaired (discussed in the next section) appear difficult to reconcile within this framework. To account for these data, the domain-specific hypothesis would likely need to be expanded so as to have independent processing modules associated with the semantic knowledge of each category for each modality, a postulation that substantially complicates the account without providing independent evidence warranting this complexity. Finally, the domain-specific hypothesis offers no insight into the qualitative differences in terms of the types of incorrect responses participants make (e.g., errors of commission vs. error of omission) when suffering from different types of semantic memory impairment.

Reductionist accounts of semantic impairments

Several attempts to account for the various semantic impairments have also been made using a reductionist approach. These theories differ in terms of whether there is an explicit semantic store (e.g., Farah & McClelland, 1991) or merely a routing hub for completing tasks that require mapping information from one sensorimotor or linguistic modality to another (e.g., Rogers et al., 2004) and whether there are innate modality-specific subdivisions of semantic knowledge (e.g., Farah & McClelland, 1991; Warrington & Shallice, 1984), a single amodal semantic store (e.g., Tyler, Moss, Durrant-Peatfield, & Levy, 2000), or some combination thereof (Simmons & Barsalou, 2003). However, all of this work shares the principle that different semantic impairments emerge as the result of an interaction between the rich statistical structure of the semantic knowledge associated with different categories and sensorimotor modalities (Cree & McRae, 2003), and basic architectural constraints in semantics – *not* from explicit category-specific semantic stores. To evaluate the plausibility of these accounts, several researchers have implemented their proposals in connectionist models which can be used to study and explore the semantic memory store, both before and after it has been subjected to simulated impairment.

The present discussion centers upon a recent theory and model of normal and impaired semantic memory outlined by Rogers et al. (2004). Though this account is not a comprehensive model of semantic impairments, it nevertheless captures many important aspects of the data and has generated interesting predictions which have advanced the empirical characterization of semantic deficits. In realizing this, the account given by Rogers et al. makes several alterations to classical theories in which semantics is an explicit knowledge storehouse, and instead characterizes semantics as an intermodal routing hub while also synthesizing important principles described in previous work – notably, the sensory-motor theory outlined by Warrington and Shallice (1984) and related computational implementation by Farah and McClelland (1991), and the notion of similarity-based organization in an amodal semantic store (Tyler et al., 2000).

The implemented model of the theory given by Rogers et al. (2004) is shown in Figure 6.1 and is organized into three main groups of features – a pool of visual feature units, a pool of semantic units, and a pool of verbal units. The verbal units are further divided into several subgroups representing different types of features: the name and the perceptual, functional, and encyclopedic features of a given

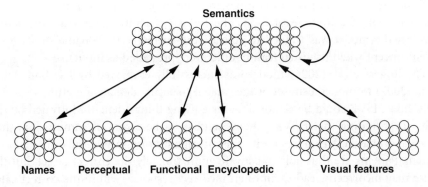

Figure 6.1 Network architecture of the model given by Rogers et al. (2004). The network was divided into three pools of units representing the visual, semantic, and verbal features of concepts. The verbal units were further partitioned to represent name, perceptual, functional, and encyclopedic features. Note that whereas the visual and verbal unit activations for a given concept were pre-specified based on normative data, the hidden unit activations were an emergent characteristic of the network as it learned to complete different tasks requiring intermodal mappings. (Adapted from Rogers et al., 2004.)

concept. Both the verbal and visual feature units can serve as either inputs or outputs to the model and are therefore considered to be "visible" units. In contrast, the states of the semantic units are "hidden" from the external environment and are determined by the activation they receive from the units with which they have connections. Rogers et al. (2004) thus instantiate the claim that rather than semantics serving as an abstract storehouse of the semantic properties we encounter in the world, it is a learned communications hub which allows for the mapping of information from one pool of units to another as required during the completion of various day-to-day tasks. It is also worth noting that in making this assumption, Rogers et al. are able to circumvent the challenging issues surrounding how and what information should be represented in the semantic storehouse (Cree & McRae, 2003). Instead, they are able to focus on the external properties of objects such as their visual features or the verbal descriptions individuals provide thereof which are more amenable to empirical research.

Recognizing the value of bringing their model in line with existing empirical data, Rogers et al. (2004) carefully crafted the input and output representations used to train their model in two main ways. First, they attempted to capture the detailed statistical structure of the different categories via an analysis of the convergent results of visual and verbal norming studies, as this structure has previously been associated with categories' respective robustness to impairment. For instance, their representations captured the finding that living thing representations tend to be more similar overall than nonliving thing representations. Second, the outputs that the model needed to produce for a given set of inputs were modeled after a series of semantic tasks analogous to those employed in testing patients: picture naming, word-to-picture matching, sorting, drawing and copying, and category-matching.

Each of these tasks consisted of employing one pool of input features to activate another pool of output features via the hidden semantic layer (e.g., in picture naming, the model was trained to activate the correct verbal "name" units for a given concept when its visual feature units were presented as input).

The Rogers et al. (2004) model was successfully employed by Lambon Ralph et al. (2007) to model a subset of the category-specific deficits literature – specifically, how HSVE could be responsible for a living things deficit. Motivated by the behavioral finding that HSVE patients tend to make errors of commission, they speculated that HSVE causes an increase in signal noise in the semantic memory system. Patients are thus able to activate approximately the correct target, but the noise may incorrectly lead them to an incorrect response within the correct category. By virtue of the high similarity between living thing exemplars, this noise would lead to a differential increase in errors for living things. Computational simulations of HSVE in which random noise was added to the values of the weights replicated this pattern of effects – the simulated patients made an increased number of commission errors, and differentially more errors were observed for the living things category.

Rogers et al. (2004) also investigated the application of another type of damage to the same model with the aim of accounting for the uniform semantic impairments associated with semantic dementia. Starting from the observation that semantic dementia patients tend to make errors of omission, Rogers et al. hypothesized that semantic dementia causes a "dimming," or reduction in size, of the weights in the semantic memory system which would decrease the overall activity therein. This would lead to insufficient semantic activity to elicit a response on a given task. Computational simulations of this hypothesis first confirmed that weight dimming caused an equal impairment to knowledge in all domains, as in semantic dementia. Furthermore, Rogers et al. noted that though the overall error rates for the different categories were identical, the types of errors that the model made were different across the living and nonliving thing categories. In particular, though errors of omission were high overall, there was a relatively greater likelihood of omitting knowledge for nonliving thing knowledge, whereas there was a relatively greater likelihood of commission errors for living thing knowledge. They attributed the former to the low similarity between nonliving thing exemplars causing each exemplar to be represented fairly separately from all others using a relatively sparse set of large-magnitude weights; a reduction in even a small portion of the weights necessary to activate a particular representation would therefore still direct the network's state towards the sparsely populated region of semantic space where that exemplar was represented, but the reduced weights were insufficiently strong to drive semantic activation above the response threshold. They attributed the latter case to the fact that living thing exemplars are highly similar to one another, and resultantly a large number of moderately sized weights therefore operate in unison to drive semantic activation above a response threshold. Dimming therefore did not lead to a substantial increase in errors of omission; however, as in the model of category-specific deficits, the reduction in magnitude of the weights in semantics led to a loss in the fine-grained distinctions between the living thing exemplars and caused an increase in errors of commission. Motivated by these unexpected findings, Rogers et al. conducted follow-up behavioral studies on patients which corroborated the model's predictions.

Taken together, the reductionist account and accompanying connectionist model outlined by Rogers et al. (2004) represents an important advance in our understanding of semantic memory deficits. This is true in two main respects: first, this work provides a highly detailed account of the patient data at a level not offered by other theories to date. Second, in addition to accounting for existing data, this model also has furthered the understanding of semantic memory impairments by producing novel predictions which were later validated via neuropsychological evaluation. Additionally, all of this work was realized within a single model which readily lends itself to parsimonious extension to other semantic memory impairments (e.g., accounting for cases wherein knowledge of a particular category and a particular modality are simultaneously impaired).

Nevertheless, several issues remain. For instance, the current modeling framework has not been applied to understanding how nonliving things could be differentially more impaired relative to living things. However, Rogers et al. (2004) speculate that adding representations for additional modalities which may be particularly salient for these domains and not others (e.g., motor representations capturing how objects are handled), combined with modality-specific biases on where simulated connection impairments occur, might allow the model to simulate this type of deficit. Past modeling work by Farah and McClelland (1991), who selectively damaged particular regions of an explicit semantic memory store, which contained architecturally separated subdivisions of sensory and functional knowledge and observed either living thing or nonliving thing deficits, lends empirical support to this intuition. The current framework also does not offer a detailed treatment of the patterning of exception categories observed in the patient literature – a key characteristic of category-specific semantic impairments – though the analysis of semantic feature norms by Cree and McRae (2003) indicates that the exception categories tend to have similar distributional characteristics as the main category of impairment; damage which affects the main category should also exert a similar pressure on the exception categories (e.g., musical instruments may group with living things in part because their auditory features are particularly useful for distinguishing amongst them).

Summary

Though neither the traditional domain-specific nor reductionist connectionist accounts of semantic memory impairments are all-encompassing at present, there appears to be additional theoretical value associated with the connectionist approach. The traditional account is able to address certain extreme patterns of data (e.g., selective impairment of nonliving things), but appears to lack a parsimonious way of extending itself to the broader semantic-memory literature, and beyond (e.g., the grammatical category deficits discussed in the following section). By virtue of being a recapitulation of the data, the traditional account also does not offer any new predictions against which we could further evaluate it and extend our empirical understanding of these phenomena.

In contrast, the reductionist connectionist account outlined by Rogers et al. (2004) is grounded in domain-general and independently verifiable principles and has directly contributed to expanding our understanding of semantic impairments. We therefore remain optimistic that future research along these lines, in conjunction with continued interleaving of neuropsychological assessment and the study of individuals who have not suffered from neural damage, will lead to the development of theories and models capable of accounting for the full gamut of deficits.

Grammatical Category Deficits

Interestingly, categorical impairments are not unique to the semantic domain; these kinds of deficits have also been reported for *grammatical* categories of words (e.g., nouns worse than verbs, De Renzi & di Pellegrino, 1995; verbs worse than nouns, Berndt, Mitchum, Haendiges, & Sandson, 1997). Paralleling the semantic category literature, these impairments have been explained either with the traditional neuropsychological logic of the double dissociation or with attempts to reduce the impairments to damage of other, underlying knowledge. But despite the successes of computational models in accounting for semantic category deficits, they have yet to impact our understanding of noun- and verb-specific impairments in the same way. The present section evaluates recent advances in the computational literature and suggests how further research in this direction will yield insights into the nature of grammatical category deficits.

Traditional accounts of grammatical category impairments

While verbs may be inherently more susceptible to loss after damage for a variety of reasons (e.g., later acquisition during development in many languages; Gentner, 1982), the existence of patients with noun-specific deficits suggests a double dissociation between these two types of knowledge (but see Mätzig, Druks, Masterson, & Vigliocco, 2009). As such, one explanation of noun/verb impairments is that grammatical category is the relevant principle of organization, either among lexical representations (Caramazza & Hillis, 1991; Hillis & Caramazza, 1995) or morphological ones (Shapiro, Shelton, & Caramazza, 2000). To account for patients whose noun or verb deficits are modality-specific (i.e., restricted to particular *linguistic* input and output modalities; e.g., a deficit for verbs only in written naming), each input or output lexicon is also assumed to have representations organized by grammatical category (Caramazza & Hillis, 1991; Hillis & Caramazza, 1995). Because some patients have no obvious semantic impairment, these grammatical distinctions are presumed to be represented independently of semantic knowledge (Caramazza, 1997). For this reason, there is no predicted effect of *semantic* similarity among the impaired words; only a word's grammatical category is relevant for predicting its loss after damage.

This explanation of noun- or verb-specific deficits can account for most of the reported patterns of data, largely because these patients motivated the theory in the first place. Nevertheless, the prediction that all words in a grammatical category should be impaired irrespective of meaning has not been confirmed. Berndt, Haendiges, Burton, and Mitchum (2002) tested patients on abstract and concrete noun and verb reading, but the results are not unequivocal: although two patients with verb deficits were indeed poorer at reading concrete *and* abstract verbs relative to nouns, no patients with noun deficits were tested, and so a difficulty effect cannot be ruled out.

Another problem with the grammatical category hypothesis is that it is inherently post hoc, motivated by the observation that some patients were worse with nouns or verbs. When modality-specific grammatical category deficits were also observed, the theory was extended to include input and output lexical representations organized by grammatical category. Together with the standard neuropsychological account of semantic category deficits, the picture that emerges is one of areas specialized for each linguistic modality and semantic and grammatical category. We find such an organization needlessly complex, especially in the absence of any complementary reasons to stipulate these subdivisions. Furthermore, the observance of new patterns of categorical deficits would not easily be accommodated by the theory – except to propose the existence of even more specialized representations.

Reductionist accounts of grammatical category impairments

The existence of a high correlation between grammatical category and semantic category suggests that there may be another explanation for noun/verb impairments. To wit, many verbs are actions, and many nouns are objects – especially the nouns and verbs used to test patients – so some researchers have proposed that noun- or verb-selective deficits are the result of semantic damage to knowledge about objects or actions (Bird, Howard, & Franklin, 2000; Gainotti, Silveri, Daniele, & Giustolisi, 1995; Vinson & Vigliocco, 2002).

One such account (Bird et al., 2000) was motivated by Warrington and Shallice's (1984) modality-specific account of semantic knowledge as well as the overlap noticed by Gainotti et al. (1995) between lesions resulting in noun and living things deficits (left temporal lobe) and verb and nonliving things deficits (left frontal and parietal lobes), respectively, (though see Capitani et al., 2003, for evidence suggesting that lesions resulting in nonlivings things deficits are more widespread). Bird et al. (2000) propose that the meanings of verbs, like those of nonliving things, are weighted more heavily towards functional semantic features relative to perceptual ones; nouns, in contrast, pattern like animate things and show the reverse weighting. Damage to sensory or functional information, then, is predicted to produce apparent category-specific deficits, and data from three patients with noun deficits who were also worse at naming living relative to nonliving things supported their hypothesis. The verb-deficit patients they tested, however, showed no grammatical category effect after the lower average imageability of verbs was taken into account, suggesting that many apparent verb deficits are the result of poorly designed testing materials.

On another reductionist account of grammatical category deficits, Vinson and Vigliocco (2002) used a computational model of semantic space to show that the meanings of words cluster by meaning and not grammatical category. Speaker-produced feature norms for nouns and verbs were used as the input to Kohonen maps, a class of connectionist models that learn without supervision to re-represent input patterns over an output "map" of lesser dimensionality (Kohonen, 1995). A winner-take-all learning procedure adjusts the weights between an input pattern and the output unit that responds maximally to it, but, critically, the weights of the winning unit's neighbors are also adjusted. After learning, similar input patterns will cluster together topographically in the output map. In Vinson and Vigliocco's (2002) model, nouns and verbs clustered according to similarity of meaning rather than grammatical category; that is, action nouns (*the bombardment*) were closer in distance to action verbs (*to bombard*) than to object nouns. Lesions to specific areas on the map or to types of semantic features (e.g. visual features) produced disproportionate object or action word deficits in the context of a mild, medium, or severe overall impairment.

Critically, many behavioral, neurophysiological, and other neuropsychological studies independently support the idea of a general object/action distinction in the brain (see Milner & Goodale, 1995, for a review). While some neuroimaging studies contrasting nouns and verbs have yielded inconsistent results (finding effects of grammatical category – Shapiro et al., 2005; Perani et al., 1999 – or not – Tyler, Russell, Fadili, & Moss, 2001), these discrepancies may also be a result of the meaning/grammatical category correlation. When nouns and verbs were matched for semantic properties (e.g., all words referred to actions), no difference between grammatical categories was found (Siri et al., 2008). Similarly, when manipulable objects and actions involving manipulation were compared, there was an effect of manipulability but not grammatical category (Saccuman et al., 2006).

However, neither traditional neuropsychological nor reductionist accounts of grammatical category deficits have adequately addressed the way in which the adult structure is learned, a research question well suited to a computational modeling approach, and to connectionist models, in particular. Because models with learned internal representations do not require prior commitment to the representational structure necessary to complete the task at hand, they provide a way to explicitly investigate the acquisition of knowledge and the learnability of a hypothesized organization. Of course, for either account, the question of learnability could be circumvented with the claim that such an organization is innate – but this claim

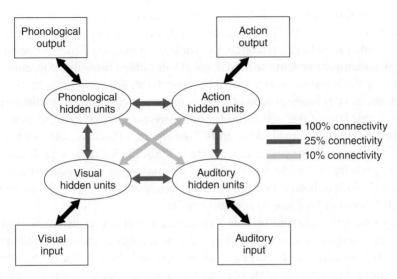

Figure 6.2 Network architecture of the Watson (2009) model. Input and output layers (26 units each) are represented by rectangles; hidden semantic layers (60 units each) are represented by ovals. The density of the connectivity between two layers is represented by the increasingly dark shades of grey: darker is equivalent to denser connectivity.

raises further questions about the selective pressures that could produce such an innately specified organization. Instead, computational models can be used to test the hypothesis that grammatical category deficits may emerge after damage to semantic knowledge shaped only by domain-general learning mechanisms, the characteristics of nouns and verbs in the environment, and the way in which people respond to them.

A connectionist model of grammatical category impairments

Watson (2009) implemented a distributed connectionist model with learned semantic representations and no explicit instruction on the grammatical category of words; the architecture of the model is shown in Figure 6.2. As in the account of semantic category deficits given by Rogers et al. (2004), "semantics" in the model (the four oval-shaped groups) was not conceived of as an amodal store of features but instead as a learned set of representations that develop under pressure to perform various linguistic and conceptual tasks successfully (see also Plaut, 2002). In this model, phonological output was required in response to the visual or auditory input associated with it (i.e., naming from vision or audition). Additionally, if the word had an action associated with it (i.e., *to kick*), the model was required to produce that action in addition to the action's name. The role of the hidden semantic units, then, was to use a domain-general learning algorithm to develop representations that enabled the model to successfully complete the tasks at hand.

These semantic representations were further shaped by a topographic bias (Jacobs & Jordan, 1992; Plaut, 2002) on the connectivity between units: units in layers close to one another were fully interconnected, while units in layers far from one another had sparser connectivity. In the model, groups of hidden units that communicated with particular input or output modalities were fully connected to them. However, the connectivity *between* groups of hidden units was constrained by distance; for instance, only 10% of the "action hidden units" were connected to the hidden group farthest from it, the "visual hidden units" (see Figure 6.2). This constraint instanti- ated computationally properties of neurons in the brain: because of size limitations, there is pressure for connections between neurons to be local rather than long- distance (Nelson & Bower, 1990). As a result, neighboring neurons will come to be strongly interconnected and to respond similarly.

Part of the motivation to include this representational pressure came from the success of a computational simulation of a different aphasic syndrome, *optic aphasia* – a selective impairment in naming visually presented objects (Plaut, 2002). In this model, imposing a topographic bias on the semantic hidden units caused units closest to particular input or output modalities to become "functionally specialized" for representing modality-specific aspects of knowledge. As a result, damage to con- nections from vision to the semantic units that were partially specialized for repre- senting phonological information produced a selective impairment for naming objects presented visually (i.e., optic aphasia).

In the context of grammatical category deficits, if nouns and verbs learn to rely on different sets of functionally specialized semantic units, damage to these units could produce disproportionate deficits for one category or the other. But how do modality-specific areas become differentially important for naming nouns or verbs? Essentially, particular input or output modalities offer sources of information that may be more or less reliable during learning, and these sources of information are hypothesized to vary between grammatical categories, on average. Previous behav- ioral (e.g., Myung, Blumstein, & Sedivy, 2006) and neuroimaging (e.g., Hauk, Johnsrude, & Pulvermüller, 2004; Martin, Haxby, Lalonde, Wiggs, & Ungerleider, 1995) data have suggested that visual and action knowledge participate in the mean- ings of nouns and verbs to differing degrees, and the representations and tasks given to the model reflected these differences. Because verbs often refer to actions, the model was required to produce both the name and the associated action during naming of a verb. Additionally, the visual representations of nouns were richer than those of verbs, reflecting the assumption that there is more detailed (e.g., color, form) and more consistent (in time and across instances) visual knowledge associ- ated with objects than with actions.

The result of using realistic tasks and representations in conjunction with the topographic bias on connectivity between semantic hidden units was that particular groups of units became more important for one grammatical category or the other – and this difference yielded grammatical category deficits after damage (Figure 6.3). In particular, the group of hidden units strongly connected to action output became specialized for representing action knowledge, and this same action knowl-

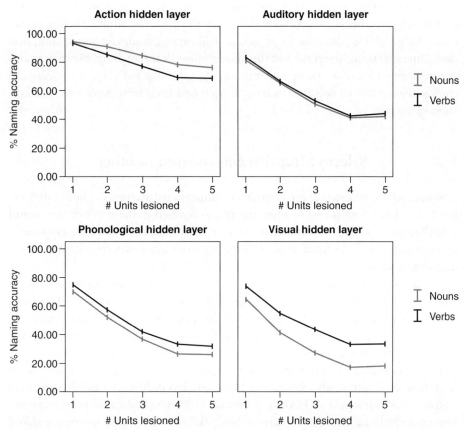

Figure 6.3 Noun and verb naming accuracy after removing individual hidden units in each semantic layer of the Watson (2009) model. Results are from naming from visual input, and only the phonological output was considered for correctness. Error bars represent +/− 1 standard error of the mean.

edge was recruited during naming. As a result, damage here produced relative verb deficits (top left panel). On the other hand, the hidden units strongly connected to visual input became specialized for representing visual knowledge. Given the richness of visual knowledge for nouns and the lack of other associated information (i.e., action), nouns were particularly affected by damage to the visual hidden units (bottom right panel). Although a difference between grammatical categories was not predicted after damage to the hidden units closest to phonological output or auditory input, a slight advantage for verbs emerged; this pattern was attributed to the higher average difficulty of nouns and was predicted to disappear if the visual representations of verbs more closely mirrored the variable and inconsistent visual input associated with actions in the world.

These modeling results support a more parsimonious and principled alternative to the view that representations must be organized by grammatical category to produce grammatical category deficits and addresses the major failing of grammatically based accounts – the problem of the way in which the adult structure comes to be. Although this domain, in particular, will benefit from continued computational investigations, the results of this model show that armed only with domain-general principles of learning and processing, grammatical category effects can emerge from a model required to learn stimuli and tasks similar to those encountered by people.

Selective Impairments in Word Reading

Semantic representations play a key role in connectionist accounts of both category-specific and grammatical-class impairments, as covered in the first two sections of this chapter. The same turns out to be true in the third domain we consider – impairments in single word reading resulting from brain damage, known as the *acquired dyslexias*.

The traditional account of oral reading is the *dual-route* model (Coltheart, 1978), which posits that there are two separate mechanisms involved in translating print to sound. The first, termed the *nonlexical* pathway, captures the systematic relationships between spelling and sound, typically in the form of grapheme–phoneme correspondence (GPC) rules (e.g., G → /g/; M → /m/; A_E → /ei/; V → /v/). Such rules generate correct pronunciations for *regular* words like GAVE, as well as for pronounceable nonwords like MAVE. However, about 20% of English words are *irregular* or *exceptions* (e.g., HAVE), in that the GPC rules yield a mispronunciation, termed a *regularization* error ("haive"). Since skilled readers can pronounce HAVE and other irregular words correctly, dual-route theories posit a second, *lexical* pathway that translates written words onto spoken words directly. However, because it relies on word-specific knowledge, the lexical pathway cannot pronounce nonwords. Thus, on a dual-route account, skilled readers need a nonlexical route to pronounce nonwords and a lexical route to pronounce irregular words. Interestingly, on most dual-route accounts, semantic representations are not directly involved in pronouncing words. The most influential computational implementation of a dual-route account is the dual-route cascaded (DRC) model of Coltheart, Rastle, Perry, Langdon, and Ziegler (2001; see also Coltheart & Kohnen, Volume 2, Chapter 43).

Traditional accounts of the acquired dyslexias

At first glance, the dual-route model would seem to receive strong support from the patterns of impairments in word reading that occur following brain damage. Patients with *phonological dyslexia* read both regular and exception words well, but make many errors on nonwords, often producing an incorrect word in response, termed a *lexicalization* error. By contrast, patients with *surface dyslexia* read regular words and pronounceable nonwords well but make regularization errors on exception words, particularly those of low frequency (e.g., PINT → "pihnt"; FLOOD → "flude"). The straightforward dual-route account is that phonological dyslexics have damage to the nonlexical pathway (impairing nonwords), whereas surface dyslexics have damage to the lexical pathway (impairing exception words).

As it turns out, the dual-route account of each of these patterns of performance runs into some difficulties. One of the challenges facing these efforts is that, as Coltheart et al. (2001) point out, "to simulate extreme versions of these two acquired dyslexias is trivial with the DRC model" (p. 242) – disabling the lexical pathway produces regularizations of *all* exception words while leaving regular words and nonwords unaffected, whereas disabling the GPC rules *eliminates* nonword reading while leaving word reading unaffected. The problem is that, although these patterns are natural to produce on a dual-route account, neither has ever been observed: impairment of exception words is always modulated by word frequency, and severe nonword reading impairment is always accompanied by some impairment to word reading.

We will focus on surface dyslexia in the remainder of this chapter as it bears more directly on the role of semantic representations in word reading; see Nickels, Biedermann, Coltheart, Saunders, and Tree, (2007) for attempts to simulate phonological dyslexia using the DRC model, and Harm and Seidenberg (1999) and Welbourne and Lambon Ralph (2007) for relevant connectionist simulations.

A connectionist account of surface dyslexia

In contrast to dual-route accounts of word reading, the "triangle" model (Harm & Seidenberg, 2004; Plaut, McClelland, Seidenberg, & Patterson, 1996; Seidenberg & McClelland, 1989) posits that word reading is supported by cooperative and competitive interactions among orthographic, phonological, and semantic representations (often depicted as the three points of a triangle; see Figure 6.4). Each type of information is encoded as patterns of activity over a group of neuron-like processing units, and the knowledge that governs their interactions is instantiated by weights on connections between them (via additional groups of "hidden" units). Within the triangle framework, there are no word-specific representations; rather, the system learns to make the orthographic, phonological, and semantic patterns for each familiar word a stable configuration over the entire network. Although interactions among orthography and phonology capture systematic spelling–sound knowledge, and interactions of each with semantics capture word-specific knowledge, the entire network participates in processing all types of stimuli: regular words, irregular words, and nonwords.

Plaut et al. (1996) presented a number of connectionist simulations in which networks based on the triangle framework learned to map from orthography to phonology for both regular and irregular words, and yet also generalized well to nonwords. These results belied dual-route claims that good performance on both irregular words and nonwords requires separate mechanisms. However, none of the

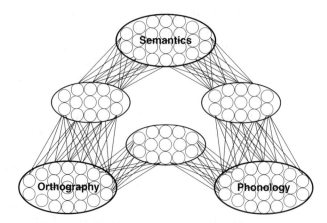

Figure 6.4   The triangle framework of word reading, in which patterns of activity in orthography, phonology, and semantics interact and mutually constrain each other (via intermediate groups of "hidden" units) in processing both words and nonwords. (Adapted from Plaut et al., 1996.)

networks, when damaged, provided a good match to surface dyslexia. A much better account was provided by more closely approximating the full triangle framework: training an orthography-to-phonology network in the context of support from semantics, and then damaging the model by progressively weakening this semantic support.

Thus, one of the main points of contention regarding surface dyslexia is whether it is due to semantic damage or, as the dual-route model claims, to lexical damage separate from semantics. Woollams, Lambon Ralph, Plaut, and Patterson (2007) presented 100 observations from 51 patients with a form of progressive semantic deterioration known as semantic dementia, and showed a systematic relationship between the severity of semantic impairment and irregular word reading (see Figure 6.5a). Critically, patients who initially showed a semantic impairment but normal exception-word reading (e.g., MA, EB) – which might seem inconsistent with the triangle model account (Blazely, Coltheart, & Casey, 2005) – went on to exhibit surface dyslexia along with the rest of the patients on further testing. Woollams et al. (2007) also showed that versions of the Plaut et al. (1996) simulation of surface dyslexia, varying in magnitude of semantic support during training, exhibited a similar distribution of performance with the progressive removal of semantics (see Figure 6.5b).

In response to Woollams et al.'s (2007) empirical findings and simulations, Coltheart, Tree, and Saunders (2010) presented DRC simulations in which they generated 40,200 versions of the model by administering all possible combinations of severity of damage to the lexical pathway (removing the X lowest-frequency orthographic word units) and the nonlexical pathway (removing the Y least-frequently used GPC rules). They then identified the 100 versions that most closely

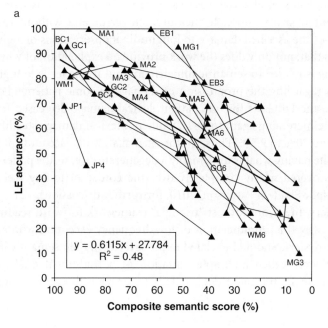

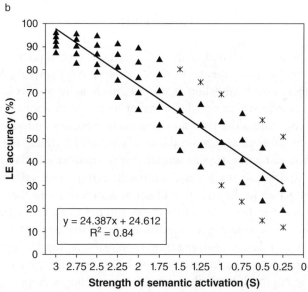

Figure 6.5 (a) Performance in reading low-frequency exception (LE) words of 100 observations of 51 patients, as a function of a measure of semantic integrity. Longitudinal observations from the same patient are connected by lines. (b) Performance of parametric variations of a connectionist simulation of word reading (varying in strength of semantic support during training) as a function of semantic damage (i.e., weakening of semantic support). (Adapted from Woollams et al., 2007.)

matched Woollams et al.'s 100 observations. Unfortunately, this data fitting was done without regard to possible measurement error and without regard to the consistency of the ascribed damage to longitudinal observations of a given patient. The result is that, not only does the work provide no explanation of why exception-word reading is related to semantic impairment, but it also leads to highly implausible claims regarding the progression of damage in some patients. For example, according to the DRC fits for one patient, lexical damage decreased from 45% to 34.5% before increasing again to 46%, while nonlexical damage steadily decreased from 47.5% to 20% to 9.5%. Thus, Coltheart et al.'s (2010) "account" of this patient is that, despite having what is undeniably a degenerate disease, the patient's nonlexical route recovered nearly completely over the course of testing (see Woollams, Lambon Ralph, Plaut, & Patterson, 2010, for further discussion).

In summary, the connectionist "triangle" framework for word reading provides insight into why the pronunciation of low-frequency exception words in patients with surface dyslexia should be related to the severity of their semantic impairment. By contrast, even when an implementation of a traditional dual-route model can be made to fit the same data, it fails to provide the same insight into the phenomenon.

Conclusion

Connectionist modeling is based on the belief that certain computational principles of neural systems are fundamental to understanding both normal and disordered cognition. The value of modeling is not so much to fit particular patterns of observed data, as to provide a vehicle for exploring the implications of a set of theoretical claims concerning the representations and processes underlying cognition, and how they are impacted by brain damage. We have illustrated the value of this approach in three domains: semantic impairments, grammatical-class impairments, and acquired dyslexia. In each case, the traditional account reifies the relevant behavioral distinction in the structure of the system itself, with the result that the account provides little insight into why the phenomena pattern as they do.

By contrast, the alternative, connectionist, accounts attempt to explain the observed patterns of data as resulting from more basic representational or processing commitments. Although the existing modeling work certainly has limitations, in each case the approach holds the promise of providing a deeper understanding of how brain processes support cognitive processes, both in neurologically intact individuals and in those who have suffered brain damage.

References

Berndt, R. S., Haendiges, A. N., Burton, M. W., & Mitchum, C. C. (2002). Grammatical class and imageability in aphasic word production: Their effects are independent. *Journal of Neurolinguistics, 15,* 353–371.

Berndt, R. S., Mitchum, C. C., Haendiges, A. N., & Sandson, J. (1997). Verb retrieval in aphasia. 1. Characterizing single word impairment. *Brain and Language, 56,* 68–106.

Bird, H., Howard, D., & Franklin, S. (2000). Why is a verb like an inanimate object? Grammatical category and semantic category deficits. *Brain and Language, 72,* 246–309.

Blazely, A. M., Coltheart, M., & Casey, B. J. (2005). Semantic impairment with and without surface dyslexia: Implications for models of reading. *Cognitive Neuropsychology, 22,* 695–717.

Capitani, E., Laiacona, M., Mahon, B., & Caramazza, A. (2003). What are the facts of semantic category-specific deficits? A critical review of the clinical evidence. *Cognitive Neuropsychology, 20,* 213–261.

Caramazza, A. (1997). How many levels of processing are there in lexical access? *Cognitive Neuropsychology, 14,* 177–208.

Caramazza, A., & Hillis, A. E. (1991). Lexical organization of nouns and verbs in the brain. *Nature, 349,* 788–790.

Caramazza, A., & Shelton, J. R. (1998). Domain-specific knowledge systems in the brain: The animate–inanimate distinction. *Journal of Cognitive Neuroscience, 10*(1), 1–34.

Coltheart, M. (1978). Lexical access in simple reading tasks. In G. Underwood (Ed.), *Strategies of information processing* (pp. 151–216). New York: Academic Press.

Coltheart, M., Rastle, K., Perry, C., Langdon, R., & Ziegler, J. (2001). DRC: A dual route cascaded model of visual word recognition and reading aloud. *Psychological Review, 108,* 204–256.

Coltheart, M., Tree, J., & Saunders, S. J. (2010). Computational modeling of reading in semantic dementia: Comment on Woollams, Plaut, Lambon Ralph and Patterson (2007). *Psychological Review, 117,* 256–272.

Cree, G. S., & McRae, K. (2003). Analyzing the factors underlying the structure and computation of the meaning of chipmunk, cherry, chisel, cheese, and cello (and many other such concrete nouns). *Journal of Experimental Psychology: General, 132,* 163–201.

De Renzi, E., & di Pellegrino, G. (1995). Sparing of verbs and preserved, but ineffectual reading in a patient with impaired word production. *Cortex, 31,* 619–36.

Farah, M. J., & McClelland, J. L. (1991). A computational model of semantic memory impairment: Modality specificity and emergent category specificity. *Journal of Experimental Psychology: General, 120,* 339–357.

Gainotti, G., Silveri, M. C., Daniele, A., & Giustolisi, L. (1995). Neuroanatomical correlates of category-specific semantic disorders: A critical survey. *Memory, 3,* 247–264.

Gentner, D. (1982). Why nouns are learned before verbs: Linguistic relativity versus natural partitioning. In S. A. Kuczaj (Ed.), *Language development: Vol. 2. Language, thought, and culture* (pp. 301–334). Hillsdale, NJ: Erlbaum.

Harm, M. W., & Seidenberg, M. S. (1999). Phonology, reading acquisition, and dyslexia: Insights from connectionist models. *Psychological Review, 106,* 491–528.

Harm, M. W., & Seidenberg, M. S. (2004). Computing the meanings of words in reading: Cooperative division of labor between visual and phonological processes. *Psychological Review, 111,* 662–720.

Hauk, O., Johnsrude, I., & Pulvermüller, F. (2004). Somatotopic representation of action words in human motor and premotor cortex. *Neuron, 41,* 301–307.

Hillis, A. E., & Caramazza, A. (1995). Representations of grammatical categories of words in the brain. *Journal of Cognitive Neuroscience, 7,* 396–407.

Jacobs, R. A., & Jordan, M. I. (1992). Computational consequences of a bias toward short connections. *Journal of Cognitive Neuroscience, 4,* 323–336.

Kohonen, T. (1995). *Self-organization maps.* New York: Springer-Verlag.

Lambon Ralph, M. A., Howard, D., Nightingale, G., & Ellis, A. W. (1998). Are living and non-living category-specific deficits causally linked to impaired perceptual or associative knowledge? Evidence from a category-specific double dissociation. *Neurocase, 4,* 311–338.

Lambon Ralph, M. A., Lowe, C., & Rogers, T. T. (2007). Neural basis of category-specific semantic deficits for living things: Evidence from semantic dementia, HSVE and a neural network model. *Brain, 130,* 1127–1137.

Magnié, M., Ferreira, C. T., Giusiano, B., & Poncet, B. (1999). Category specificity in object agnosia: Preservation of sensorimotor experiences related to objects. *Neuropsychologia, 37,* 67–74.

Martin, A., & Chao, L. L. (2001). Semantic memory and the brain: Structure and processes. *Current Opinion in Neurobiology, 11,* 194–201.

Martin, A., Haxby, J. V., Lalonde, F. M., Wiggs, C. L., & Ungerleider, L. G. (1995). Discrete cortical regions associated with knowledge of color and knowledge of action. *Science, 270,* 102–105.

Mätzig, S., Druks, J., Masterson, J., & Vigliocco G. (2009). Noun and verb differences in picture naming: Past studies and new evidence. *Cortex, 45,* 738–758.

Milner, A. D., & Goodale, M. A. (1995). *The visual brain in action.* Oxford: Oxford University Press.

McCarthy, R. A., & Warringon, E., K. (1988). Evidence for modality-specific meaning systems in the brain. *Nature, 334,* 428–430.

Myung, J., Blumstein, S. E., & Sedivy, J. C. (2006). Playing on the typewriter, typing on the piano: Manipulation knowledge of objects. *Cognition, 98,* 223–43.

Nelson, M. E., & Bower, J. M. (1990). Brain maps and parallel computers. *Trends in Neurosciences, 13,* 403–408.

Nickels, L., Biedermann, B., Coltheart, M., Saunders, S., & Tree, J. J. (2007). Computational modelling of phonological dyslexia: How does the DRC model fare? *Cognitive Neuropsychology, 25,* 165–193.

Noppeny, U., Patterson, K., Tyler, L. K., Moss, H., Stamatakis, E. A., Bright, P., et al. (2007). Temporal lobe lesions and semantic impairment: a comparison of herpes simplex virus encephalitis and semantic dementia. *Brain, 130,* 1138–1147.

Perani, D., Cappa, S. F., Schnur, T., Tettamanti, M., Collina, S., Rosa, M. M., et al. (1999). The neural correlates of verb and noun processing: A PET study. *Brain, 122,* 2337–2344.

Plaut, D. C. (2002). Graded modality-specific specialization in semantics: A computational account of optic aphasia. *Cognitive Neuropsychology, 19,* 603–639.

Plaut, D. C., McClelland, J. L., Seidenberg, M. S., & Patterson, K. (1996). Understanding normal and impaired reading: Computational principles in quasi-regular domains. *Psychological Review, 103,* 56–105.

Pulvermüller, F. (1999). Words in the brain's language. *Behavioral and Brain Sciences, 22,* 253–336.

Pulvermüller, F., Härle, M., & Hummel, F. (2001). Walking or talking?: Behavioral and electrophysiological correlates of action verb processing. *Brain and Language, 78,* 143–168.

Rogers, T. T., Lambon Ralph, M. A., Garrard, P. A., Bozeat, S., McClelland, J. L., Hodges, J. R., et al. (2004). Structure and deterioration of semantic memory: A neuropsychological and computational investigation. *Psychological Review, 111*, 205–235.

Saccuman, M. C., Cappa, S. F., Bates, E. A., Arevalo, A., Della Rosa, P., Danna, M., et al. (2006). The impact of semantic reference on word class: An fMRI study of action and object naming. *NeuroImage, 32*, 1865–1878.

Santos, L. R., & Caramazza, A. (2002). The domain-specific hypothesis: A developmental and comparative perspective on category-specific deficits. In E. M. E. Forde & G. W. Humphreys (Eds.), *Category specificity in brain and mind* (1–23). New York: Psychology Press.

Sartori, G., & Job, R. (1988). The oyster with four legs: A neuropsychological study on the interaction of visual and semantic information. *Cognitive Neuropsychology, 5*, 105–132.

Seidenberg, M. S., & McClelland, J. L. (1989). A distributed, developmental model of word recognition and naming. *Psychological Review, 96*, 523–568.

Shapiro, K. A., Mottaghy, F. M., Schiller, N. O., Poeppel, T. D., Fluss, M. O., Müller, H. W., et al. (2005). Dissociating neural correlates for nouns and verbs. *NeuroImage, 24*, 1058–1067.

Shapiro, K., Shelton, J., & Caramazza, A. (2000). Grammatical class in lexical production and morphological processing: Evidence from a case of fluent aphasia. *Cognitive Neuropsychology, 17*, 665–682.

Simmons, K., & Barsalou, L. W. (2003). The similarity in topography principle: Reconciling theories of conceptual deficits. *Cognitive Neuropsychology, 20*, 451–486.

Siri, S., Tettamanti, M., Cappa, S. F., Della Rosa, P., Saccuman, C., Scifo, P., et al. (2008). The neural substrate of naming events: Effects of processing demands but not of grammatical class. *Cerebral Cortex, 18*, 171–177.

Tyler, L. K., Moss, H. E., Durrant-Peatfield, M. R., & Levy, J. P. (2000). Conceptual structure and the structure of concepts: A distributed account of category-specific deficits. *Brain and Language, 75*, 195–231.

Tyler, L. K., Russell, R., Fadili, J., & Moss, H. E. (2001). The neural representation of nouns and verbs: PET studies. *Brain, 124*, 1619–1634.

Vigliocco, G., Vinson, D. P., Lewis, W., & Garrett, M. F. (2004). Representing the meanings of object and action words: The featural and unitary semantic space hypothesis. *Cognitive Psychology, 48*, 422–488.

Vinson, D. P., & Vigliocco, G. (2002). A semantic analysis of grammatical class impairments: Semantic representations of object nouns, action nouns and action verbs. *Journal of Neurolinguistics, 15*, 317–351.

Warrington, E. K., & McCarthy, R. A. (1983). Category specific access dysphasia. *Brain, 106*, 859–878.

Warrington, E. K., & McCarthy, R. A. (1987). Categories of knowledge: Further fractionations and an attempted integration. *Brain, 110*, 1273–1296.

Warrington, E. K., & Shallice, T. (1984). Category specific semantic impairments. *Brain, 107*, 829–854.

Watson, C. E. (2009). *Computational and behavioral studies of normal and impaired noun/verb processing* (Unpublished doctoral dissertation). Department of Psychology, Carnegie Mellon University.

Welbourne, S. R., & Lambon Ralph, M. A. (2007). Using PDP models to simulate phonological dyslexia: The key role of plasticity-related recovery. *Journal of Cognitive Neuroscience, 19*, 1125–1139.

Woollams, A. M., Lambon Ralph, M. A., Plaut, D. C., & Patterson, K. (2007). SD-squared: On the association between semantic dementia and surface dyslexia. *Psychological Review, 114*, 316–339.

Woollams, A. M., Lambon Ralph, M. A., Plaut, D. C., & Patterson, K. (2010). SD-squared revisited: Reply to Coltheart, Tree, & Saunders (2010). *Psychological Review, 117*, 273–281.

7

Neural Network Models of Speech Production

Matthew Goldrick

The ability to translate thoughts into articulatory gestures – resulting in sounds that others can perceive – is a critical part of human behavior. Concepts from neural or connectionist networks have played an important role in the development of theories in this domain. Following Smolensky (1999), this chapter focuses on three core principles of connectionist theories of speech production:

- *Mental representations are distributed, graded patterns of activation.* Mental representations are realized as gradient numerical patterns of activation over simple processing units.
- *Cognitive processing is the spread of activation.* Cognitive processes are realized by transformations of activity patterns by numerical connections.
- *Cognitive processing reflects the statistical structure of the environment.* The structure of cognitive processes reflects the ongoing modification of the spread of activation based on the statistics of the environment.

Following a brief introduction to connectionist networks, the impact of each of these principles on psycholinguistic theories of speech production is reviewed. The next section then examines how learning-based modification of spreading activation may (or may not) lead to novel theories of cognitive processes.

At the outset, it should be noted that connectionist networks are best thought of not as networks of realistic models of neurons but rather as neurally *inspired* networks. Although the principles of connectionist computation are broadly consistent with what is known regarding neuronal computational principles, connectionist processing mechanisms represent considerable abstractions from actual

The Handbook of the Neuropsychology of Language, First Edition. Edited by Miriam Faust.
© 2012 Blackwell Publishing Ltd. Published 2012 by Blackwell Publishing Ltd.

neurobiological mechanisms. Connectionist researchers see this as a virtue; such networks provide an appropriate theoretical vocabulary for bridging cognitive- and neural-level explanations (Smolensky, 2006). This chapter aims to illustrate how the integration of cognitive concepts with neuronal processing principles has served to enhance theory development in the domain of speech production.

A Connectionist Primer

A connectionist network is a computational device composed of simple processing units linked by numerical connections or weights. The processing units are associated with a numerical quantity referred to as activation. Processing occurs via the propagation of activation along the numerical connections. This allows activation from one unit to "flow" to others, allowing one unit to influence the activation of others.

In many domains, cognitive processes can be conceptualized as input–output mappings – a relation between two sets of mental representations. For example, Palmer and Kimchi (1986, p. 40) define the components of cognitive psychological theories as "informational events" consisting of "the *input information* (what it starts with), the *operation* performed on the input (what gets done to the input) and the *output information* (what it ends up with) [emphasis original]." In a connectionist network realizing or modeling a cognitive process, mental representations are instantiated via patterns of activation over sets of units. The input to the cognitive process is realized by imposing an activation pattern over one set of units (the input units). Activation then spreads via connections to other units (instantiating the operation performed on the input). This results in a pattern of activation over a set of output units; the mental representation corresponding to this pattern of activity is the output.

To provide a concrete illustration of this framework, consider the simple network illustrated in Figure 7.1. This implements a cognitive process that maps conceptual representations to lexical representations. These representations are realized via patterns of activation over two sets of processing units. This example follows many

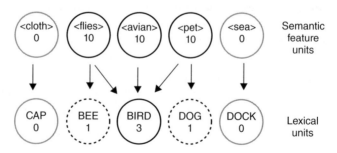

Figure 7.1   Illustration of the spread of distributed patterns of activation. All connections have strength 0.1. Activations are shown below unit labels.

connectionist theories of speech production (e.g., Dell, 1986) by making use of localist representations. In strictly local representations, each distinct mental representation is realized by a single processing unit (e.g., each word has an independent unit such as <BIRD> [angle brackets (< , >) denote the content of the mental representation instantiated by the unit]). In feature-based or semi-local representations a set of processing units realizes each distinct mental representation (e.g., each concept is encoded by a set of semantic features such as <avian>). In contrast, in a distributed representational framework there is not a strict relationship between elements of mental representations and processing units; individual processing units participate in the realization of many distinct mental representations (see Vousden, Brown, & Harley, 2000, for an example within phonological processing in speech production).

In this example, the concept "a flying avian pet" is provided as input to this cognitive process by activating the semantic feature units corresponding to this concept. Here they are assigned the arbitrary activation level of 10 (other features remain inactive). Activation then spreads along the connections between semantic features and lexical items. The amount of activation flowing to each lexical item is simply the sum over all incoming connections of the connections' weight times the activation of the sending unit. For example, the amount of activation flowing to <BEE> is 0.1 times the activation of <flies> ($10 * .1 = 1$). In simple linear networks, the activation of the unit is simply equal to this value. In more complex networks, the activation of the unit is a nonlinear function of the amount of incoming activation (Rumelhart, Hinton, & Williams, 1986).

Note that the output of this process does not simply specify a single representation. It contains a blend of several partially activated lexical items. Although <BIRD> (the target) is the most strongly activated, its semantic neighbors are partially activated as well. Since activation levels can vary gradiently, connectionist networks allow multiple representations to simultaneously contribute to processing. Note that in this example the cognitive process is structured such that only semantically related items are co-activated; words with nonoverlapping semantic representations (e.g., CAP and DOCK for BIRD) are not activated.

As illustrated above, the structure of a cognitive process – the output generated for a given input – is determined by the spread of activation within the network. In some cases, this is completely specified by the theorist. A cognitive process is hypothesized to have a certain structure; a set of representations, connections, and connection weights is then specified to realize this structure (e.g., Dell, 1986). In other cases, some aspects of the structure of the cognitive process are determined via a learning procedure (e.g., Warker & Dell, 2006).

In networks utilizing a learning procedure, the theorist typically hypothesizes the structure of input and output representations along with the pattern of connectivity within the network (e.g., a set of semantic features fully connected with a set of localist lexical representations). The flow of activation is left unspecified; the network is initialized with a set of random connection weights. The network therefore fails to produce the appropriate output for each input (e.g., given "flying avian pet" it will activate a set of random lexical items – not "bird" and its semantic neighbors). To allow the network to acquire the correct input–output mapping, the theorist specifies a set of examples of correct mappings between input and output representations (e.g., <flies> <avian> <pet>; <BIRD>). A learning rule uses these data to modify the spread of activation within the network such that after training the network will produce the correct output for each input. As discussed in more detail below, these learning rules typically aim to approximate the covariance between elements of input and output patterns (i.e., the activation over input and output units; van Orden, Pennington, & Stone, 1990). Thus, over the course of learning, connectionist networks acquire the statistical structure of their environment.

Theories of speech production have deployed these general connectionist computational mechanisms to account for a wide variety of empirical patterns in spoken language processing. The following sections examine a few such cases that serve to illustrate the importance of each core connectionist principle.

Gradient Activation in Theories of Speech Production

In connectionist networks, mental representations are realized via gradient patterns of activation over simple processing units. As summarized in Table 7.1, this principle has played a key role in connectionist accounts of an array of empirical phenomena.

Table 7.1 Illustration of Principle 1: mental representations are gradient patterns of activation.

Empirical phenomenon	Connectionist account
During phonological spell-out, errors with a mixed semantic-phonological relationship to the target occur at rates greater than chance.	
Words phonologically related to synonyms of the target show reduced reaction times relative to controls.	Lexical representations of semantic neighbors (including translation equivalents) are gradiently activated during lexical retrieval; this partial activation cascades to phonological spell-out, facilitating retrieval of their phonological representations.
In bilingual production, cognate words (sharing form and meaning across languages) show reduced reaction times relative to noncognates.	
Phonetic properties of speech errors reflect a trace of the intended target.	Phonological representations of targets remain gradiently activated during production of errors; this partial activation cascades to subsequent phonetic processes, influencing the phonetic realization of the target.

Based on evidence from wide variety of sources, including speech errors (Garrett, 1980), chronometric (reaction time), electrophysiological, and neuroimaging studies (Levelt, 2001), theories of speech production generally assume that there are two major stages of cognitive processing that map meaning (e.g., "flying avian pet") onto the long-term memory representation of its spoken form (the sound sequence /b/ /ɚ/ /d/). The first, lexical selection, is driven primarily by considerations of meaning and grammatical structure. In the context of single word production, this stage involves the selection of a (syntactically appropriate) lexical item to express the intended meaning (e.g., "bird" for "a flying avian pet.") The second stage, phonological spell-out, involves retrieval of the spoken form of this lexical item (e.g., recalling that "bird" contains the sound sequence /b/ /ɚ/ /d/).

Although a large body of evidence suggests these two processing stages form independent components of the cognitive system underlying language production, there is also ample evidence suggesting some degree of interaction between them. One dimension of interaction concerns the activation of semantically related words during phonological spell-out processes. This is supported by the *mixed error effect*. During phonological spell-out processes, errors that have a mixed semantic and phonological relationship to the target (e.g., "shirt" → "skirt") are found to occur more often than predicted based on the rates of purely semantic (e.g., "shirt" → "pants") or purely phonological errors (e.g., "shirt" → "hurt"). This has been documented in speech errors arising spontaneously (Dell & Reich, 1981) or due to acquired impairments to phonological spell-out (Rapp & Goldrick, 2000). This is unexpected if lexical selection and phonological spell-out are completely independent stages of processing. If these two processing stages do not interact, semantic factors should only influence lexical selection – not phonological spell-out. Mixed errors should therefore be no more likely to occur during spell-out than purely phonological errors.

To account for this pattern, theorists have appealed to the connectionist principle of gradient activation (but see Roelofs, 2004). Following the example above (Figure 7.1), assume lexical selection is implemented by a mapping from semantic features to lexical units. Phonological spell-out is implemented by a mapping from lexical to phoneme units. Spreading activation allows multiple semantically related words to become activated during the course of lexical selection. As illustrated above, this causes the output of lexical selection to reflect not just the activation of the target but the partial activation of its semantic neighbors. For example, although the target <SHIRT> will be most strongly activated, the semantic neighbor <SKIRT> will be partially activated (in contrast, the purely phonologically related word <HURT> will be inactive). The spread of activation from the partially activated representations into phonological spell-out processes is referred to as cascading activation. One consequence of this cascade is the activation of the phonological representations of semantically related words. For example, cascading activation from <SKIRT> will activate its constituent sounds. This will boost the activation of the nontarget initial cluster /sk/. In contrast, the nontarget initial consonant /h/ will not receive a similar benefit; "shirt" → "*skirt*" will therefore be more likely than "shirt" → "*hurt*." Connectionist simulation studies (Rapp & Goldrick, 2000) show that these mechanisms are sufficient to yield a mixed error effect within phonological spell-out processes.

Cascade from gradiently activated nontarget representations has also been used to account for patterns in chronometric studies (see Goldrick, 2006, for a review). For example, Peterson and Savoy (1998) found faster naming latencies for words phonologically related to the synonyms of target pictures. For example, after presentation of a target picture "couch," facilitation was observed in the subsequent latency for reading aloud words phonologically similar to the synonym "sofa" (e.g., "soda"). Cascading activation provides a ready account of this effect. If the lexical representation <SOFA> is partially activated during processing of the target <COUCH>, cascading activation will provide a boost to its phonological representations (e.g., /s/, /a/). This facilitates processing of words overlapping in form (e.g., "soda").

The cascade of gradient activation of nontarget items has been used to account for a wide range of empirical data. For example, Costa, Caramazza, and Sebastian-Galles (2000) report that bilingual individuals have shorter naming latencies for cognate words (sharing form and meaning across the two languages) relative to noncognates. They attribute this to gradient activation of the lexical representation of the translation equivalent in the nontarget language. Since cognates share the target's phonology, cascading activation from the lexical representation of the translation equivalent facilitates access to the sounds of the target word. For example, for a Spanish–English bilingual the co-activation of <GUITAR> and <GUITARRA> will facilitate access to shared phonological structures (e.g., /g/). In contrast, noncognates provide no support for the target's sounds. For example, <TABLE> and <MESA> do not share sounds; their co-activation will therefore not facilitate retrieval of the target's sounds.

More recent studies have utilized gradient activation to account for interactions between phonological spell-out and subsequent postlexical phonetic processes. Phonetic processes specify the details of how sounds are articulated (e.g., specifying that in English an initial /ba/ is produced by closing the lips, releasing them, and then a short time later allowing the vocal folds to vibrate). As demonstrated by both acoustic (Goldrick & Blumstein, 2006) and articulatory data (McMillan, Corley, & Lickley, 2009), phonetic properties of speech errors reflect properties of both the intended target and the error outcome. For example, when the intended target "big" is replaced by an error "pig" (written as "big" → "pig"), the [p]'s phonetic properties are different than correctly produced instances of "pig." Specifically, in errors resulting in [p] the voice onset time (roughly, the amount of time between the opening of the lips and the beginning of vocal fold vibration) is shorter – more similar to that of [b] – compared to correct productions. This pattern can be attributed to gradient activation of the target's representation during phonological spell-out. The phonological representation of the sound /b/ remains partially active during production of a /b/ → [p] error. This partial activation cascades to postlexical phonetic processing, distorting the articulation of the [p] error to reflect a "trace" of the intended target's phonetic properties. This account illustrates how gradient activation is a general principle of theories of speech production processing, crossing levels of representation and linguistic populations.

The gradient nature of activation has also allowed researchers to examine not just the simple presence versus absence of interaction but also varying degrees of interaction between cognitive processes. By limiting the relative activation of nontarget representations, it is possible to minimize the degree to which they can influence subsequent processes. This reduces interactive effects, allowing processing to be more discrete. Limiting interaction in this manner allows theories to better account for the full range of speech production data (Goldrick, 2006; Rapp & Goldrick, 2000). For example, chronometric studies have found strong phonological activation only for words that are highly semantically related to the target (e.g., synonyms; Peterson & Savoy, 1998). This pattern can be understood by postulating strong limits on the activation of nontarget items. Only those lexical representations that are strongly activated via spreading activation from semantic representations will be able to influence subsequent processing. Other lexical representations will be too weakly activated to influence phonological spell-out processes – limiting the presence of interactive effects. To implement these limitations on interaction, a number of selection mechanisms have been proposed. They include boosting the target's activation (Dell, 1986) as well as inhibiting nontarget representations (Harley, 1995). Either of these serve to enhance the relative activation of the target versus competing lexical representations.

Spreading Activation in the Speech Production System

The generation of output representations based on input representations is instantiated by the spread of activation between simple processing units. Spreading activation critically interacts with the core representational principles of connectionist networks. Excepting strictly local representations, each processing unit participates in the realization of multiple distinct mental representations. The spread of activation from overlapping representations automatically leads to the activation of a set of related representations. Following the lexical selection example above, overlap in semantic features causes the automatic activation of not just the target "bird" but its semantic neighbors "dog" and "bee" as well. This automatic activation of representations with overlapping representational components has been used to account for a wide array of empirical observations. Table 7.2 provides an overview of accounts utilizing the principles that are reviewed in the section below.

One very general observation regarding errors in speech production is that they tend to result in representations that share structure with the target. For example, errors arising in lexical selection during single word naming tend to share semantic features with the target (e.g., "tiger" → "lion"; Rapp & Goldrick, 2000). Lexical selection errors involving items from the sentence context tend to share grammatical category (e.g., "This *spring* has a *seat* in it"; Garrett, 1980). Similar effects are

Table 7.2   Illustration of Principle 2: cognitive processing as spreading activation.

Empirical phenomenon	*Connectionist account*
Errors tend to result in representations that share structure with the target.	Spreading activation from overlapping processing units automatically boosts the activation of representations that share structure with the target.
During lexical selection, errors with a mixed semantic-phonological relationship to the target occur at rates greater than chance. Phonological errors result in words at rates greater than chance. Phonetic properties of speech errors reflect less of a trace of the intended target when the outcome is a word.	Spreading activation from phonological representations facilitates the activation of lexical representations that share the target's phonology. This enhanced activation cascades to phonological and phonetic levels.
Compared to words that share structure with few lexical items, words that share phonological structure with many lexical items are retrieved more quickly and accurately. Compared to words that share structure with few lexical items, words that share phonological structure with many lexical items are produced with more extreme articulations.	Spreading activation from phonological representations facilitates the activation of lexical representations that share the target's phonology. These lexical representations re-activate the phonological structure of the target, boosting its activation. This enhanced activation cascades throughout the production system.

seen at smaller grain sizes; phoneme-level exchanges tend to involve similar sounds (e.g., "made possible" → "*p*ade *m*ossible"; Shattuck-Hufnagel & Klatt, 1979). Spreading activation offers a natural account of this general phenomenon. Since representations that share structure with the target are automatically activated by spreading activation, they have an inherent advantage over unrelated representations. When processing is disrupted (as in the circumstances that give rise to production errors), this activation advantage means that related forms will be more likely to dominate processing. Following the example of Figure 7.1, during processing of the target "bird," the higher activation of semantically related "bee" means that it is more likely to be mis-selected than the unrelated word "cap."

Goldrick (2008) offers a formal analysis of the conditions under which this account of errors holds. In feature-based or semi-local representational frameworks (such as the semantic features in Figure 7.1), error probability will always reflect representational overlap. Interestingly, in distributed representational frameworks this is not necessarily true. If the distance between the patterns of activation realizing mental representations does not reflect the degree to which their cognitive representations overlap, errors will not respect similarity (see Goldrick, 2008, for further discussion). For example, if the semantic representations for "bird" and "bee" are realized by activation patterns that are further apart than the patterns for "bird" and "cap," errors may be more likely to produce the unrelated form "cap" than the related form "bee." This highlights the critical interrelationship between spreading activation and representational structure (at both cognitive and connectionist levels of representation) in accounting for the influence of similarity on errors.

Spreading activation has also played a critical role in understanding interactions between stages of processing in speech production. The preceding section discussed how cascading activation from gradiently activated lexical representations allowed semantic relationships to influence phonological processing. Allowing the reciprocal spread of activation – from phonological to lexical representations – allows phonological similarity to influence lexical selection. This mechanism can account for the observation of mixed error effects during lexical selection.

Rapp and Goldrick (2000) report such an effect in the errors of P. W., an individual with an acquired deficit to speech production processes. Although his semantic processing is intact, P. W.'s spoken errors are all semantically related (e.g., naming a picture of a tiger "lion"). This pattern is not predicted by damage to phonological processing; as confirmed by simulation analyses, disruptions to this level would result in purely phonologically related words and nonwords. Rapp and Goldrick therefore attribute P. W.'s errors to a disruption of lexical selection processes. Critically, P. W.'s semantic errors have a higher degree of phonological overlap than would be predicted by random substitutions of words within a semantic category. This suggests that errors sharing both phonological and semantic structure – mixed errors – are more likely to occur than purely semantically related errors.

This pattern can be accounted for by allowing activation to spread from phonological to lexical representations. This feedback from "late" to "early" processing stages boosts the activation of mixed errors during lexical selection. For example, the target "bird" activates the phoneme /b/. Feedback from this boosts the activation of the mixed semantically and phonologically related word "bee," producing an activation advantage for it over the purely semantically related word "dog." This activation advantage leads to a mixed error effect following disruptions to lexical selection (Rapp & Goldrick, 2000).

Spreading activation from phonological representations also provides a mechanism to account for the influence of purely phonologically related lexical representations (e.g., for target "mitten," <MUFFIN>). These are frequently referred to as *neighbors* of the target. In the absence of feedback, such words would not become active; semantically driven activation from the speaker's intended message would only activate words that share the target's meaning. Feedback from shared phonological structure is required to activate the lexical representations of these purely phonologically related neighbors.

Cascade from the lexical representations of neighbors enhances the activation of their phonological representations. This provides an advantage for phonological representations corresponding to words over those corresponding to nonwords. For example, for target "bird" the lexical representation of the neighbor <HERD> will be strongly activated by feedback by the shared phonemes /ɚ/ and /d/. The lexical representation <HERD> will then enhance the activation of /h/. In contrast, the phonological representation of the nonword outcome "zerd" will receive little support; there is no lexical representation *<ZERD> to provide strong activation to the phoneme /z/. This accounts for the *lexical bias effect*, the observation that phonological errors are more likely to result in words than predicted by chance (Dell, 1986; but see Levelt, Roelofs, & Meyer, 1999).

This strengthening of word error outcomes persists into subsequent phonetic processes. As discussed above, phonetic properties of speech errors reflect properties of both the intended target and the error outcome (e.g., the [p] in the error "big" → "pig" exhibits a phonetic trace of the intended target /b/). The influence of the intended target is significantly smaller for word versus nonword error outcomes. For example, the [p] in "bid" → "pid" will exhibit a greater trace of the target /b/ than the [p] in "big" → "pig" (Goldrick & Blumstein, 2006; McMillan et al., 2009).

Spreading activation from phonological representations serves not only to strengthen nontarget representations; it also facilitates access to the target. Specifically, words that are similar to many lexical items show a processing advantage relative to those that are similar to few words. Words with many neighbors are produced with shorter latencies than words with few neighbors (Vitevitch, 2002). Following acquired deficits affecting phonological spell-out, words with few neighbors are produced less accurately than words with many neighbors (Goldrick, Folk, & Rapp, 2010). Additionally, words with many neighbors are less likely to fall into tip-of-the-tongue (TOT) states (Harley & Bown, 1998). The enhanced activation of words with many neighbors manifests itself not just in speed and accuracy but also in articulation. Relative to words with few neighbors, words with many neighbors are produced with more extreme articulations (consonants: Baese-Berk & Goldrick, 2009; vowels: Wright, 2004).

Feedback-driven activation of lexical representations provides an account of the facilitatory influence of neighbors. After the lexical representations of neighbors are activated by feedback, they in turn reactivate the phonological structure they share with the target. Feedback allows this enhanced activation to strengthen the lexical representation of the target (Dell & Gordon, 2003). Cascade then serves to strengthen processing of the target at phonological and phonetic processing levels. For example, target <BIRD> activates <HERD> via feedback from the shared phonemes /ɚ/ and /d/. <HERD> in turn reactivates /ɚ/ and /d/; via feedback, these provide an additional boost to the target <BIRD>. Via cascade, the heightened activation of <BIRD> influences processing of its phonological and phonetic structure – enhancing the speed and accuracy of retrieval and leading to more extreme articulations.

Acquiring the Statistical Structure of the Environment

The preceding discussion has shown how spreading activation is a central principle of connectionist explanation. The final principle examined here focuses on what

Table 7.3   Illustration of Principle 3: cognitive processes are structured via statistical learning.

Empirical phenomenon	*Connectionist account*
Speech errors tend to not result in sequences of sounds that are infrequent within an experimental context.	Spreading activation is continuously updated to reflect the statistical structure of sound sequences. Infrequent sound sequences are therefore less activated than frequent sequences.
Picture naming is slower and less accurate following the retrieval of semantically related items.	Spreading activation is continuously updated to reflect the covariance of semantic features and lexical representations. Recently produced lexical items are therefore more strongly reactivated by their semantic features.

determines the flow of activation. In the majority of theories reviewed above, the spread of activation is stipulated by the theorist. The theorist specifies one or more hypotheses regarding the structure of some cognitive process and then implements this hypothesis using spreading activation. In contrast, the research reviewed below uses statistical learning algorithms to address the origin of this structure. Table 7.3 provides an overview of these contributions.

Warker and Dell's (2006) proposal provides an illustration of this approach. They focus on the linking of segmental units or phonemes (retrieved during phonological spell-out) with prosodic structure (specifically syllables). On the basis of speech error and chronometric data, most current theories of speech production (e.g., Levelt et al., 1999) assume that such information is not linked together in long-term memory. The output of phonological spell-out specifies the linear order of a set of segments; these must be associated with prosodic structure before they can engage articulatory planning and execution processes. Warker and Dell therefore postulate a syllabification process that takes as an input a set of phonemes and a specification of their linear order; it generates as output an association of segments to syllable positions (e.g., /b/-onset /ɚ/-nucleus /d/-coda for "bird").

To realize this process as a connectionist network, Warker and Dell (2006) construct two semi-local levels of representation. The input representation has a single unit for each segment, followed by a unit representing the linear order of those segments. For example, for "cat" the representation would be: /æ/ /k/ /t/ <k-1 æ-2 t-3>. For "zat" it would be /æ/ /t/ /z/ <z-1 æ-2 t-3>. The output representation has a single unit for each segment within each syllable position. For example, the "cat" representation would be </k/-ONSET> </æ/-VOWEL> </t/-CODA>.

Rather than specify how activation spreads within the network, Warker and Dell (2006) allowed the network to acquire structure through learning. Initially the connections are seeded with random values. The network is then presented with a series of correct input–output representation pairs. The input is presented and the network generates an output. This is compared to the correct output. If the network's response is different than the target output, the weights throughout the network are slightly adjusted (using the algorithm in Rumelhart et al., 1986) such that the next time the input is presented the network is more likely to generate the correct output. Critically, the algorithm learns to perform this mapping by encoding the statistical structure of the training set – specifically, the covariance between the activation of input and output units (van Orden et al., 1990).

Warker and Dell's (2006) network also incorporates a set of *hidden* units that intervene between the input and output representations. These are hidden in the sense that they do not interface with processing "external" to the syllabification process; furthermore, their activation values are not specified by the theorist. The activation patterns over these units emerge as a consequence of the learning algorithm that adjusts the spread of activation. Incorporating such units greatly increases the range of input–output mappings that connectionist networks can compute (Rumelhart et al., 1986), making them a standard feature of connectionist theories incorporating learning.

After the learning rule has adjusted the weights for several thousand input–output pairs (reflecting the full range of English monosyllables), Warker and Dell's (2006) network assigns a strong activation to the correct segment–syllable position bindings and low activation to the incorrect outputs. For example, for syllables like "cat" it assigns 0.9 to /k/-onset but only 0.05 to /k/-coda. This shows that this network can acquire the correct structure to compute the syllabification process. Of greater interest, however, is the network's ability to encode the statistical regularities that hold across this set of syllables. For example, when presented with an /h/ as input, the network should strongly activate /h/-onset but not /h/-coda. The latter never appears in any English syllables (e.g., there are English words like "him" but none like *"mih"). In fact, Warker and Dell report that for target "hing," the error /h/-coda has an activation of only 0.002. In contrast, for target "kaf," the error /k/-coda has an activation of 0.05 (much closer to the 0.9 activation level of the correct segment–syllable position bindings). The weaker activation of /h/-coda reflects the network's encoding of the statistical structure of English.

This learning mechanism provides an account for the tendency of speech errors to respect phonotactic regularities (statistical regularities in sound sequences). As noted above, in English no syllables end in /h/. When English speakers make speech errors, the errors rarely result in the production of /h/ in coda position (i.e., very few errors resemble "head lock" → "head lo*h*"; Vousden et al., 2000). Assuming that relative activation reflects production probability, Warker and Dell's (2006) proposal provides an account of how syllabification processes come to respect these phonotactic regularities (see Goldrick, 2007, for a more formal analysis of this proposal). Because spreading activation reflects the statistical structure of the environment, the errors produced during processing will be sensitive to the distributional properties of sound sequences.

Warker and Dell (2006) propose that this learning mechanism can also account for speakers' sensitivity to shifts in the statistical structure of their environment. Dell, Reed, Adams, and Meyer (2000) document such a shift by showing that participants can acquire novel phonotactic regularities. In Dell et al.'s study, participants read aloud sets of tongue twisters that exhibited novel phonotactic regularities. For example, in contrast to the participant's native language (English), /f/ appeared only in the onset of syllables, never in the coda (e.g., syllables like "feg" were presented, but "geff" was not). Other segments respected their normal distribution in English, appearing in both onset and coda position. The participant's speech errors reflected these novel regularities. When a segment was restricted to one position, errors overwhelmingly favored producing the segment in that position. For example, when /f/ was restricted to the onset of syllables, onset errors such as "feg kem" → "feg fek" made up 97% of errors resulting in /f/. In contrast, for segments that appeared in both onset and coda, errors appeared in both syllable positions. For example, /m/ appeared in both onset and coda; errors such as "meg kef" → "meg mef" made up approximately 70% of errors involving this segment.

Warker and Dell (2006) account for the acquisition of these novel regularities by appealing to the continual operation of the learning mechanism outlined above. To model the experience of the experiment, following exposure to all of the syllables of English the connectionist network received additional training on the experimental syllables. The network was therefore exposed to many syllables in which /f/ was associated to onset, but no syllables where /f/ was associated to coda. Similar to the phonotactic regularities observed in the training set as a whole, spreading activation within the network changed to reflect these new statistical regularities. For example, if the target was "feg," the error /f/-coda had an activation of 0.02. In contrast, following this additional training the error /g/-coda (for input "gef") had an activation of 0.04. Through continual operation of a statistical learning procedure, network processing has adapted to reflect the statistical structure of the environment – providing an account for the flexible nature of syllabification processes in speech production.

Furthermore, Warker and Dell's (2006) connectionist learning mechanism provides an account of the relative difficulty of acquiring different statistical regularities. Warker and Dell report behavioral findings that show more complex regularities (e.g., /f/ is onset when the vowel is /i/, but is the coda when the vowel is /e/) require more time for participants to learn than simple segment–syllable position regularities (e.g., /f/ is always in onset). The connectionist learning mechanism exhibits this same pattern; it requires greater training to acquire the more complex phonotactic regularities (see Goldrick, 2007, for further discussion).

Dell, Oppenheim, and Kittredge (2008) adopt a similar learning-based perspective to account for the dynamics of lexical selection. Behavioral studies have shown that the difficulty of lexical selection can vary depending on the relationship between items that have been recently processed. When participants are asked to name a series of pictures from a single semantic category, they are slower and less accurate compared to trials where the same pictures are named in mixed sets. For example, naming a picture of a fox in the context of a tiger, dog, and owl is slower and less accurate than naming the same picture in the context of a chair, star, and hammer. Because this interference effect is not observed in reading aloud of the same items (a task which does not require access to semantic representations), this effect has been attributed to semantically driven lexical selection processes (Damian, Vigliocco, & Levelt, 2001). Specifically, context is assumed to enhance competition from semantically related items. As discussed above, spreading activation automatically activates semantic neighbors of the target during lexical selection. If these already-active words are further boosted by the context, they will induce significant competition during lexical selection.

How does context enhance the activation of lexical items? One account is based around priming; prior access to a lexical representation temporarily increases its activation. Such an account has difficulty explaining why the strength of interference is not influenced by the temporal lag between presentation of semantically related items (Howard, Nickels, Coltheart, & Cole-Virtue, 2006). A temporary, activation-based mechanism would be expected to show decay over time.

Dell et al. (2008) offer a learning-based alternative in the same spirit as Warker and Dell (2006). They assume that spreading activation between semantic features and lexical units is driven by a covariant learning rule; furthermore, this learning rule continues to update spreading activation during adult processing. This allows spreading activation to be influenced by the statistical structure of recent trials. Prior presentation of a lexical item strengthens the connections between the corresponding semantic features and lexical unit. This leads the lexical unit to become more active when another item sharing its features is presented – inducing increased semantic interference. Furthermore, because this mechanism changes the structure of lexical selection processes (modifying the flow of activation), it is not subject to a purely temporal decay process; it persists until a sufficiently large number of intervening trials have altered the statistical structure of the input–output mapping. To demonstrate the adequacy of this account, Dell et al. (2008) present a series of simulations showing this approach provides a qualitative match to both latency and error data from this experimental paradigm.

In sum, connectionist theories assume that the structure of cognitive processes – the way in which activation spreads between simple processing units – reflects the statistical structure of the environment. The continuous operation of learning algorithms that allow networks to encode this statistical structure allows connectionist researchers to account for the dynamic, context-dependent nature of speech production processes.

Learning and the Emergence of Structure

Acquiring the structure of cognitive processes via learning algorithms means that connectionist networks are not simply devices for instantiating cognitive theories. They also offer the possibility of developing novel theoretical accounts – acquiring internal structure that differs in substantive ways from existing proposals. To illustrate this approach, the discussion below focuses on the work of Dell, Juliano, and Govindjee (1993), which aimed to develop a new framework for phonological spell-out processes via a statistical learning with simple recurrent networks (Elman, 1990; Jordan, 1986).

Dell et al. (1993) began with a set of slightly different representational assumptions than the processing architecture discussed in previous sections. First, they assumed that input representations consisted of a distributed pattern of activation encoding lexical identity (rather than strictly local lexical representations). Instead of phoneme units, they assumed the output was a set of phonological features. Finally, and most critically, rather than generating all phonological elements of a word in parallel, the network was trained to sequentially generate the features of each segment. The simple recurrent network architecture provides an appropriate connectionist mechanism for this task. Specifically, in Dell et al.'s networks, the activation of hidden and output units was influenced by the activation of these units at the previous point in time – allowing for recurrent activation flow. Allowing previous states of the network to influence processing endows the network with a "memory" of what occurred previously; this gives simple recurrent networks the capacity to produce sequences of output representations.

The aim of Dell et al.'s (1993) simulations was to develop an alternative to existing accounts of phonological spell-out. These existing accounts make use of frame representations – explicit representations of structure that serve to guide the selection of phonological representations. For example, Dell (1986) assumes a syllabic frame representation consisting of a set of abstract consonant and vowel units. These guide selection of phonemes in the appropriate sequence to generate syllables (e.g., ensuring that for target "bird" the first segment selected is an onset consonant). Critically, these representations form a set of mechanisms distinct from spreading activation from lexical to phoneme units. The structure of the syllable (its consonant/vowel organization) is therefore processed separately from its content (the specific segments that occur in each structural position). (Note, however, that structure processing occurs in parallel with retrieval of content; see below for further discussion.) In contrast to this frame-based model, Dell et al.'s (1993) simple recurrent network utilizes a single set of hidden and context units to both activate the appropriate phonological representations and produce them in the correct sequence. A single set of processing mechanisms therefore implements both structure and content processing.

Dell et al. (1993) find that this network is able to capture empirical patterns that have been attributed to the influence of the syllabic frame. For example, speech errors tend to respect syllabic constituency. Theories of English syllable structure (Venneman, 1988) have postulated that syllables are composed of two constituents, the onset (roughly, all segments preceding the vowel) and the rime (roughly, the vowel and all following segments). Speech errors respect this division; errors involving the replacement of the vowel and coda (e.g., "read" → "rope") are more frequent than errors involving the replacement of the vowel and onset (e.g., "read" → "load"; Stemberger, 1983). This has typically been attributed to the influence of an explicit structural frame that includes a representation of onset–rime structure (Sevald, Dell, & Cole, 1995). However, Dell et al.'s simulations exhibited the same pattern;

the authors take this to suggest that phonological spell-out processes do not need to incorporate explicit structural representations.

Some theorists have questioned whether this account can capture the full range of speech production data (Sevald et al., 1995). Assuming that the proposal is in fact empirically adequate, the challenge is to precisely articulate the content of the connectionist proposal. What is the nature of the network's solution to the problem? Until this has been established to a sufficient level of detail, it is unclear what specific elements of previous theoretical approaches are challenged by these findings (McCloskey, 1991). The complexity of connectionist networks – the distribution of computation over many units and connections – has made such analyses difficult. However, simple recurrent networks have been extensively analyzed in the context of sentence processing using the prediction task (for recent reviews, see Elman, 2009; Tabor, 2009). The task of these networks is to generate predictions regarding the next word in a sentence, given the preceding word (e.g., given the English sequence "The dog bites the . . ." the network should predict a noun will appear). In many cases, these networks converge on a solution where the structural position of elements is encoded by regions within the space of hidden unit activations. The dynamics of the network – how it transitions from one region of the hidden unit space to another – encode the relations between these structural positions (e.g., the serial order or dependencies such as subject/verb number agreement). The regions that define structural positions are themselves structured to encode the particular element that occurs within this position. These analyses suggest that it is possible that Dell et al.'s (1993) networks developed an internal structure that reflected the distinction between structure and content. Structure reflects the high-level dynamical organization of the network's trajectory through hidden unit space; content is reflected by its fine-grained structure. At one level, this agrees with a central property of frame-based models; namely, that structure and content are distinctly represented within the production system. In fact, it is possible that Dell et al.'s networks converged upon a dynamical organization that closely approximated the frame-based proposals – where content and structure are processed in parallel yet independent processing streams.

Research in sentence production has underscored the fact that connectionist networks must acquire sufficient distinctions between structure and content to account for the full range of empirical data. Chang (2002) compared several sentence production architectures built around simple recurrent networks. The architecture analogous to that of Dell et al.'s (1993) phonological spell-out model mapped from a static representation of the speaker's message to a sequence of words. Among other issues, this model failed to exhibit sufficient (and appropriate) generalization from its training set. For example, it had difficulty producing combinations of adjectives and nouns that had not occurred in its training set (e.g., although it could produce *silly dog* and *good cake*, it could not produce *silly cake* – a nonsensical but syntactically legitimate string). In order to acquire an appropriate internal structure that supported generalization, Chang adopted representational and architectural assumptions that built on previous frame-based production theories. First, he adopted compositional semantic representations; these distinguished event roles (e.g., <agent>) from the lexical concepts that filled those roles (e.g., <man>). In essence, this creates an abstract semantic frame. The second set of assumptions was architectural. Chang assumed that two interacting pathways were involved in the generation of the next word in a sentence. A meaning system mapped directly from the conceptual representation of the sentence. A second sequencing system was a simple recurrent network; it made use of additional sets of hidden units to develop representations that abstract over word categories (much like a syntactic frame). These assumptions enabled the network to exhibit proper generalization and account for a wide range of data from speech production (see also Chang, Dell, & Bock, 2006, for discussion). Critically, analysis of the network's internal structure (Chang, 2002) reveals that this success is made possible in part by developing representations and mechanisms that make robust distinctions between structure (i.e., syntactic role) and content (i.e., lexical items).

Although these architectures do incorporate key insights of more traditional frame-based models, at finer-grained levels of analysis they may be capable of accounting for empirical data that cannot be modeled by traditional frame-based theories. For example, research in sentence processing (Elman, 2009) and in routine sequential actions more generally (Botvinick & Plaut, 2004) have examined how simple recurrent networks exhibit greater expressive power than models built around simple abstract frames. Simple recurrent networks can also capture "quasi-hierarchical" patterns of performance, wherein dependencies between items in a sequence are not limited to relations between categories. For example, Lee and Goldrick (2008) found that English speakers are sensitive not only to onset–rime structure (holding over all onset consonants) but also to relationships between *particular* onset consonants and vowels. In a strict consonant–vowel frame-based framework (as in Dell, 1986), such dependencies could not be represented; the frame collapses all onset consonants into a single entity.

Utilizing connectionist networks and learning algorithms to develop novel theoretical accounts such as those based around quasi-hierarchical structure is very much an open area of speech production research. As shown by the discussion above, detailed analysis of connectionist processing is required. Although they can acquire internal structure that differs in substantive ways from existing proposals, connectionist networks can only contribute to theory development if their internal structure and processing principles are fully explicated.

Conclusion

Connectionist principles have played an integral role in the development of theories of speech production. From semantically driven lexical selection processes to phonetic processes, researchers have accounted for empirical patterns by appealing to connectionist computational mechanisms. In many ways, these mechanisms represent a theoretical vocabulary more powerful than purely symbolic computational mechanisms. Rather than being limited to digital symbolic representations, connectionist networks can express gradient blends of multiple representational states. Furthermore, as discussed in the preceding sections, connectionist networks offer a procedure for developing internal representations; in contrast, many symbolic architectures are forced to postulate representational structure a priori.

An important challenge for connectionist theories is to rein in this expressive power. This chapter touched on two such points. Gradient activation flow and the spread of activation must be restricted; empirical evidence suggests there are strong limitations on the strength of interactions between stages of spoken production (Rapp & Goldrick, 2000). Although digital representations are too restrictive, they may in fact represent a close approximation of the state of many stages of processing. The second issue reviewed above suggests a similar conclusion. The work of Chang and colleagues (Chang, 2002; Chang et al., 2006) underscores the need for abstract, symbol-like representations to account for many of our speech production abilities. Again, symbolic representations may provide a good approximation for the structure of cognitive processes. The connectionist challenge is to explain the constraints on learning, processing, and behavior that give rise to this structure.

Note

Thanks to Melissa Baese-Berk for helpful comments. Preparation of this chapter was supported by NIH grant NIDCD DC007977 and NSF grant BCS-0846147.

References

Baese-Berk, M., & Goldrick, M. (2009). Mechanisms of interaction in speech production. *Language and Cognitive Processes, 24,* 527–554.

Botvinick, M., & Plaut, D. C. (2004). Doing without schema hierarchies: A recurrent connectionist approach to normal and impaired routine sequential action. *Psychological Review, 111,* 395–429.

Chang, F. (2002) Symbolically speaking: A connectionist model of sentence production. *Cognitive Science, 26,* 609–51.

Chang, F., Dell, G. S., & Bock, K. (2006). Becoming syntactic. *Psychological Review, 113,* 234–272.

Costa, A., Caramazza, A., & Sebastian-Galles, N. (2000). The cognate facilitation effect: Implications for models of lexical access. *Journal of Experimental Psychology: Learning, Memory, and Cognition, 26,* 1283–1296.

Damian, M. F., Vigliocco, G., & Levelt, W. J. M. (2001). Effects of semantic context in the naming of pictures and words. *Cognition, 81,* B77–B86.

Dell, G. S. (1986). A spreading activation theory of retrieval in sentence production. *Psychological Review, 93,* 283–321.

Dell, G. S., & Gordon, J. K. (2003). Neighbors in the lexicon: Friends or foes? In N. O. Schiller & A. S. Meyer (Eds.), *Phonetics and phonology in language comprehension and production: Differences and similarities*. New York: Mouton de Gruyter.

Dell, G. S., Juliano, C., & Govindjee, A. (1993). Structure and content in language production: A theory of frame constraints in phonological speech errors. *Cognitive Science, 17*, 149–95.

Dell, G. S., Oppenheim, G. M., & Kittredge, A. K. (2008). Saying the right word at the right time: Syntagmatic and paradigmatic interference in sentence production. *Language and Cognitive Processes, 23*, 583–608.

Dell, G. S., Reed, K. D., Adams, D. R., & Meyer, A. S. (2000). Speech errors, phonotactic constraints, and implicit learning: A study of the role of experience in language production. *Journal of Experimental Psychology: Learning, Memory, and Cognition, 26*, 1355–1367.

Dell, G. S. & Reich, P. A. (1981). Stages in sentence production: An analysis of speech error data. *Journal of Verbal Learning and Verbal Behavior, 20*, 611–629.

Elman, J. L. (1990). Finding structure in time. *Cognitive Science, 14*, 179–211.

Elman, J. L. (2009). On the meaning of words and dinosaur bones: Lexical knowledge without a lexicon. *Cognitive Science, 33*, 547–582.

Garrett, M. F. (1980). Levels of processing in sentence production. In B. Butterworth (Ed.), *Language production: Speech and talk* (vol. 1, pp. 177–220). New York: Academic Press.

Goldrick, M. (2006). Limited interaction in speech production: Chronometric, speech error, and neuropsychological evidence. *Language and Cognitive Processes, 21*, 817–855.

Goldrick, M. (2007). Constraint interaction: A lingua franca for stochastic theories of language. In C. T. Schütze & V. S. Ferreira (Eds.), *The state of the art in speech error research: Proceedings of the LSA Institute workshop* (MITWPL vol. 53, pp. 95–114). Cambridge, MA: MIT Working Papers in Linguistics.

Goldrick, M. (2008). Does like attract like? Exploring the relationship between errors and representational structure in connectionist networks. *Cognitive Neuropsychology, 25*, 287–313.

Goldrick, M., & Blumstein, S. E. (2006). Cascading activation from phonological planning to articulatory processes: Evidence from tongue twisters. *Language and Cognitive Processes, 21*, 649–683.

Goldrick, M., Folk, J., & Rapp, B. (2010). Mrs Malaprop's neighborhood: Using word errors to reveal neighborhood structure. *Journal of Memory and Language, 62*, 113–134.

Harley, T. A., (1995). Connectionist models of anomia: A comment on Nickels. *Language and Cognitive Processes, 10*, 47–58.

Harley, T. A., & Bown, H. E. (1998). What causes a tip-of-the-tongue state? Evidence for lexical neighbourhood effects in speech production. *British Journal of Psychology, 89*, 151–174.

Howard, D., Nickels, L., Coltheart, M., & Cole-Virtue, J. (2006). Cumulative semantic inhibition in picture naming: Experimental and computational studies. *Cognition, 100*, 464–482.

Jordan, M. I. (1986). *Serial order: A parallel distributed processing approach*. Institute for Cognitive Science Report 8604. University of California, San Diego. Reprinted (1997) in J. W. Donahoe & V. P. Dorsel (Eds.), *Neural-network models of cognition: Biobehavioral foundations* (pp. 221–277). Amsterdam: Elsevier.

Lee, Y., & Goldrick, M. (2008). The emergence of sub-syllabic representations. *Journal of Memory and Language, 59,* 155–168.

Levelt, W. J. M. (2001). Spoken word production: A theory of lexical access. *Proceedings of the National Academy of Sciences, 98,* 13464–13471.

Levelt, W. J. M., Roelofs, A., & Meyer, A. S. (1999). A theory of lexical access in speech production. *Behavioral and Brain Sciences, 22,* 1–75.

McCloskey, M. (1991). Networks and theories: The place of connectionism in cognitive science. *Psychological Science, 2,* 387–395.

McMillan, C., Corley, M., & Lickley, R. (2009). Articulatory evidence for feedback and competition in speech production. *Language and Cognitive Processes, 24,* 44–66.

Palmer, S. E., & Kimchi, E. (1986). The information processing approach to cognition. In T. J. Knapp & L. C. Roberts (Eds.), *Approaches to cognition: Contrasts and controversies* (pp. 37–77). Hillsdale, NJ: Erlbaum.

Peterson, R. R., & Savoy, P. (1998). Lexical selection and phonological encoding during language production: Evidence for cascaded processing. *Journal of Experimental Psychology: Learning, Memory, and Cognition, 24,* 539–557.

Rapp, B. & Goldrick, M. (2000). Discreteness and interactivity in spoken word production. *Psychological Review, 107,* 460–499.

Roelofs, A. (2004). Error biases in spoken word planning and monitoring by aphasic and nonaphasic speakers: Comment on Rapp and Goldrick (2000). *Psychological Review, 111,* 561–572.

Rumelhart, D. E., Hinton, G. E., & Williams, R. J. (1986). Learning internal representations by error propagation. In D. E. Rumelhart, J. L. McClelland, & the PDP Research Group *Parallel distributed processing: Explorations in the microstructure of cognition* (vol. 1, Foundations, pp. 318–62). Cambridge, MA: MIT Press.

Sevald, C. A., Dell, G. S., & Cole, J. (1995). Syllable structure in speech production: Are syllables chunks or schemas? *Journal of Memory and Language, 34,* 807–820.

Shattuck-Hufnagel, S., & Klatt, D. (1979). The limited use of distinctive features and markedness in speech production: Evidence from speech errors. *Journal of Verbal Learning and Verbal Behavior, 18,* 41–55.

Smolensky, P. (1999). Grammar-based connectionist approaches to language. *Cognitive Science, 23,* 589–613.

Smolensky, P. (2006). Computational levels and integrated connectionist/symbolic explanation. In P. Smolensky & G. Legendre *The harmonic mind: From neural computation to optimality-theoretic grammar* (vol. 2, Linguistic and philosophical implications, pp. 503–592). Cambridge, MA: MIT Press.

Stemberger, J. (1983). *Speech errors and theoretical phonology: A review.* Unpublished manuscript, Carnegie-Mellon University. Distributed by the Indiana University Linguistics Club, Bloomington, IN.

Tabor, W. (2009). Dynamical insight into structure in connectionist models. In J. P. Spencer, M. S. C. Thomas, & J. L. McClelland (Eds.), *Towards a unified theory of development: Connectionism and dynamical systems theory reconsidered* (pp. 165–181). Oxford: Oxford University Press.

Van Orden, G. C., Pennington, B. F., & Stone, G. O. (1990). Word identification in reading and the promise of subsymbolic psycholinguistics. *Psychological Review, 97,* 488–522.

Venneman, T. (1988). *Preference laws for syllable structure and the explanation of sound change.* Berlin: Mouton de Gruyter.

Vitevitch , M. S. (2002). The influence of phonological similarity neighborhoods on speech production. *Journal of Experimental Psychology: Learning, Memory, and Cognition, 28,* 735–747.

Vousden, J. I., Brown, G. D. A., & Harley, T. A. (2000). Serial control of phonology in speech production: A hierarchical model. *Cognitive Psychology, 41,* 101–75.

Warker, J. A., & Dell, G. S. (2006). Speech errors reflect newly learned phonotactic constraints. *Journal of Experimental Psychology: Learning, Memory, and Cognition, 32,* 387–398.

Wright, R. A. (2004). Factors of lexical competition in vowel articulation. In J. J. Local, R. Ogden, & R. Temple (Eds.), *Laboratory Phonology VI* (pp. 26–50). Cambridge: Cambridge University Press.

8

Word Learning as the Confluence of Memory Mechanisms: Computational and Neural Evidence

Prahlad Gupta

In this article, I review evidence for the proposal that the processing and learning of words can usefully be understood as lying at the intersection of a variety of memory mechanisms. I begin with consideration of the temporally dynamic and serially ordered nature of human spoken language, focusing particularly on spoken word forms, and discuss the computational consequences of these properties and how they constrain the manner in which certain critical aspects of language are likely to be processed in the brain. In the second part, I discuss another fundamental property of language – its *arbitrariness* – and discuss how this once again is a functional characteristic that has important implications for how language must be processed in the mind/brain. Relevant neuroscientific evidence is briefly reviewed along with each of these discussions. The third part of the article brings together these ideas in a framework that integrates functional and computational considerations in word processing and word learning. I also discuss how this functionally and computationally derived proposal is quite consistent with other recent architectural suggestions derived from less computational and more neurophysiological points of view (further discussion on natural vocabulary acquisition is provided in de Groot, Volume 1, Chapter 23, and Ellis, Volume 2, Chapter 31). The present article thus provides an integration of various sources of evidence that bear on word-level processing and word learning.

Serial Ordering in Spoken Language

Spoken language is processed over time. Unlike written language, in which a unit such as a word is present throughout the process of reading, and is present in its

The Handbook of the Neuropsychology of Language, First Edition. Edited by Miriam Faust.
© 2012 Blackwell Publishing Ltd. Published 2012 by Blackwell Publishing Ltd.

entirety at the conclusion of a writing event, a spoken word is never present in its entirety during listening, nor is there any point during production when the spoken form is present in its entirety. At every point during spoken language processing (both listening and producing), all that is present as a stimulus is the currently spoken/heard piece of the speech stream.

This essential characteristic of spoken language is so obvious that it may appear uninteresting and/or inconsequential – emphasizing it might seem much like saying that cars run on wheels, which does not provide much insight into how cars work. In fact, however, the evanescence of spoken language has profound implications for how it must be processed in the mind/brain. A useful starting point in thinking about these implications is the fact that a novel word form, on first exposure, is a novel sequence of sounds. The task of repeating such a stimulus immediately after exposure to it requires the listener to encode the serial order of this sequence during its presentation, and then replicate this serial order when the stimulus is no longer present. That is, immediate repetition of a novel word form requires the encoding and retrieval of a novel serial ordering of constituent sounds. What are the mechanistic underpinnings of such a serial ordering task?

Twenty years ago, Jordan (1986) pointed out that, despite the fundamental importance of serially ordered action to human behavior, no general theory of serial ordering had emerged. Nor is any such generally accepted theory available today. However, many mathematically and/or computationally specified accounts have been developed of various aspects of serially ordered behavior (many of them in the context of the immediate serial recall task, e.g., Botvinick & Plaut, 2006; Brown, Preece, & Hulme, 2000; Burgess & Hitch, 1992, 1999; Gupta, 1996; Hartley & Houghton, 1996; Page & Norris, 1998). Although these accounts differ in numerous respects, they do all converge on one notion: in all of these accounts, producing a serially ordered sequence has the computational requirement of maintaining *state* or *context* information. For example, in order to replicate the sequence "BACDAB," a system must disambiguate the first and second occurrences of "A," so as to be able to produce "C" following the first "A," but "B" following the second "A." This requires maintenance of state or context information – information about where the system currently is in producing the sequence, and, in particular, information that distinguishes the state of "currently producing A" for the two instances of A. Thus in *all* computational accounts of serial ordering, the system must maintain some kind of state information.[1] That is, computational analysis indicates that a serial ordering task such as nonword repetition cannot be performed without a serial ordering mechanism, which in turn requires maintenance of state information.[2]

But maintenance of such state information is nothing if not *memory* for sequential information, as will be discussed in greater detail below. Computational analysis thus indicates that encoding and repeating a novel sequence requires some kind of serial ordering memory. This, then, provides a clear answer to our question of what is required computationally for repetition of a novel word form or nonword: it indicates the computational necessity in nonword repetition of *serial ordering*, and of a serial ordering *memory* mechanism. Importantly, this requirement follows directly from the temporally dynamic and serially ordered nature of spoken language – in this case, of word forms.

Over the last two decades, the relationship between phonological short-term memory (PSTM) and language processing (and especially phonological vocabulary learning – i.e., the learning of novel phonological word forms) has become a major focus of investigation in psychological research, generating extensive bodies of study in the traditional domains both of memory research and of language research (e.g., Dollaghan, 1987; Gathercole & Baddeley, 1989; Gathercole, Service, Hitch, Adams, & Martin, 1999; Gathercole, Willis, Emslie, & Baddeley, 1992; Gupta, MacWhinney, Feldman, & Sacco, 2003; Martin & Saffran, 1997; Martin, Saffran, & Dell, 1996; Montgomery, 2002; Saffran, 1990; for review, see Baddeley, Gathercole, & Papagno, 1998; Gathercole, 2006). Among the results that initiated these bodies of research were the findings that novel word repetition ability (i.e., the ability to immediately repeat possible but nonoccurring word forms, also termed nonwords) is correlated with immediate serial list recall ability on the one hand, and with vocabulary achievement on the other, in normally developing children (Gathercole & Baddeley, 1989) and in children with specific language impairment (SLI; Gathercole & Baddeley, 1990a). Since these initial reports, an overwhelming amount of further evidence has documented the existence of a relationship between vocabulary size and/or new word learning, nonword repetition, and immediate serial recall (e.g., Atkins & Baddeley, 1998; Baddeley, 1993; Baddeley, Papagno, & Vallar, 1988; Gathercole & Baddeley, 1990b; Gathercole et al., 1999; Gathercole et al., 1992; Gathercole, Hitch, Service, & Martin, 1997; Gupta, 2003; Gupta et al., 2003; Michas & Henry, 1994; Papagno, Valentine, & Baddeley, 1991; Papagno & Vallar, 1992; Service, 1992; Service & Kohonen, 1995).

What has remained unexplained, however, is the nature of the observed relationships between PSTM and the processing and learning of novel word forms. The computational analysis outlined above suggests a formal reason why the dynamic and serially ordered nature of spoken language (in this case, of spoken word forms) should necessitate a reliance on short-term memory. In recent work, Gupta and Tisdale (2009) concretized this analytic formulation in the form of a computational model. Gupta and Tisdale (2009) constructed a model that was exposed to word forms represented as input phonological sequences, and that attempted to repeat each word form immediately after presentation. The model incorporated the ability to learn from each such exposure. Over many exposures to many word forms, the model learned about the corpus of word forms to which it was being exposed, and thus acquired a *phonological vocabulary*. Gupta and Tisdale (2009) were then able to examine various aspects of the model's behavior and functioning, including: factors that affected its phonological vocabulary learning; its ability to repeat unlearned sequences (i.e., its nonword repetition) as well as factors that affected this ability; and, of greatest relevance for the present chapter, how the model instantiated PSTM.

The structure (*architecture*) of the model is shown in Figure 8.1a, and is an adaptation of an architecture introduced by Botvinick & Plaut (2006). The model has

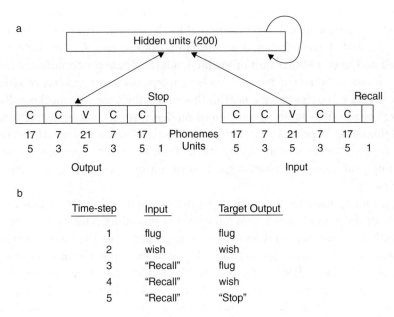

Figure 8.1 (a) Architecture of the model. (b) Processing regimen in the model, illustrated for the word form *flugwish*.

an input layer at which a representation of an entire syllable is presented, and an output layer that uses the same representation scheme, at which the model's output is produced. The representation of a syllable, at both the input and the output layers, is in terms of a CCVCC (i.e., consonant-consonant-vowel-consonant-consonant) template. That is, a syllable is represented at the input layer across a set of units that are divided into five slots. Activation of units in the first slot denotes the first C (if any) of the syllable, activation of units in the second slot denotes the second C (if any) of the syllable, activation of units in the third slot denotes the V of the syllable, and so on. Within each of these slots, the various phonemes that are legal for that slot for English are represented as different patterns of activations across a set of units. For example, for the encoding scheme used, there are 17 different phonemes of English that are legal for the first C slot. These phonemes were represented as different patterns of activation across five units constituting the first C slot. Similarly, the 21 phonemes that are possible in the V slot were represented as different patterns of activation across a set of five units constituting the V slot; and so on for the various slots shown at the input and output layers in Figure 8.1a.

The model also has an intermediate layer of 200 units. Such an intermediate layer, which does not directly receive the model's input or directly produce the model's output, is usually termed a *hidden layer* in such models, and therefore the units it contains are typically termed *hidden units*, as shown in Figure 8.1a. All units in the input layer project to all units in the hidden layer, and all units in the hidden layer project to all units in the output layer, as is common in such connectionist models of cognitive phenomena. An additional aspect of the architecture is the self-connections on the hidden layer (indicated by the circular arrow from the hidden layer back to itself), which denote a connection from every unit in the hidden layer to itself and to every other unit in the hidden layer. These connections are termed *recurrent* connections. The model's task is to accept as input a *sequence* of syllables, and to produce as output a *sequence* (for this model, the same sequence) of syllables. It is well established that for connectionist models that perform sequential processing of this kind, the presence of recurrent connections is critical. Thus, the recurrent connections in the present model are crucial for it to be able to perform the task of inputting and repeating phonological word forms presented as sequences of syllables.

Figure 8.1b illustrates the regimen of presentation and desired output in the model, for the example word form *flugwish*. The procedure is the same irrespective of whether or not the word form has been presented to the model previously. Following presentation of the first syllable *flug* at the input, the model's task is to produce that same syllable at the output. The model's actual output may or may not be correct. Either way, after the model has produced an output, the activation pattern at the hidden layer is transmitted across the recurrent connections, thus transmitting information to *itself* that will arrive at the next time-step, so that when the second syllable *wish* is presented, the model's hidden layer actually receives input from two sources: the input representing *wish*, and input from its own previous state. When presented with this second syllable at the input, the model's task, as for the first syllable, is to produce the input syllable at the output. Again, the output may or may not be correct. Again, the hidden layer activation pattern is transmitted across the recurrent connections to be available at the next time-step. The input at this next step is actually an indication of the end of input, denoted by activation of the Recall unit in the input layer. At this point the model's task is to produce at the output layer the *entire* sequence of syllable representations previously presented at the input layer, i.e., *flug* followed by *wish*, and then activate the Stop unit at the output layer, to signify the end of production of the word form. As this repetition must be performed in the absence of any external input representing the word form, the network must necessarily have encoded some internal memory representation of the word form to allow it to now produce it in correct sequence (i.e., to perform immediate serial recall of the word form). At each point during recall, the model's hidden layer receives input from activation of the Recall unit, and from its own state at the previous time-step. (Note that the activation of the Recall unit is only a cue, and carries no information about the specific word form that was presented, because this same unit is activated as a cue for *all* word forms). Thus overall, the model attempts to match its own production (i.e., repetition) of a syllable sequence constituting a word form with the observed linguistic sequence provided by the environment. At the end of presentation and repetition of one word form, the model's connections weights are adjusted using a learning procedure for neural networks with recurrent connections that is known as *back propagation through time*, whose details are beyond the scope of this article (for further discussion, see Botvinick & Plaut, 2006; Gupta & Tisdale, 2009; Rumelhart, Hinton, & Williams, 1986).

The essence of what this model does is to encode the serially ordered sequence of constituents comprising a word form, and then, after input has ended, to reproduce that serially ordered sequence, in the absence of any further informative input. That is, the model performs the task of serially ordered production of word forms. The model's serial ordering capability is critically dependent on the recurrent connections on the hidden layer; as described above, they provide the ability for the model to know where it is in producing the current word form, by providing information about what had already been produced. Gupta and Tisdale (2009) pointed out that this information is information about the *past*, and thus indubitably constitutes *memory* information, and that this information is overwritten when a subsequent word form sequence is produced, so that it is *short-term memory information*. They were also able to show that it can be regarded as phonological short-term memory information. Thus, the mechanisms in the model that provided this information provided PSTM functionality. This in turn indicated that PSTM functionality was crucial to serially ordered word form production in the model. Gupta and Tisdale (2009) also demonstrated that impairment of this functionality is severely disruptive to novel word from repetition as well as learning. The Gupta and Tisdale (2009) model thus provided a concrete demonstration of how the temporally dynamic and serially ordered nature of spoken language has implications for its processing in the mind/brain: it necessitates a reliance on short-term memory.

There is a fair amount of evidence regarding the neural substrates of such PSTM functionality, which appears to map onto an interactive neural system that is importantly dependent on temporoparietal cortex but that also encompasses anterior perisylvian regions. For instance, patients with posterior damage in general appear to suffer from span deficits (Risse, Rubens, & Jordan, 1984). Furthermore, in reviewing the neuropsychological syndrome of "pure STM" deficit, which involves reduced auditory-verbal short-term memory in the absence of other major language and cognitive deficits, Shallice and Vallar (1990) conclude that the condition reflects impairment to a short-term "input phonological store," and, based on clinical-anatomical correlations, that the anatomical region compromised in this deficit is left inferior parietal cortex (angular gyrus and supramarginal gyrus). In patients with preserved span abilities, these areas seem quite consistently spared (Shallice & Vallar, 1990). This suggests that subsets of left temporoparietal cortex (e.g., left inferior parietal cortex) may be particularly specialized for the temporary storage of phonological information, and thus particularly crucial for verbal short-term memory. Supporting evidence that areas of temporoparietal cortex play a role in the temporary maintenance of information comes from single-cell recordings in primates, which showed memory-related planning activity in posterior parietal cortex (Gnadt & Anderson, 1988); and from a positron emission tomography (PET) study involving a verbal short-term memory task which revealed a supramarginal focus of activation, which the authors interpreted as the locus of phonological storage involved in the verbal short-term memory task (Paulesu, Frith, & Frackowiak,

1993). Furthermore, Baddeley et al. (1988) have described a patient, P. V., who has a pure short-term memory deficit. P. V. was able to learn meaningful paired associates in a familiar language. However, she was unable to learn to associate an unfamiliar word (in an unfamiliar language) with a familiar word in a familiar language, which is akin to learning a new vocabulary item. The fact that P. V. was a pure short-term memory patient suggests that the critical damage in her case was to left inferior parietal cortex. This in turn indicates that this area of cortex does play a role in vocabulary acquisition. So, one part of the neural substrate commonly underlying PSTM and vocabulary acquisition appears to be left inferior parietal cortex. Beyond this, it appears that the encoding and retrieval of verbal sequences may be subserved by regions of inferior/posterior parietal cortex (especially BA 40, but also BA 39 and BA 7), while active maintenance and rehearsal are subserved by regions of (pre) frontal cortex, especially Broca's area (BA 44/45), premotor and supplementary motor cortex (BA 6), and dorsolateral prefrontal cortex (BA 9/46; Awh et al., 1996; Gupta & MacWhinney, 1997; Paulesu et al., 1993; Risse et al., 1984; Shallice & Vallar, 1990). However, other studies have failed to find inferior parietal activation during verbal short-term memory tasks (e.g., Chein & Fiez, 2001; Fiez et al., 1996; Grasby et al., 1993), and a clear consensus has not as yet emerged regarding the role of various neural regions in sub-aspects of PSTM tasks, although there is a fair consensus on the overall involvement of inferior/posterior parietal cortex.

The Arbitrariness of Language

Virtually every introductory textbook on language points out that language is *arbitrary*. That is, the mapping of phonological forms onto meanings does not follow any identifiable pattern within a language (much less across languages). For example, in English, the fact that the phonological form *hat* maps onto the meaning "something to wear on the head," cannot be taken to predict that the similar phonological form *rat* will map onto a meaning that is similar to that of *hat*. Morphology provides exceptions to this arbitrariness, so that, for example, the presence of an -*s* at the end of a noun of English does fairly consistently indicate plurality, and hence arguably something about meaning. There are also submorphological regularities, such as, for instance, similarities in meaning that are signaled by initial segment clusters such as *sn-*, as in *sneer*, *snigger*, and *snide*. Despite these exceptions, it is quite clear that the form–meaning mapping incorporates a high degree of arbitrariness in human languages; hence the definitional nature of this arbitrariness. Once again, this property of language is so fundamental that emphasizing it might appear to be uninformative. In fact, however, the arbitrariness of language is once again a functional characteristic that has important implications for how language must be processed in the mind/brain.

These implications arise from the integration of a number of ideas, which are worth clarifying here. The first of these ideas pertains to the distinction between *systematic mappings* and *arbitrary mappings*. A systematic mapping can be defined as a *function* (in the mathematical sense of a transformation of a set of inputs into a corresponding set of outputs) in which inputs that are similar on some specifiable dimension are mapped to outputs that are similar on some specifiable dimension. An example of a systematic mapping is a function whose input is the orthographic representation of a word and whose output is the reversed spelling of the same word. In this mapping, the similar orthographic forms *BUTTER* and *BETTER* map onto the also similar orthographic forms *RETTUB* and *RETTEB*. As another example, the function mapping the length of a bar of mercury in a thermometer onto temperature is systematic, in that numerically similar lengths map onto numerically similar temperatures. An arbitrary mapping, in contrast, is a function in which inputs that are similar on some specifiable dimension are mapped to outputs that are not necessarily similar on any specifiable dimension. For example, the mapping between the names of countries and the names of their capital cities is arbitrary: phonologically similar country names (e.g., Canada, Panama) do not map onto capital city names that are consistently similar phonologically or on any other identifiable dimension (Ottawa, Panama City). As another example, the mapping between human proper names and the personality characteristics of those bearing them is arbitrary within a particular gender and culture. That is, the phonologically similar names John and Don do not map onto personality types that are more similar on any identifiable dimension than the personality types associated with the phonologically dissimilar names John and Fred. The property of arbitrariness discussed above for human languages is an instantiation of precisely this type of arbitrary mapping between the forms and meaning of words.

The second idea is that connectionist networks are devices that instantiate mappings. When an input is provided, such a network transforms the input stimulus into an output response, thus instantiating a mapping. The distinction between systematic and arbitrary mappings thus becomes relevant to such networks, and, in particular, to the nature of learning that can occur in connectionist networks whose input and output representations allow for measurement of similarity – i.e., which employ *distributed representations* at the input and output. The defining characteristic of such representations is that a stimulus is represented as a pattern of activation that is *distributed* across a pool of units, with each unit in the pool representing a feature that comprises the entity; there is no individual unit that represents the whole entity. The most important characteristic of distributed representations is that they enable similar stimuli to have similar representations. If such a connectionist system instantiates a systematic mapping, presentation of a novel input stimulus leads to production of a correct or close-to-correct output response simply by virtue of generalization based on prior knowledge: because the representations are distributed, the network will respond to the novel input in a manner that is similar to the response for previous similar inputs; because the mapping is systematic, this will be approximately the correct response. Little or no learning (adjustment of connection weights) is therefore needed for production of a correct response to a novel stimulus. Thus even though distributed connectionist networks incorporate incremental weight adjustment together with a slow learning rate (because fast learning rates can lead to unstable learning and/or interference with previously established weights – what McCloskey & Cohen, 1989, termed *catastrophic interference*), if the mapping that such a network instantiates is systematic, then learning the correct response to a novel input can be fast, requiring only a few exposures to the novel input–output pairing (because, even on first exposure, the response is close to correct).

The situation is different, however, where a mapping is arbitrary. In a distributed connectionist network that instantiates an arbitrary mapping, presentation of a novel input stimulus is unlikely to lead to production of a near-correct response: previous learning does not help, precisely because the mapping is arbitrary. Learning to produce the correct response will require considerable weight change. Therefore, because weight change is made only incrementally in a distributed connectionist network, learning a new input–output pairing in an arbitrary mapping can only occur gradually, over many exposures, at each of which the weights are adjusted slightly. However, the learning of arbitrary associations of items of information such as those comprising episodes and new facts can occur swiftly in humans, often within a single encounter, and without catastrophic interference. Gradual weight change in distributed connectionist networks thus cannot offer an account of such learning behavior. Such learning would, however, be possible in a connectionist system that employed orthogonal or localist representations (which do not overlap and hence do not interfere with each other) together with a faster learning rate.

These points suggest a functional requirement for two types of networks: one employing distributed representations that incorporates the desirable property of generalizing appropriately for novel inputs, which also enables it to quickly learn new entries in a systematic mapping; and one that employs orthogonal representations and a faster learning rate. McClelland, McNaughton, and O'Reilly (1995) proposed that these two functional requirements are indeed provided by the human brain, in the form of what have respectively been termed the procedural memory system and the declarative memory system. The procedural memory system, which provides for the learning and processing of motor, perceptual, and cognitive skills, is believed to be subserved by learning that occurs in nonhippocampal structures such as neocortex and the basal ganglia (e.g., Cohen & Squire, 1980; McClelland et al., 1995; Mishkin, Malamut, & Bachevalier, 1984; Squire, Knowlton, & Musen, 1993), and can be thought of as operating like distributed connectionist networks (Cohen & Squire, 1980; McClelland et al., 1995). The declarative memory system is believed to be subserved by the hippocampus and related medial temporal lobe structures (we will refer to this loosely as "the hippocampal system"); these structures provide for the initial encoding of memories involving arbitrary conjunctions, and also for their eventual consolidation and storage in neocortex (e.g., Cohen & Squire, 1980; Mishkin et al., 1984; Squire et al., 1993). It can be thought of as a system that converts distributed representations into localist non-overlapping ones, and swiftly establishes associations between such converted representations (Cohen & Eichenbaum, 1993; McClelland et al., 1995). That is, the hippocampal system performs fast learning, based on orthogonalized representations, thus constituting the second necessary type of network and providing a basis for the swift encoding of arbitrary associations of the kind that comprise episodic and factual information. Neocortex and the hippocampal system thus perform complementary learning functions, and these functions constitute the essence of procedural and declarative memory, respectively. McClelland et al. (1995) marshaled a variety of arguments and evidence to support these proposals. Their framework offers a means of reconciling the weaknesses of distributed connectionist networks with the human capacity for fast learning of arbitrary associations as well as with neurophysiological data.

It should be noted that different learning tasks are not viewed as being routed to one or other learning system by some controller based on whether each task is better suited to declarative or procedural learning. Rather, both learning systems are engaged in all learning behavior. However, for any given learning task, components of the task that constitute arbitrary mappings will be ineffectively acquired by the procedural system, and will only be effectively acquired by the declarative system, with later consolidation into the procedural system then being necessary. Any components of the task that constitute systematic mappings may be acquired by the declarative system but can also be effectively acquired directly by the procedural system, so that their declarative learning and later consolidation does not add much benefit. McClelland et al.'s (1995) framework has been widely influential, and constitutes the third idea that Gupta and Dell (1999; Gupta & Cohen, 2002) incorporated.

Gupta and Dell (1999; Gupta & Cohen, 2002) noted that phonology incorporates a systematic mapping, in that similar input phonology representations map onto similar output phonology representations; and that in contrast, the mapping between word forms and meanings is largely arbitrary as discussed above, with similar phonological word form representations not being guaranteed to map onto similar meanings. Furthermore, in humans, learning a new word can in general occur relatively rapidly, which implies that learning can occur relatively rapidly for both the systematic phonology of a novel word, and its links with semantics. Based on these observations and the assumption that the human lexical system employs distributed representations, Gupta and Dell (1999; Gupta & Cohen, 2002) suggested that the fast learning of new distributed representations of phonological word forms in the systematic input–output phonology mapping can be accomplished by a distributed connectionist-like procedural learning system even if it incorporates incremental weight adjustment. However, the swift establishment of the expressive and receptive links (i.e., learning associations between distributed phonological and semantic representations, which are in an arbitrary mapping) cannot be accomplished via incremental weight adjustment alone, and necessitates a computational mechanism employing orthogonal representations and a faster learning rate – i.e., a hippocampus-like system.

This hypothesis is consistent with the kinds of impairments observed in hippocampal amnesics. Such patients are virtually unable to learn new word meanings (e.g., Gabrieli, Cohen, & Corkin, 1988; Grossman, 1987), which is an indication of their impairment in declarative memory. However, these same patients exhibit intact repetition priming for both known and novel words (e.g., Haist, Musen, & Squire, 1991), which is an indication of their relatively spared procedural memory. More recently, it has been reported that some children who suffered early damage to limited parts of the hippocampal system nevertheless achieve vocabulary levels in the low normal range by early adulthood (Vargha-Khadem et al., 1997). While the broader implications of this finding have been the matter of debate (Mishkin, Vargha-Khadem, & Gadian, 1998; Squire & Zola, 1998), the results are not inconsistent with the present hypothesis. They may indicate that not all parts of the hippocampal system are equally critical for learning of associations between word meanings and word forms, but remain consistent with the larger body of evidence indicating that parts of the hippocampal system are critical for normal learning of such associations (and for semantic memory more generally). Gupta and Dell's (1999; Gupta & Cohen, 2002) proposal regarding the differential engagement of procedural and declarative memory systems in word learning thus appears to be consistent with computational analysis of the requirements of word learning as well as with neuropsychological data. The distinction between the roles of procedural and declarative learning is similar to a view proposed by Ullman (2001, 2004), who also suggests that these two types of learning play specific roles in language learning, but who suggests that they underlie the distinction between syntax and the lexicon, rather than underlying different aspects of word learning.

Thus once again, computational analysis of fundamental properties of language (in this case, arbitrariness and systematicity) leads to constraints on how language must be processed in the mind/brain. Interestingly, we are once again led to a dependence of novel word processing/learning on *memory* systems.

Word Learning as a Confluence of Memory Systems: An Integrated View

The ideas outlined above can be seen as offering the beginnings of an integration of the domains of input phonology and output phonology in the lexical domain. As is clear from Figure 8.1a, input-side processing in the model incorporates a key element of what is required for spoken word recognition, in that a sequence of sublexical elements is transduced into an internal word form representation. The model also, of course, incorporates a key element of word production: an internal representation is transformed into a sequence of output phonological representations. In the model, the input and output phonology processes are tightly integrated, and are subserved by the same internal representation. In this sense, the model offers a tentative integration of the domains of spoken word recognition and spoken word production, or input and output phonology.

Because its learning algorithms constitute procedural learning, the model also incorporates Gupta and Dell's (1999; Gupta & Cohen, 2002) proposal that the learning of phonological forms is accomplished via procedural memory/learning.

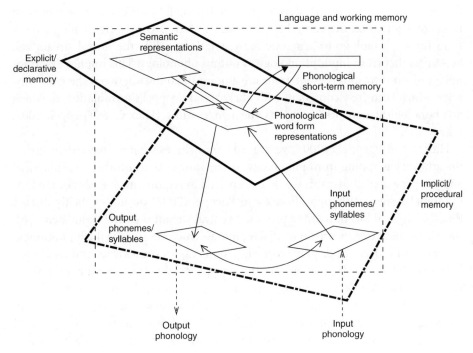

Figure 8.2 Word learning as a confluence of memory systems.

Because the model does not simulate semantic processing or the linking of semantic with phonological representations, it does not speak to the second aspect of Gupta's proposal, viz. that the linking of word form representations to semantic representations requires declarative memory/learning. To the extent that the proposal is correct, however, we are led to a view of word learning in which the seemingly simple process of learning a new word is a rich confluence of short-term, procedural, and declarative memory systems. This view is sketched in Figure 8.2, which illustrates the interaction of PSTM, procedural learning, and declarative learning in providing for novel word learning. It should be clear that the implemented model of Gupta and Tisdale (2009) constitutes the phonological processing subset of this integrated architecture.

Neuroscientific Evidence for the Integrated View

We have already surveyed neuroscientific evidence relevant to the individual ideas presented above. It is important to note, however, that recent integrative views about the neural substrates of language processing/learning also fit quite well with the overall functional/computational scheme laid out above. Hickok and Poeppel (2007), for instance, have proposed two streams of speech-related processing, in which a ventral stream processes speech signals for comprehension, and a dorsal stream maps acoustic speech signals to frontal lobe articulatory networks. In terms of Figure 8.2, the ventral stream can be seen as consisting of the pathway from input phonology to semantic representations, while the dorsal stream can be seen as that from input phonology to output phonology. This implies that phonological word form representations are a point of contact between the two pathways, which is entirely consistent with Hickok and Poeppel's formulation, in which a "phonological network" connects the two streams (Hickok & Poeppel, 2007; Figure 8.1).

Hickok and Poeppel's (2007) ventral stream includes what we have identified as the arbitrary mapping from phonology to semantics. Based on the computational analysis presented above, this would be expected to require involvement of the hippocampal system. Although Hickok and Poeppel (2007) do not explicitly discuss this, the physical location of the proposed ventral stream is entirely consistent with the engagement of subcortical medial temporal structures such as the hippocampal system. And indeed, Rodriguez-Fornells, Cunillera, Mestres-Misse, and de Diego-Balaguer (2009), building on Hickok and Poeppel's (2007) formulation, posit three pathways that are relevant to language learning: (1) a *dorsal audio-motor interface*, corresponding with Hickok and Poeppel's (2007) dorsal stream; (2) a *ventral meaning integration interface*, corresponding to Hickok and Poeppel's (2007) ventral stream; and (3) an *episodic-lexical interface*. Rodriguez-Fornells et al. (2009) explicitly characterize this third pathway as incorporating declarative learning structures such as the hippocampal system.

Rodriguez-Fornells et al. (2009) also posit an integrative role for the basal ganglia, noting their importance to sequential tasks. As we noted earlier, the basal ganglia and neocortex are regarded as important substrates that incorporate procedural learning (e.g., Cohen & Squire, 1980; McClelland et al., 1995; Mishkin et al., 1984; Squire et al., 1993), and can be thought of as operating like distributed connectionist networks (Cohen & Squire, 1980; McClelland et al., 1995). In the conceptualization shown in Figure 8.2, the operation of such procedural learning is pervasive throughout the system. Thus, consistently with the formulation of Rodriguez-Fornells et al. (2009), it does indeed play an integrative role. The two streams that Rodriguez-Fornells et al. (2009) add to Hickok and Poeppel's (2007) formulation can thus be seen as the complementary operation of declarative and procedural memory discussed in this article and depicted in Figure 8.2.

The present chapter's integrated view of word processing and learning as lying at the confluence of several memory systems is thus in considerable consonance with current thinking in integrative neurophysiology. Furthermore, the present formulation offers an analysis of the functional architecture that is derived from computational consideration of fundamental characteristics of language. The combination of such integrative approaches from behavioral, computational, and neurophysiological perspectives appears particularly well suited to furthering our understanding of language, and the present chapter has aimed to review evidence that word processing and word learning are domains of language that are well amenable to such integrative treatment.

Notes

1 Maintenance of state information is necessary, but not sufficient, for a system to be able to produce specific serially ordered sequences of output. There must also be a sequential control policy that specifies, among other things: (1) how the current state of the system is determined (it is usually here that the state information is required); (2) how the output is determined from the current state; and (3) how the output maps onto the sequential elements of the desired sequential behavior. For example, in accounts of serial ordering that employ a time-varying context signal (e.g., Burgess & Hitch, 1992, 1999; Brown et al., 2000; Gupta, 1996; Hartley & Houghton, 1996), the procedure that updates the context signal is an aspect of the sequential control policy, as is the specification of how the updated context signal is translated into an output representing a sequence element. In a simple recurrent (SRN; e.g., Elman, 1990), the procedure that merges the "context layer" activation with the current input is part of the sequential control policy, as is the specification of the target sequence element to be produced at each point in time. Thus having and executing a sequential control policy, together with maintenance of state information, are the necessary and sufficient conditions for serially ordered sequential behavior. For the present discussion, the most directly relevant of these requirements is the maintenance of state information, and we therefore do not provide further analysis of the sequential control policy. It may be noted, however, that such analysis would be closely related to the theory of formal languages, automata, and computation (Hopcroft & Ullman, 1979).

2 In some accounts, the maintenance of state information is more implicit, but is nevertheless critical to the production of a serially ordered sequence. For instance, in some models, the serial ordering is encoded directly by the structure of the representations such as linguistic syntactic frames or slot-filler representations (Dell, 1986; Dell, Schwartz, Martin, Saffran, & Gagnon, 1997; Kuehne, Gentner, & Forbus, 2000; Levelt, Roelofs, & Meyer, 1999; Warker & Dell, 2006) or storage structures such as arrays (e.g. Nairne, 1990; Nairne & Neumann, 1993) themselves. In such accounts, it is assumed that some process unpacks this structurally encoded serial ordering (e.g., Dell et al., 1997). But this requires maintenance of context: During sequence production, such a process (which instantiates the sequential control policy) would need to keep track of which structural element of the frame or array was currently being accessed, which is functionally identical to maintaining state or context information.

References

Atkins, P. W. B., & Baddeley, A. D. (1998). Working memory and distributed vocabulary learning. *Applied Psycholinguistics, 19*, 537–552.

Awh, E., Jonides, J., Smith, E. E., Schumacher, E. H., Koeppe, R. A., & Katz, S. (1996). Dissociation of storage and rehearsal in verbal working memory: Evidence from positron emission tomography. *Psychological Science, 7*, 25–31.

Baddeley, A. D. (1993). Short-term phonological memory and long-term learning: A single case study. *European Journal of Cognitive Psychology, 5*, 129–148.

Baddeley, A. D., Gathercole, S. E., & Papagno, C. (1998). The phonological loop as a language learning device. *Psychological Review, 105*, 158–173.

Baddeley, A. D., Papagno, C., & Vallar, G. (1988). When long-term learning depends on short-term storage. *Journal of Memory and Language, 27*, 586–595.

Botvinick, M., & Plaut, D. (2006). Short-term memory for serial order: A recurrent neural network model. *Psychological Review, 113*, 201–233.

Brown, G. D. A., Preece, T., & Hulme, C. (2000). Oscillator-based memory for serial order. *Psychological Review, 107*, 127–181.

Burgess, N., & Hitch, G. J. (1992). Toward a network model of the articulatory loop. *Journal of Memory and Language, 31*, 429–460.

Burgess, N., & Hitch, G. J. (1999). Memory for serial order: A network model of the phonological loop and its timing. *Psychological Review, 106*, 551–581.

Chein, J. M., & Fiez, J. A. (2001). Dissociation of verbal working memory system components using a delayed serial recall task. *Cerebral Cortex, 11*, 1003–1014.

Cohen, N. J., & Eichenbaum, H. (1993). *Memory, amnesia, and the hippocampal system.* Cambridge, MA: MIT Press.

Cohen, N. J., & Squire, L. R. (1980). Preserved learning and retention of pattern analyzing skill in amnesia: Dissociation of knowing how and knowing that. *Science, 210*, 207–209.

Dell, G. S. (1986). A spreading activation theory of retrieval in sentence production. *Psychological Review, 93*, 283–321.

Dell, G. S., Schwartz, M. F., Martin, N., Saffran, E. M., & Gagnon, D. A. (1997). Lexical access in normal and aphasic speakers. *Psychological Review, 104*, 801–838.

Dollaghan, C. (1987). Fast mapping in normal and language-impaired children. *Journal of Speech and Hearing Disorders, 52*, 218–222.

Elman, J. L. (1990). Finding structure in time. *Cognitive Science, 14*, 179–211.

Fiez, J. A., Raife, E. A., Balota, D. A., Scwarz, J. P., Raichle, M. E., & Petersen, S. E. (1996). A positron emission tomography study of the short-term maintenance of verbal information. *Journal of Neuroscience, 16*, 808–822.

Gabrieli, J. D. E., Cohen, N. J., & Corkin, S. (1988). The impaired learning of semantic knowledge following bilateral medial temporal-lobe resection. *Brain, 7*, 157–177.

Gathercole, S. E. (2006). Nonword repetition and word learning: The nature of the relationship. *Applied Psycholinguistics, 27*, 513–543.

Gathercole, S. E., & Baddeley, A. D. (1989). Evaluation of the role of phonological STM in the development of vocabulary in children: A longitudinal study. *Journal of Memory and Language, 28*, 200–213.

Gathercole, S. E., & Baddeley, A. D. (1990a). Phonological memory deficits in language-disordered children: Is there a causal connection? *Journal of Memory and Language, 29*, 336–360.

Gathercole, S. E., & Baddeley, A. D. (1990b). The role of phonological memory in vocabulary acquisition: A study of young children learning arbitrary names of toys. *British Journal of Psychology, 81*, 439–454.

Gathercole, S. E., Hitch, G. J., Service, E., & Martin, A. J. (1997). Short-term memory and new word learning in children. *Developmental Psychology, 33*, 966–979.

Gathercole, S. E., Service, E., Hitch, G. J., Adams, A.-M., & Martin, A. J. (1999). Phonological short-term memory and vocabulary development: Further evidence on the nature of the relationship. *Applied Cognitive Psychology, 13*, 65–77.

Gathercole, S. E., Willis, C., Emslie, H., & Baddeley, A. D. (1992). Phonological memory and vocabulary development during the early school years: A longitudinal study. *Developmental Psychology, 28*, 887–898.

Gnadt, J. W., & Anderson, R. A. (1988). Memory related motor planning activity in posterior parietal cortex of macaque. *Experimental Brain Research, 70,* 216–220.

Grasby, P. M., Frith, C. D., Friston, K. J., Bench, C., Frackowiak, R. S. J., & Dolan, R. J. (1993). Functional mapping of brain areas implicated in auditory-verbal memory function. *Brain, 116,* 1–20.

Grossman, M. (1987). Lexical acquisition in Alcoholic Korsakoff psychosis. *Cortex, 23,* 631–644.

Gupta, P. (1996). Word learning and verbal short-term memory: A computational account. In G. W. Cottrell (Ed.), *Proceedings of the eighteenth annual meeting of the Cognitive Science Society* (pp. 189–194). Mahwah, NJ: Erlbaum.

Gupta, P. (2003). Examining the relationship between word learning, nonword repetition, and immediate serial recall in adults. *Quarterly Journal of Experimental Psychology (A), 56,* 1213–1236.

Gupta, P., & Cohen, N. J. (2002). Theoretical and computational analysis of skill learning, repetition priming, and procedural memory. *Psychological Review, 109,* 401–448.

Gupta, P., & Dell, G. S. (1999). The emergence of language from serial order and procedural memory. In B. MacWhinney (Ed.), *The emergence of language,* 28th Carnegie Mellon Symposium on Cognition. Mahwah, NJ: Erlbaum.

Gupta, P., & MacWhinney, B. (1997). Vocabulary acquisition and verbal short-term memory: Computational and neural bases. *Brain and Language, 59,* 267–333.

Gupta, P., MacWhinney, B., Feldman, H., & Sacco, K. (2003). Phonological memory and vocabulary learning in children with focal lesions. *Brain and Language, 87,* 241–252.

Gupta, P., & Tisdale, J. (2009). Does phonological short-term memory causally determine vocabulary learning? Toward a computational resolution of the debate. *Journal of Memory and Language, 61,* 481–502.

Haist, F., Musen, G., & Squire, L. R. (1991). Intact priming of words and nonwords in amnesia. *Psychobiology, 19,* 275–285.

Hartley, T., & Houghton, G. (1996). A linguistically constrained model of short-term memory for nonwords. *Journal of Memory and Language, 35,* 1–31.

Hickok, G., & Poeppel, D. (2007). The cortical organization of speech processing. *Nature Reviews Neuroscience, 8,* 393–402.

Hopcroft, J. E., & Ullman, J. D. (1979). *Introduction to automata theory, languages, and computation.* Redwood City, CA: Addison-Wesley.

Jordan, M. I. (1986). *Serial order: A parallel distributed processing approach* (Report 8604). La Jolla, CA: Institute for Cognitive Science, University of California, San Diego.

Kuehne, S. E., Gentner, D., & Forbus, K. D. (2000). Modeling infant learning via symbolic structural alignment. In *Proceedings of the twenty-second annual conference of the Cognitive Science Society* (pp. 286–291). Mahwah, NJ: Erlbaum.

Levelt, W. J. M., Roelofs, A., & Meyer, A. S. (1999). A theory of lexical access in speech production. *Behavioral and Brain Sciences, 22,* 1–75.

Martin, N., & Saffran, E. (1997). Language and auditory-verbal short-term memory impairments: Evidence for common underlying processes. *Cognitive Neuropsychology, 14,* 641–682.

Martin, N., Saffran, E. M., & Dell, G. S. (1996). Recovery in deep dysphasia: Evidence for a relation between auditory-verbal STM capacity and lexical errors in repetition. *Brain and Language, 52,* 83–113.

McClelland, J. L., McNaughton, B. L., & O'Reilly, R. C. (1995). Why there are complementary learning systems in the hippocampus and neocortex: Insights from the successes and failures of connectionist models of learning and memory. *Psychological Review, 102,* 419–457.

McCloskey, M., & Cohen, N. J. (1989). Catastrophic interference in connectionist networks: The sequential learning problem. In G. H. Bower (Ed.), *The psychology of learning and motivation,* (vol. 24, pp. 109–165). New York: Academic Press.

Michas, I. C., & Henry, L. A. (1994). The link between phonological memory and vocabulary acquisition. *British Journal of Developmental Psychology, 12,* 147–164.

Mishkin, M., Malamut, B., & Bachevalier, J. (1984). Memories and habits: Two neural systems. In G. Lynch, J. McGaugh, & N. Weinberger (Eds.), *Neurobiology of learning and memory* (pp. 65–77). New York: Guilford.

Mishkin, M., Vargha-Khadem, F., & Gadian, D. G. (1998). Amnesia and the organization of the hippocampal system. *Hippocampus, 8,* 212–216.

Montgomery, J. W. (2002). Understanding the language difficulties of children with specific language impairments: Does verbal working memory matter? *American Journal of Speech-Language Pathology, 11,* 77–91.

Nairne, J. S. (1990). A feature model of immediate memory. *Memory and Cognition, 18,* 251–269.

Nairne, J. S., & Neumann, C. (1993). Enhancing effects of similarity on long-term memory for order. *Journal of Experimental Psychology: Learning, Memory, and Cognition, 19,* 329–337.

Page, M. P. A., & Norris, D. (1998). The primacy model: A new model of immediate serial recall. *Psychological Review, 105,* 761–781.

Papagno, C., Valentine, T., & Baddeley, A. D. (1991). Phonological short-term memory and foreign-language learning. *Journal of Memory and Language, 30,* 331–347.

Papagno, C., & Vallar, G. (1992). Phonological short-term memory and the learning of novel words: The effects of phonological similarity and item length. *Quarterly Journal of Experimental Psychology, 44A,* 47–67.

Paulesu, E., Frith, C. D., & Frackowiak, R. S. J. (1993). The neural correlates of the verbal component of working memory. *Nature, 362,* 342–345.

Risse, G. L., Rubens, A. B., & Jordan, L. S. (1984). Disturbance of long-term memory in aphasic patients: A comparison of anterior and posterior lesions. *Brain, 107,* 605–617.

Rodriguez-Fornells, A., Cunillera, T., Mestres-Misse, A., & de Diego-Balaguer, R. (2009). Neurophysiological mechanisms involved in language learning in adults. *Philosophical Transactions of the Royal Society B, 364,* 3711–3735.

Rumelhart, D., Hinton, G., & Williams, R. (1986). Learning internal representations by error propagation. In D. Rumelhart & J. McClelland (Eds.), *Parallel distributed processing* (vol. 1, *Foundations,* pp. 318–362). Cambridge, MA: MIT Press.

Saffran, E. M. (1990). Short-term memory impairment and language processing. In A. Caramazza (Ed.), *Cognitive neuropsychology and neurolinguistics.* Mahwah, NJ: Erlbaum.

Service, E. (1992). Phonology, working memory, and foreign-language learning. *Quarterly Journal of Experimental Psychology, 45A,* 21–50.

Service, E., & Kohonen, V. (1995). Is the relation between phonological memory and foreign language learning accounted for by vocabulary acquisition? *Applied Psycholinguistics, 16,* 155–172.

Shallice, T., & Vallar, G. (1990). The impairment of auditory-verbal short-term storage. In G. Vallar & T. Shallice (Eds.), *Neuropsychological impairments of short-term memory.* Cambridge: Cambridge University Press.

Squire, L. R., Knowlton, B., & Musen, G. (1993). The structure and organization of memory. *Annual Review of Psychology, 44,* 453–495.

Squire, L. R., & Zola, S. M. (1998). Episodic memory, semantic memory, and amnesia. *Hippocampus, 8,* 205–211.

Ullman, M. T. (2001). The declarative/procedural model of lexicon and grammar. *Journal of Psycholinguistic Research, 30,* 37–69.

Ullman, M. T. (2004). Contributions of memory circuits to language: The declarative/ procedural model. *Cognition, 92,* 231–270.

Vargha-Khadem, F., Gadian, D. G., Watkins, K. E., Connely, A., van Paesschen, W., & Mishkin, M. (1997). Differential effects of early hippocampal pathology on episodic and semantic memory. *Science, 277,* 376–380.

Warker, J. A., & Dell, G. S. (2006). Speech errors reflect newly learned phonotactic constraints. *Journal of Experimental Psychology: Learning, Memory, and Cognition, 32,* 387–398.

Part III

Neural Correlates of Language Production and Comprehension

9

Neural Correlates of Semantic Processing in Reading Aloud

William W. Graves, Jeffrey R. Binder,
Mark S. Seidenberg, and Rutvik H. Desai

For over a century, beginning at least as early as Cattell (1886), experimental psychologists have investigated the mental processes involved in reading single words aloud. For writing systems such as English, the task is challenging because of the many inconsistencies in the correspondences between spelling and sound. Early investigations into the neural systems supporting this task relied on autopsy studies, which established some of the critical brain regions responsible for acquired alexia (Déjerine, 1892). Integration of experimental and anatomical data, on the other hand, began comparatively recently, spurred in particular by the advent of noninvasive functional brain imaging. Reading aloud is thought to involve a combination of orthographic (visual word form), phonological (word sound), and perhaps semantic (word meaning) information processing. Although the necessity for orthographic and phonological processing is undisputed, the degree to which semantic information is recruited to aid in reading aloud is a matter of debate. One possibility is that, for example, words with unusual correspondences between spelling and sound (e.g., YACHT, COLONEL) might benefit more from the collateral recruitment of semantic codes than words with more regular spelling–sound correspondences (Plaut, McClelland, Seidenberg, & Patterson, 1996).

Although there is agreement that semantic information is not always necessary for single-word reading aloud, two major cognitive and computational models posit very different roles for semantic processing in this task. Dual-route models, such as the dual-route cascaded (DRC) model, propose two separate pathways, one that implements a set of grapheme–phoneme correspondence (GPC) rules for mapping letter combinations to sound combinations (Coltheart, Curtis, Atkins, & Haller, 1993; Coltheart, Rastle, Perry, Langdon, & Ziegler, 2001; see also Coltheart &

The Handbook of the Neuropsychology of Language, First Edition. Edited by Miriam Faust.
© 2012 Blackwell Publishing Ltd. Published 2012 by Blackwell Publishing Ltd.

Kohnen, Volume 2, Chapter 43). Words with mappings that do not follow such rules are processed through a "lexical" route, in which the word's orthographic and phonological forms are matched with corresponding whole-word structural (i.e., non-semantic) representations in a lexicon. Output from both pathways is passed to a response buffer for overt speech. Although a role for semantic processing is sketched as an offshoot of the lexical pathway, any such role is considered incidental, and no dual-route model has attempted to model the influence of semantics on reading aloud (Coltheart et al., 2001; Perry, Ziegler, & Zorzi, 2007).

Parallel distributed processing (PDP) models (e.g., Harm & Seidenberg, 2004; Plaut et al., 1996; Seidenberg & McClelland, 1989; see also Watson, Armstrong, & Plaut, Volume 1, Chapter 6), on the other hand, propose a single mechanism for processing all words, which involves multiple constraint satisfaction in a neural network composed of simple neuron-like units. In this system, distributed representations of orthographic, phonological, and semantic information are recruited to varying degrees depending on the properties of the individual word. For example, reading aloud words with highly consistent spelling–sound mappings is determined primarily by mappings between orthography and phonology. This is particularly true for high-consistency words that appear often in the language (i.e., high-frequency words). For well-sampled training corpora, such words would be presented more often during training, leading to a strengthening of associations (connection weights) between orthographic and phonological information for higher-frequency words. This leads to the prediction, borne out in the experimental data, that high-frequency, high-consistency words are processed more efficiently (in terms of faster response times and lower error rates) than words of lower frequency and consistency (Seidenberg, Waters, Barnes, & Tanenhaus, 1984).

Conversely, low-frequency, low-consistency words have relatively weak connections between orthography and phonology. However, the connections between orthographic and semantic information, on the one hand, and semantic and phonological information, on the other, should not be affected by spelling–sound consistency. This leads to the prediction that low-consistency words, for which orthography–phonology mappings are less robust, rely more on activation of semantic information than do high-consistency words. Thus, the PDP framework specifies a role for semantic information in reading aloud, and predicts stimulus conditions for which that role will be more or less prominent. A specific experimental prediction is that reading aloud words for which semantic information is expected to play a role should be modulated by semantic variables such as imageability. Support for this prediction is provided by behavioral studies in which low-consistency, low-frequency words are read aloud faster if they are of high compared to low imageability (Shibahara, Zorzi, Hill, Wydell, & Butterworth, 2003; Strain & Herdman, 1999; Strain, Patterson, & Seidenberg, 1995; Woollams, 2005).

In discussing the neurobiological basis of semantic processing in reading aloud, relevant behavioral and hemodynamic neuroimaging studies will be presented in terms of three variables thought to influence the degree of semantic processing in reading aloud: imageability, spelling–sound consistency, and word frequency. In addition to the neural localization results provided by such studies, the question of when semantic processing occurs in reading aloud is addressed in the section on chronometry. In the final section we attempt to clarify the different contributions of neural systems supporting semantic processing in reading aloud with reference to patterns of symptoms and pathology in several neurological disorders.

Hemodynamic Functional Neuroimaging Studies

Imageability

A word's imageability is the degree to which it evokes a mental image, as judged by subjective ratings averaged across a group of participants (Bird, Franklin, & Howard, 2001; Clark & Paivio, 2004; Cortese & Fugett, 2004; Gilhooly & Logie, 1980; Paivio, Yuille, & Madigan, 1968; Toglia & Battig, 1978). Semantic representations for highly imageable words are thought to be richer or more easily accessed (Paivio, 1991; Schwanenflugel, 1991; Shallice, 1988). As with the demonstrated effects of imageability on behavioral performance in reading aloud, functional imaging studies showing effects of imageability on brain activation can provide evidence for the use of semantics in helping to compute phonological output from orthographic input. Two recent functional magnetic resonance imaging (fMRI) studies from our lab investigated imageability effects on blood oxygen level dependent (BOLD) signal during reading aloud (Binder, Medler, Desai, Conant, & Liebenthal, 2005; Graves, Desai, Humphries, Seidenberg, & Binder, 2010). Using separate datasets, both studies found reading aloud of higher-imageability words to be associated with increased neural activity in bilateral angular gyrus (AG) and posterior cingulate/precuneus (PC). These were among the areas found to be reliably activated when comparing semantically rich to semantically impoverished conditions across more than 100 studies in a recent meta-analysis (Binder, Desai, Graves, & Conant, 2009). Thus, it appears that imageability effects can be used both as a behavioral indicator of semantic involvement in reading aloud and as a means of revealing neural systems that support this semantic access.

Additional insight into the interpretation and consistency of such findings can be gained by comparison with results from other reading-related studies. Interpreting divergent findings across studies using different tasks, however, is potentially problematic, as task demands can differ in multiple ways, the import of which is not always clear. For example, in one fMRI study that examined imageability effects (Hauk, Davis, Kherif, & Pulvermüller, 2008), participants read single words silently and no performance measures were collected. Positive correlations between imageability and BOLD signal were reported in the fusiform gyrus bilaterally but not in AG or PC regions. The divergence of these results from those discussed previously could be due, for example, to the shorter display time used by Hauk et al. (100 ms) compared to that of Binder et al. (2000 ms) and Graves et al. (1000 ms), or to a lesser degree of task engagement during passive reading compared to reading aloud.

Convergent findings for imageability, on the other hand, come from studies using tasks that emphasize comprehension, such as lexical decision or semantic decision (e.g., similarity matching). Four such studies found activation in AG and PC for highly imageable compared to less imageable words (Bedny & Thompson-Schill, 2006; Binder, Westbury, McKiernan, Possing, & Medler, 2005; Jessen et al., 2000; Sabsevitz, Medler, Seidenberg, & Binder, 2005). Although divergent findings have also been reported (Fiebach & Friederici, 2003; Pexman, Hargreaves, Edwards, Henry, & Goodyear, 2007), the more general convergence of activation in these areas across a large number of lexical semantic processing studies (Binder et al., 2009), and specifically in studies investigating effects of imageability, points to a highly reliable association of the AG and PC regions with semantic processing.

Consistency

Spelling–sound consistency relates to the computation of phonology from orthography, and can be defined in terms of a word's "friends" and "enemies." Friends of a word share the spelling and pronunciation of its rime (vowel nucleus and coda), whereas enemies share the same rime spelling but differ in pronunciation. Words with low spelling–sound consistency (e.g., PINT has many enemies such as LINT, HINT, and MINT, but no friends) generally elicit longer response times (RTs) than high-consistency words (Andrews, 1982; Baron & Strawson, 1976; Glushko, 1979; Jared, 1997, 2002; Taraban & McClelland, 1987). Other types of overlap (e.g., BAT, BAG) also affect processing to a much lesser degree (Kessler & Treiman, 2001) and so tend to be excluded from neighborhood calculations.

Functional brain imaging studies investigating the effects of spelling–sound consistency during single-word reading (either silently or aloud) typically report activation for low- compared to high-consistency words in left lateral prefrontal and medial premotor areas such as the inferior frontal gyrus (IFG) and anterior insula (Binder, Medler, et al., 2005; Fiez, Balota, Raichle, & Petersen, 1999; Graves et al., 2010; Herbster, Mintun, Nebes, & Becker, 1997; Mechelli et al., 2005). In studies of reading aloud, additional activations for low- compared to high-consistency words were found at the junction of the inferior and precentral sulci (inferior frontal junction, IFJ), and the supplementary motor area (SMA; Binder, Medler, et al., 2005; Fiez et al., 1999; Graves et al., 2010). Positive correlations between RT and BOLD signal are found in these areas during both reading aloud (Binder, Medler, et al., 2005; Graves et al., 2010) and lexical decision (Binder, Westbury, et al., 2005). These areas also show activation under conditions of high compared to low demands on working memory (Owen, McMillan, Laird, & Bullmore, 2005) and cognitive control (Derrfuss, Brass, Neumann, & Yves von Cramon, 2005). The co-occurrence of activation for low-consistency words with activations related to increased demands on working memory and cognitive control raises the possibility that activation in these areas may not be due specifically to lexical processing.

An increased reliance on semantic processing for reading low-consistency words is predicted by PDP models, but findings of a reliable association between reading low-consistency words and activation in temporal or parietal areas typically associated with lexical semantics, rather than more general processes such as those related to working memory, have been scarce. Initial evidence that such a pattern might obtain in the left middle temporal gyrus (MTG) was reported by Frost et al. (2005), who manipulated consistency along with word frequency and imageability in reading aloud. Using a region-of-interest (ROI) approach restricted to left IFG, MTG, and angular gyrus, they found activation for low-consistency, high-imageability words in the MTG. ROI-based approaches are advantageous in that they increase the power to detect subtle effects in hypothesized areas. They are also disadvantageous in that they de-emphasize strict control over false positives and are silent regarding contributions from neural areas outside the ROI. Using a whole-brain analysis, we recently found activation for reading aloud low- compared to high-consistency words in an area similar to the MTG ROI used by Frost et al. (2005), spanning the middle part of the MTG and inferior temporal gyrus (ITG; Graves et al., 2010). Together these findings point to a role for the MTG/ITG in accessing semantic information to aid in mapping orthographic input to phonological output. This is in contrast to the pattern of activation found in AG and PC, which showed positive correlations of BOLD signal with imageability, but no correlation with spelling–sound consistency (Graves et al., 2010). Such a pattern suggests a distinction between the processing that occurs in MTG/ITG and AG/PC during reading aloud.

Word frequency

Effects of word frequency tend to be quite robust in both behavioral and functional neuroimaging studies. Words of lower frequency elicit longer RTs compared to those of higher frequency, with other factors equated. Most functional imaging studies report neural effects of word frequency in the direction of activation for reading low- compared to high-frequency words (Fiez et al., 1999; Hauk, Davis, & Pulvermüller, 2008; Joubert et al., 2004; Kronbichler et al., 2004). Similar frequency effects are reported in studies using picture naming tasks (Graves, Grabowski, Mehta, & Gordon, 2007; S. M. Wilson, Isenberg, & Hickok, 2009). For reading, these activations tend to occur in left IFG/anterior insula, IFJ, and SMA – areas similar to those activated for low- compared to high-consistency words (Binder, Medler, et al., 2005; Fiez et al., 1999; Herbster et al., 1997; Mechelli et al., 2005) – and in areas showing activation for increasing demands on working memory (Owen et al., 2005) and cognitive control (Derrfuss et al., 2005).

We recently investigated the degree and location of this overlap in a study of reading aloud in which word frequency, consistency, imageability, bigram frequency, biphone frequency, and number of letters were orthogonally manipulated (Graves et al., 2010). Positive correlations between BOLD signal and RT, and negative correlations between BOLD signal and imageability, consistency, and word frequency all overlapped in the left IFJ, a region strongly associated with cognitive control processes (Derrfuss et al., 2005). Positive correlations of RT and negative correlations of consistency and word frequency with BOLD signal were also found in the left IFG and anterior insula. The consistent pattern of overlap for these disparate effects in left inferior frontal areas across multiple studies and within the same study suggests that these regions may be responding to more general processing demands rather than demands specifically related to lexical processing.

Effects of word frequency in the opposite direction (activation for high- compared to low-frequency words) are relatively rare and, with the exception of our recent study (Graves et al., 2010), have only been reported in neuroimaging studies using silent reading (Yarkoni, Speer, Balota, McAvoy, & Zacks, 2008) or lexical decision (Carreiras, Riba, Vergara, Heldmann, & Münte, 2009; Prabhakaran, Blumstein, Myers, Hutchison, & Britton, 2006). That this pattern of activation has primarily been reported for lexical decision is notable because semantic variables such as imageability and lexical variables such as word frequency tend to show greater effect sizes with lexical decision compared to reading aloud (Balota, Cortese, Sergent-Marshall, Spieler, & Yap, 2004; Balota, Ferraro, & Connor, 1991; Forster & Chambers, 1973; Schilling, Rayner, & Chumbley, 1998). Evidence that word frequency could modulate semantic processing comes from findings that high-frequency words elicit retrieval of more features (McRae, Cree, Seidenberg, & McNorgan, 2005) and more associations with other words compared to low-frequency words (Nelson & McEvoy, 2000), and are found in more numerous and diverse contexts (Adelman, Brown, & Quesada, 2006). Thus, while word frequency effects can arise at multiple levels of the lexical system (for a review see Monsell, 1991), activations for high- compared to low-frequency words could in part reflect a more extensive and rapid access to semantic information in the case of high-frequency words. This component should be distinguishable from other aspects of lexical processing to the extent that it spatially overlaps effects of variables such as imageability that are thought to be more specifically related to lexical semantics. In our recent study of reading aloud (Graves et al., 2010), such an overlap was found in bilateral PC and AG. These areas were also found in a large-scale meta-analysis (Binder et al., 2009) to be reliably associated with lexical semantic processing. Thus, the overall pattern of overlapping positive correlations of word frequency and imageability with BOLD signal in areas implicated in lexical semantic processing suggests that the PC and AG support semantic processing in reading aloud. Unlike the MTG/ITG, however, the AG/PC was not found to be modulated by spelling–sound consistency. Together with the finding that activation in the AG/PC region was positively associated with imageability and frequency, this pattern suggests that the MTG/ITG activation may reflect recruitment of semantic information during computation of a pronunciation, whereas activation in the AG/PC may reflect another process such as word comprehension.

Chronometry

Information on the time course of activation within the lexical system should help determine whether semantic information is accessed alongside orthographic and phonological information, as predicted by PDP models, or whether its access is incidental, perhaps following both orthographic and phonological access, as compatible with DRC models. Two widely used methods for time course investigations with resolution on the order of milliseconds are electroencephalography studies analyzed in terms of event-related potentials (ERP), and magnetoencephalography (MEG).

MEG is a particularly promising technique in that it combines exquisite temporal resolution with spatial resolution that, while not as fine-grained as fMRI, can detect locations of distinct cortical activity. Compared to fMRI, there are relatively few research groups using MEG, and although the number of MEG centers is expanding, so far there have been few MEG studies of reading aloud. An exception is a study by Simos et al. (2002), in which an area of the MTG was shown to be more active for low-consistency words than pronounceable nonwords. This result is very close to the area showing a negative correlation between BOLD signal and consistency for reading words aloud in fMRI (Graves et al., 2010). Although this convergence of findings across MEG and fMRI experiments is encouraging, temporal specificity was sacrificed by merging the data into two large time bins (150–300 and 300–1000 ms), and it is not clear that the MEG result is specific to low-consistency words. One line of study that would be useful in clarifying the role of semantic processing in reading aloud would be to examine the neural effects of factors such as word frequency and imageability as they unfold in time and space. Although we are aware of no such study of reading aloud, there are several relevant studies of word recognition (also discussed in Lee & Federmeier, Volume 1, Chapter 10).

ERP and MEG studies report lexical and semantic effects occurring in both relatively early (~150 ms) and late (~400 ms) time-frames. As summarized in two recent reviews, effects of word frequency and lexicality (differences between words and nonwords) are present by 150 ms post-stimulus-onset (Dien, 2009; Pulvermüller, Shtyrov, & Hauk, 2009). A recent lexical decision ERP study replicated the finding of early effects of word frequency and further showed that they subside over about 100 ms then re-emerge as a sustained difference lasting up to 500 ms post-stimulus (Hauk, Davis, Ford, Pulvermüller, & Marslen-Wilson, 2006). This study also investigated a variable called "semantic coherence," a measure of the number of contexts in which a word occurs, which was significantly correlated with word frequency. Effects of this variable occurred by 160 ms post-stimulus, subsided, then re-emerged at 425 ms, suggesting the presence of separate early and late stages of semantic processing. If words and word-like nonwords differ primarily in degree of meaningfulness, and high-frequency words have more associations with other words in the language, then it seems plausible that early temporally overlapping effects of word frequency, lexicality, and semantic coherence reflect initial activation of semantic features.

Regarding effects of imageability, a study using a concrete/abstract judgment task compared differences in MEG activity to abstract and concrete words and found differences peaking around 400 ms post-stimulus-onset (Dhond, Witzel, Dale, & Halgren, 2007). Cortical sources of effects arising in this time-frame were identified that showed greater activity for concrete compared to abstract words in right AG and bilateral PC. Activations in these regions for concrete compared to abstract words have also been found in fMRI studies using similar tasks (Bedny & Thompson-Schill, 2006; Binder, Westbury, et al., 2005; Sabsevitz et al., 2005). Although imageability effects peaked at around 400 ms, they began to diverge in the PC as early as 330 ms. Considering that the abstract words, while significantly less imageable than the concrete ones, were still quite imageable (the mean imageability was 401 for their abstract words and 576 for concrete words, on a scale from 100 to 700), it may be the case that differences across levels of imageability would have arisen even earlier had the levels been more clearly separated.

Imageability effects have also been investigated using ERP. For example, Holcomb and colleagues compared the time courses for concrete (highly imageable) and abstract (less imageable) words both in isolation and in sentence contexts. During lexical and semantic decisions to individual words, differences between word types emerged by 300 ms but not within the earlier 150–300 ms time window (Kounios & Holcomb, 1994). Similar results were found for making semantic or imagery decisions to sentence-final words. That is, differences between word types emerged by around 300 ms but not earlier (West & Holcomb, 2000). Another study by the same group, however, did find differences between concrete and abstract sentence-final words during a meaningfulness judgment task that emerged within an early 150–300 ms window (Holcomb, Kounios, Anderson, & West, 1999). Thus, evidence for imageability effects occurring early during lexical access is somewhat equivocal. Additionally, none of the specific studies discussed here examined the time course of imageability effects during reading aloud, leaving open the question of whether or not semantic processing occurs in parallel with early orthographic and phonological processing.

Distinct Neural Substrates

Before proposing a set of neural regions supporting semantic processing in reading aloud, it is important to note that several regions are good candidates for supporting direct mapping from orthography to phonology, including the left posterior superior temporal sulcus, supramarginal gyrus, and midfusiform gyrus. A discussion of the possible roles of these regions in reading aloud is beyond the scope of this chapter, and we refer the interested reader to other studies that address this topic (Binder, Medler, et al., 2005; Graves et al., 2010; Richlan, Kronbichler, & Wimmer, 2009).

The pattern of results described above points to two spatially and possibly functionally distinct regions supporting semantic processing during reading aloud. One involves the angular gyrus and posterior cingulate/precuneus, for which overlapping effects in the direction of greater activity for higher values of imageability and word frequency have been found. The other involves a more anterior region in the middle part of the MTG/ITG, for which increasing activity was found for reading words of decreasing spelling–sound consistency (Graves et al., 2010). We propose that this MTG/ITG area, compared to the AG and PC, plays a more central role in mapping from semantics to phonology for the purpose of generating a phonological code. Consistent with this interpretation are results from a meta-analysis of word production studies (Indefrey & Levelt, 2004), in which the mapping from lexical semantic to phonological codes is suggested to occur along the MTG.

Activation in the AG and PC regions, on the other hand, may reflect integration or activation of conceptual/semantic information, perhaps in a manner similar to that described in accounts of convergence zones. According to relevant aspects of the Damasio (1989) account, first-order convergence zones integrate information from adjacent early sensory cortex. This somewhat abstracted but still modality-dependent information is further abstracted by higher-order convergence zones located in multimodal association cortex. Due to their anatomical locations and patterns of connectivity, as summarized in more detail elsewhere (Binder et al., 2009), the AG and PC regions may be considered higher-order convergence zones for integration of multimodal information relevant to lexical semantics. Such representations contribute to word comprehension but may play a smaller role in computation of phonology. A schematic diagram of the proposed posterior left hemisphere pathways for reading aloud is provided in Figure 9.1.

The AG and PC are prominent components of the "default-mode" network (Gusnard & Raichle, 2001). As discussed in more detail elsewhere (Binder et al., 2009), these areas are part of a larger semantic system that appears to be active during resting and other passive states. One implication of this is that studies comparing conditions of interest to a resting baseline are likely to miss activations in these regions. In fact, several functional neuroimaging studies that examined effects of word frequency restricted their analyses to areas that were more active for words compared to a resting baseline (Carreiras, Mechelli, & Price, 2006; Fiez et al., 1999; Kronbichler et al., 2004). This practice may help explain the paucity of activation findings for reading high- compared to low-frequency words.

Evidence from acquired dyslexia

Independent evidence for distinct roles for semantic processing in the AG/PC on the one hand, and the middle MTG/ITG on the other, comes from studies of acquired dyslexia. Semantic dementia (SD) is a clinical variant of frontotemporal

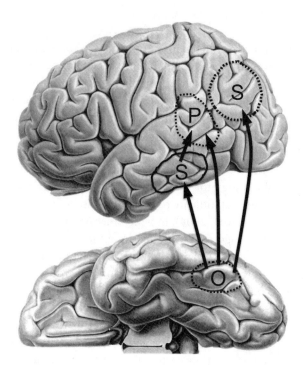

Figure 9.1   A neuroanatomical model of posterior left hemisphere pathways involved in reading aloud. Orthographic information (letter and letter string identity) is processed in the posterolateral fusiform gyrus and adjacent occipitotemporal sulcus ("O"). This information is mapped directly onto phonological representations in the posterior superior temporal region, including superior temporal sulcus and supramarginal gyrus ("P"). Low spelling–sound consistency produces enhanced activation of semantic representations in the middle and inferior temporal gyri (area "S" marked by solid line), which in turn provide input to P that assists in correct phonological retrieval. All words activate semantic representations in the angular gyrus (area "S" marked by dotted line). This latter area is modulated by word frequency and imageability but not by spelling–sound consistency, suggesting that semantic processing here supports word comprehension rather than pronunciation.

lobar degeneration, associated with both loss of semantic knowledge and atrophy of the anterior middle and inferior temporal lobes (Neary et al., 1998). SD patients tend to exhibit surface dyslexia, producing regularized pronunciations of low-consistency words (e.g., pronouncing "deaf" to rhyme with "leaf"; Patterson & Hodges, 1992). The association of surface dyslexia with the pattern of brain damage in SD is highly reliable, with the severity of surface dyslexia increasing with overall degree of semantic impairment (Woollams, Lambon Ralph, Plaut, & Patterson, 2007). Although SD patients have primarily anterior temporal lobe damage (Brambati, Ogar, Neuhaus, Miller, & Gorno-Tempini, 2009; Nestor, Fryer, & Hodges, 2006; S. M. Wilson, Brambati, et al., 2009), the posterior extent of this damage in the left hemisphere includes the middle MTG/ITG (Rohrer et al., 2009), an area found by Graves et al. (2010) to show increasing activity for reading aloud words of decreasing spelling–sound consistency.

Patients with Alzheimer's disease (AD), by comparison, show widespread pathology in temporal and parietal lobe areas that prominently include the medial temporal lobe, posterior cingulate/precuneus, and lateral posterior temporoparietal regions such as angular gyrus (Arnold, Hyman, Flory, Damasio, & van Hoesen, 1991), with comparative sparing of ventral and lateral anterior temporal regions (Buckner et al., 2005). In addition to this partially distinct pattern of pathology distribution, these patient groups also differ symptomatically. As discussed above, SD patients exhibit surface dyslexia. Although surface dyslexia may occur in later stages of AD (Strain, Patterson, Graham, & Hodges, 1998), AD patients more typically show preserved reading of low-consistency words (Noble, Glosser, & Grossman, 2000). Like SD patients, however, AD patients have been shown to exhibit impairment on tasks related to semantic knowledge. Specifically, AD patients produce more shared compared to distinct features for concrete concepts (Alathari, Ngo, & Dopkins, 2004), and loss of knowledge about distinguishing features may lead to a characteristic "hyperpriming" phenomenon (Chertkow, Bub, & Seidenberg, 1989; Giffard et al., 2001; Martin, 1992). Additional evidence for the erosion of distinctive relative to shared features in AD comes from the finding that AD patients show greater naming impairment for categories such as animals with many shared features, compared to objects with relatively few shared features (Whatmough et al., 2003). AD patients also show greater impairment on semantic compared to phonemic fluency tasks, despite the comparable executive control processes required by these tasks (Henry, Crawford, & Phillips, 2004; Salmon, Butters, & Chan, 1999; see also Pekkala, Volume 2, Chapter 30). Thus, although deficits in semantic processing are evident in both SD and AD, damage in SD includes the middle MTG/ITG region found by Graves et al. (2010) to be associated with consistency effects in reading aloud, and damage to this region results in surface dyslexia symptoms not typically seen in AD.

To our knowledge, only two studies have examined surface dyslexia in cases of focal brain damage. A longitudinal study of recovery from acquired dyslexia by B. A. Wilson (1994) included two cases of herpes simplex encephalitis who exhibited surface dyslexia. Although no information was given about their lesion locations, damage associated with herpes simplex encephalitis tends to concentrate in the anteromedial and ventral temporal lobes. These patients were the only two of the entire group of seven who were specifically diagnosed with surface dyslexia. A recent study by Jefferies, Rogers, Hopper, and Lambon Ralph (2010) included 13 patients with strokes that impaired semantic processing. This study examined effects of consistency and word frequency on reading aloud in both stroke and SD cohorts, finding a greater proportion of errors for less consistent and lower-frequency words in both groups. An interaction between consistency and word frequency, with a larger difference in error rate between low- and high–consistency words for those of lower frequency, was, however, found only in the SD group. Brief verbal descriptions of approximate lesion location were provided for 9 of the 13 stroke patients, indicating widespread damage in frontal, occipital, temporal, parietal, and subcortical areas. However, no lesion-deficit analyses were performed, leaving open the question of whether the differing response profiles were due, for example, to the stable versus progressive nature of the damage, or to the disruption of different neural structures in the patients with stroke compared to SD.

Conclusion

Although the role of semantic processing in reading aloud is controversial and is likely to remain so for some time, recent evidence from functional neuroimaging, considered alongside existing behavioral and computational studies, suggests an integral role for semantic processing in reading aloud. A set of neural areas including bilateral angular gyrus, posterior cingulate/precuneus, and left middle MTG/ITG appears to support semantic processing in several tasks, including reading aloud. Based on recent parametric and chronometric studies of reading aloud, we suggest that immediately following the initial decoding of a word's orthographic information, and likely before such decoding is completed, processing in the angular gyrus and posterior cingulate/precuneus serves to support automatic comprehension of the word, perhaps through integration and/or retrieval of its semantic features. Processing in the middle MTG/ITG, on the other hand, serves to map the retrieved semantic information onto a corresponding phonological representation for production.

References

Adelman, J. S., Brown, G. D. A., & Quesada, J. F. (2006). Contextual diversity, not word frequency, determines word-naming and lexical decision times. *Psychological Science, 17*(9), 814–823.

Alathari, L., Ngo, C. T., & Dopkins, S. (2004). Loss of distinctive features and a broader pattern of priming in Alzheimer's disease. *Neuropsychology, 18*(4), 603–612.

Andrews, S. (1982). Phonological recoding: Is the regularity effect consistent? *Memory and Cognition, 10*(6), 565–575.

Arnold, S. E., Hyman, B. T., Flory, J., Damasio, A. R., & van Hoesen, G. W. (1991). The topographical and neuroanatomical distribution of neurofibrillary tangles and neuritic plaques in the cerebral cortex of patients with Alzheimer's disease. *Cerebral Cortex, 1,* 103–116.

Balota, D. A., Cortese, M. J., Sergent-Marshall, S. D., Spieler, D. H., & Yap, M. J. (2004). Visual word recognition of single-syllable words. *Journal of Experimental Psychology: General, 133*(2), 283–316.

Balota, D. A., Ferraro, F. R., & Connor, L. T. (1991). On the early influence of meaning in word recognition: A review of the literature. In P. J. Schwanenflugel (Ed.), *The psychology of word meanings* (pp. 187–222). Hillsdale, NJ: Erlbaum.

Baron, J., & Strawson, C. (1976). Use of orthographic and word-specific knowledge in reading words aloud. *Journal of Experimental Psychology: Human Perception and Performance, 2*(3), 386–393.

Bedny, M., & Thompson-Schill, S. L. (2006). Neuroanatomically separable effects of imageability and grammatical class during single-word comprehension. *Brain and Language, 98*, 127–139.

Binder, J. R., Desai, R. H., Graves, W. W., & Conant, L. L. (2009). Where is the semantic system? A critical review and meta-analysis of 120 functional neuroimaging studies. *Cerebral Cortex, 19*, 2767–2796.

Binder, J. R., Medler, D. A., Desai, R., Conant, L. L., & Liebenthal, E. (2005). Some neurophysiological constraints on models of word naming. *NeuroImage, 27*, 677–693.

Binder, J. R., Westbury, C. F., McKiernan, K. A., Possing, E. T., & Medler, D. A. (2005). Distinct brain systems for processing concrete and abstract concepts. *Journal of Cognitive Neuroscience, 17*(6), 905–917.

Bird, H., Franklin, S., & Howard, D. (2001). Age of acquisition and imageability ratings for a large set of words, including verbs and function words. *Behavior Research Methods, Instruments, and Computers, 33*(1), 73–79.

Brambati, S. M., Ogar, J., Neuhaus, J., Miller, B. L., & Gorno-Tempini, M. L. (2009). Reading disorders in primary progressive aphasia: A behavioral and neuroimaging study. *Neuropsychologia, 47*, 1893–1900.

Buckner, R. L., Snyder, A. Z., Shannon, B. J., LaRossa, G., Sachs, R., Fotenos, A. F., et al. (2005). Molecular, structural, and functional characterization of Alzheimer's disease: Evidence for a relationship between default activity, amyloid, and memory. *The Journal of Neuroscience, 25*(34), 7709–7717.

Carreiras, M., Mechelli, A., & Price, C. J. (2006). Effect of word and syllable frequency on activation during lexical decision and reading aloud. *Human Brain Mapping, 27*, 963–972.

Carreiras, M., Riba, J., Vergara, M., Heldmann, M., & Münte, T. F. (2009). Syllable congruency and word frequency effects on brain activation. *Human Brain Mapping, 30*(9), 3079–3088.

Cattell, J. M. (1886). The time it takes to see and name objects. *Mind, 11*, 63–65.

Chertkow, H., Bub, D., & Seidenberg, M. S. (1989). Priming and sematic memory loss in Alzheimer's disease. *Brain and Language, 36*, 420–446.

Clark, J. M., & Paivio, A. (2004). Extensions of the Paivio, Yuille, and Madigan (1968) norms. *Behavior Research Methods, Instruments, and Computers, 36*(3), 371–383.

Coltheart, M., Curtis, B., Atkins, P., & Haller, M. (1993). Models of reading aloud: Dual-route and parallel-distributed-processing approaches. *Psychological Review, 100*, 589–608.

Coltheart, M., Rastle, K., Perry, C., Langdon, R., & Ziegler, J. (2001). DRC: A dual route cascaded model of visual word recognition and reading aloud. *Psychological Review, 108*(1), 204–256.

Cortese, M. J., & Fugett, A. (2004). Imageability ratings for 3,000 monosyllabic words. *Behavior Research Methods, Instruments, and Computers, 36*(3), 384–387.

Damasio, A. R. (1989). Time-locked multiregional retroactivation: A systems-level proposal for the neural substrates of recall and recognition. *Cognition, 33*(1–2), 25–62.

Déjerine, J. (1892). Contribution à l'étude anatomo-pathologique et clinique des différentes variétés de cécité verbale. *Computes Rendus des Séances de la Société de Biologie, 44*, 61–90.

Derrfuss, J., Brass, M., Neumann, J., & Yves von Cramon, D. (2005). Involvement of the inferior frontal junction in cognitive control: Meta-analyses of switching and stroop studies. *Human Brain Mapping, 25*, 22–34.

Dhond, R. P., Witzel, T., Dale, A. M., & Halgren, E. (2007). Spatiotemporal cortical dynamics underlying abstract and concrete word reading. *Human Brain Mapping, 28*, 355–362.

Dien, J. (2009). The neurocognitive basis of reading single words as seen through early latency ERPs: A model of converging pathways. *Biological Psychology, 80*, 10–22.

Fiebach, C. J., & Friederici, A. D. (2003). Processing concrete words: fMRI evidence against a specific right-hemisphere involvement. *Neuropsychologia, 42*, 62–70.

Fiez, J. A., Balota, D. A., Raichle, M. E., & Petersen, S. E. (1999). Effects of lexicality, frequency, and spelling-to-sound consistency on the functional anatomy of reading. *Neuron, 24*, 205–218.

Forster, K. I., & Chambers, S. M. (1973). Lexical access and naming time. *Journal of Verbal Learning and Verbal Behavior, 12*, 627–635.

Frost, S. J., Mencl, W. E., Sandak, R., Moore, D. L., Rueckl, J. G., Katz, L., et al. (2005). A functional magnetic resonance imaging study of the tradeoff between semantics and phonology in reading aloud. *NeuroReport, 16*(6), 621–624.

Giffard, B., Desgranges, B., Nore-Mary, F., Lalevée, C., de la Sayette, V., Pasquier, F., et al. (2001). The nature of semantic memory deficits in Alzheimer's disease: New insights from hyperpriming effects. *Brain, 124*, 1522–1532.

Gilhooly, K. J., & Logie, R. H. (1980). Age-of-acquisition, imagery, concreteness, familiarity, and ambiguity measures for 1,944 words. *Behavior Research Methods and Instrumentation, 12*(4), 395–427.

Glushko, R. J. (1979). The organization and activation of orthographic knowledge in reading aloud. *Journal of Experimental Psychology: Human Perception and Performance, 5*(4), 674–691.

Graves, W. W., Desai, R., Humphries, C., Seidenberg, M. S., & Binder, J. R. (2010). Neural systems for reading aloud: A multiparametric approach. *Cerebral Cortex, 20*, 1799–1815.

Graves, W. W., Grabowski, T. J., Mehta, S., & Gordon, J. K. (2007). A neural signature of phonological access: Distinguishing the effects of word frequency from familiarity and length in overt picture naming. *Journal of Cognitive Neuroscience, 19*(4), 617–631.

Gusnard, D. A., & Raichle, M. E. (2001). Searching for a baseline: Functional imaging and the resting brain. *Nature Reviews Neuroscience, 2*, 685–694.

Harm, M. W., & Seidenberg, M. S. (2004). Computing the meanings of words in reading: Cooperative division of labor between visual and phonological processes. *Psychological Review, 111*(3), 662–720.

Hauk, O., Davis, M. H., Ford, M., Pulvermüller, F., & Marslen-Wilson, W. D. (2006). The time course of visual word recognition as revealed by linear regression analysis of ERP data. *NeuroImage, 30*, 1383–1400.

Hauk, O., Davis, M. H., Kherif, F., & Pulvermüller, F. (2008). Imagery or meaning? Evidence for a semantic origin of category-specific brain activity in metabolic imaging. *European Journal of Neuroscience, 27*, 1856–1866.

Hauk, O., Davis, M. H., & Pulvermüller, F. (2008). Modulation of brain activity by multiple lexical and word form variables in visual word recognition: A parametric fMRI study. *NeuroImage, 42*, 1185–1195.

Henry, J. D., Crawford, J. R., & Phillips, L. H. (2004). Verbal fluency performance in dementia of the Alzheimer's type: a meta-analysis. *Neuropsychologia, 42*, 1212–1222.

Herbster, A. N., Mintun, M. A., Nebes, R. D., & Becker, J. T. (1997). Regional cerebral blood flow during word and nonword reading. *Human Brain Mapping, 5*, 84–92.

Holcomb, P. J., Kounios, J., Anderson, J. E., & West, W. C. (1999). Dual-coding, context-availability, and concreteness effects in sentence comprehension: An electrophysiological investigation. *Journal of Experimental Psychology: Learning, Memory, and Cognition, 25*(3), 721–742.

Indefrey, P., & Levelt, W. J. M. (2004). The spatial and temporal signatures of word production components. *Cognition, 92*(1–2), 101–144.

Jared, D. (1997). Spelling–sound consistency affects the naming of high-frequency words. *Journal of Memory and Language, 36*, 505–529.

Jared, D. (2002). Spelling–sound consistency and regularity effects in word naming. *Journal of Memory and Language, 46*, 723–750.

Jefferies, E., Rogers, T. T., Hopper, S., & Lambon Ralph, M. A. (2010). "Pre-semantic" cognition revisited: Critical differences between semantic aphasia and semantic dementia. *Neuropsychologia, 48*, 248–261.

Jessen, F., Heun, R., Erb, M., Granath, D.-O., Klose, U., Papassotiropoulos, A., et al. (2000). The concreteness effect: Evidence for dual-coding and context availability. *Brain and Language, 74*(1), 103–112.

Joubert, S., Beauregard, M., Walter, N., Bourgouin, P., Beaudoin, G., Leroux, J.-M., et al. (2004). Neural correlates of lexical and sublexical processes in reading. *Brain and Language, 89*, 9–20.

Kessler, B., & Treiman, R. (2001). Relationships between sounds and letters in English monosyllables. *Journal of Memory and Language, 44*, 592–617.

Kounios, J., & Holcomb, P. J. (1994). Concreteness effects in semantic processing: ERP evidence supporting dual-encoding theory. *Journal of Experimental Psychology: Learning Memory and Cognition, 20*, 804–823.

Kronbichler, M., Hutzler, F., Wimmer, H., Mair, A., Staffen, W., & Ladurner, G. (2004). The visual word form area and the frequency with which words are encountered: Evidence from a parametric fMRI study. *NeuroImage, 21*, 946–953.

Martin, A. (1992). Degraded knowledge representations in patients with Alzheimer's disease: Implications for models of semantic and repetition priming. In L. R. Squire & N. Butters (Eds.), *Neuropsychology of memory* (pp. 220–232). New York: Guilford Press.

McRae, K., Cree, G. S., Seidenberg, M. S., & McNorgan, C. (2005). Semantic feature production norms for a large set of living and nonliving things. *Behavior Research Methods, Instruments, and Computers, 37*(4), 547–559.

Mechelli, A., Crinion, J. T., Long, S., Friston, K. J., Lambon Ralph, M. A., Patterson, K., et al. (2005). Dissociating reading processes on the basis of neuronal interactions. *Journal of Cognitive Neuroscience, 17*(11), 1753–1765.

Monsell, S. (1991). The nature and locus of word frequency effects in reading. In D. Besner & G. W. Humphreys (Eds.), *Basic processes in reading: Visual word recognition* (pp. 148–197). Hillsdale, NJ: Erlbaum.

Neary, D., Snowden, J. S., Gustafson, L., Passant, U., Stuss, D., Black, S., et al. (1998). Frontotemporal lobar degeneration: A consensus on clinical disgnostic criteria. *Neurology, 51*, 1546–1554.

Nelson, D. L., & McEvoy, C. L. (2000). What is this thing called frequency? *Memory and Cognition, 28*(4), 509–522.

Nestor, P. J., Fryer, T. D., & Hodges, J. R. (2006). Declarative memory impairments in Alzheimer's disease and semantic dementia. *NeuroImage, 30*, 1010–1020.

Noble, K., Glosser, G., & Grossman, M. (2000). Oral reading in dementia. *Brain and Language,* *74,* 48–69.

Owen, A. M., McMillan, K. M., Laird, A. R., & Bullmore, E. (2005). N-back working memory paradigm: A meta-analysis of normative functional neuroimaging studies. *Human Brain Mapping, 25,* 46–59.

Paivio, A. (1991). Dual coding theory: Retrospect and current status. *Canadian Journal of Psychology, 45*(3), 255–287.

Paivio, A., Yuille, J. C., & Madigan, S. A. (1968). Concreteness, imagery, and meaningfulness values for 925 nouns. *Journal of Experimental Psychology Monograph Supplement, 76*(1, Pt. 2), 1–25.

Patterson, K., & Hodges, J. R. (1992). Deterioration of word meaning: Implications for reading. *Neuropsychologia, 30,* 1025–1040.

Perry, C., Ziegler, J., & Zorzi, M. (2007). Nested incremental modeling in the development of computational theories: The CDP+ model of reading aloud. *Psychological Review, 114*(2), 273–315.

Pexman, P. M., Hargreaves, I. S., Edwards, J. D., Henry, L. C., & Goodyear, B. G. (2007). Neural correlates of concreteness in semantic categorization. *Journal of Cognitive Neuroscience, 19*(8), 1407–1419.

Plaut, D. C., McClelland, J. L., Seidenberg, M. S., & Patterson, K. (1996). Understanding normal and impaired word reading: Computational principles in quasi-regular domains. *Psychological Review, 103*(1), 56–115.

Prabhakaran, R., Blumstein, S. E., Myers, E. B., Hutchison, E., & Britton, B. (2006). An event-related fMRI investigation of phonological–lexical competition. *Neuropsychologia, 44,* 2209–2221.

Pulvermüller, F., Shtyrov, Y., & Hauk, O. (2009). Understanding in an instant: Neurophysiological evidence for mechanistic language circuits in the brain. *Brain and Language, 110,* 81–94.

Richlan, F., Kronbichler, M., & Wimmer, H. (2009). Functional abnormalities in the dyslexic brain: A quantitative meta-analysis of neuroimaging studies. *Human Brain Mapping, 30*(10), 3299–3308.

Rohrer, J. D., Warren, J. D., Modat, M., Ridgway, G. R., Douiri, A., Rossor, M. N., et al. (2009). Patterns of cortical thinning in the language variants of frontotemporal lobar degeneration. *Neurology, 72,* 1562–1569.

Sabsevitz, D. S., Medler, D. A., Seidenberg, M., & Binder, J. R. (2005). Modulation of the semantic system by word imageability. *NeuroImage, 27,* 188–200.

Salmon, D. P., Butters, N., & Chan, A. S. (1999). The deterioration of semantic memory in Alzheimer's disease. *Canadian Journal of Experimental Psychology, 53*(1), 108–116.

Schilling, H. H., Rayner, K., & Chumbley, J. I. (1998). Comparing naming, lexical decision, and eye fixation times: Word frequency effects and individual differences. *Memory and Cognition, 26*(6), 1270–1281.

Schwanenflugel, P. J. (1991). Why are abstract concepts hard to understand? In P. J. Schwanenflugel (Ed.), *The psychology of word meanings* (pp. 223–250). Hillsdale, NJ: Erlbaum.

Seidenberg, M. S., & McClelland, J. L. (1989). A distributed, developmental model of word recognition and naming. *Psychological Review, 96*(4), 523–568.

Seidenberg, M. S., Waters, G. S., Barnes, M., & Tanenhaus, M. K. (1984). When does irregular spelling or pronunciation influence word recognition? *Journal of Verbal Learning and Verbal Behavior, 23,* 383–404.

Shallice, T. (1988). *From neuropsychology to mental structure*. New York: Cambridge University Press.

Shibahara, N., Zorzi, M., Hill, M. P., Wydell, T., & Butterworth, B. (2003). Semantic effects in word naming: Evidence from English and Japanese Kanji. *Quarterly Journal of Experimental Psychology, 56A*(2), 263–286.

Simos, P. G., Breier, J. I., Fletcher, J. M., Foorman, B. R., Castillo, E. M., & Papanicolaou, A. C. (2002). Brain mechanisms for reading words and pseudowords: An integrated approach. *Cerebral Cortex, 12*, 297–305.

Strain, E., & Herdman, C. M. (1999). Imageability effects in word naming: An individual differences analysis. *Canadian Journal of Experimental Psychology, 53*(4), 347–359.

Strain, E., Patterson, K., Graham, N., & Hodges, J. R. (1998). Word reading in Alzheimer's disease: cross-sectional and longitudinal analyses of response time and accuracy data. *Neuropsychologia, 36*(2), 155–171.

Strain, E., Patterson, K., & Seidenberg, M. S. (1995). Semantic effects in single-word naming. *Journal of Experimental Psychology: Learning Memory and Cognition, 21*, 1140–1154.

Taraban, R., & McClelland, J. L. (1987). Conspiracy effects in word recognition. *Journal of Memory and Language, 26*, 608–631.

Toglia, M. P., & Battig, W. F. (1978). *Handbook of semantic word norms*. Hillsdale, NJ: Erlbaum.

West, W. C., & Holcomb, P. J. (2000). Imaginal, semantic, and surface-level processing of concrete and abstract words: An electrophysiological investigation. *Journal of Cognitive Neuroscience, 12*(6), 1024–1037.

Whatmough, C., Chertkow, H., Murtha, S., Templeman, D., Babins, L., & Kelner, N. (2003). The semantic category effect increases with worsening anomia in Alzheimer's type dementia. *Brain and Language, 84*, 134–147.

Wilson, B. A. (1994). Syndromes of acquired dyslexia and patterns of recovery: A 6- to 10-year follow-up study of seven brain-injured people. *Journal of Clinical and Experimental Neuropsychology, 16*(3), 354–371.

Wilson, S. M., Brambati, S. M., Henry, R. G., Handwerker, D. A., Agosta, F., Miller, B. L., et al. (2009). The neural basis of surface dyslexia in semantic dementia. *Brain, 132*, 71–86.

Wilson, S. M., Isenberg, A. L., & Hickok, G. (2009). Neural correlates of word production stages delineated by parametric modulation of psycholinguistic variables. *Human Brain Mapping, 30*, 3596–3608.

Woollams, A. M. (2005). Imageability and ambiguity effects in speeded naming: Convergence and divergence. *Journal of Experimental Psychology: Learning Memory and Cognition, 31*(5), 878–890.

Woollams, A. M., Lambon Ralph, M. A., Plaut, D. C., & Patterson, K. (2007). SD-squared: On the association between semantic dementia and surface dyslexia. *Psychological Review, 114*(2), 316–339.

Yarkoni, T., Speer, N. K., Balota, D. A., McAvoy, M. P., & Zacks, J. M. (2008). Pictures of a thousand words: Investigating the neural mechanisms of reading with extremely rapid event-related fMRI. *NeuroImage, 42*, 973–987.

10

In a Word: ERPs Reveal Important Lexical Variables for Visual Word Processing

Chia-lin Lee and Kara D. Federmeier

Words are a language system's building blocks, making the apprehension and recognition of words one of the most fundamental language skills. Because words encapsulate different kinds of information, successful comprehension involves bringing online and integrating a number of diverse processes, such as analyzing the physical features of the incoming string, retrieving meaning representations and grammatical usages, and, eventually, relating the appropriate meaning and grammatical function to the larger discourse context. Given the complexity of these interwoven processes and their critical role in language comprehension, it is not surprising that word processing has been one of the most intensively studied topics in psycholinguistics.

In the psycholinguistic literature, a number of lexical features – including frequency, word class, concreteness, and ambiguity, among others – have been recognized for their robust influences on the process of recognizing words. Although such variables are often treated as independent and unitary, in this chapter we will review research using electrophysiological methods that expands this view by showing that some classic lexical effects documented in uni-dimensional behavioral measurements like response time or accuracy actually consist of multiple sub-effects. In particular, this body of work suggests that individual lexical features impact multiple aspects of the temporally distributed process of word recognition. Furthermore, these features are not independent dimensions, as they importantly modulate one another's influences.

The measurement of brain electrophysiology offers an importantly different perspective on word recognition because it provides a temporally precise, continuous, and multidimensional view of cognitive and neural processing. Event-related

The Handbook of the Neuropsychology of Language, First Edition. Edited by Miriam Faust.
© 2012 Blackwell Publishing Ltd. Published 2012 by Blackwell Publishing Ltd.

potentials (ERPs) measure brain electrical activity (derived from the continuous electroencephalogram or EEG) that is time-locked to a particular sensory, cognitive, or motor event (Fabiani, Gratton, & Federmeier, 2007). Because they are a direct assessment of brain activity and can track that activity on a millisecond level, ERPs provide the opportunity to continuously monitor processing and to measure temporally transient effects. ERPs are also a multidimensional measure, indexing multiple features (including amplitude, latency, and distribution) of multiple components linked to different aspects of neurocognitive functioning. Thus, ERPs offer the opportunity to observe different types of effects that may not be distinguishable in behavioral measures and/or that may occur too quickly to be captured by most other methods (for more details on this method, see Kutas, Kiang, & Sweeney, Volume 2, Chapter 26).

In this chapter, we review four widely recognized lexical features in turn: lexical frequency, word class (with a focus on the noun/verb distinction), linguistic concreteness, and lexical semantic ambiguity. Within the discussion for each lexical feature, we first provide a brief overview of the relevant behavioral and eye-tracking literature, then relate these findings to ERP studies that reveal the multifaceted nature of the effect in question, and finally discuss how the sub-effects highlighted by ERP studies may be influenced by information from other lexical features or from the larger language context. Taken together, these studies highlight the multidimensionality of the organization of the mental lexicon. They also tend to align well with more interactive views of lexical processing, in suggesting that word recognition is a flexible and dynamic process that is sensitive to features within the lexical item itself as well as to information in the surrounding linguistic context.

Lexical Frequency

Word frequency refers to the probability of occurrence of a given word in a language and reflects the accumulated experience one is likely to have had with that word. To estimate the frequency of a word, most studies have relied on calculating the number of occurrences of a certain written word form in a published corpus (e.g., Francis & Kucera, 1982). Although these can sometimes be dissociated, the frequency of a given word form oftentimes highly correlates with the frequency of its referent concept.

Effects of frequency are well documented and, accordingly, frequency has gained a prominent place in various models of word recognition (e.g., Becker, 1980; Morton, 1969; Norris, 1986). Overall, it has been found that higher-frequency words are associated with a number of processing advantages. Relative to lower-frequency words, readers tend to spend less time gazing at higher-frequency words (Just & Carpenter, 1980; Rayner & Sereno, 1994), and higher-frequency words can be named more quickly (Schilling, Rayner, & Chumbley, 1998), responded to faster in lexical decision tasks (Rubenstein, Garfield, & Millikan, 1970), and identified with shorter exposures (Solomon & Howes, 1951).

In the ERP literature, frequency has been found to modulate electrical brain responses at multiple time points during the course of word recognition. Effects of lexical frequency (or of the frequency of letter combinations; e.g., bigram and trigram frequency) have sometimes been reported within the first 200 ms after word presentation (e.g., Bles, Alink, & Jansma, 2007; Hauk, Davis, Ford, Pulvermüller, & Marslen-Wilson, 2006; Proverbio, Vecchi, & Zani, 2004), as amplitude modulations of sensory evoked responses. Word frequency has also been shown to affect the latency of a left lateralized anterior negativity between 200 and 400 ms (frequency sensitive negativity, FSN, or lexical processing negativity, LPN; King & Kutas, 1998; Munte et al., 2001; Osterhout, Bersick, & McKinnon, 1997) and the amplitude of the N400 between about 250 and 550 ms (for example, Bentin, McCarthy, & Wood, 1985; Rugg, 1990; van Petten & Kutas, 1990). Consistent with the more general sensitivities of these components to physical or semantic aspects of word processing, these frequency effects have been demonstrated to be differentially modulated by information related to physical or semantic aspects of a word.

Early frequency effects

Several studies have noted early ERP effects of lexical frequency or of the frequency of letter combinations (e.g., bigram and trigram frequency). Proverbio et al. (2004), for example, measured responses to real words, pseudowords and nonwords as participants performed a phoneme monitoring task. The results showed that word frequency modulated the response of the central-parietal P150, with more positive responses to higher- than lower-frequency words. Interestingly, this frequency effect was NOT sensitive to the lexical status of the stimuli: P150 amplitudes did not differ between low-frequency real words and well-formed pseudowords. Similar results were found by Hauk and colleagues (2006), who used a regression approach to examine the effects of frequency along with word length, orthographic n-gram frequency, and lexicality. They reported frequency effects as early as 110 ms, with decreased amplitudes for higher-frequency words. Effects of other surface variables such as length and n-gram frequency were similarly early, whereas the lexicality effect started at around 160 ms.

These early effects tend to be less robust and more variable across studies compared to later frequency effects. When they occur, they are usually associated with aspects of the brain response that are common to stimulus types other than words and that have been closely linked to sensory analysis and attention. For example, the P150 is elicited by images resembling any well-learned visual category and is particularly prominent for faces (Schendan, Ganis, & Kutas, 1998). Furthermore, the fact that these responses are typically similar for words and pseudowords suggests that they reflect some aspect of perceptual fluency driven by readers' experience with orthographic patterns in their language rather than by lexical frequency per se.

Frequency sensitive negativity (FSN)

Another lexical frequency effect has been observed in a slightly later time window over anterior electrode sites. Osterhout and colleagues (1997), looking at the response to words embedded in congruent or randomized prose passages, found an early negativity immediately followed the Nl-P2 complex that was sensitive to frequency, with higher-frequency words eliciting an earlier peaking negativity. This frequency effect was shown to be insensitive to the semantic congruency of the passage in which the words were embedded, but was found to interact with another physical feature of words, namely length: for words presented in both coherent text and randomized prose, the negativity's peak latency was negatively correlated with word frequency but positively correlated with length. Interactions between word frequency and word length on early effects have also been reported in other studies (Assadollahi & Pulvermüller, 2003).

A similar negativity (termed the frequency sensitive negativity, FSN, or lexical processing negativity, LPN) was also examined in King and Kutas (1998). With words presented in normal sentence contexts, King and Kutas observed a frontally distributed negativity whose peak latency varied as a function of lexical frequency, ranging between 280 and 340 ms postword onset. To isolate this early negativity from temporally overlapping slow potentials, King and Kutas obtained peak latencies from high-pass filtered ERPs. Regressions showed a negative linear correlation between the latency of the FSN and normalized word frequency, with high-frequency words (>10,000 per million) peaking at around 280 ms postword onset, medium-frequency words (~500 per million) at around 310 ms, and low-frequency words (<10 per million) at around 340 ms. King and Kutas found that after high-pass filtering, this negativity was not modulated by word length. However, similar to what was found in Osterhout et al. (1997), this high-pass filtered negativity was insensitive to higher-order word properties, such as the open/closed word class distinction (see Munte et al., 2001, for similar findings). Thus, effects of frequency within the first 300 or so milliseconds of word processing, although sometimes found to interact with other physical features of a word, have been largely shown to be separable from lexical class differences (e.g., open vs. closed class words) and syntactic/semantic processing.

N400 frequency effect

Various studies have found that the amplitude of the N400 is smaller in response to high- than low-frequency words (e.g., Rugg, 1990; Smith & Halgren, 1987; van Petten & Kutas, 1990), a pattern that suggests that more experience with a given word form facilitates semantic access. However, this particular frequency effect has been shown to interact with a variety of other factors that influence the ease of semantic processing, including word repetition (Rugg, 1990), ordinal word position in semantically congruent sentences (van Petten, 1993; van Petten & Kutas, 1990, 1991), and the predictability of a word in its context (Dambacher, Kliegl, Hofmann, & Jacobs, 2006).

For example, although lower-frequency words occurring near the beginning of sentences elicit larger N400s compared to higher-frequency words, this effect diminishes quickly over the course of a semantically congruent sentence (van Petten, 1993; van Petten & Kutas, 1990, 1991). Indeed, the N400s elicited by lower- and higher-frequency words are no longer statistically distinguishable beyond the fifth word of congruent sentences (van Petten, 1993). The N400 frequency effect is also reduced or eliminated when semantic access is facilitated by repetition, both in word lists and in sentence contexts (Besson, Kutas, & van Petten, 1992; Rugg, 1990; Smith & Halgren, 1987). Interestingly, however, the N400 word frequency effect appears to be insensitive to syntactic constraints, as it persists throughout the course of word streams that maintain legal syntactic structure without providing coherent semantic information (van Petten, 1993; van Petten & Kutas, 1991). Thus, frequency continues to affect processing at stages in which word forms are being mapped onto meaning, but its import is diminished in the face of other factors that affect the accessibility of semantic information.

Summary

Taken together, these studies suggest that accumulated language experience, as indexed by word frequency, affects processing throughout word recognition. It facilitates word perception in a number of ways, as indexed by changes in the amplitude of sensory-related components such as the P150, as well as reductions in the latency of the FSN. It also seems to be one of many factors that can ease semantic access, as indexed by N400 amplitude reductions.

Noun/Verb Word Class Distinction

Different kinds of words play different kinds of roles in language, making syntactic word class (e.g. nouns, verbs, adjectives, etc.) a critical factor for word processing. In particular, among content words, the distinction between nouns and verbs has been intensively studied and has been shown to play out in important ways in a variety of language and memory processes, including children's early lexical development (Gentner, 1982), memory performance (Reynolds & Flagg, 1976), and patterns of language deficits (McCarthy & Warrington, 1985; Miceli, Silveri, Nocentini, & Caramazza, 1988; Myerson & Goodglass, 1972).

In general, nouns and verbs differ along various dimensions, including average frequency, age of acquisition, lexical neighborhood density, number of semantic associates, and mutability of meanings (Gentner, 1981; Szekely et al., 2005). Much research has been devoted to singling out a critical dimension to account for the behavioral differences elicited by the two word classes. Some work has focused on the grammatical characteristics of these two word classes, such as the pivotal role of verbs for sentence construction (Berndt, Haendiges, Mitchum, & Sandson, 1997; Saffran, Schwartz, & Marin, 1980; Shapiro, Zurif, & Grimshaw, 1987) or the heavier morphological loading of verbs (Longe, Randall, Stamatakis, & Tyler, 2007). Other work has highlighted the differences in the semantic features associated with prototypical nouns and verbs, arguing that nouns and verbs tend to differ in their conceptual complexity, their degree of concreteness (Berndt et al., 1997; Williams & Canter, 1987), or their perceptual and functional/associative features (Bird, Howard, & Franklin, 2000; Marshall, Pring, Chiat, & Robson, 1996). All of these factors may well be important, and, indeed, noun/verb word class effects in behavior may be a composite manifestation of multiple kinds of processing differences.

For example, in a series of ERP studies, we have examined the processing of nouns and verbs in syntactically well-specified contexts (Federmeier, Segal, Lombrozo, & Kutas, 2000; Lee & Federmeier, 2006). To avoid potential limitations in generalizing to word class differences from more restricted subtypes of words (e.g., action verbs vs. object nouns), these studies included a wide range of nouns and verbs (including concrete and abstract nouns as well as action and nonaction verbs) matched for important lexical features and amount of preceding context. In light of the prevalence of word class ambiguity and the modulations of noun/verb effects by word class ambiguity that have been documented in the lesion literature (Jonkers & Bastiaanse, 1998; Kemmerer & Tranel, 2000), word class ambiguous words were treated as a separate category. Thus, effects could be assessed specifically for words that are exclusively or predominantly used as either nouns or verbs (e.g., word class unambiguous nouns like "beer" and word class unambiguous verbs like "eat"), and these could be compared with effects on word class ambiguous words used as nouns or verbs (e.g., "to drink" vs. "the drink"). Word class was cued by sentential (e.g., "Jane wanted to/the . . ."; Federmeier et al., 2000) or phrasal (e.g., "to/the . . ."; Lee & Federmeier, 2006) contexts that also served to specify the grammatical category for the ambiguous words. The results of these studies revealed two major noun/verb effects.

N400 word class effect

For both ambiguous and unambiguous words, nouns elicited more negative N400 responses (between 250 and 450 ms over central/posterior sites) than did verbs (Federmeier et al., 2000; Lee & Federmeier, 2006); see Figure 10.1. This is consistent with N400 response differences observed between nouns and verbs occurring in natural short passages (Osterhout et al., 1997) as well as for pairs of nouns and verbs in a lexical decision task (Rosler, Streb, & Haan, 2001). The fact that class ambiguous words also showed this pattern is in line with previous findings showing that, in the presence of disambiguating syntactic information, the

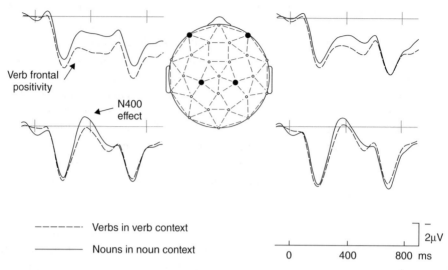

- - - - -	Verbs in verb context	
————	Nouns in noun context	

Figure 10.1   Noun/verb word class effects for word class unambiguous items. For this and all subsequent figures, data are shown at a subset of representative electrode sites indicated by enlarged circles on the head diagram. In the anterior region, verbs used in a verb-predicting context elicited an enhanced frontal positivity (200–400 ms post-stimulus-onset) relative to nouns used in a noun-predicting context. In the central/posterior region, nouns elicit more negative amplitudes than verbs on the N400 component. Data reported in Federmeier et al. (2000).

processing of these words tends to align with whatever word class the context indicates (e.g., Brown, Lehmann, & Marsh, 1980; Caramazza & Hillis, 1991). Overall, the fact that these noun/verb effects are seen in the form of amplitude – but *not* topographic (Gomes, Ritter, Tartter, Vaughan, & Rosen, 1997; Khader, Scherag, Streb, & Rösler, 2003) – shifts on the N400, a component elicited by all open class words, suggests that at this stage processing differences between nouns and verbs are quantitative rather than qualitative in nature, perhaps reflecting the number or type of semantic features associated with these word classes (or, in the case of ambiguous words, called up in response to the same word form when it is used as a noun or a verb).

Frontal positivity effect

In addition to quantitative processing differences on the N400, a frontally distributed positivity in response to verbs was evident between 200 and 400 ms post-stimulus-onset (Federmeier et al., 2000; Lee & Federmeier, 2006); see Figure 10.1. Unlike the effect pattern on the N400, this frontal positivity was seen only for word class unambiguous verbs and not for ambiguous words used as verbs (i.e., "Jane wanted to *drink* . . ." did not elicit this effect). Furthermore, the effect was seen only when the word class unambiguous verbs were in grammatically appropriate, verb-predicting contexts; the same lexical items did not elicit this effect when used in syntactically anomalous contexts, such as "Tom liked the *eat* . . .". The results thus extended previous observations of verb-specific frontal positivities with subsets of nouns and verbs (Dehaene, 1995: action verbs vs. animal names and proper names; Preissl, Pulvermüller, Lutzenberger, & Birbaumer, 1995: concrete nouns vs. action verbs) and further revealed that this processing difference reflects both the long-term and immediate syntactic environment in which a word occurs.

Summary

Together, these results suggest that the distinction between nouns and verbs encompasses a constellation of linguistic features and functions, which trigger different patterns of neurological responses over the course of word recognition. Behavioral processing differences are thus likely to arise from multiple sources, including both differences in the amount or type of semantic information accessed from nouns and verbs, as reflected by the N400 word class effect, and differences in the grammatical functions that these words can play and are playing within a particular context, as indicated by the frontal positivity to unambiguous verbs.

Linguistic Concreteness

Linguistic concreteness – i.e., the extent to which an expression describes a concept that can be perceived by the senses – has also been shown to have robust effects on language processing, in addition to various other cognitive processes such as free recall, recognition memory, and paired-associate learning (see the review by Paivio, Yuille, & Madigan, 1968). With respect to language processing, it has been found that concrete words are responded to more quickly in lexical decision tasks (Schwanenflugel, Harnishfeger, & Stowe, 1988) and are read aloud with higher accuracy and fewer semantic errors by deep dyslexic patients (Gerhand & Barry, 2000). The benefits of linguistic concreteness are also seen at the sentence processing level: concrete sentences are comprehended more quickly and accurately than are abstract sentences (Haberlandt & Graesser, 1985; Schwanenflugel & Shoben, 1983) and are responded to faster in tasks involving judging meaningfulness (Holmes & Langford, 1976) and truthfulness (Belmore, Yates, Bellack, Jones, & Rosenquist, 1982).

 Several hypotheses have been put forward to account for the behavioral processing advantages observed for concrete words; among the more prominent of these are the dual-coding theory and the context availability theory. In his dual-coding theory, Paivio (1969, 1991) hypothesized that imagery is a critical determinant of concreteness-based processing differences. In particular, dual-coding theory posits that concrete words accrue a processing advantage because they can be accessed via both the imagery system and the verbal system (also used to store and process abstract words). In contrast, unitary semantic system accounts, such as the context availability theory (Schwanenflugel, 1991; Schwanenflugel et al., 1988) argue that the concreteness advantage comes from the richer availability of contextual information for concrete words. Support for this account comes from observations that the robust effects of concreteness seen for words presented in isolation or deprived of contextual information (e.g. in random sentential/paragraph contexts) are attenuated when words are repeated or are encountered in richer, semantically coherent contexts (Marschark, 1985; Paivio, Clark, & Khan, 1988; Schwanenflugel & Shoben, 1983).

Recent ERP studies, however, have instead uncovered data patterns suggestive of an account that combines elements of both views. Holcomb and colleagues (Holcomb, Kounios, Anderson, & West, 1999; Kounios & Holcomb, 1994; West & Holcomb, 2000) found that concrete words were associated with more negative-going potentials, beginning in the time window of the N400 component and continuing to up to 800 ms. Unlike the central/posterior focus for typical N400 effects, this concreteness-based difference was most pronounced over frontal scalp sites. The effect was more robust for tasks that tap more heavily into semantic processing (Kounios & Holcomb, 1994; West & Holcomb, 2000) but was strongly attenuated when concrete and abstract words were put into predictive sentence contexts (Holcomb et al., 1999) or were repeated (Kounios & Holcomb, 1994).

On the one hand, the scalp distributional differences between concrete and abstract words support dual-coding accounts in suggesting that different neural resources are involved in processing the two categories of words. On the other hand, however, the fact that the differences are observed in the time window of the N400 – a component that has been strongly linked to semantic processing (Kutas & Federmeier, 2000) – is suggestive that concreteness effects may be at least partially based on the richness of the words' semantic associations. Moreover, that the effect diminishes when semantic access is facilitated also makes clear that, as predicted by context availability theory, contextual manipulations can modulate concreteness-based processing differences. Based on their findings, therefore, Holcomb and colleagues have proposed the "context extended dual-coding hypothesis," which states that a complete account of concreteness effects must include not only multiple semantic codes for representing and processing the two different word types, to account for the topographic differences, but also a contextual component, to account for the context-based modulations (Holcomb et al., 1999).

The hypothesis that the impact of concreteness is mediated through multiple neurocognitive mechanisms is further corroborated by recent findings suggesting that the ERP concreteness effect itself is made up of dissociable subcomponents. In particular, the increased negativity to concrete words seems to reflect separable responses over central/posterior and frontal electrode sites, which are differentially sensitive to linguistic and task manipulations and have different neurophysiological sources.

Posterior concreteness effect

The posterior concreteness effect between 250 and 450 ms has been linked to modulations of the classical N400 component, with more negative amplitudes to concrete than to abstract words, when these words are encountered out of context. The effect is consistent across word classes, including nouns, verbs, and adjectives (Huang, Lee, & Federmeier, 2010; Lee & Federmeier, 2008), as well as words with different variations of lexical ambiguities, such as word class ambiguity (e.g. "to vote" vs. "the vote") and semantic ambiguity (e.g. "to watch" vs. "the watch"; Lee & Federmeier, 2008); see Figure 10.2. Given what is known about the functional sensitivity of the N400 (Federmeier & Laszlo, 2009), it seems likely that these processing differences arise from general semantic properties of words, such as the richness of the featural information that they evoke, and are mediated through basic mechanisms

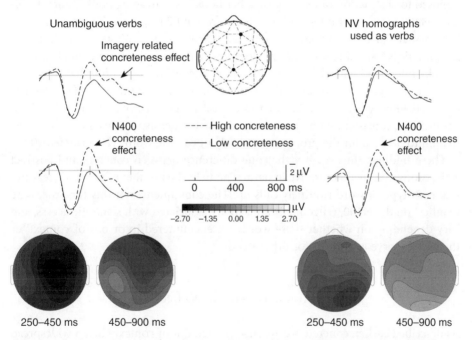

Figure 10.2 Concreteness effects for unambiguous verbs (left) and ambiguous words used as verbs (right). Unambiguous high concreteness verbs are more negative than low concreteness verbs. The negativity at central/posterior sites peaks around 400 ms (N400), whereas at frontal sites the difference due to concreteness extends to later parts of the epoch. Ambiguous words used as verbs show a similar concreteness effect over posterior but *not* frontal sites. The separability of the frontal and posterior effects is also shown in the isopotential voltage maps (bottom). For unambiguous verbs, the concreteness effect is widespread between 250 and 450 ms, and restricted to the anterior region between 450 and 900 ms. For ambiguous verbs, however, the effect is only apparent in the posterior region, in the earlier time window. Data reported in Lee & Federmeier (2008).

of semantic access. The hypothesis that highly concrete words may be associated with a richer set of semantic associations than less concrete words is supported by findings from a recurrent connectionist model (Plaut & Shallice, 1993) that defines concreteness as the number of associated semantic features and thereby successfully simulates the classic concreteness effect in deep dyslexia.

If the posterior concreteness effect seen to words out of context reflects differential effort involved in accessing words with many (concrete) as opposed to fewer (abstract) semantic features, then this effect should be attenuated in the presence of congruent context information that could serve to preactivate those features. Indeed, when concrete and abstract nouns are embedded in semantically constraining contexts, the posterior concreteness effect is attenuated or eradicated (Holcomb et al., 1999; Swaab, Baynes, & Knight, 2002). Furthermore, the same difference in richness of semantic feature information that makes concrete expressions harder to access out of context might render them more constraining contexts for words that follow them. Huang et al. (2010) showed that nouns preceded by concrete as opposed to abstract modifiers (e.g. "leather book" vs. "engaging book") elicit facilitated N400 responses (along with enhanced frontal P2 responses, a pattern that has been associated with increased contextual constraint; e.g., Wlotko & Federmeier, 2007). This N400 reduction was limited to cases in which the noun could be meaningfully integrated with the preceding adjectival context, suggesting that it was the activation of specific features of the nouns that was important. The effect was also observed only when processing of the critical nouns was biased toward the left hemisphere, consistent with views that only the left hemisphere uses context information to prepare for the processing of likely upcoming words (Federmeier, 2007).

These findings thus suggest that one difference between concrete and abstract expressions may be quantitative in nature: namely, the number of semantic features that each type of word routinely calls up. The consequences of this for processing manifest on the N400, reflecting brain activity associated with semantic access, and vary depending on whether these words are encountered in or out of context, or themselves serve as context for other words.

Frontal concreteness effect

As described earlier, concrete words encountered out of context elicit a widespread negativity relative to less concrete words. The concreteness-related negativity, however, is more long lasting over frontal scalp sites; for example, as seen in Figure 10.2, it is evident between 250 and 900 ms post-word-onset in Lee and Federmeier (2008). Similar frontally distributed negative potentials are also elicited in studies of mental imagery (taking into account differences in reference site; Farah, Weisberg, Monheit, & Peronnet, 1989). In addition, although this effect can arise without instructions or task demands that would bias participants to image (Huang et al., 2010), it has been shown to be enhanced by tasks that encourage mental imagery (West & Holcomb, 2000). Consequently, the frontal concreteness effect has been taken to reflect the mental simulation of sensory experience triggered by the meaning of a word, something that is perhaps exclusively available for concrete expressions.

Unlike the posterior concreteness effect, the frontal concreteness effect is not attenuated by supportive contextual information. Swaab et al. (2002) compared ERPs to highly imageable and less imageable words when these were preceded by related context (e.g., "pig" – "leopard"; "atom" – "molecule") or unrelated context (e.g., "wheat" – "slipper"; "pace" – "dispute"). Brain responses to the target (second) words were more negative over frontal electrode sites between 350 and 650 post-word-onset for highly imageable than less imageable words, irrespective of semantic relatedness. Whereas context does not eliminate this effect, it can modulate it – for example, in the case of words that can be understood with either a more concrete or a more abstract interpretation (e.g., the physical sense and the intellectual sense of the word "book"). In the Huang et al. (2010) study, polysemous nouns preceded by modifiers inducing a concrete reading (e.g., "hilly farm") elicited a frontal nega-tivity (500–900 ms) compared to the same nouns preceded by modifiers inducing an abstract meaning (e.g., "productive farm"). Interestingly, this effect was only observed when processing was biased towards the right hemisphere, and only when the modifier could be meaningfully integrated with the noun. The fact that the frontal effect seems to arise from right hemisphere processing mechanisms is con-sistent with more general data linking the right hemisphere to imagery processes (e.g., Ehrlichman & Barrett, 1983; Kosslyn, 1987) and provides a strong dissociation between this effect and concreteness effects over posterior regions, which were associated with left-hemisphere-biased processing.

Thus, the elicitation of concrete conceptual information from a word or phrase seems to trigger the simulation of sensory experience (imagery), reflected in frontal negativity (see Bergen, Lindsay, Matlock, & Narayanan, 2007, for similar findings with behavioral measures). This predicts that, under certain circumstances, the frontal concreteness effect may be delayed or even suppressed if the prerequisite conceptual activation is difficult or prolonged – for example, if words are associated with multiple meanings, such that ambiguity needs to be resolved before imagery can take place. This prediction is born out in a study examining how concreteness interacts with semantic/syntactic ambiguity, comparing the processing of unam-biguous words (e.g., "desk," "eat"), words with syntactic ambiguity only (e.g., "taste," which has related noun and verb senses), and words with both syntactic and seman-tic ambiguity (e.g., "register," which has unrelated noun and verb senses), in the context of a grammatical cue (e.g., "to" or "the") specifying the word class of the ambiguous words (Lee & Federmeier, 2008). The frontal concreteness effect was seen for all nouns regardless of ambiguity type (e.g., "the desk/plan/bat") and for verbs without semantic ambiguity (e.g., "to eat/plan"). Strikingly, however, this effect was *not* seen for syntactically and semantic ambiguous items used as verbs (e.g. "to register"); see Figure 10.2. Similar results have also been found in the behavioral literature. For example, Eviatar, Menn, and Zaidel (1990), using a lexical decision task, found that word class ambiguous verbs (with some degree of semantic ambiguity) failed to show the concreteness-based facilitation effect. Given that the meaning of verbs seems to be more context dependent, ambiguity resolution may be more difficult and/or take longer when a lexical item is used as a verb.

Summary

Collectively, the studies reviewed in this section suggest that linguistic concreteness has impacts on multiple aspects of neurocognitive processing – reflecting, for example, both the richness of associated semantic information as well as the possibility/efficacy of imagery processes. Whereas the central/posterior (N400) concreteness effect is a modulation of a process that is elicited by both concrete and abstract words and across word types, the frontal, imagery-related concreteness effect seems to involve an extra process that may be induced only by concrete items. Both effects are sensitive to the availability of semantic information, as modulated by context, albeit in different ways.

Lexical Semantic Ambiguity

Yet another factor that has been shown to greatly affect word processing is ambiguity. Ambiguity is a central feature of language at many processing levels; at the level of words, it is well documented that a single spelling or pronunciation is oftentimes associated with multiple meaning senses. In English, for example, 44% of a random sampling of words and 85% of a sample of high-frequency words had more than one meaning (Twilley, Dixon, Taylor, & Clark, 1994). Among lexically ambiguous words, some are associated with closely related meanings, such as "twist" and "hammer," whereas others are associated with unrelated meanings, such as "organ" and "watch." And, as demonstrated by these examples, alternative meanings can belong to the same or to different parts of speech. Depending on the relationship among the alternative meanings available for a particular word form, lexical ambiguity has been categorized as either polysemous, when meanings are related, or homonymous, when unrelated. Although ambiguity is graded, for words that are at one or the other end of this spectrum and thus are easy to classify, polysemy and homonymy have been shown to have differing effects on reading behaviors. Whereas related meanings have been shown to facilitate word recognition, unrelated meanings have been found to slow processing times (e.g., Rodd, Gaskell, & Marslen-Wilson, 2002).

Processing costs for homonymous words, in the form of delayed reaction times or increased gaze measures, have been found even in the presence of syntactically disambiguating information (Seidenberg, Tanenhaus, Leiman, & Bienkowski, 1982; Tanenhaus, Leiman, & Seidenberg, 1979) or semantically biasing information, especially when context picks out nondominant interpretations (e.g., Duffy, Morris, & Rayner, 1988; Rayner, Pacht, & Duffy, 1994). Collectively, this literature suggests that multiple meanings are often activated even in the presence of contextual constraints.

Several theoretical accounts of the mechanisms of semantic ambiguity resolution have been put forward (e.g., Duffy, Kambe, & Rayner, 2001; Hogaboam & Perfetti, 1975; Paul, Kellas, Martin, & Clark, 1992; Rayner & Frazier, 1989). These theories vary in their assumptions about the autonomy of lexical activation and the general role of context in word recognition and language comprehension, but most, if not all, treat the processing costs that have been observed for ambiguous words as if they are unitary in nature and thus the same for ambiguous words encountered in different types of contextual environments. Whether different contextual information sources can critically alter how lexically ambiguous words are processed and what neural mechanisms are thus engaged is something that has rarely been discussed.

However, there are reasons to believe that different types of context information may affect lexical ambiguity resolution in different ways. First, semantic and syntactic contextual constraints differ in nature: syntactic constraints are oftentimes definitive but semantic constraints are more graded. For example, a sentence beginning "Paul liked the . . ." requires a noun phrase and thus would seem to rule out the verb use and meaning of an upcoming noun/verb (NV-) homograph such as "duck." In contrast, a sentence beginning "Mary searched in the bushes for the . . ." may favor the "tool" meaning of a subsequent ambiguous word "spade," but cannot rule out a continuation like ". . . spade, which had blown off the card table." On the other hand, syntactic constraints are likely to be considerably more general (e.g., requiring a noun but providing very little information about its features), whereas semantic constraints can be more specific. Semantic and syntactic information sources also differ in how they accrue across words and over time. Whereas semantic constraints build up incrementally over the course of a context, syntactic constraints seem more likely to operate locally. Semantically constraining contexts have been shown to lead to progressively faster word monitoring latencies and increasing N400 reduction over the course of sentences, but such accumulative effects were not found for syntactic contexts (e.g., Marslen-Wilson & Tyler, 1980; van Petten & Kutas, 1991). This difference between syntactic and semantic contextual constraints affects general word processing differently and thus could conceivably provide differential aids for lexical ambiguity resolution as well.

To examine this, we compared the influences of syntactic and semantic disambiguating information on ambiguity resolution for homographs whose meaning varies across word class (NV-homographs; Lee & Federmeier, 2009). We examined ERP responses to NV-homographs at the end of congruent sentences, which provide both a well-specified syntactic structure and constraining semantic information (e.g., "My grandpa said he hadn't played that game since he was a *kid*"), and embedded in syntactic prose, which offers identical syntactic cues but is semantically incoherent (e.g., "My board said he hadn't called that volcano since he was a *kid*"). The ERPs time-locked to the critical ambiguous words were then compared with those to matched unambiguous words in each type of context (e.g., "His

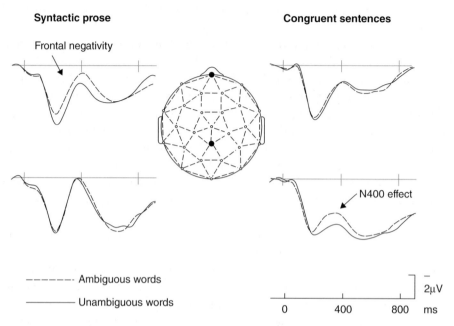

Figure 10.3 Ambiguity effects in congruent and syntactic prose sentences. In syntactic prose sentences (left), responses to ambiguous words (e.g. "the season/to season") are more negative than those to unambiguous words (e.g. "the logic/to eat") over frontal channels (200–700 ms). In congruent sentences (right), there is no enhanced frontal negativity. Instead, ambiguous words are more negative over central/posterior sites in the N400 time window (250–500 ms). Data reported in Lee & Federmeier (2009).

job at the store was his only source of *income*"; "His lot at the submarine was his big pet of *income*"). The results revealed qualitatively different processing consequences for homographs preceded by disambiguating syntactic versus semantic information.

Ambiguity resolution in the context of syntactic constraints

In the syntactic prose condition (left panel of Figure 10.3), NV-homographs elicited a prolonged frontal negativity (200–700 ms) relative to unambiguous words. This frontal effect replicates patterns in other studies, such as when NV-homographs are in midsentence positions of syntactically congruent but semantically unconstraining sentences (e.g., "Jeremy wanted to/the *watch* even though . . ."; Federmeier et al., 2000) or follow a single, syntactically constraining cue (e.g., "to/the watch"; Lee & Federmeier, 2006). The effect is not simply due to syntactic ambiguity, since word class ambiguous items whose meanings are very similar across their noun and verb senses (e.g., "drink") do not elicit this response (Lee & Federmeier, 2006). Similar effects have also been seen in cases that do not involve syntactic ambiguity, such as when there are multiple possible referents for a pronoun (van Berkum, Brown, Hagoort, & Zwitserlood, 2003; van Berkum, Hagoort, & Brown, 1999). Thus, the frontal negativity appears to be linked to processes of selecting among alternative referents, and is seen under conditions in which syntactic but *not* semantic constraints are available to aid with ambiguity resolution.

The idea that the frontal negativity indexes a controlled selection process receives support from several sources. Similar sustained frontal negativities have been observed in conjunction with working memory demands (King & Kutas, 1995) and the need to maintain and select among candidate items during recollection (Rugg, Allan, & Birch, 2000). Moreover, data from other imaging methods point to frontal lobe sources for selection-related brain activity. A number of hemodynamic imaging studies have reported frontal activation (for example, in the inferior frontal gyrus, either bilaterally or with a left hemisphere focus) associated with the resolution of lexical ambiguity (e.g., Mason & Just, 2007; Rodd, Davis, & Johnsrude, 2005; Zempleni, Renken, Hoeks, Hoogduin, & Stowe, 2007). In particular, Gennari, MacDonald, Postle, and Seidenberg (2007) used a design very similar to that of Lee and Federmeier (2006), with NV-homographs embedded in minimal syntactic phrases (e.g., "to/the bowl"), and found activations in the left inferior frontal gyrus that they linked to selection among competing semantic attributes. In turn, the conclusions of these hemodynamic imaging studies of ambiguity resolution are supported by more general results from the neuropsychological literature, which link frontal lobe damage to deficits in selecting relevant representations among competitors, including – but not limited to – tasks involving semantic ambiguity resolution (Metzler, 2001; Robinson, Blair, & Cipolotti, 1998; Thompson-Schill et al., 1998). This body of data thus suggests that selecting among alternative meanings of ambiguous words sometimes involves the recruitment of (possibly domain-general) frontal lobe control processes, and that this is a mechanism engaged when such words are encountered in circumstances that demand selection (i.e., in the presence of syntactic constraints) but that provide little semantic support.

Ambiguity resolution in the context of semantic constraints

The presence of constraining semantic context information greatly reduces the N400 to both ambiguous and unambiguous sentence final words (right panel of Figure 10.3). Strikingly, in the context of this general facilitation for word processing, there is no reliable evidence of frontal negativity for the NV-homographs. In other words, during the processing of a constraining, congruent sentence, the accumulated (pre)activation of semantic information seems to mitigate the need for recruitment of the kind of controlled selection mechanisms indexed by the frontal negativity.

However, this does not mean that ambiguous and unambiguous words are now processed identically. As can be seen in Figure 10.3, N400 responses to ambiguous words are less facilitated by context than are those to unambiguous words, despite careful matching of the two conditions for lexical properties and, critically, context-based predictability as indexed by cloze probability (Taylor, 1953). A follow-up experiment (Experiment 2 of Lee & Federmeier, 2009) showed that this ambiguity-related N400 difference was limited to cases in which the context picked out an ambiguous word's nondominant meaning (whereas responses to homographs in dominant-biased contexts fully converged with those to unambiguous words). This pattern is thus consistent with behavioral findings of processing costs for ambiguous words even in the presence of the disambiguating semantic information, when nondominant meanings are selected (Rayner et al., 1994; Duffy et al., 2001). What the ERP data make clear, however, is that the processing costs seen in these circumstances and those incurred when ambiguous words are processed in syntactically well-specified but semantically neutral contexts are qualitatively different.

In both cases, the processing costs seen in behavioral measures (e.g., increased response times) have typically been linked to competition between simultaneously activated meanings. For example, the reordered access model (see Duffy et al., 2001, for a review) assumes that, out of context, multiple meanings of ambiguous words become active, to a degree proportional to their meaning dominance. Context information can then "reorder" the meanings by changing their relative activation strengths. Strong activation, and hence rapid access, of the dominant meaning would be expected when high meaning frequency is buttressed by contextual support, allowing processing to approximate that for unambiguous words (as seen in Lee & Federmeier, 2009). However, subordinate-biased contexts will boost non-dominant meaning activation, making the activation levels of the two meanings more similar; thus, both when ambiguous words are encountered with little contextual support and when semantic context information is available but picks out a nondominant meaning, it is assumed that additional processes must be brought online to resolve the resultant competition.

The ERP data, however, tell a different story in suggesting that controlled selection mechanisms, linked to frontal brain activity, are necessary when semantic constraints are absent but *not* when nondominant meanings are picked out in the presence of semantically constraining context information. Although in the latter case there are residual processing differences between ambiguous and unambiguous words – which could have behavioral consequences – those ambiguity effects are of a qualitatively different nature. The larger N400 for ambiguous words in subordinate-biased contexts likely reflects a contextual mismatch created by residual activation of dominant meaning features. Importantly, however, it seems clear that the preactivation of subordinate-associated features from constraining semantic context information allows a sufficiently stable activation state to arise that the need for additional selection-related resources is mitigated, even in the face of residual automatic activation of dominant-associated meaning features. Thus, selection of a given sense of an ambiguous word need not entail fully selective access, in the form of activation limited to a single meaning.

Summary

The results across this pair of experiments are thus coherent with the behavioral literature in showing that neither syntactically nor semantically constraining context information can completely prevent the activation of alternative meanings of ambiguous words in all circumstances. Extending this literature, however, this set of data further suggests that similar behavioral processing costs (lengthened response times) for ambiguity resolution in different context types can arise from qualitatively different underlying neural mechanisms. When no biasing semantic constraints are available, arriving at the correct meaning of an ambiguous homograph (e.g., the one that fits a specified syntactic frame) involves the recruitment of (frontal lobe) selection-related resources, which manifest in the ERP signal in the form of a sustained frontal negativity. In contrast, when the context provides constraining semantic information, which facilitates semantic access, demands for these resources are reduced or eliminated. However, under these circumstances, contextually inappropriate meaning features may still become active to some extent, leading to reduced N400 facilitation for ambiguous as compared to unambiguous words, similar to patterns seen for unambiguous words that contain features that are unpredictable within a given context.

General Discussion

In this chapter, we reviewed electrophysiological research that highlights the multidimensional organization of the mental lexicon and the composite nature of word recognition. These studies show that a variety of attributes, including word frequency, word class, linguistic concreteness and lexico-semantic ambiguity, not only individually and jointly affect word recognition, but themselves consist of multiple sub-effects that impact multiple aspects of the temporally and spatially distributed processes of word recognition.

Recognizing a visual word involves mapping patterns of lines and curves onto stored knowledge of a given word form's associated semantic features, past experience with how that word form can be and is typically used in language, and the incrementally built representation of the current context in which the word form appears. It is thus not surprising that many different factors can render that mapping process easier or more difficult. For example, ease of semantic access, as indexed by the amplitude of the N400 component of the ERP, is affected by all of the variables discussed in the present chapter – not only by the richness and consistency of the semantic features associated with the word (concreteness and ambiguity), but also by whether the word form is being used as a noun or a verb, whether it is predictable in its context, and how often the connection between that letter string and its corresponding semantic features has been practiced, as in the case of higher-frequency words.

Indeed, the data make clear that the brain carefully tracks language experience on multiple levels, noting not only how often a given string has been processed (as indexed by frequency) but also specific aspects of how it has previously been used both syntactically and semantically. For example, if, in one's reading experience, a certain orthographic pattern has always been used as a verb, then verb-related information (as indexed by the verb frontal positivity) can be readily instantiated upon apprehending that word. However, if a given word form has previously been used as multiple word classes, this process is strikingly affected – even when context renders its current use unambiguous. Similarly, for words that have multiple discrete meaning senses, the more frequently a word is used in a context that supports a particular sense, the more dominant this sense will come to be. Later encounters, then, are highly shaped by this accumulated meaning dominance, such that, depending on the sense being picked out by the context, the recognition of an ambiguous word may be either indistinguishable from or more taxing than that for words with single meanings.

Furthermore, whereas some aspects of word processing seem fairly ubiquitous and are affected by a wide range of variables, as evidenced by patterns on the N400, other aspects of processing are more specific and brought online under particular circumstances. For example, the apprehension of concrete words is associated with imagery generation processes, which likely involve the automatic re-enactment of perceptual and motor states. However, a stable semantic state (one which seems more difficult to achieve for ambiguous words used as verbs), appears to be required before these processes can be initiated. In contrast, other processes are initiated by the *lack* of a stable semantic representation – such as those indexed by the frontal negativity associated with ambiguity, observed when semantic contextual constraints are unavailable to resolve the conflicting bottom-up information.

Given the diversity of the processes that could potentially be (and often are) involved in recognizing a word, a pivotal issue is how these processes are coordinated over time. The studies reviewed here suggest that although the involvement of some processes, such as imagery and controlled selection, is contingent on the (in)stability of the semantic state, the temporal onset of those effects nevertheless coincides with when information about a word's meaning features is just beginning to become available (as suggested by the timing of the N400). Thus, these processes seem to be initiated fairly rapidly and do not wait for meaning access to be completed but rather are carried out in parallel with it. Indeed, the data suggest that, perhaps due to the inherent time pressure created by the rapidity of normal language input, some processes simply do not occur if they are not initiated in time. Both the lack of a verb frontal positivity for word class ambiguous words and the lack of image-related negativity for doubly ambiguous words used in a verb context suggest that complications and/or delays in some aspects of word processing can lead to omissions of – or at least substantial delays in – other processes.

ERP data thus paint a picture of word recognition that is both more multifaceted and more dynamic than is sometimes assumed. We have shown that many lexical variables affect multiple aspects of word processing and that their effects are rarely independent of one another, or of the larger context in which a word occurs. In fact, although frequency, concreteness, word class, semantic ambiguity, and context effects seem very different linguistically, at least part of their influence on word recognition emerges from a common language processing mechanism – i.e., their respective effects on the N400, a component that seems to reflect a critical point in the temporally extended processing stream of word recognition, when many sources of information have simultaneous, interactive effects. More generally, the data show that what determines how lexical variables interact, what influence(s) they have, and even whether they have effects at all, is *time* . . . as successful and efficient word recognition requires that multifaceted and diverse information be brought together both over time and in time.

References

Assadollahi, R., & Pulvermüller, F. (2003). Early influences of word length and frequency: A group study using MEG. *Neuroreport, 14*(8), 1183–1187.

Becker, C. A. (1980). Semantic context effects in visual word recognition: An analysis of semantic strategies. *Memory and Cognition, 8*, 493–512.

Belmore, S. M., Yates, J. M., Bellack, D. R., Jones, S. N., & Rosenquist, S. E. (1982). Drawing inferences from concrete and abstract sentences. *Journal of Verbal Learning and Verbal Behavior, 21*, 338–351.

Bentin, S., McCarthy, G., & Wood, C. C. (1985). Event-related potentials, lexical decision and semantic priming. *Electroencephalography Clinical Neurophysiology, 60*(4), 343–355.

Bergen, B. K., Lindsay, S., Matlock, T., & Narayanan, S. (2007). Spatial and linguistic aspects of visual imagery in sentence comprehension. *Cognitive Science, 31*(5), 733–764.

Berndt, R. S., Haendiges, A. N., Mitchum, C. C., & Sandson, J. (1997). Verb retrieval in aphasia. 2. Relationship to sentence processing. *Brain and Language, 56*(1), 107–137.

Besson, M., Kutas, M., & van Petten, C. (1992). An event-related potential (ERP) analysis of semantic congruity and repetition effects in sentences. *Journal of Cognitive Neuroscience, 4*(2), 132–149.

Bird, H., Howard, D., & Franklin, S. (2000). Why is a verb like an inanimate object? Grammatical category and semantic category deficits. *Brain and Language, 72*(3), 246–309.

Bles, M., Alink, A., & Jansma, B. M. (2007). Neural aspects of cohort-size reduction during visual gating. *Brain Research, 1150*(30), 143–154.

Brown, W. S., Lehmann, D., & Marsh, J. T. (1980). Linguistic meaning related differences in evoked potential topography: English, Swiss-German, and imagined. *Brain and Language, 11*(2), 340–353.

Caramazza, A., & Hillis, A. E. (1991). Lexical organization of nouns and verbs in the brain. *Nature, 349*, 788–790.

Dambacher, M., Kliegl, R., Hofmann, M., & Jacobs, A. M. (2006). Frequency and predictability effects on event-related potentials during reading. *Brain Research, 1084*, 89–103.

Dehaene, S. (1995). Electrophysiological evidence for category-specific word processing in the normal human brain. *Neuroreport, 6*(16), 2153–2157.

Duffy, S. A., Kambe, G., & Rayner, K. (2001). The effect of prior disambiguating context on the comprehension of ambiguous words: Evidence from eye movements. In D. S. Gorfein (Ed.), *On the consequences of meaning selection – Perspectives on resolving lexical ambiguity* (pp. 27–44). Washington, DC: American Psychological Association.

Duffy, S. A., Morris, R. K., & Rayner, K. (1988). Lexical ambiguity and fixation times in reading. *Journal of Memory and Language, 27*(4), 429–446.

Ehrlichman, H., & Barrett, J. (1983). Right hemispheric specialization for mental imagery: A review of the evidence. *Brain and Cognition, 2*(1), 55–76.

Eviatar, Z., Menn, L., & Zaidel, E. (1990). Concreteness: Nouns, verbs, and hemispheres. *Cortex, 26*(4), 611–624.

Fabiani, M., Gratton, G., & Federmeier, K. D. (2007). Event-related brain potentials: Methods, theory, and application. In J. T. Cacioppo, L. Tassinary, & G. Berntson (Eds.), *Handbook of psychophysiology* (3rd edn., pp. 85–119). Cambridge: Cambridge University Press.

Farah, M. J., Weisberg, L. L., Monheit, M. A., & Peronnet, F. (1989). Brain activity underlying mental imagery: Event-related potentials during mental image generation. *Journal of Cognitive Neuroscience, 1*(4), 302–316.

Federmeier, K. D. (2007). Thinking ahead: The role and roots of prediction in language comprehension. *Psychophysiology, 44*, 491–505.

Federmeier, K. D., & Laszlo, S. (2009). Time for meaning: Electrophysiology provides insights into the dynamics of representation and processing in semantic memory. In B. Ross (Ed.), *Psychology of learning and memory* (Vol. 51). Amsterdam: Elsevier.

Federmeier, K. D., Segal, J. B., Lombrozo, T., & Kutas, M. (2000). Brain responses to nouns, verbs and class-ambiguous words in context. *Brain, 123*(12), 2552–2566.

Francis, W. N., & Kucera, H. (1982). *Frequency analysis of English usage: Lexicon and grammar* Boston: Houghton Mifflin.

Gennari, S. P., MacDonald, M. C., Postle, B. R., & Seidenberg, M. S. (2007). Context-dependent interpretation of words: Evidence for interactive neural processes. *NeuroImage, 35*(3), 1278–1286.

Gentner, D. (1981). Some interesting differences between verbs and nouns. *Cognition and Brain Theory, 4*, 161–178.

Gentner, D. (1982). Why nouns are learned before verbs: Linguistic relativity versus natural partitioning. In S. A. Kuczaj (Ed.), *Language development. Language, thought and culture* (Vol. 2, pp. 301–334). Hillsdale, NJ: Erlbaum.

Gerhand, S., & Barry, C. (2000). When does a deep dyslexic make a semantic error? The roles of age-of-acquisition, concreteness, and frequency. *Brain and Language, 74*(1), 26–47.

Gomes, H., Ritter, W., Tartter, V. C., Vaughan, H. G., & Rosen, J. J. (1997). Lexical processing of visually and auditorily presented nouns and verbs: Evidence from reaction time and N400 priming data. *Cognitive Brain Research, 6*(2), 121–134.

Haberlandt, K. F., & Graesser, A. C. (1985). Component processes in text comprehension and some of their interactions. *Journal of Experimental Psychology: General, 114*, 357–375.

Hauk, O., Davis, M. H., Ford, M., Pulvermüller, F., & Marslen-Wilson, W. D. (2006). The time course of visual word recognition as revealed by linear regression analysis of ERP data. *Neuroimage, 30*(4), 1383–1400.

Hogaboam, T. W., & Perfetti, C. A. (1975). Lexical ambiguity and sentence comprehension. *Journal of Verbal Learning and Verbal Behavior, 14*(3), 265–272.

Holcomb, P. J., Kounios, J., Anderson, J. E., & West, W. C. (1999). Dual-coding, context-availability, and concreteness effects in sentence comprehension: An electrophysiological investigation. *Journal of Experimental Psychology: Learning Memory and Cognition*, *25*(3), 721–742.

Holmes, V. M., & Langford, J. (1976). Comprehension and recall of abstract and concrete sentences. *Journal of Verbal Learning and Verbal Behavior*, *15*(5), 559–566.

Huang, H. W., Lee, C. L., & Federmeier, K. D. (2010). Imagine that! ERPs provide evidence for distinct hemispheric contributions to the processing of concrete and abstract concepts. *NeuroImage*.

Jonkers, R., & Bastiaanse, R. (1998). How selective are selective word class deficits? Two case studies of action and object naming. *Aphasiology*, *12*(3), 245–256.

Just, M. A., & Carpenter, P. A. (1980). A theory of reading: From eye fixations to comprehension. *Psychological Review*, *87*, 329–354.

Kemmerer, D., & Tranel, D. (2000). Verb retrieval in brain-damaged subjects: 1. Analysis of stimulus, lexical, and conceptual factors. *Brain and Language*, *73*, 347–392.

Khader, P., Scherag, A., Streb, J., & Rösler, F. (2003). Differences between noun and verb processing in a minimal phrase context: A semantic priming study using event-related brain potentials. *Cognitive Brain Research*, *17*(2), 293–313.

King, J. W., & Kutas, M. (1995). Who did what and when? Using word- and clause-level ERPs to monitor working memory usage in reading. *Journal of Cognitive Neuroscience*, *7*(376–395).

King, J. W., & Kutas, M. (1998). Neural plasticity in the dynamics of human visual word recognition. *Neuroscience Letters*, *244*(2), 61–64.

Kosslyn, S. M. (1987). Seeing and imagining in the cerebral hemispheres: A computational approach. *Psychological Review*, *94*(2), 148–175.

Kounios, J., & Holcomb, P. J. (1994). Concreteness effects in semantic processing: ERP evidence supporting dual-coding theory. *Journal of Experimental Psychology: Learning, Memory, and Cognition*, *20*(4), 804–823.

Kutas, M., & Federmeier, K. D. (2000). Electrophysiology reveals semantic memory use in language comprehension. *Trends in Cognitive Sciences*, *4*(12), 463–470.

Lee, C. L., & Federmeier, K. D. (2006). To mind the mind: An event-related potential study of word class and semantic ambiguity. *Brain Research*, *1081*(1), 191–202.

Lee, C. L., & Federmeier, K. D. (2008). To watch, to see, and to differ: An event-related potential study of concreteness effects as a function of word class and lexical ambiguity. *Brain and Language*, *104*(2), 145–158.

Lee, C. L., & Federmeier, K. D. (2009). Wave-ering: An ERP study of syntactic and semantic context effects on ambiguity resolution for noun/verb homographs. *Journal of Memory and Language*.

Longe, O., Randall, B., Stamatakis, E. A., & Tyler, L. K. (2007). Grammatical categories in the brain: The role of morphological structure. *Cerebral Cortex*, *17*(8), 1812–1820.

Marschark, M. (1985). Imagery and organization in recall of prose. *Journal of Memory and Language*, *24*, 734–745.

Marshall, J., Pring, T., Chiat, S., & Robson, J. (1996). Calling a salad a federation: An investigation of semantic jargon – Part 1: Nouns. *Journal of Neurolinguistics*, *9*, 237–250.

Marslen-Wilson, W., & Tyler, L. K. (1980). The temporal structure of spoken language understanding. *Cognition*, *8*, 1–71.

Mason, R. A., & Just, M. A. (2007). Lexical ambiguity in sentence comprehension. *Brain Research*, *1146*, 115–127.

McCarthy, R., & Warrington, E. K. (1985). Category specificity in an agrammatic patient: The relative impairment of verb retrieval and comprehension. *Neuropsychologia, 23,* 709–727.

Metzler, C. (2001). Effects of left frontal lesions on the selection of context-appropriate meanings. *Neuropsychology, 15*(3), 315–328.

Miceli, G., Silveri, M. C., Nocentini, U., & Caramazza, A. (1988). Patterns of dissociations in comprehension and production of nouns and verbs. *Aphasiology, 2*(351–358).

Morton, J. (1969). The interaction of information in word recognition. *Psychological Review, 76,* 165–178.

Munte, T. F., Wieringa, B. M., Weyerts, H., Szentkuti, A., Matzke, M., & Johannes, S. (2001). Differences in brain potentials to open and closed class words: Class and frequency effects. *Neuropsychologia, 39*(1), 91–102.

Myerson, R., & Goodglass, H. (1972). Transformational grammars of three agrammatic patients. *Language and Speech, 15,* 40–50.

Norris, D. (1986). Word recognition: Context effects without priming. *Cognition* (22), 93–136.

Osterhout, L., Bersick, M., & McKinnon, R. (1997). Brain potentials elicited by words: Word length and frequency predict the latency of an early negativity. *Biological Psychology, 46*(2), 143–168.

Paivio, A. (1969). Mental imagery in associative learning and memory. *Psychological Review, 76,* 241–263.

Paivio, A. (1991). Dual coding theory: Retrospect and current status. *Canadian Journal of Psychology, 45,* 255–287.

Paivio, A., Clark, J. M., & Khan, M. (1988). Effects of concreteness and semantic relatedness on composite imagery ratings and cued recall. *Memory and Cognition, 16*(5), 422–430.

Paivio, A., Yuille, J. C., & Madigan, S. A. (1968). Concreteness, imagery, and meaningfulness values for 925 nouns. *Journal of Experimental Psychology: Monograph Supplement, 76*(1), 1–25.

Paul, S. T., Kellas, G., Martin, M., & Clark, M. B. (1992). Influence of contextual features on the activation of ambiguous word meanings. *Journal of Experimental Psychology: Learning, Memory and Cognition, 18*(4), 703–717.

Plaut, D. C., & Shallice, T. (1993). Deep dyslexia: A case study of connectionist neuropsychology. *Cognitive Neuropsychology, 10,* 377–500.

Preissl, H., Pulvermüller, F., Lutzenberger, W., & Birbaumer, N. (1995). Evoked potentials distinguish between nouns and verbs. *Neuroscience Letters, 197*(1), 81–83.

Proverbio, A. M., Vecchi, L., & Zani, A. (2004). From orthography to phonetics: ERP measures of grapheme-to-phoneme conversion mechanisms in reading. *Journal of Cognitive Neuroscience, 16*(2), 301–317.

Rayner, K., & Frazier, L. (1989). Selection mechanisms in reading lexically ambiguous words. *Journal of Experimental Psychology: Learning, Memory, and Cognition, 15*(5), 779–790.

Rayner, K., Pacht, J. M., & Duffy, S. A. (1994). Effects of prior encounter and global discourse bias on the processing of lexically ambiguous words: Evidence from eye fixations. *Journal of Memory and Language, 33*(4), 527–544.

Rayner, K., & Sereno, S. C. (1994). Eye movements in reading: Psycholinguistic studies. In M. Gernsbacher (Ed.), *Handbook of psycholinguistics* (pp. 57–81). New York: Academic Press.

Reynolds, A., & Flagg, P. (1976). Recognition memory for elements of sentences. *Memory and Cognition, 4*, 422–432.

Robinson, G., Blair, J., & Cipolotti, L. (1998). Dynamic aphasia: An inability to select between competing verbal responses? *Brain, 121*(1), 77–89.

Rodd, J., Gaskell, G., & Marslen-Wilson, W. (2002). Making sense of semantic ambiguity: Semantic competition in lexical access. *Journal of Memory and Language, 46*(2), 245–266.

Rodd, J. M., Davis, M. H., & Johnsrude, I. S. (2005). The neural mechanisms of speech comprehension: fMRI studies of semantic ambiguity. *Cerebral Cortex, 15*(8), 1261–1269.

Rosler, F., Streb, J., & Haan, H. (2001). Event-related brain potentials evoked by verbs and nouns in a primed lexical decision task. *Psychophysiology, 38*(4), 694–703.

Rubenstein, H., Garfield, L., & Millikan, J. (1970). Homographic entries in the internal lexicon. *Journal of Verbal Learning and Verbal Behavior, 9*, 487–494.

Rugg, M. D. (1990). Event-related brain potentials dissociate repetition effects of high- and low-frequency words. *Memory and Cognition, 18*(4), 367–379.

Rugg, M. D., Allan, K., & Birch, C. S. (2000). Electrophysiological evidence for the modulation of retrieval orientation by depth of study processing. *Journal of Cognitive Neuroscience, 12*(4), 664–678.

Saffran, E. M., Schwartz, M. F., & Marin, S. M. (1980). Evidence from aphasia: Isolating the components of a production model. In B. Butterworth (Ed.), *Language production* (Vol. 1, pp. 221–241). London: Academic Press.

Schendan, H. E., Ganis, G., & Kutas, M. (1998). Neurophysiological evidence for visual perceptual categorization of words and faces within 150 ms. *Psychophysiology, 35*, 240–251.

Schilling, H. E. H., Rayner, K., & Chumbley, J. I. (1998). Comparing naming, lexical decision, and eye fixation times: Word frequency effects and individual differences. *Memory and Cognition, 26*(6), 1270–1281.

Schwanenflugel, P. (1991). Why are abstract concepts hard to understand? In P. Schwanenflugel (Ed.), *The psychology of word meanings* (pp. 223–250). Hillsdale, NJ: Erlbaum.

Schwanenflugel, P. J., Harnishfeger, K. K., & Stowe, R. W. (1988). Context availability and lexical decisions for abstract and concrete words. *Journal of Memory and Language, 27*, 499–520.

Schwanenflugel, P. J., & Shoben, E. J. (1983). Differential context effects in the comprehension of abstract and concrete verbal materials. *Journal of Experimental Psychology: Learning, Memory, and Cognition, 9*(1), 82–102.

Seidenberg, M. S., Tanenhaus, M. K., Leiman, J. M., & Bienkowski, M. (1982). Automatic access of the meanings of ambiguous words in context: Some limitations of knowledge-based processing. *Cognitive Psychology, 14*(4), 489–537.

Shapiro, L., Zurif, E., & Grimshaw, J. (1987). Sentence processing and the mental representation of verbs. *Cognition, 27*(3), 219–246.

Smith, M. E., & Halgren, E. (1987). Event-related potentials during lexical decision: Effects of repetition, word frequency, pronounceability, and concreteness. *Electroencephalography and Clinical Neurophysiology, Supplement, 40*, 417–421.

Solomon, R. L., & Howes, D. H. (1951). Word frequency, personal values and visual duration thresholds. *Psychological Review, 58*, 256–270.

Swaab, T. Y., Baynes, K., & Knight, R. T. (2002). Separable effects of priming and imageability on word processing: An ERP study. *Cognitive Brain Research, 15*(1), 99–103.

Szekely, A., D'Amico, S., Devescovi, A., Federmeier, K., Herron, D., Iyer, G., et al. (2005). Timed action and object naming. *Cortex, 41*(1), 7–25.

Tanenhaus, M. K., Leiman, J. M., & Seidenberg, M. S. (1979). Evidence for multiple stages in the processing of ambiguous words in syntactic contexts. *Journal of Verbal Learning and Verbal Behavior, 18,* 427–440.

Taylor, W. L. (1953). "Cloze procedure": A new tool for measuring readability. *Journalism Quarterly, 30,* 415–433.

Thompson-Schill, S. L., Swick, D., Farah, M. J., D'Esposito, M., Kan, I. P., & Knight, R. T. (1998). Verb generation in patients with focal frontal lesions: A neuropsychological test of neuroimaging findings. *Proceedings of the National Academy of Sciences USA, 95*(26), 15855–15860.

Twilley, L. C., Dixon, P., Taylor, D., & Clark, K. (1994). University of Alberta norms of relative meaning frequency for 566 homographs. *Memory and Cognition, 22*(1), 111–126.

Van Berkum, J. J., Brown, C. M., Hagoort, P., & Zwitserlood, P. (2003). Event-related brain potentials reflect discourse-referential ambiguity in spoken language comprehension. *Psychophysiology, 40*(2), 235–248.

Van Berkum, J. J., Hagoort, P., & Brown, C. M. (1999). Semantic integration in sentences and discourse: Evidence from the N400. *Journal of Cognitive Neuroscience, 11*(6), 657–671.

Van Petten, C. (1993). A comparison of lexical and sentence-level context effects in event-related potentials. *Language and Cognitive Processes, 8*(4), 485–531.

Van Petten, C., & Kutas, M. (1990). Interactions between sentence context and word frequency in event-related brain potentials. *Memory and Cognition, 18*(4), 380–393.

Van Petten, C., & Kutas, M. (1991). Influences of semantic and syntactic context on open- and closed-class words. *Memory and Cognition, 19*(1), 95–112.

West, W. C., & Holcomb, P. J. (2000). Imaginal, semantic, and surface-level processing of concrete and abstract words: An electrophysiological investigation. *Journal of Cognitive Neuroscience, 12*(6), 1024–1037.

Williams, S. E., & Canter, G. J. (1987). Action-naming performance in four syndromes of aphasia. *Brain and Language, 32*(1), 124–136.

Wlotko, E. W., & Federmeier, K. D. (2007). Finding the right word: Hemispheric asymmetries in the use of sentence context information. *Neuropsychologia, 45*(13), 3001–3014.

Zempleni, M.-Z., Renken, R., Hoeks, J. C. J., Hoogduin, J. M., & Stowe, L. A. (2007). Semantic ambiguity processing in sentence context: Evidence from event-related fMRI. *NeuroImage, 34*(3), 1270–1279.

11

Hemodynamic Studies
of Syntactic Processing

Peter Indefrey

Introduction

Over the last twenty years, hemodynamic techniques for measuring brain activation have completely changed the scientific investigation of neural correlates of syntactic processing. Before these techniques became available, the only way to obtain information about the involvement of brain structures in the production and comprehension of grammar was the study of impairments of grammatical processing ("agrammatism") resulting from brain lesions. These studies showed that there must be neural substrates of syntactic processing, because, across patients, problems with syntactic processing were found not to be inevitably coupled to other types of general cognitive or language processing problems. This basic finding meant that there had to be brain structures that were of particular importance for syntactic processing. To some degree it was also possible to say something about where in the brain such structures might be. Taking other symptoms, such as motor deficits, into account, neurologists could infer that agrammatism resulted from lesions of the dominant, i.e., in right-handers the left, hemisphere of the brain. Postmortem examinations of brains of agrammatic patients showed that brain regions close to the left Sylvian fissure were affected. Nonetheless, even after the invention of computerized tomography which allowed for the first time an exact in vivo delineation of brain lesions in agrammatic patients, one fundamental problem remained: the localization and extent of lesions was determined by their causes, not by their consequences. Lesions as a result of stroke, for example, reflect the anatomy of the blood supply, not the functional role of the affected brain tissue.

The Handbook of the Neuropsychology of Language, First Edition. Edited by Miriam Faust.
© 2012 Blackwell Publishing Ltd. Published 2012 by Blackwell Publishing Ltd.

In this respect, the invention of hemodynamic techniques, first positron emission tomography (PET) then functional magnetic resonance imaging (fMRI), promised the possibility of a wholly different approach. Researchers could in principle manipulate brain function by asking their subjects to perform certain cognitive tasks, such as reading a sentence, and study the localization and extent of the resulting brain activation. This possibility relies on a basic physiological mechanism: the activity of nerve cells in a part of the brain leads to an increase in the blood supply of just this part, not of the whole brain. It is not yet fully understood how the electrical activity of neurons triggers the dilation of supplying blood vessels – the release of a certain mediator substance plays a major role – but no matter how, the mechanism ensures that the detection of local cerebral blood flow (CBF) changes allows conclusions about local nerve cell activity. Note that whereas nerve cell activity implies blood flow changes, the reverse is not true: there are many other possible causes of blood flow changes, for example changes in blood pressure or breathing rate. Fortunately (for functional imaging research), they tend to affect the whole brain so that measurements of local CBF can be corrected for such global blood flow changes.

PET and fMRI differ in how they measure blood flow changes. With PET, blood flow is measured by injecting a weakly radioactive tracer molecule (usually water or butanol, a type of alcohol) into the bloodstream and recording the amount of radiation from different parts of the brain. Compared to a baseline measurement, activation of a brain area during a cognitive task results in a local increase of radiation indicating the increased local blood flow. Magnetic resonance imaging (MRI) measures an electrical signal that is produced by hydrogen nuclei (protons) rotating in a magnetic field. The strength of the signal depends on the strength of the magnetic field and on the coordination of the rotation. Functional MRI exploits the fact that the blood flow increase induced by neural activity is stronger than necessary to meet the oxygen demands of active nerve cells. As a result, not all of the additional oxygen carried by the blood hemoglobin is used up and the amount of oxygen-carrying hemoglobin (oxyhemoglobin) is increased in the small veins of active brain regions. Using a radio frequency pulse, fMRI causes protons in a part of the brain to rotate in synchrony ("in phase") thus emitting an electrical signal. Because oxyhemoglobin disturbs the magnetic field (and hence proton rotation) less than deoxyhemoglobin (hemoglobin that has delivered its oxygen load to the brain tissue), the proton rotation remains synchronized longer in an active compared to an inactive brain region, resulting in a stronger signal.

PET and fMRI thus have in common that they do not directly measure the activity of nerve cells in the brain but make use of the fact that neural activity in a particular brain region induces a local blood flow increase to this region. This means that they also have in common that their temporal resolution is determined by the time course of the blood flow changes. Due to the fact that the blood flow change starts only several seconds after the neural activity (and other limitations), the methods do not provide good information about the timing of cognitive processes.

By contrast, with a spatial resolution of a few millimeters, they provide quite information about where in the brain nerve cells are activated.

Keeping in mind a certain weakness with respect to detecting the time cour. neural activation, hemodynamic methods are thus indeed well suited to detect brain regions that contain a sufficient number of nerve cells that are activated when the brain performs the cognitive operations involved in processing a sentence. After a first wave of studies presenting participants with sentences in one condition and asking them to relax and not to do anything in another condition ("rest"), research- ers soon discovered that very many brain regions become activated when reading or listening to a sentence and it is far from easy to isolate the neural correlate of a single cognitive operation, such as syntactic processing, in such a complex brain activation pattern.

Depending on the input modality, processing a simple sentence like "Peter is eating an apple" comprises visual or auditory processing, letter or phoneme recogni- tion, word recognition, and sentence-level phonemic (intonation) and semantic processing. It is known that reading (but possibly also listening to speech) engages motor planning, because even skilled readers articulate subvocally to some extent. The necessary maintenance and manipulation of symbols and mental representa- tions recruit working memory resources. Finally, the meaning extracted from the words and the sentence as a whole, may trigger a visualization of someone eating an apple and, as we know from recent work, even triggers motor activity related to eating. All these processes have their neural correlates that show up as brain activa- tion in a hemodynamic activation measurement.

To identify a single processing component of interest, in this case syntactic processing, researchers soon started using two main experimental strategies. The first one is to keep using sentence stimuli in one condition but use stimuli that share some of the "uninteresting" properties with the sentences in the control condition. In this way, brain activation related to the "uninteresting" properties can be sub- tracted from the brain activation elicited by sentences, and the resulting activation reflects only the additional properties of sentences. In visual sentence processing studies, researchers have used control conditions such as presenting a fixation cross, strings of meaningless symbols, strings of consonants, and strings of words. In auditory sentence processing studies, they have used tones, environmental sounds, speech sounds, reversed speech or speech that was made unintelligible in some other way, and spoken word lists. Obviously each of these stimuli controlled for some aspect of sentence processing but none for all nonsyntactic aspects. The same basic strategy has also been used in a handful of studies investigating syntactic processing in speech production. The first studies (Indefrey, Brown, et al., 2001; Indefrey, Hellwig, Herzog, Seitz, & Hagoort, 2004) used a scene description paradigm, in which participants described the actions of colored geometrical figures either in full sentences ("The red square is pushing the green triangle away") or in ordered lists of syntactically unrelated words ("square, red, triangle, green, push away"). Participants were instructed to always name the "agent" of an action first to keep the visual and conceptual processing of the scenes constant across conditions. More recent studies elicited sentences by presenting one or more words from which sentences had to be generated. Control conditions typically required reading the stimulus words.

The second strategy consisted in making the processing component of interest, i.e., syntactic processing, more demanding in some sentences and use syntactically less demanding sentences in the control condition. Higher syntactic processing demands were achieved, for example, by making the sentences structurally more complex. Two studies that introduced the structural complexity manipulation (Just, Carpenter, Keller, Eddy, & Thulborn, 1996; Stromswold, Caplan, Alpert, & Rauch, 1996) used different types of relative clauses that had been shown to be of different processing difficulty in psycholinguistic studies. The sentence "The juice that the child spilled stained the rug" takes longer to process than the sentence "The child spilled the juice that stained the rug." (Stromswold et al., 1996), although they refer to roughly the same event, because in the first sentence the syntactic roles of *juice* differ between main clause (subject) and relative clause (object) and the main clause is separated by a center-embedded relative clause, so that one has to wait until the end of the sentence before it becomes clear what predicate goes with the subject. Because the higher complexity is due to syntactic properties, this approach assumes that brain structures that process syntax will have to work harder and hence will be more strongly activated.

Another way to manipulate the load of syntactic processing has been to present sentences that contain syntactic violations. Using syntactic violations to increase the syntactic processing demands has a slightly different rationale. This approach assumes that the brain structures processing syntax will also be (among) the ones detecting syntactic violations. Consider the sentence "Peter is eating an apple." The syntactic feature *number = singular* establishes agreement between the subject noun "Peter" and the verb "is" and this information is used in building up a sentence representation. When processing the sentence "Peter are eating an apple" we may still build up a sentence representation but the lack of subject–verb agreement will make it more difficult to link the subject to its predicate and will trigger additional reanalysis processes. Obviously, extra work needs to be done in more than one processing component, so that it is arguably less clear than in the case of higher structural complexity what the additional hemodynamic response elicited by syntactic violations reflects.

Using syntactically less demanding control sentences has the advantage that brain activation due to most or even all nonsyntactic processing components can be subtracted out, because the control sentences can be made very similar in meaning and nonsyntactic complexity. A disadvantage is that at least some activation related to syntactic processing is also subtracted out, because the control sentences require some degree of syntactic processing as well.

In the next section I will present the results of a systematic analysis of the findings of more than 80 hemodynamic studies on sentence processing that used one or the other of the two basic designs: comparing sentences to a below-sentence-level control condition (nonsyntactic control) or comparing syntactically more demanding sentences to less demanding sentences (syntactic control). I will analyze the pattern of reported findings according to the following heuristic: Brain regions that are reliably found with both types of design and irrespective of whether subjects read or listened to the stimulus sentences can be assumed to be involved in syntactic processing, because they do not reflect activation due to modality-specific perceptual processes, activation due to language processing below the sentence level, or general cognitive activation due to the difficulty of syntactically demanding sentences.

In further sections I will discuss how current neurocognitive models explain the data (not all assume that brain regions involved in syntactic processing actually perform syntactic processing) and introduce recent findings from a few hemodynamic studies using a novel and very promising approach called repetition suppression.

Reliable Findings: A Meta-Analysis

Sentence comprehension has been studied in a large number of hemodynamic studies with or without the aim to isolate the neural correlates of syntactic processing. For a review this is both a curse and a blessing. A curse, because it is obviously impossible to discuss them all in detail or even discuss all aspects of study design that have an impact on the outcome. A blessing, because a large number of studies allows for an assessment of the degree to which results have been replicated across studies and thus can be considered reliable. A large number of studies also provides a sufficient basis to compare the reliable findings in the two presentation modalities obtained with the different strategies mentioned above.

Reliability of findings is an issue as serious in hemodynamic studies as in behavioral studies of sentence processing. In fact even more so, because the dependent variable, hemodynamic brain activation, is sensitive to more aspects of the measurement situation and procedures than reaction times are. To anticipate two results of the meta-analysis: *no* brain region (except for Broca's area when collapsing findings in the pars opercularis and the pars triangularis of the left posterior inferior frontal gyrus) was found activated in more than half of the 79 experiments on sentence comprehension analyzed here and *more than half* of all brain regions were reported activated in at least one study. The latter result indicates that a reliability assessment is necessary to exclude spurious findings that are due to irrelevant experiment-specific factors. The former result indicates that hemodynamic studies are susceptible to a number of factors that may cause null findings and lack of overlap between studies. Among these are technical issues (lack of sensitivity in some brain regions, state-of-the-art of scanning devices), anatomical and physiological issues (anatomical variability between participants, physiological "noise," such as heartbeat, blood pressure, and breathing rate differences), and an issue that is most relevant for the question of syntactic processing: listeners and readers may not always perform a full syntactic analysis (parsing) of a sentence and there is evidence that the depth of syntactic processing varies depending on the requirements of the task at hand (Indefrey et al., 2004). These are good reasons not to expect every single study to detect all brain regions involved in syntactic processing. One can nonetheless identify brain regions that are found so often that the agreement between studies is unlikely to come about by chance.

Procedure

Seventy-nine hemodynamic sentence comprehension experiments and six sentence production experiments that reported activated brain regions with Talairach coordinates or Montreal Neurological Institute (MNI) coordinates were analyzed. The activation foci were coded in a descriptive reference system of 112 regions (see Indefrey & Levelt, 2004, for details). In this system, the cerebral lobes were divided into two or three rostro-caudal or mediolateral segments of roughly equal size. The regions within this gross division were defined in terms of gyri and subcortical structures following Talairach and Tournoux (1988). Due to the particular relevance of the left posterior inferior frontal gyrus (Broca's area) for syntactic processing, this region was further subdivided into three regions labeled descriptively Brodmann areas (BA) 44, 45, and 47 in the stereotaxic atlas of Talairach and Tournoux (1988). Activation foci located near the border of two adjacent regions were coded in both regions.

Reliability estimate

The studies included in this meta-analysis were not given any weights reflecting differences due to design or size. This means that the overlap of activations between studies that was considered reliable should not be interpreted as statistically significant. Nonetheless, the notion of "reliability" was not totally arbitrary, but based on the following quasi-statistical estimate: the average number of activated regions reported per experiment divided by the number of regions (112) equals the probability for any particular region to be reported in an experiment, if reports were randomly distributed over regions. Assuming this probability, the chance level for a region to be reported as activated in a number of experiments is given by a binomial distribution. The possibility that the agreement of reports about a certain region was coincidental was rejected if the chance level was less than 5%. Assuming, for example, an average number of 6 activated regions per study, this reliability criterion corresponded to a minimum agreement of 2 studies for regions covered by 2–7 studies, a minimum agreement of 3 studies for regions covered by 8–18 studies, and so forth (4 out of 19–31; 7 out of 61–76). In this way, the reliability threshold controlled for the fact that due to the heterogeneity of techniques and analysis procedures (for example, analyzing only a set of regions of interest) not all studies covered the whole brain. The procedure also controlled for the fact that in studies comparing sentences to nonsyntactic control conditions, the number of activated regions that were found was typically higher than in studies comparing syntactically demanding to less demanding sentences, so that the chances of coincidental agreements of findings between studies were also higher.

Results

Figure 11.1a–d shows the reliably activated regions for the four basic types of sentence comprehension studies described above. The numbers in the regions give the proportion of studies reporting a particular region as being activated relative to the number of studies that looked into that region. As already mentioned above, there are few regions that were found activated in more than half of the cases. Nonetheless, quite a number of regions can be considered reliably replicated. This holds even for a region like the left posterior middle temporal gyrus that has been reported only by 4 out of 26 sentence reading studies with sentence-level control (see Figure 11.1a). The reason for this is that in a set of studies that reported on average 4.5 out of 112 possible regions it is unlikely that more than 3 find the same area by chance ($p = 0.019$; for a validation of the reliability estimate, see Indefrey & Levelt, 2004).

When participants read or listen to syntactically demanding sentences (Figures 11.1a and 11.1c), the pars opercularis (BA 44) and the pars triangularis (BA 45) of the left posterior inferior frontal gyrus (together often referred to as Broca's area) and the posterior parts of the superior and middle temporal gyri are more strongly activated than when they read or listen to simpler sentences. For reading, there is additional activation of the right hemispheric homologue of Broca's area. For listening, there is additional activation in the lower motor cortex and the more anterior parts of the temporal lobe. Figures 11.2a and 11.2b show the separate results for studies that increased syntactic demands by presenting sentences containing syntactic violations and studies that increased syntactic demands by higher grammatical complexity (collapsed over reading and listening). Both paradigms elicit activation of Broca's area, but sentences of higher structural complexity activate a larger region of the posterior temporal lobe than syntactic violations.

Activation of Broca's area and the left posterior temporal lobe is also reliably found when reading or listening to sentences is compared to control conditions below the sentence level (Figures 11.1b and 11.1d). In addition, the pars orbitalis (BA 47) of the left posterior inferior frontal gyrus, bilateral more anterior parts of the middle temporal gyrus, and the left upper motor cortex are activated for both reading and listening. These regions thus might reflect some modality-independent aspect of language processing below the sentence level, for example lexical processing, or they might be involved in a sentence level process that is not modulated by increased syntactic demands. To distinguish between these two possibilities, one can look into the findings of a subset of studies that compared visual or auditory sentence processing to the processing of word lists. In these studies lexical or sublexical

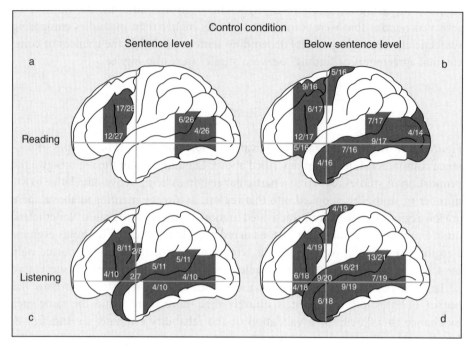

Figure 11.1 Schematic representations of left hemispheric brain regions that are activated in hemodynamic sentence comprehension studies. Numbers in regions give the proportion of studies reporting a particular region as being activated relative to the number of studies that looked into that region. (a) Reliable activations across 30 studies (marked [1] in the reference list) with an average number of 11.6 participants reading syntactically more demanding sentences compared to less demanding sentences. On average 4.5 regions were reported as being more strongly activated for demanding sentences. (b) Reliable activations across 17 studies (marked [2] in the reference list) with an average number of 12.1 participants reading sentences compared to lower level control conditions. On average 7.6 regions were reported as being more strongly activated for sentences. (c) Reliable activations across 11 studies (marked [3] in the reference list) with an average number of 11.7 participants listening to syntactically more demanding sentences compared to less demanding sentences. On average 4.6 regions were reported as being more strongly activated for demanding sentences. (d) Reliable activations across 21 studies (marked [4] in the reference list) with an average number of 10.8 participants listening to sentences compared to lower-level control conditions. On average 7.5 regions were reported as being more strongly activated for sentences.

processing should be controlled for. Nonetheless, as shown in Figure 11.2c, activation of BA 47 and of the left anterior middle temporal gyrus are still reliably found (left motor cortex and the right middle temporal gyrus are not), suggesting that they are involved in some modality-independent aspect of sentence processing.

Other regions show modality-specific activation. For reading, these are the Broca homologue, the left posterior middle frontal gyrus, and the left occipital cortex, the

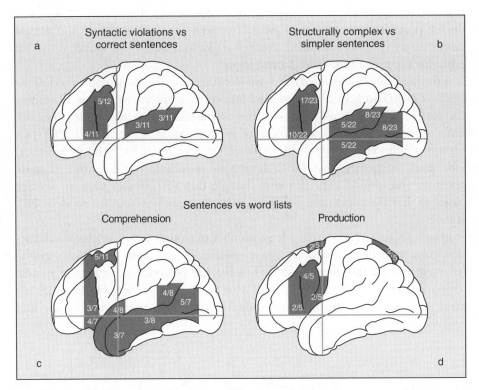

Figure 11.2 Schematic representations of left hemispheric brain regions that are activated in hemodynamic sentence comprehension studies. Numbers in regions give the proportion of studies reporting a particular region as being activated relative to the number of studies that looked into that region. (a) Reliable activations across 12 studies (marked [5] in the reference list) with an average number of 13.5 participants reading or listening to sentences with syntactic violations compared to correct sentences. On average 4.3 regions were reported as being more strongly activated for sentences with syntactic violations. (b) Reliable activations across 24 studies (marked [6] in the reference list) with an average number of 11.5 participants reading or listening to structurally complex compared to simpler sentences. On average 5.4 regions were reported as being more strongly activated for complex sentences. (c) Reliable activations across 8 studies (marked [7] in the reference list) with an average number of 14.1 participants reading or listening to sentences compared to word lists. On average 7.5 regions were reported as being more strongly activated for sentences. (d) Reliable activations across 5 studies (marked [8] in the reference list) with an average number of 16.8 participants producing sentences compared to word lists. On average 6.5 regions were reported as being more strongly activated for sentences.

latter most likely reflecting insufficient control of visual stimulus properties. For listening, this is bilateral activation of the anterior and mid superior temporal gyrus, reflecting insufficient control of acoustic stimulus properties.

The pattern of activations found in studies investigating syntactic encoding by comparing sentence production to the production of syntactically unrelated words

Peter Indefrey

is shown in Figure 11.2d. The majority of studies reported activation of BA 44 of the left posterior inferior frontal gyrus. Two adjacent regions (BA 45 and ventral motor cortex) are also activated. Further activations have been found in the left posterior superior frontal and parietal lobes.

A further analysis addressed the possible influence of the measurement technique (PET or fMRI) on activations observed for sentence processing. Across all studies, the pattern of results obtained with the two measurement techniques does not differ. However, the average number of regions found activated with PET (4.4 regions) was lower than with fMRI (6.9 regions). This result also holds for temporal lobe areas, suggesting that fMRI despite its inevitable scanner noise is more sensitive. One should keep in mind, though, that PET studies were on average older, so that the conclusion of lower sensitivity may not hold for modern PET scanners.

In sum (Figure 11.3), across a large number of studies using the classic subtraction paradigm, Broca's area, i.e., pars opercularis and pars triangularis of the left posterior inferior frontal gyrus, and the left posterior superior and middle temporal gyrus (together at least part of what is commonly referred to as Wernicke's area) show reliable modality-independent activation for simple sentences and

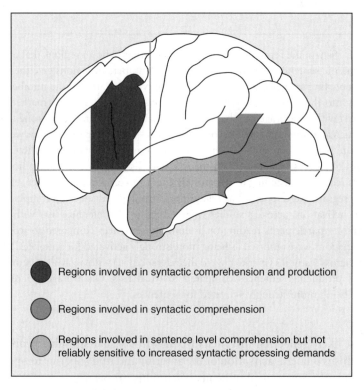

Figure 11.3   Schematic representation of left hemispheric brain regions that are activated in hemodynamic sentence processing studies.

respond to increased syntactic demands. These regions are most likely involved in syntactic processing in comprehension. As indicated by clinical data, both these regions are also necessary for syntactic comprehension. (Note that hemodynamic data alone can never demonstrate that a region is necessary for a particular function: regions may be active even if their activity is redundant.) Caplan, Hildebrandt, and Makris (1996) showed that the proportion of syntactic comprehension deficits in aphasic patients did not differ between frontal and temporal/inferior parietal lesions.

Interestingly, Wernicke's area shows no reliable activation for syntactic production in this type of study. I will come back to this issue when discussing the function of Wernicke's area in syntactic processing.

Modality-independent sentence processing responses that do not increase with syntactic demands are found in the left BA 47 and in anterior parts of the left temporal lobe. These regions, thus, could be involved in syntactic processing, but an involvement in other sentence-level processes, for example, semantic or prosodic processes, is also possible.

I will now turn to more recent types of analysis of fMRI data that have, so far, only been used by very few studies, but seem to be able to provide valuable complementary evidence for the functional characterization of some of the regions found in the previous set of studies.

The Time Course Of Hemodynamic Responses to Sentence Stimuli

As mentioned above, hemodynamic methods have a relatively bad temporal resolution. In addition, the time course of the local blood flow response in different parts of the brain differs and, hence, is not directly comparable. In consequence, fMRI data are normally not used to obtain any time course information on sentence processing. Nonetheless, differences in the onset and the duration of hemodynamic responses *within* one region can in principle be related to corresponding differences in neural activation. Haller, Klarhöfer, Radue, Schwarzbach, and Indefrey (2007) exploited this possibility by investigating how the onset of the blood flow response was affected by sentence complexity in different regions. They found that dorsal (upper) parts of the left inferior frontal gyrus (BA 44 and 45) showed a later onset of the blood flow response for complex compared to simpler sentences but BA 47 and the left posterior superior temporal gyrus did not. These observations suggest that Broca's area subserves a process that (1) does not start immediately upon sentence presentation and (2) starts even later when a complex sentence is presented. Obviously, sublexical and lexical processes do start immediately when the first word comes in, so that the delayed activation onset in Broca's area points to a sentence-level process. This process may be delayed for complex sentences that contain more words, because it does not start with the first word but "waits" for a bit more input from earlier lexical or sublexical processes. Note, however, that the observed onset delay in Broca's area was far shorter than the increase in activation duration observed for BA 47 and the left posterior superior temporal gyrus when reading complex sentences. So, if these regions are involved in (sub)lexical processing and provide input to a sentence-level process, then this process starts before they have finished: in other words, the system operates in a cascaded manner.

Another study investigating temporal properties of the hemodynamic response to sentences was conducted by Bahlmann, Rodriguez-Fornells, Rotte, and Münte (2007). These authors observed a delayed onset of a stronger blood flow response to noncanonical object-first compared to subject-first sentences when the initial noun phrase was not case marked. In this case, readers had to wait until a later case-marked noun phrase disambiguated the sentence structure as canonical or not. This result is very interesting, because it provides evidence for an immediate commitment to a preferred structure (here: subject-first) in structurally ambiguous sentences. This commitment is later revised when contradictory evidence comes in.

A Novel Approach: Repetition Suppression

Whereas time course analyses still rely on the basic design principle to elicit a stronger hemodynamic response in the condition of interest compared to a control or baseline condition, this is no longer the case in so-called fMRI adaptation or "repetition suppression" studies. In these studies, researchers are interested in an attenuation of the blood flow response that is observed when stimuli are repeated. The reduced hemodynamic response is linked to less activity in a population of neurons that are involved in processing the stimulus. The exact mechanism (whether all neurons of the population become less active or only a subset) is not yet clear. Nonetheless, repetition suppression opens fascinating perspectives, because unlike the blood flow response in the classic approach which reflects the summated activity of *all* neurons in a region, repetition suppression measures a blood flow response that reflects the (decrease of) activity of only those neurons that actually process a particular stimulus. This also means that it is not necessary for the whole stimulus to be repeated. If some interesting aspect of a stimulus, for example its syntactic structure, is repeated, then neurons processing this aspect should show reduced activity, leading to attenuated blood flow in the part of brain where they are situated. First studies using this paradigm have been conducted. Noppeney and Price (2004) found syntactic repetition suppression in the left anterior temporal lobe for the comprehension of English sentences. In a study with bilingual German–English participants, Weber and Indefrey (2009) found syntactic repetition suppression within and between languages in Broca's area, the left premotor cortex, and the left posterior temporal lobe. The same areas showed syntactic repetition suppression for sentence production in a recent study by Menenti, Segaert, and Hagoort (under review).

The Function of Brain Regions Involved in Syntactic Processing

Encoding a syntactic structure in language production and syntactic parsing in comprehension require a range of processes or cognitive components, each of which may be underlying the hemodynamic activations (or processing deficits in the case of lesions) observed. With respect to the role of Broca's area in syntactic comprehension, a number of hypotheses have been proposed that are compatible with stronger Broca's area activation when comparing object-extracted relative clauses to simpler sentences. These proposals (and the neurocognitive models from which they are derived) can be sorted according to the degree of specificity for syntax they assume for brain activation during syntactic processing. The most specific and explicit assumptions are made by two models relating different neural substrates to different syntactic operations (Bornkessel & Schlesewsky, 2006; Grodzinsky & Friederici, 2006). Both models distinguish between the function of the deep frontal operculum (a cortical region in the depth of the left posterior inferior frontal gyrus covering the insula) and BA 44, assigning the first processing step of syntactic constituent building to the operculum. Grodzinsky and Friederici (2006) assume BA 44 to be involved in the computation of syntactic movement, whereas Bornkessel and Schlesewsky (2006) assume this region to be involved in the processing of argument hierarchies. For the left posterior temporal cortex, the two models assume a role in syntactic integration or linking arguments to verbs.

Other models assign less specific, yet still language-related compositional functions to Broca's area. Hagoort (2005) suggests different roles for frontal and temporal perisylvian regions, with Broca's area performing syntactic (but also semantic and phonological) unification operations and posterior temporal cortex being the storage site for lexical syntactic information. Confirmation for the differential role of these regions comes from a recent study by Snijders et al. (2009) who showed that Dutch words of ambiguous syntactic category status (noun or verb) elicited stronger activation of posterior Broca's area only when they were presented in sentences but stronger activation of the left posterior middle temporal gyrus also when they were presented in a nonsyntactic context.

Chen, West, Waters, and Caplan (2006) reanalyzed a number of previous studies reporting stronger activation of Broca's area by object-extracted compared to subject relative clauses. They showed that activation increases are only observed when the subject of the relative clause is inanimate and the subject of the main clause animate (e.g., "The golfer that the lightning struck") and not for syntactically identical sentences with animate relative clause subjects. They argue that this finding rules out hypotheses based on syntactic structure complexity and rather suggests that Broca's area activation reflects the relative difficulty of thematic role assignment, with inanimate referents being dispreferred agents and animate referents dispreferred patients (see also Kuperberg, Sitnikova, & Lakshmanan, 2008).

Other authors do not assume activation of Broca's area to reflect a compositional function but rather emphasize the impact of the syntactic working memory load required by syntactic relationships of distant elements in complex sentences (Cooke et al., 2001; Fiebach, Schlesewsky, & Friederici, 2001).

Finally, there are models whose authors do not see a language-specific, let alone syntax-specific, role for Broca's area at all. Novick, Trueswell, and Thompson-Schill (2005) attribute a cognitive control function to this region and interpret its activation in the comprehension of complex sentences as due to the resolution of a conflict between competing representation similar to those elicited by garden-path sentences (see Vissers, Chwilla, & Kolk, 2006, for a similar view).

To date, none of these hypotheses is able to account for all available hemodynamic activation data. While it is true that many of the syntactically complex sentences that have been used involved movement of syntactic constituents, it is not true that Broca's area is only activated when there is movement. The meta-analysis data show that it is also reliably activated for sentences containing syntactic violations and even for simple correct sentences. One might argue that in these studies at least BA 44 activation is entirely due to word or phonemic level processing, because it is not reliably activated in a subset of studies where simple sentences were compared to word lists (see Figure 11.2c). Note, however, that BA 44 is the most reliably found region for the same comparison in syntactic production (Figure 11.2d), so that a specific involvement of this region in syntactic movement is still unlikely. The finding of Chen et al. (2006) that the animacy of noun phrase referents determines Broca's area activation in the most frequently used type of syntactically complex sentences is difficult to explain not only for a movement account but also for accounts emphasizing the role of working memory load for Broca's area activation. Also data from a study reporting that Broca's area activation was not affected by participants' working memory capacity (Waters, Caplan, Alpert, & Stanczak, 2003) are problematic in this respect.

By contrast, Chen et al.'s (2006) conclusion that Broca's area is involved in thematic role assignment is compatible with the proposals of Bornkessel and Schlesewsky (2006), Hagoort (2005), and Kuperberg et al. (2008), and thus seems a promising avenue for further research. In particular, it would be necessary to find evidence distinguishing between an initial thematic role assignment only (as postulated by Bornkessel & Schlesewsky, 2006) and thematic role assignment in general, and to find evidence distinguishing between thematic role assignment and more general control, reanalysis or monitoring functions, which are quite plausibly more strongly recruited in case of difficulty with thematic role assignment.

An as yet underestimated issue is the relationship between syntactic comprehension and production. Note that a thematic role assignment account of Broca's area activation leaves activation of the same region in syntactic production unaccounted for: when producing sentences, speakers know the thematic roles even before they encode the syntactic structure. If this region is involved in mapping syntactic to thematic roles in comprehension and in mapping thematic to syntactic roles in production, its function is probably better characterized as one of structure-building similar to the notion of "unification" suggested by Hagoort (2005).

While not as much in the focus of the discussion between proponents of different models as the role of Broca's area, the proposed functional characterizations of the left posterior temporal lobe in sentence processing are as difficult to reconcile with the available evidence. A role in the storage of lexical syntactic information does not explain why this region is more strongly activated for object relative clause compared to subject relative clause sentences containing the same words. It also doesn't explain why this region is not (or at least much less) active in syntactic production. A role in syntactic integration or argument linking might explain these results better, but is not easily reconciled with the abovementioned finding of Snijders et al. (2009) that this region did not respond differentially for category-ambiguous words presented in sentences and syntactically unrelated word lists. It also remains to be seen whether future syntactic repetition suppression studies confirm a sensitivity of this region to syntactic structure.

Conclusion

There is good and largely consistent evidence for Broca's area and the left posterior temporal lobe as neural substrates of syntactic processing in sentence comprehension and production. The question is which aspect of syntactic processing they actually reflect. For comprehension, Broca's area rather plays a role in thematic role assignment than in building a syntactic structure per se. A better characterization also capturing its function in syntactic production may be that Broca's area is involved in the bidirectional mapping of thematic and syntactic structures.

References

Numbers in square brackets relate to the identification of studies in Figure 11.1 and Figure 11.2.

Bahlmann, J., Rodriguez-Fornells, A., Rotte, M., & Münte, T. F. (2007). An fMRI study of canonical and noncanonical word order in German. *Human Brian Mapping, 28,* 940–949.

Bavelier, D., Corina, D., Jezzard, P., Clark, V., Karni, A., Lalwani, A., et al. (1998). Hemispheric specialization for English and ASL: Left invariance right variability. *Neuroreport, 9,* 1537–1542. [2]

Bavelier, D., Corina, D., Jezzard, P., Padmanabhan, S., Clark, V. P., Karni, A., et al. (1997). Sentence reading: A functional MRI study at 4 tesla. *Journal of Cognitive Neuroscience, 9,* 664–686. [2]

Ben-Shachar, M., Hendler, T., Kahn, I., Ben-Bashat, D., & Grodzinsky, Y. (2003). The neural reality of syntactic transformations: Evidence from functional magnetic resonance imaging. *Psychological Science, 14,* 433–440. [3] [6]

Ben-Shachar, M., Palti, D., & Grodzinsky, Y. (2004). Neural correlates of syntactic movement: Converging evidence from two fMRI experiments. *NeuroImage, 21*, 1320–1336. [3] [6]

Bornkessel, I., & Schlesewsky, M. (2006). The extended argument dependency model: A neurocognitive approach to sentence comprehension across languages. *Psychological Review, 113*, 787–821.

Bottini, G., Corcoran, R., Sterzi, R., Paulesu, E., Schenone, P., Scarpa, P., et al. (1994). The role of the right-hemisphere in the interpretation of figurative aspects of language – A positron emission tomography activation study. *Brain, 117*, 1241–1253. [2] [7]

Capek, C. M., Bavelier, D., Corina, D., Newman, A. J., Jezzard, P., & Neville, H. J. (2004). The cortical organization of audio-visual sentence comprehension: An fMRI study at 4 Tesla. *Cognitive Brain Research, 20*, 111–119. [2] [4]

Caplan, D., Alpert, N., & Waters, G. (1998). Effects of syntactic structure and propositional number on patterns of regional cerebral blood flow. *Journal of Cognitive Neuroscience, 10*, 541–552. [1] [6]

Caplan, D., Alpert, N., & Waters, G. (1999). PET studies of syntactic processing with auditory sentence presentation. *NeuroImage, 9*, 343–351. [3] [6]

Caplan, D., Alpert, N., Waters, G., & Olivieri, A. (2000). Activation of Broca's area by syntactic processing under conditions of concurrent articulation. *Human Brain Mapping, 9*, 65–71. [1] [6]

Caplan, D., Hildebrandt, N., & Makris, N. (1996). Location of lesions in stroke patients with deficits in syntactic processing in sentence comprehension. *Brain, 119*, 933–949.

Chee, M. W. L., Caplan, D., Soon, C. S., Sriram, N., Tan, E. W. L., Thiel, T., et al. (1999). Processing of visually presented sentences in Mandarin and English studied with fMRI. *Neuron, 23*, 127–137. [2]

Chen, E., West, W. C., Waters, G., & Caplan, D. (2006). Determinants of bold signal correlates of processing object-extracted relative clauses. *Cortex, 42*, 591–604. [1] [6]

Constable, R. T., Pugh, K. R., Berroya, E., Mencl, W. E., Westerveld, M., Ni, W. J., et al. (2004). Sentence complexity and input modality effects in sentence comprehension: An fMRI study. *NeuroImage, 22*, 11–21. [2] [4]

Cooke, A., Grossman, M., DeVita, C., Gonzalez-Atavales, J., Moore, P., Chen, W., et al. (2006). Large-scale neural network for sentence processing. *Brain and Language, 96*, 14–36. [1] [5]

Cooke, A., Zurif, E. B., DeVita, C., Alsop, D., Koenig, P., Detre, J., et al. (2001). Neural basis for sentence comprehension: Grammatical and short-term memory components. *Human Brain Mapping, 15*, 80–94. [1] [6]

Dapretto, M., & Bookheimer, S. Y. (1999). Form and content: Dissociating syntax and semantics in sentence comprehension. *Neuron, 24*, 427–432. [3] [6]

Embick, D., Marantz, A., Miyashita, Y., O'Neil, W., & Sakai, K. L. (2000). A syntactic specialization for Broca's area. *Proceedings of the National Academy of Sciences of the United States of America, 97*, 6150–6154. [1] [5]

Fiebach, C. J., Schlesewsky, M., & Friederici, A. D. (2001). Syntactic working memory and the establishment of filler-gap dependencies: Insights from ERPs and fMRI. *Journal of Psycholinguistic Research, 30*, 321–338.

Fiebach, C. J., Schlesewsky, M., Lohmann, G., von Cramon, D. Y., & Friederici, A. D. (2005). Revisiting the role of Broca's area in sentence processing: Syntactic integration versus syntactic working memory. *Human Brain Mapping, 24*, 79–91. [1] [6]

Friederici, A. D., Meyer, M., & von Cramon, D. Y. (2000). Auditory language comprehension: An event-related fMRI study on the processing of syntactic and lexical information. *Brain and Language, 74*, 289–300. [4] [7]

Giraud, A. L., Truy, E., Frackowiak, R. S. J., Gregoire, M. C., Pujol, J. F., & Collet, L. (2000). Differential recruitment of the speech processing system in healthy subjects and reha-bilitated cochlear implant patients. *Brain, 123*, 1391–1402. [4]

Golestani, N., Alario, F. X., Meriaux, S., Le Bihan, D., Dehaene, S., & Pallier, C. (2006). Syntax production in bilinguals. *Neuropsychologia, 44*, 1029–1040. [8]

Grodzinsky, Y. & Friederici, A. D. (2006). Neuroimaging of syntax and syntactic processing. *Current Opinion in Neurobiology, 16*, 240–246.

Grossman, M., Cooke, A., DeVita, C., Alsop, D., Detre, J., Chen, W., et al. (2002). Age-related changes in working memory during sentence comprehension: An fMRI study. *NeuroImage, 15*, 302–317. [1] [6]

Hagoort, P. (2005). On Broca, brain, and binding: A new framework. *Trends in Cognitive Sciences, 9*, 416–423.

Haller, S., Klarhöfer, M., Radue, E. W., Schwarzbach, J., & Indefrey, P. (2007). Temporal analysis of fMRI data on word and sentence reading. *European Journal of Neuroscience, 26*, 2074–2084.

Haller, S., Radue, E. W., Erb, M., Grodd, W., & Kircher, T. (2005). Overt sentence production in event-related fMRI. *Neuropsychologia, 43*, 807–814. [8]

Hashimoto, R., & Sakai, K. L. (2002). Specialization in the left prefrontal cortex for sentence comprehension. *Neuron, 35*, 589–597. [2]

Hoen, M., Pachot-Clouard, M., Segebarth, C., & Dominey, P. F. (2006). When Broca experi-ences the Janus syndrome: An ER-fMRI study comparing sentence comprehension and cognitive sequence processing. *Cortex, 42*, 605–623. [1] [5]

Homae, F., Hashimoto, R., Nakajima, K., Miyashita, Y., & Sakai, K. L. (2002). From perception to sentence comprehension: The convergence auditory and visual information of lan-guage in the left inferior frontal cortex. *NeuroImage, 16*, 883–900. [4]

Humphries, C., Love, T., Swinney, D., & Hickok, G. (2005). Response of anterior temporal cortex to syntactic and prosodic manipulations during sentence processing. *Human Brain Mapping, 26*, 128–138. [4]

Humphries, C., Willard, K., Buchsbaum, B., & Hickok, G. (2001). Role of anterior temporal cortex in auditory sentence comprehension: An fMRI study. *Neuroreport, 12*, 1749–1752. [4] [7]

Indefrey, P., Brown, C. M., Hellwig, F., Amunts, K., Herzog, H., Seitz, R. J., et al. (2001). A neural correlate of syntactic encoding during speech production. *Proceedings of the National Academy of Sciences of the United States of America, 98*, 5933–5936. [8]

Indefrey, P., Hagoort, P., Herzog, H., Seitz, R. J., & Brown, C. M. (2001). Syntactic processing in left prefrontal cortex is independent of lexical meaning. *NeuroImage, 14*, 546–555. [2]

Indefrey, P., Hellwig, F., Herzog, H., Seitz, R. J., & Hagoort, P. (2004). Neural responses to the production and comprehension of syntax in identical utterances. *Brain and Language, 89*, 312–319. [4] [7] [8]

Indefrey, P., & Levelt, W. J. M. (2004). The spatial and temporal signatures of word produc-tion components. *Cognition, 92*, 101–144.

Inui, T., Otsu, Y., Tanaka, S., Okada, T., Nishizawa, S., & Konishi, J. (1998). A functional MRI analysis of comprehension processes of Japanese sentences. *Neuroreport, 9*, 3325–3328. [1] [6]

Just, M. A., Carpenter, P. A., Keller, T. A., Eddy, W. F., & Thulborn, K. R. (1996). Brain activation modulated by sentence comprehension. *Science, 274*, 114–116. [1] [6]

Kang, A. M., Constable, R. T., Gore, J. C., & Avrutin, S. (1999). An event-related fMRI study of implicit phrase-level syntactic and semantic processing. *NeuroImage, 10*, 555–561. [1] [5]

Kinno, R., Kawamura, M., Shioda, S., & Sakai, K. L. (2008). Neural correlates of noncanonical syntactic processing revealed by a picture–sentence matching task. *Human Brain Mapping, 29*, 1015–1027. [1] [6]

Kuperberg, G. R., Holcomb, P. J., Sitnikova, T., Greve, D., Dale, A. M., & Caplan, D. (2003). Distinct patterns of neural modulation during the processing of conceptual and syntactic anomalies. *Journal of Cognitive Neuroscience, 15*, 272–293. [1] [5]

Kuperberg, G. R., McGuire, P. K., Bullmore, E. T., Brammer, M. J., Rabe-Hesketh, S., Wright, I. C., et al. (2000). Common and distinct neural substrates for pragmatic, semantic, and syntactic processing of spoken sentences: An fMRI study. *Journal of Cognitive Neuroscience, 12*, 321–341. [1] [4] [5] [7]

Kuperberg, G. R., Sitnikova, T., & Lakshmanan, B. M. (2008). Neuroanatomical distinctions within the semantic system during sentence comprehension: Evidence from functional magnetic resonance imaging. *NeuroImage, 40*, 367–388.

Love, T., Haist, F., Nicol, J., & Swinney, D. (2006). A functional neuroimaging investigation of the roles of structural complexity and task-demand during auditory sentence processing. *Cortex, 42*, 577–590. [3]

Mazoyer, B. M., Tzourio, N., Frak, V., Syrota, A., Murayama, N., Levrier, O., et al. (1993). The Cortical Representation of Speech. *Journal of Cognitive Neuroscience, 5*, 467–479. [4]

Menenti, L., Segaert, K., & Hagoort, P. (under review). The neuronal infrastructure of speaking.

Meyer, M., Alter, K., & Friederici, A. (2003). Functional MR imaging exposes differential brain responses to syntax and prosody during auditory sentence comprehension. *Journal of Neurolinguistics, 16*, 277–300. [4]

Meyer, M., Alter, K., Friederici, A. D., Lohmann, G., & von Cramon, D. Y. (2002). FMRI reveals brain regions mediating slow prosodic modulations in spoken sentences. *Human Brain Mapping, 17*, 73–88. [4]

Meyer, M., Friederici, A. D., & von Cramon, D. Y. (2000). Neurocognition of auditory sentence comprehension: Event-related fMRI reveals sensitivity to syntactic violations and task demands. *Cognitive Brain Research, 9*, 19–33. [3] [5]

Michael, E. B., Keller, T. A., Carpenter, P. A., & Just, M. A. (2001). fMRI investigation of sentence comprehension by eye and by ear: Modality fingerprints on cognitive processes. *Human Brain Mapping, 13*, 239–252. [1] [3] [6]

Moro, A., Tettamanti, M., Perani, D., Donati, C., Cappa, S. F., & Fazio, F. (2001). Syntax and the brain: Disentangling grammar by selective anomalies. *NeuroImage, 13*, 110–118. [1] [5]

Müller, R. A., Rothermel, R. D., Behen, M. E., Muzik, O., Mangner, T. J., & Chugani, H. T. (1997). Receptive and expressive language activations for sentences: A PET study. *Neuroreport, 8*, 3767–3770. [4]

Naito, Y., Tateya, I., Fujiki, N., Hirano, S., Ishizu, K., Nagahama, Y., et al. (2000). Increased cortical activation during hearing of speech in cochlear implant users. *Hearing Research, 143*, 139–146. [4]

Nakai, T., Matsuo, K., Kato, C., Matsuzawa, M., Okada, T., Glover, G. H., et al. (1999). A functional magnetic resonance imaging study of listening comprehension of languages in human at 3 tesla-comprehension and activation of the language areas. *Neuroscience Letters, 263,* 33–36. [4]

Nathaniel-James, D. A., Fletcher, P., & Frith, C. D. (1997). The functional anatomy of verbal initiation and suppression using the Hayling Test. *Neuropsychologia, 35,* 559–566. [2]

Neville, H. J., Bavelier, D., Corina, D., Rauschecker, J., Karni, A., Lalwani, A., et al. (1998). Cerebral organization for language in deaf and hearing subjects: Biological constraints and effects of experience. *Proceedings of the National Academy of Sciences of the United States of America, 95,* 922–929. [2]

Newman, S. D., Just, M. A., Keller, T. A., Roth, J., & Carpenter, P. A. (2003). Differential effects of syntactic and semantic processing on the subregions of Broca's area. *Cognitive Brain Research, 16,* 297–307. [1] [6]

Ni, W., Constable, R. T., Mencl, W. E., Pugh, K. R., Fulbright, R. K., Shaywitz, S. E., et al. (2000). An event-related neuroimaging study distinguishing form and content in sentence processing. *Journal of Cognitive Neuroscience, 12,* 120–133. [4]

Nichelli, P., Grafman, J., Pietrini, P., Clark, K., Lee, K. Y., & Miletich, R. (1995). Where the brain appreciates the moral of a story. *Neuroreport, 6,* 2309–2313. [1] [5]

Noguchi, Y., Takeuchi, T., & Sakai, K. L. (2002). Lateralized activation in the inferior frontal cortex during syntactic processing: Event-related optical topography study. *Human Brain Mapping, 17,* 89–99. [1]

Noppeney, U., & Price, C. J. (2004). An fMRI study of syntactic adaptation. *Journal of Cognitive Neuroscience, 16,* 702–713.

Novick, J. M., Trueswell, J. C., & Thompson-Schill, S. L. (2005). Cognitive control and parsing: Re-examining the role of Broca's area in sentence comprehension. *Cognitive, Affective, and Behavioral Neuroscience, 5,* 263–281.

Ozawa, F., Matsuo, K., Kato, C., Nakai, T., Isoda, H., Takehara, Y., et al. (2000). The effects of listening comprehension of various genres of literature on response in the linguistic area: An fMRI study. *Neuroreport, 11,* 1141–1143. [4]

Peck, K. K., Wierenga, C. E., Moore, A. B., Maher, L. M., Gopinath, K., Gaiefsky, M., et al. (2004). Comparison of baseline conditions to investigate syntactic production using functional magnetic resonance imaging. *NeuroImage, 23,* 104–110. [8]

Peelle, J. E., McMillan, C., Moore, P., Grossman, M., & Wingfield, A. (2004). Dissociable patterns of brain activity during comprehension of rapid and syntactically complex speech: Evidence from fMRI. *Brain and Language, 91,* 315–325. [3] [6]

Rapp, A. M., Leube, D. T., Erb, M., Grodd, W., & Kircher, T. T. J. (2004). Neural correlates of metaphor processing. *Cognitive Brain Research, 20,* 395–402. [2]

Robertson, D. A., Gernsbacher, M. A., Guidotti, S. J., Robertson, R. R. W., Irwin, W., Mock, B. J., et al. (2000). Functional neuroanatomy of the cognitive process of mapping during discourse comprehension. *Psychological Science, 11,* 255–260. [2]

Röder, B., Stock, O., Neville, H., Bien, S., & Rösler, F. (2002). Brain activation modulated by the comprehension of normal and pseudo-word sentences of different processing demands: A functional magnetic resonance imaging study. *NeuroImage, 15,* 1003–1014. [3] [6]

Rüschemeyer, S. A., Zysset, S., & Friederici, A. D. (2006). Native and non-native reading of sentences: An fMRI experiment. *NeuroImage, 31,* 354–365. [1][5]

Salvi, R. J., Lockwood, A. H., Frisina, R. D., Coad, M. L., Wack, D. S., & Frisina, D. R. (2002). PET imaging of the normal human auditory system: Responses to speech in quiet and in background noise. *Hearing Research, 170,* 96–106. [4]

Schlosser, M. J., Aoyagi, N., Fulbright, R. K., Gore, J. C., & McCarthy, G. (1998). Functional MRI studies of auditory comprehension. *Human Brain Mapping, 6*, 1–13. [4]

Scott, S. K., Blank, C. C., Rosen, S., & Wise, R. J. S. (2000). Identification of a pathway for intelligible speech in the left temporal lobe. *Brain, 123*(12), 2400–2406. [4]

Snijders, T. M., Vosse, T., Kempen, G., van Berkum, J. J. A., Petersson, K. M., & Hagoort, P. (2009). Retrieval and unification of syntactic structure in sentence comprehension: An fMRI study using word-category ambiguity. *Cerebral Cortex, 19*, 1493–1503. [1] [2] [7]

Stowe, L. A., Broere, C. A. J., Paans, A. M. J., Wijers, A. A., Mulder, G., Vaalburg, W., et al. (1998). Localizing components of a complex task: Sentence processing and working memory. *Neuroreport, 9*, 2995–2999. [1] [6]

Stowe, L. A., Paans, A. M. J., Wijers, A. A., & Zwarts, F. (2004). Activations of "motor" and other non-language structures during sentence comprehension. *Brain and Language, 89*, 290–299. [1]

Stowe, L. A., Wijers, A. A., Willemsen, A., Reuland, E., Paans, A. M. J., & Vaalburg, W. (1994). PET studies of language – An assessment of the reliability of the technique. *Journal of Psycholinguistic Research, 23*, 499–527. [2]

Stromswold, K., Caplan, D., Alpert, N., & Rauch, S. (1996). Localization of syntactic comprehension by positron emission tomography. *Brain and Language, 52*, 452–473. [1] [6]

Suh, S., Yoon, H. W., Lee, S., Chung, J. Y., Cho, Z. H., & Park, H. (2007). Effects of syntactic complexity in L1 and L2; An fMRI study of Korean–English bilinguals. *Brain Research, 1136*, 178–189. [1] [6]

Suzuki, K., & Sakai, K. L. (2003). An event-related fMRI study of explicit syntactic processing of normal/anomalous sentences in contrast to implicit syntactic processing. *Cerebral Cortex, 13*, 517–526. [3]

Talairach, J., & Tournoux, P. (1988). *Co-planar stereotaxic atlas of the human brain*. Stuttgart: Georg Thieme Verlag.

Vissers, T. W. M., Chwilla, D. J., & Kolk, H. H. J. (2006) Monitoring in language perception: The effect of misspellings of words in highly constrained sentences. *Brain Research, 1106*, 150–163.

Wang, S. P., Zhu, Z. D., Zhang, J. X., Wang, Z. X., Xiao, Z. W., Xiang, H. D., et al. (2008). Broca's area plays a role in syntactic processing during Chinese reading comprehension. *Neuropsychologia, 46*, 1371–1378. [1] [5]

Wartenburger, I., Heekeren, H. R., Burchert, F., De Bleser, R., & Villringer, A. (2003). Grammaticality judgments on sentences with and without movement of phrasal constituents – An event-related fMRI study. *Journal of Neurolinguistics, 16*, 301–314. [1] [5]

Waters, G., Caplan, D., Alpert, N., & Stanczak, L. (2003). Individual differences in rCBF correlates of syntactic processing in sentence comprehension: Effects of working memory and speed of processing. *NeuroImage, 19*, 101–112. [1] [6]

Weber, K., & Indefrey, P. (2009). Syntactic priming in German–English bilinguals during sentence comprehension. *NeuroImage, 46*, 1164–1172. [2]

Wong, D., Miyamoto, R. T., Pisoni, D. B., Sehgal, M., & Hutchins, G. D. (1999). PET imaging of cochlear-implant and normal-hearing subjects listening to speech and nonspeech. *Hearing Research, 132*, 34–42. [4] [7]

Xu, J., Kemeny, S., Park, G., Frattali, C., & Braun, A. (2005). Language in context: Emergent features of word, sentence, and narrative comprehension. *NeuroImage, 25*, 1002–1015. [2] [7]

12

The Neurobiology of Structure-Dependency in Natural Language Grammar

Marco Tettamanti and Daniela Perani

Introduction

Human linguistic communication, be it spoken or signed, is characterized by a property that allows infinite possibilities of expression: a finite number of linguistic signs can be combined by a finite number of structure-dependent rules in an infinite number of ways. Signs – such as speech sounds, words, or phrases – can be combined into larger entities by means of structure-dependent computational processes, thus generating hierarchical structures. Likewise, larger entities of hierarchical structure can be decomposed in a structure-dependent manner into elementary units that can be learned, processed, and stored.

The aim of this chapter is to present evidence from a wide host of empirical studies showing, at a behavioral, cognitive, and neural level, how structure-dependent regularities are represented in the human brain for the purpose of higher cognitive functions, with a special focus on language.

The chapter starts by examining structure-dependency in linguistic theories, showing how the language grammar, and syntax in particular, is based on structure-dependent, recursive hierarchical computation. We will then consider developmental studies showing how structure dependencies are acquired throughout the early lifespan. The main section of the chapter will then be dedicated to a review of the literature on the neural correlates of structure-dependence processing in humans. Special attention will be devoted to sign language, which shows unique properties integrating linguistic, motor and visuospatial functions. These unique properties emphasize the degree of modality-independent computation of hierarchical structural principles in humans. Throughout the different sections of the chapter, evidence in humans will be complemented, if available, by

The Handbook of the Neuropsychology of Language, First Edition. Edited by Miriam Faust.
© 2012 Blackwell Publishing Ltd. Published 2012 by Blackwell Publishing Ltd.

evidence in nonhuman primates and other vertebrates, to provide a phylogenetic perspective on the neural correlates of such a fundamental computational ability that attains an unrivaled degree of complexity in the human species.

Structure-Dependency in Linguistic Theories

Language is a hierarchical communication system that maps multidimensional conceptual relationships onto sequences of physical vectors. In generative linguistic models (e.g., minimalist program, Shannon & Weaver, 1949; head driven phrase structure grammar, Pollard & Sag, 1994; parallel constraint-based theories, Jackendoff, 2003), the term "hierarchical" is broadly taken to indicate that higher-level structures (e.g., sentence-level clauses such as "The yellow fog that rubs its back upon the window panes" (T. S. Eliot)) consist of a combination of lower-level constituents (e.g., phrases such as "the yellow fog" or "upon the window panes"), which in turn can be composed of lower-level entities (e.g., determiners such as "the," adjectives such as "yellow," nouns such as "fog"). Higher-level constituent combinations can be further hierarchically embedded in even more complex structures. Basically, this structure-dependent recursive process can be reiterated infinitely, generating complex linguistic structures featuring long-distance dependencies among constituents. A formal description of the algorithm of recursion is provided by phrase structure grammars (PSG) of the form A^nB^n, generating embedded sequences such as A_1B_1, $A_1A_2B_2B_1$, $A_1A_2A_3B_3B_2B_1$, and so on (Chomsky, 1957).

The hierarchical syntactic organization, as reflected in phrase structure, is based on lexical categories such as nouns, verbs, adjectives, or adverbs. The words belonging to these lexical categories are represented in a mental lexicon. The mental lexicon specifies, in addition to a word's meaning, information pertaining to its phonological form and its syntactic properties, including inflectional and positional information.

Hierarchical structuring principles are found at all linguistic levels: phonological, syntactic, morphosyntactic, and semantic. At the phonological level, phonemes form syllables, which in turn form words. With a finite number of phonemes, a virtually infinite number of words can be generated. The syllable structure itself is hierarchically organized, with a "nucleus" that forms the sonorous core of the syllable, which together with an optional "coda" is grouped as a "rime." The nucleus itself may be preceded by other phonological material, which is then called "onset." At the syntactic level, constituents, such as heads and modifiers, are grouped together into phrases, and at a higher level phrases are grouped into clauses. At the morpho-syntactic level, word formation is governed by rules specifying how particular morphemes can be combined according to hierarchical tree structures (e.g., the verb "perturb" and the suffix "able" forming the adjective "perturbable," which can be further combined with the prefix "im," yielding "imperturbable"). At the semantic level, concepts are hierarchically organized into subordinate and superordinate categories (such as [[[cat] felines] animals]) and, although with considerable disagreement among linguists, sentences are formed by embedded conceptual constituents (such as "the little star," in which, apart from the conceptual relation established between the object "star" and its property "little" and a definite quantity "the," object and property may each have further internal conceptual structure: e.g., "little" specifies that the size of the object is smaller than a pragmatically determined norm) (Jackendoff, 2003).

The generation of the set of all the well-formed linguistic expressions, and only these, is strictly constrained by structural relations that can operate nonlinearly and nonlocally at long distances. In other words, the distribution of linguistic elements into composite sequences is not determined by specification rules that map elements to cardinal positions along a linear segment or by rules that predict the position of a certain element as a function of the preceding one (e.g., in terms of linear order or local transition probabilities). Quite the contrary, the position of elements in higher-order units is specified by context-sensitive boundaries marked by phrase structure that can be extended by inserting an undetermined number of further elements. These boundaries also constrain the number of positions that a particular element can take to a specific subset. For example, depending on whether a sentence has an active or passive form, a particular word will take two different contextually constrained well-defined positions, which are associated with distinct grammatical functions.

Nevertheless, due to the physical constraints of human linguistic communication, hierarchical structures must be linearized into sequences of words for language production. An interesting hypothesis that has been recently proposed by linguists is that the mapping of linguistic abstract structures onto linear physical strings of sounds requires that linguistic symbols be linked by hierarchical syntactic relations, in order to adequately (univocally and without error) convey a vast number of concepts (Jackendoff, 1999). Hierarchy in language helps to solve the problem of reconstructing the intended conceptual meaning from the linear sequence of speech, a problem that, without hierarchical organization, would not have unequivocal solutions. Some mathematical models of evolutionary dynamics have been developed, showing that in the course of cultural evolution an increase in the number of relevant concepts that humans adopted may have guided the transition from nonsyntactic to hierarchical syntactic forms of expression (Nowak, Plotkin, & Jansen, 2000; Nowak & Komarova, 2001). The use of nonsyntactic communication (i.e., the use of elementary signals, such as single words, to refer to entire events) with a large lexicon inevitably leads to a high number of errors in message production and comprehension. Given that signals cannot vary unboundedly (i.e., they must be small in size, in order to be memorable), a large lexicon with many different signals of limited size makes the signals physically similar, such that they are easily confounded. On a more complex level of nonsyntactic communication, on which different elementary signals are combined to form complex signals, the lack of hierarchical phrase structure – a stage that has been termed as "protolanguage" (Bickerton, 1990) – allows for unambiguous message communication, however only in cases in which interpretation is driven by the pragmatics of the words involved (e.g., "eat apple Fred," in which only "Fred" can be the agent of the action "to eat"). In the absence of pragmatic cues (e.g., "kiss John Mary," where agent and patient are not univocally defined) ambiguities arise (Jackendoff, 1999).

It is possible that among the different properties of hierarchical structure-dependency illustrated above, syntactic recursion occupies a prominent position, both at the theoretical and at the evolutionary level. Hauser, Chomsky, & Fitch (2002) proposed the definition of a so-called "faculty of language in the narrow sense" (FLN) included within a more general "faculty of language in the broad sense" (FLB). While FLB consists of the conceptual and sensorimotor faculties exploited by human language, FLN incorporates, as a distinguishing feature, the computational system of recursion. The authors also proposed that FLN is a uniquely human computational mechanism, which qualitatively distinguishes us from nonhuman primates and all other species. On this view, the evolution of language in phylogenesis may be strictly linked to the evolution of FLN.

Acquisition of Structure-Dependent Grammatical Skills in Early Ontogeny

As discussed above, human natural language is organized according to multiple levels of structure-dependent hierarchical relationships at the phonological, morphological, and syntactic levels, and in a broader sense also at the conceptual-semantic level. However, only a subset of these hierarchical properties is transparent at the surface structure level of language, i.e., at the level of language production and perception. Most hierarchical relations are established at a deep abstract level and are not obviously mirrored by surface structures. The fact that complex hierarchical principles are not physically manifest at the language surface level poses intriguing questions about the mechanisms underlying language acquisition. Children are not given instructions as to the properties that human language must conform to, yet most of them develop the capacity to properly use and understand language in their first few years of life. It is plausible that certain universal properties of human language emerged or were selected as a consequence of specific constraints imposed by the general learning capacities that become available to infants with an ontogenetically determined chronological progression (Saffran, 2001).

At the surface structural level, a crucial problem that every child is faced with is to segment fluent speech such that the boundaries that separate adjacent words can be identified. The sensitivity to the phonemic properties of spoken language might be attained very early during development, possibly even before birth (Jusczyk, Friederici, Wessels, Svenkerud, & Jusczyk, 1993). Neonates as young as 4 days are capable of discriminating sentences in their native language from native speech played backward (Bertoncini et al., 1989; Dehaene-Lambertz & Houston, 1998; Mehler et al., 1988). Event-related potentials (ERP) and functional magnetic resonance imaging (fMRI) studies have shown that 3- to 6-month-old babies dispose of left-perisylvian neural structures in the temporoparietal and frontal cortex that respond selectively to the phonemic and prosodic contours of the infants' native language (Cheour et al., 1998; Dehaene-Lambertz & Dehaene, 1994; Dehaene-Lambertz, Dehaene, & Hertz-Pannier, 2002). The capacity to perform phonemic and prosodic discriminations does not seem to be human-specific, given that it has been demonstrated also in a number of nonhuman species, and might reflect general-domain auditory processing mechanisms (Kuhl, 2000).

The sensitivity to the phonemic and prosodic contours of natural languages is assumed to guide infants in determining the segmental transitions across words. This is a difficult learning process, as word boundaries in fluent speech are inconsistently marked by acoustic cues such as pauses, contrary to clause boundaries that tend to be systematically marked by pauses and other prosodic cues, and which can be exploited by 6-month-old infants to detect clause boundaries in a language specific manner (Hirsh-Pasek et al., 1987; Jusczyk, 1997). Nevertheless, not later than at 7 months of age, children are able to identify single words (Jusczyk, 1997). One possible mechanism by which children learn which sound combinations are words is the extraction of statistical (probabilistic and distributional) regularities from linguistic input, i.e., by the detection of consistent sequential patterns of sounds. This is in principle possible because the probability that a particular syllable follows another one tends to be higher when the two syllables belong to the same word than when they are each part of one of two subsequent words. Thus, children can compute sequential statistics from speech to determine which syllable sequences form potential words.

It has indeed been shown that 8-month-old infants can detect and use syllabic distribution information to segment words they have never encountered before, after no more than 2 minutes of exposure (Aslin, Saffran, & Newport, 1998; Saffran, Aslin, & Newport, 1996). Another set of experiments (Marcus, Vijayan, Bandi Rao, & Vishton, 1999) with 7-month-old infants demonstrated that, apart from picking up statistical information, children are also capable of learning abstract rules, in the form of algebraic representations (e.g., adjacent, nonhierarchical rules of the type ABA, or AAB). In these experiments the words presented during familiarization never occurred in the test phase. Performance in the test phase was interpreted as reflecting a generalization of the learned abstract rules. Similar findings were obtained in a nonlinguistic version of this task (Saffran, Pollak, Seibel, & Shkolnik, 2007). These results, however, have led to opposing interpretations as to whether the infants were indeed using abstract rules to make generalizations or were instead relying on statistical information (McClelland & Plaut, 1999). Interestingly, children aged 1–6 days have been shown to be able to detect and recognize adjacent repetitions within phonological syllable sequences, based on some automatic perceptual mechanisms (Gervain, Macagno, Cogoi, Peña, & Mehler, 2008). Using optical brain imaging, Gervain, Macagno et al. (2008) demonstrated enhanced neurophysiological responses in temporal and left frontal brain regions when newborns listened to adjacent repetition ABB sequences compared to random control ABC sequences. In turn, no evidence of discrimination was found when newborns listened to nonadjacent repetition ABA sequences compared to, again, random control ABC sequences.

Transition probabilities between subsequent syllables are based on adjacent, non-hierarchical properties of surface structures. To understand and produce well-formed sentences in their native language, children must also learn to assign words to grammatical categories – such as nouns, determiners or verbs – and to combine words into phrases and phrases into clauses. This requires knowledge of the underlying abstract hierarchical principles of the grammar. The mechanisms by which they learn such nonadjacent structural dependencies are still largely unknown.

Several observations are concordant in suggesting that grammatical categories may be assigned to words by detecting their co-occurrence regularities (Cartwright & Brent, 1997), by detecting phonological cues that systematically occur with some categories and not with others (Shi, Werker, & Morgan, 1999), and perhaps also prosodic and morphological cues and the different distribution frequencies of function versus content words (Gervain, Nespor, Mazuka, Horie, & Mehler, 2008). Function words distribution is a salient marker of edges between syntactic units, and it may underlie the acquisition of syntactic categories. Once grammatical categories have been acquired, the distributional behavior of grammatical categories may in principle be used to determine how words form phrases by learning predictive dependencies, for example by learning that the appearance of a determiner (such as "the" in English) in a sentence predicts that, with high probability, a noun will appear later on (whereas the reverse prediction is less probable) or by learning that words that make up phrases move together within and across sentences. Once the basic phrase structure has been learned, other dependencies may be more easily discovered, such as the relationship between transitive verbs and object noun phrases, or between prepositions and noun phrases (Saffran, 2001). Lany and Gómez (2008) found that experience with regularities based on adjacency can bootstrap the infants' ability to track nonadjacent dependencies. Saffran (2001), however, showed that children between 6 and 9 years of age possess limited abilities to detect such nonadjacent predictive dependencies and use these only to acquire relatively simple syntactic rules. This suggests that in children, the acquisition of syntactic properties, in particular those of higher hierarchical complexity, cannot be reduced to statistical learning. Children may possess either some kind of neurobiological predisposition or other types of learning abilities that enable them to detect and incorporate linguistic information without explicit guidance, thus developing full language competence.

In addition to the study by Gervain, Macagno, et al. (2008) discussed above, only a few studies to date have directly investigated the neurophysiological correlates of structural dependencies processing at early ontogenetic stages, but their results do already allow rough delineation of the timing and the anatomy of some relevant developmental maturation processes undergoing in the brain during the first years of life, and how these processes could be deranged in pathological language acquisition. Oberecker, Friedrich, and Friederici (2005) used ERPs to compare the neurophysiological responses to syntactic local phrase-structure violations in adults with those in children from 31 to 34 months of age. Similar to adults, children displayed a biphasic ERP pattern, with an early left-hemispheric anterior negativity (LAN), thought to reflect first-pass, preliminary syntactic parsing (Friederici, 2002), followed by a centro-parietal positivity (P600), thought to reflect a second-pass, more controlled syntactic reanalysis (Friederici, 2002). However, both ERP components presented delayed latencies and lasted longer in children compared to adults, suggesting that the neural mechanisms of phrase-structure computation are already present at such an early age, but that maturation processes in perisylvian language areas are still underway. This view is reinforced by evidence showing that in children that are only a few months younger (24 months of age), local phrase-structure violations only elicit a P600-like neurophysiological response, but no LAN (Oberecker & Friederici, 2006). This may suggest that 2-year-old children are still not fully capable of computing first-pass phrase-structure dependencies, but instead more heavily rely on indirect cues, such as lexical semantics, during second-pass syntactic reanalysis (Friederici, 2006). Morphosyntactic processing also seems to be affected by neurophysiological maturation processes in early ontogeny, as demonstrated in 30-month-olds (Silva-Pereyra, Klarman, et al., 2005) and in 36- to 48-month-olds (Silva-Pereyra, Rivera-Gaxiola, et al., 2005).

Evidence on children with specific language impairment (SLI) further emphasizes the importance of anterior left-hemispheric brain maturation processes for the full development of syntactic processing capabilities. Function words, which are known to elicit a LAN response in normally developing children, evoked a more bilateral or even right-lateralized negativity in SLI children (Neville, Coffey, Holcomb, & Tallal, 1993). Similarly, LAN responses to nonlocal phrase-structure violations were found to be strongly delayed and more posteriorly distributed in 12- to 14-year-old children with the grammatical variant of SLI – N400 responses to lexical semantics being comparable to normally developing children (Fonteneau & van der Lely, 2008).

Finally, preliminary results of a neuroanatomical comparison between adults and 7-year-old children, using a magnetic resonance imaging-based measure of white matter myelination (fractional anisotropy), indicate that the fibers forming the arcuate fasciculus and the superior longitudinal fasciculus may not be fully myelinized in children at this developmental stage, who in parallel also present a not fully developed syntactic competence (Friederici, 2009). These two dorsal white matter pathways play a crucial role in connecting the posterior inferior frontal gyrus (IFG) and the posterior superior temporal lobe, i.e., two brain regions that seem to play a crucial role in the processing of long-distance syntactic dependencies (see next section).

A highly relevant issue with respect to the language-specificity of the ontogenetic acquisition processes of structural dependencies regards the existing correlations in infancy between the linguistic developmental stages and the stages attained in other cognitive domains, in particular the correlation between speech and gestural production. Gestures are particularly relevant to the study of hierarchical structure dependencies as they consist of a wide range of motor acts that reflect a hierarchical (though sequential) organization (Lashley, 1951) and often convey communicative intentions. Parallels between early language development and manual communicative gestures have been recognized, reinforcing the view that linguistic and nonlinguistic symbolic communication may be correlated (see Bates & Dick, 2002, for a review).

In the development of gestures, children progress from a stage in which gestures display rudimentary structures to stages in which gestural sequences of a higher structural complexity are produced. This is illustrated by the fact that, for example, the onset of vocal babbling coincides with the onset of rhythmic hand banging or clapping (Ejiri & Masataka, 2001). In 12- to 18-month-old infants the first instances of naming and gesturing are positively correlated (Shore, Bates, Bretherton, Beeghly, & O'Connell, 1990). At this stage, the produced gestures, just as names, symbolize a particular concept (e.g., mimicking the action of putting a phone to the ear with a clear communicative intent). Somewhat later, two-item combinations are produced: the first two-word combinations are accompanied or slightly preceded by gesture–word (e.g., pointing to an object while uttering its name) and gesture–gesture combinations (e.g., mimicking the action of stirring with a spoon and then drinking from a cup; Capirci, Iverson, Pizzuto, & Volterra, 1996). At 24 to 30 months of age, children produce syntactically complex utterances rich in function words and inflections, and are able to remember and imitate arbitrary sequences of manual actions, the two developments again being positively correlated (Bates and Dick, 2002).

In the lack of specific neuroimaging or neuropsychological data, these early ontogenetic correlations may be attributed to partially overlapping anatomo-functional maturational processes in the left frontotemporoparietal cortex of the kind reviewed above, accompanying both language and sensorimotor learning. On the other hand, later on in ontogenesis, the language system, but less so the gestural repertoire, further expands the typology and complexity of the hierarchical structures used, giving rise to the full linguistic competence of adult human subjects. This points to a plausible differentiation into, at least in part, distinct neural systems.

Structure-Dependency Acquisition and Processing in Adults

While, as we have seen in the previous section, children between 6 and 9 years of age seem to possess limited abilities to detect nonadjacent structural dependencies (Saffran, 2001), the situation with respect to grammatical learning in adults may be somewhat different. Saffran (2001) administered the same artificial grammar learning task to a group of adults. The authors noticed that, compared to the group of children, adults showed significantly better performances in acquiring the same set of simple syntactic rules. They concluded that adult learners can detect phrasal units by just relying on predictive dependencies, i.e., by making inferences on the regularities governing the grouping of word classes into phrases. Accordingly, covariance analyses showed that the hierarchical syntactic structure of natural language cannot be acquired by solely extracting distributional properties of surface cues, such as syllabic or graphemic transitions, and generalizing these properties into rules.

In a different set of related experiments (Peña, Bonatti, Nespor, & Mehler, 2002), it was shown that, at least in adults, language structure acquisition may be driven by two different computational processes, i.e., statistical computations and nonstatistical grammatical rule generalizations. Subjects were presented with streams of continuous synthesized speech composed of syllables. The succession of syllables was governed by nonadjacent transition probabilities, according to which syllables could be grouped into discrete trisyllabic segments (i.e., "words"), as transition probabilities were stronger within segments than across segments. Nonadjacent relations of the type used here (A_iXC_i, where A_i, X, C_i are different syllables, and A_i predicts the appearance of C_i with a probability of 1), although of a simple nature, are compatible with the hierarchical structure of human language. Furthermore, the "words" delimited by such probabilistic constraints all conformed to an underlying abstract rule (of the type A_iXC_i). In a first experiment, after listening to a 10-minute-long familiarization speech stream, subjects were required to choose from a test word pair the word that resembled more closely words present in the speech stream (target words indeed appeared in the familiarization speech stream). The results showed that chunking of fluent speech into single words could indeed be carried out by statistical computation on the basis of nonadjacent transition probabilities. However, in a second experiment, subjects were confronted with word pairs, in which the item congruent with generalization had not appeared in the familiarization set (a rule word). In this second experiment, testing rule generalization, subjects responded at chance, suggesting that they had failed to infer the underlying grammatical rule (A_iXC_i). In a further experiment, however, in the presence of subliminal pauses of 25 ms duration between words, subjects did show generalization to novel items according to the rule, indicating a computational switch from a statistical to a nonstatistical mode. Under these conditions, more closely reflecting natural languages, rule acquisition was found after only 2 minutes of exposure. These data suggest that to discover grammatical regularities, words acquired through statistical information serve as the basis for projecting, nonstatistically, abstract structural generalizations.

Only in recent years, thanks in particular to the progress of neuroimaging techniques, have the neuroanatomical correlates subserving the acquisition of structure-dependency in natural languages begun to be elucidated. Even though, as we have mentioned in our first section, hierarchical structuring principles can be posited at all levels of the language grammar, much of the relevant work in this new field has focused on the acquisition of syntactic structure-dependency. A complete review of the studies that have been devoted to the investigation of the neural bases of syntactic processing is out of the scope of the present chapter (the reader may refer to, e.g., Bookheimer, 2002; Demonet, Thierry, & Cardebat, 2005; see also Indefrey, Volume 1, Chapter 11). More specifically, although it is obvious that the syntactic language component intrinsically reflects hierarchical structuring, we believe that the specific question of structure-dependency in the language grammar can be best addressed by studies that selectively compared hierarchical versus nonhierarchical syntactic structures. In the following we will therefore summarize the major findings that directly pertain to the question of syntactic structure-dependency.

With a high degree of consistency, neuroimaging studies have demonstrated a strong correlation between activations within and around the left inferior frontal cortex (broadly corresponding to the anatomical region that is traditionally defined as Broca's area) and syntactic processing. One of the first experimental approaches employed consisted of varying the level of syntactic complexity, resulting in differential demands on verbal working memory resources that modulated the activity of Broca's area (e.g., Caplan, Alpert, & Waters, 1998; Stromswold, Caplan, Alpert, & Rauch, 1996). Only more recently, convincing evidence was provided that dissociates the working memory load related to syntactic complexity from purely syntactic computational processes: using a two-way factorial manipulation that allowed them to independently test hierarchical center-embedding of clauses and working memory load, Makuuchi, Bahlmann, Anwander, and Friederici (2009) have elegantly demonstrated that structural syntactic processing depends on the pars opercularis of Broca's area, whereas working memory load modulates the activity of the left inferior frontal sulcus. Furthermore, the two anatomical regions were shown to be interconnected through neuronal fiber tracts by magnetic resonance diffusion tensor imaging, and to increase their functional coupling during the processing of complex, hierarchically structured sentences.

A different experimental approach has consisted of directly manipulating syntactic structure dependencies by using syntactically anomalous sentences (Embick, Marantz, Miyashita, O'Neil, & Sakai, 2000; Meyer, Friederici, & von Cramon, 2000; Ni et al., 2000). A drawback of such an approach, however, was that violations at the syntactic level concomitantly disturb semantic interpretation at the sentence level (such as in "All the eaten have eagles snakes"). To eliminate such confounding semantic effects, Moro and colleagues (2001) also used a syntactic violation detection task, but one in which syntax was isolated from lexical semantics, by replacing lexical word roots by phonologically legal pseudowords (such as in "The gulk has ganfed the flust"). In this study, syntactic processing was associated with activation in the circular sulcus, a deep component of Broca's area, in the right IFG, in the left insula, and in the left caudate nucleus.

In addition to left inferior frontal cortical and subcortical regions, the processing of syntactic structure dependencies seems to also engage the left temporal cortex, including in particular the anterior and posterior superior temporal gyrus (STG). The anterior STG may act together with the left frontal operculum (i.e., the cortical band between the crown of the pars opercularis of Broca's area and the anterior insula) in dealing with local phrase structure, whereas the posterior STG may underlie the integration of thematic role assignment and syntactic information to achieve understanding of "who is doing what to whom." The anterior and posterior components of the left STG seem to be differentially interconnected through neuronal fiber tracts to these distinct portions of the frontal cortex: the anterior STG via the uncinate fasciculus to the left frontal operculum, and the posterior STG via the superior longitudinal fasciculus to the pars opercularis of Broca' s area (see Friederici, 2009, for a review).

Specifically, the pars opercularis of Broca's area has been consistently implicated in the processing of linguistic hierarchical structure-dependency, in experimental tasks comparing the acquisition of grammatical rules governed by "nonrigid" syntactic structural dependencies based on hierarchical phrase structure (i.e., the core type of dependencies found in the syntax of all natural languages) to "rigid" syntactic structural dependencies established between words at fixed cardinal positions along the linear word order (i.e., syntactic dependencies that are never found in human languages). Tettamanti and colleagues (2002) let native speakers of Italian acquire novel syntactic rules reflecting hierarchical versus linear syntactic dependencies during fMRI. Based on the work of Moro et al. (2001), the novel syntactic rules were generated by selectively manipulating word order in a synthetic version of Italian, in which open-class word roots were replaced by pseudowords. Hierarchical, but not linear, syntactic rule acquisition selectively activated left perisylvian regions, including Broca's area pars opercularis, the ventral and dorsal premotor cortex, the insula, the posterior STG, and the angular gyrus. The implications of these results have received support by a fMRI study of Musso and colleagues (2003), showing that the acquisition of hierarchical syntactic rules, compared to invented linear rules, can modulate activity in Broca's area across a wide range of typological grammatical variations, such as found between Japanese and Italian. More recently, Broca's area, among other cortical and subcortical brain regions (including, bilaterally, the ventral premotor cortex, the insula, and the basal ganglia), has been shown to selectively subserve the processing of long-distance hierarchical dependencies established by a PSG (A^nB^n), as opposed to local transitions established by a finite state grammar $(AB)^n$ (Bahlmann, Schubotz, & Friederici, 2008; Friederici, Bahlmann, Heim, Schubotz, & Anwander, 2006). A similar contrast between distance-related syntactic dependencies has provided congruent fMRI evidence of an involvement of Broca's area pars opercularis in long-distance dependencies and of the left ventral premotor cortex and bilateral hippocampus in local phrase structure dependencies (Opitz & Friederici, 2007).

As can be gathered from this brief summary, while the involvement of other cortical and subcortical brain regions may vary depending on the type of task and data analysis, Broca's area has been found to be consistently implicated in the acquisition of syntactic dependencies based on recursive hierarchical rules in all the fMRI studies cited above. With the exception of one study, which found an effect localized to the pars triangularis (Musso et al., 2003), all other studies reviewed above found it localized to the pars opercularis of Broca's area. Most studies also converge in showing an increase of activation in Broca's area that correlates with the temporal course (Tettamanti et al., 2002) and with the attained level of proficiency (Musso et al., 2003) in hierarchical rule learning. This pattern of signal increase in Broca's area (paralleled by a signal decrease in the left posterior hippocampus) was also found in a fMRI study on the acquisition of a miniature artificial grammar based on phrase structure (Opitz & Friederici, 2003).

Although traditionally based on Markovian finite state grammars that do not conform to the recursive hierarchical structure dependencies found in natural languages, studies focusing on the acquisition of artificial grammars will be briefly considered here in relation to a further interesting finding of some of the fMRI studies reviewed so far. The right hemispheric homologous region of Broca's area, i.e., the right IFG, was also found to be activated in relation to the detection of violations of hierarchical syntactic dependencies (Moro et al., 2001; Musso et al., 2003; Tettamanti et al., 2002). Bahlmann et al. (2008) found a similar effect, but in the slightly more posterior adjacent rim of the right ventral premotor cortex. Broca's area and its right-hemispheric homologous appear to be part of a larger system of anatomically and functionally interconnected frontoparietal and anterior cingulate cortical regions (Tettamanti et al., 2002) that play a role in rule-based memory. This system was first revealed by a fMRI study on the acquisition of a finite state artificial grammar (Fletcher, Buchel, Josephs, Friston, & Dolan, 1999). The study by Fletcher and colleagues (1999) demonstrated that right IFG activations were associated to the episodic encoding of item-specific letter strings generated by the artificial grammar, rather than to the acquisition of the underlying rules. Furthermore, the right IFG displayed strong functional interconnections with the right inferior parietal lobule at the beginning of the rule acquisition task, whereas these interconnections became weaker once the rule system had been learned. The functional connectivity between Broca's area and the left inferior parietal lobule presented the temporally reversed pattern. A better understanding of such a pattern of right IFG involvement was made possible by a follow-up fMRI study (Fletcher et al., 2005), which showed that right IFG activation subserving item-specific explicit encoding was inversely correlated with implicit learning-related changes, as an increase of right IFG activation induced an activity attenuation in the medial temporal lobe and the thalamus. To summarize, the right IFG may play a relevant role in the initial stages of the acquisition and in the detection of violations of hierarchical syntactic dependencies (congruently with Hampshire, Chamberlain, Monti, Duncan, & Owen, 2010), by supporting the explicit encoding of individual items from the administered repertoire of linguistic utterances. The right IFG may thus operate synergistically with the left IFG (Broca's area), where the encoded individual items may be transcoded into the underlying grammatical rules.

A crucial issue that has been much debated in the literature regards the language-specificity of Broca's area: again, an extensive review of this issue is out of the scope of the present chapter, but it may suffice to emphasize the involvement of this area in a wide host of cognitive and sensorimotor functions (for recent accounts, see Keller, Crow, Foundas, Amunts, & Roberts, 2009; Koechlin & Jubault, 2006; Lindenberg, Fangerau, & Seitz, 2007). More central to the present analysis is the issue of whether the computational properties of the left IFG that code for hierarchical structural dependencies are confined to the processing of the linguistic code or whether they may be exploited also in relation to other cognitive domains (Tettamanti & Weniger, 2006). With respect to theoretical linguistics, it is worth noting that the idea that all components of grammar are language-specific has been challenged (Hauser et al., 2002). Hierarchical structure dependencies, at least in simple form, are not unique to language; parallels can be found in other cognitive domains, including music (Patel, 2003), gestures (see above), action control (Conway & Christiansen, 2001; Greenfield, 1991), and visuospatial processing (Greenfield, 1991). These instances of sequential behavior rely on hierarchical cognitive control and structuring (Byrne & Russon, 1998; Greenfield, 1991; Lashley, 1951). These control mechanisms are required for manageability of complexity, sequence and outcome predictions, and repair; they contribute to the organization of simple subunit-chunks into higher-order assemblies of increasing hierarchical complexity (Byrne and Russon, 1998; Conway and Christiansen, 2001). The grouping of elements into subunit-chunks according to feature and contextual similarity and the linkage of subunits into more complex hierarchical structures, are both flexible processes based on relative (nonrigid) rather than fixed sequential dependencies (Conway and Christiansen, 2001).

Several types of evidence concur in suggesting that common, basic neural and computational mechanisms may underlie both language and nonlinguistic hierarchical processing. In a recent ERP experiment (Lelekov-Boissard & Dominey, 2002), the detection of violations in hierarchical sequences of nonlinguistic symbols was compared with the detection of violations in linguistic syntactic structures. Violations in both types of stimulus materials elicited a late positive electrophysiological component (P600). However, the topographical cortical distribution in the two conditions overlapped only partially, the linguistic structures producing effects more lateralized to the left hemisphere, and nonlinguistic structures producing effects more lateralized to the right hemisphere. As more recent ERP and fMRI experiments suggest, however, the state of affairs may be more complex, and the processing of nonlinguistic hierarchical structures may be subserved by the left hemisphere as well. A neurophysiological study found left anterior negativity effects for the processing of both linguistic and nonlinguistic rule-based sequences (Hoen & Dominey, 2000). Using fMRI, Hoen, Pachot-Clouard, Segebarth, & Dominey (2006) showed that both linguistic and nonlinguistic rule-based sequences activate the frontolateral cortex, bilaterally. A subsequent fMRI study by Tettamanti and colleagues (2009) was specifically aimed at testing the hypothesis of whether the same distinction between "nonrigid" syntactic rules based on hierarchical structure dependency and "rigid" rules based on linear order that was previously investigated in the language domain (see above) led to the selective activation of Broca's area in the visuospatial domain. The acquisition of "nonrigid" but not of "rigid" structural dependencies established within strings of visuospatial nonlinguistic symbols was shown to selectively depend on the activation of the pars opercularis of the left IFG. A formal comparison between the linguistic and nonlinguistic fMRI data corroborated the view of a domain-independent computational role of Broca's area, a kind of "grammar without words" that may serve several cognitive functions. These results were confirmed by another fMRI study (Bahlmann, Schubotz, Mueller, Koester, & Friederici, 2009), in which analogues of a PSG (A^nB^n) and a finite state grammar $(AB)^n$ were implemented in the visuospatial domain.

As we have seen in above, it has been proposed that the "faculty of language in the narrow sense" (FLN) is biologically relevant in distinguishing humans from nonhuman primates (Hauser et al., 2002). Nonhuman primates readily learn to master finite state grammars, based on adjacent linear relations, but seem incapable of spontaneously acquiring PSGs establishing hierarchical relations (Fitch & Hauser, 2004; Jackendoff, 1999; Terrace, Petitto, Sanders, & Bever, 1979). This does not imply that nonhuman primates could not be taught simple PSGs by massive training, as suggested by recent findings showing that a species of common songbirds, European starlings, can learn to classify stimuli that are compatible with context-free PSGs after massive training (Gentner, Fenn, Margoliash, & Nusbaum, 2006; but see Perruchet & Rey, 2005, for an alternative view). Spontaneous acquisition of natural language grammars, however, has never been attested in nonhuman species. This limitation does not appear to be restricted to grammar acquisition: nonhuman primates lack the capacity to cope with hierarchically organized cognitive processes that give rise to nonrigid sequences of actions, such as in the spontaneous imitation of motor actions (Byrne & Russon, 1998; Conway & Christiansen, 2001; Premack, 2004). Altogether, these observations suggest that the human brain has some distinctive traits by which it is capable of encoding hierarchical structure dependencies across diverse higher cognitive functions. With this respect, Broca's area appears to play a central role.

Structure-Dependency in Sign Language

There is general agreement that, compared to spoken language, sign language presents the same distinctive characteristics that are universally recognized to be essential to the human language faculty. In contrast to spoken language based on auditory–oral input–output, sign language is produced by means of manual and facial gestures and is perceived visually. Spoken and signed languages thus provide the opportunity to investigate abstract linguistic structures irrespective of the input–output modality. Sign language, just like spoken language, is characterized by a set of grammatical features that regulate the relationships between concepts (as specified by lexical entries), at the phonological, the morphological, and the syntactic level (Klima & Bellugi, 1979; Petitto et al., 2000). At the phonological level, signs are formed by combining a finite set of meaningless, sublexical elements that can vary along four different dimensions: hand shape, movement, location in space, and palm orientation. These sublexical elements are assembled into units of higher structural complexity, namely syllables, which constitute the basic perceptual unit of sign language. Syllables, in turn, are assembled into signs. Signs have comparable linguistic properties to words in spoken language. At the morphological level, regular changes in form across classes of signs mark both inflectional and derivational changes in meaning; inflections mark such grammatical categories as person, number, distributional and temporal aspect. In sign language, a sign and its inflectional marker may co-occur in time, as for instance in American Sign Language (Klima & Bellugi, 1979). The possibility to express different linguistic symbols simultaneously, rather than just one at a time as in spoken language, is due to the hand-motor and spatial properties exploited by sign language, which offer more degrees of freedom than the oral–auditory modality of speech (Studdert-Kennedy & Lane, 1980). Finally, at the syntactic level, the relations among lexical items are determined by a combination of sign order and manipulation of sign forms in space, modifying the argumental structure of signs, and a small set of facial expressions that indicate particular syntactic forms, as for example questions or topicalized sentences (Liddell, 1980).

Studies in both profoundly deaf and hearing infants acquiring, respectively, signed language only and both signed and spoken language, have shown remarkable parallels in the mechanisms underlying the acquisition of signed language and spoken language. These parallels are equally consistent if compared to hearing babies who acquire spoken language only. There is abundant evidence that deaf babies acquire signed language along the same maturational time schedule as spoken language (Petitto, 1987; Petitto, Katerelos, et al., 2001). Deaf babies spontaneously start producing babbles in the manual modality between 6 and 8 months of age – at the same age when hearing babies produce their first vocal babbles. Manual babbling is characterized by a specific low-frequency rhythmic hand activity at around 1 Hz, differing from other types of nonlinguistic gestures observed in both signing and speaking children which present a higher frequency of approximately 2.5 Hz (Petitto, Holowka, Sergio, & Ostry, 2001).

In deaf and hearing children, the first sign and, respectively, the first word appear at 10–12 months of age. Typically, this first word or sign is produced from the pool of "phonetic" sublexical unit types rehearsed during the babbling phase. By 12–14 months of age deaf infants produce babbling sequences, which resemble whole sentences, in that they display characteristic patterns of rhythm and duration, but are devoid of meaning. Similar sentence-like vocal babbling is produced by hearing infants at this age (Petitto & Marentette, 1991). These observations suggest, above and beyond the linguistic modality used, that there is a predisposition for infants exposed to language to discover on their own the temporal and abstract hierarchical structure of natural language phonology.

The fact that hierarchical structure dependencies are intrinsic to human language grammar, independently of modality, becomes even more evident when considering the results of another set of studies. As Goldin-Meadow and Mylander (1998) report, congenitally deaf children exposed only to spoken language and thus being deprived not only of vocal linguistic input but also of signed linguistic input, nevertheless spontaneously produce syntactically organized sequences of gestures.

The syntactic structures of the sequences of gestures are of a different type than those found in the vocal languages spoken by their parents (English and Mandarin). Furthermore, the mothers produced complex sequences of gestures to a significantly lesser proportion than their deaf children, and with different syntactic characteristics. It is therefore unlikely that these children learned to produce syntactically organized gestures by mere exposure to their parents' speech and gestures. Similarly, before special schools were introduced and Nicaraguan Sign Language emerged, deaf children in Nicaragua until the 1980s faced an analogous linguistically deprived environment. The analysis of the signs produced by Nicaraguan children revealed that their utterances were governed by grammatical regularities not to be found in their input (Senghas & Coppola, 2001). In the last two decades, with the spread of Nicaraguan Sign Language, its grammar has been subject to constant enrichment. The syntactic constructions of today's adults are based solely on sign ordering, whereas those of adolescents, being a generation younger, exploit both sign ordering and spatial relations (Saffran, Senghas, & Trueswell, 2001).

These data support the hypothesis that human infants spontaneously develop learning abilities that guide them in the acquisition of the complex hierarchical structure dependencies displayed by human natural languages, and that these mechanisms are independent of the linguistic modalities adopted. In contrast to spoken language, however, where speech is physically conveyed by streams of sounds with rapid changes of frequency in time, in sign language manual signs are characterized by rhythmic gestural patterns that are realized in space. This characteristic provides an additional parameter along which hierarchical relations can be established, namely a 3-dimensional space – so-called signing space – that lies in front of the signing person and extends approximately from waist to forehead and where signs can be articulated. Grammatical syntactic relations in signed language are established by using the signing space. In particular, noun phrases are assigned arbitrary reference points in a horizontal plane of the signing space, while verb phrases and, more in general, grammatical relations are realized by hand movements between such reference points (Bavelier, Corina, & Neville, 1998). This use of the signing space is symbolic and not iconic, as illustrated by the fact that it can convey wholly abstract concepts, such as "Experiences can influence beliefs." Such a visuospatial grammatical organization is hierarchical: signs can be linked together by syntactic and morphosyntactic markings, thus forming sign phrases that can be embedded incrementally one into another and give rise to clauses with several levels of hierarchical complexity. This system is often referred to as "spatialized syntax" (Poizner, Klima, & Bellugi, 1987). Iconic spatial reference represents a totally distinct phenomenon (referred to as the "classifier system") and it is used to represent nonhierarchically the spatial relations holding among real-world objects (Emmorey et al., 2002).

Given the hierarchical linguistic use of space specific to sign language, one would expect specific brain regions – typically not recruited by spoken language – to be activated during the processing of sign language. Isolated cases of deficits affecting spatialized syntax in native signers following right hemisphere lesions have been reported (Corina, 1998). However, these patients were generally also impaired in their visuo-constructive and visuo-perceptual abilities and their deficits may thus not have been of a linguistic nature proper. In a neuroimaging study, Newman, Bavelier, Corina, Jezzard, & Neville (2001) investigated differences in brain activation during sign language comprehension between a group of native sign users and a group of signers who had learned sign language in early adulthood. Only native signers showed activations in the right angular gyrus, and to a lesser extent also the right precentral gyrus. These regions might thus be related to the processing of the hierarchical spatial relations that are specific to sign language grammar, and be only activated in highly proficient subjects that acquired sign language from early childhood. These results are complemented by a recent ERP study (Capek et al., 2009), that specifically investigated the neurophysiological correlates of spatialized syntax, by using sign language stimuli with syntactic violations determined by altered hand movements for verb phrases with respect to noun phrases reference points. Movements that did not proceed to any of the reference points and violated the hierarchical relations established in space were associated to a LAN that was maximal over right lateral frontal electrodes and a P600 over medial central and parietal electrodes.

In conclusion, sign language, just as spoken language, is a hierarchically organized system. Compared to spoken language, however, sign language possesses at least an additional domain in which hierarchical linguistic relations can be expressed, namely the signing space. This does not imply per se that sign language is more intricately structured than spoken language. On the contrary, the fact that linguistic relations can be mapped onto hand and arm movements in space and time, as opposed to the essentially linearly concatenated vocalizations produced in spoken language, may, to some extent, pose fewer constraints on the sign language system. While in sign language real-world space–time relations can be represented in a stylized version in a quasi-isomorphic linguistic space–time domain, in spoken language, elaborate structural solutions, such as word ordering and affixing have to be adopted (Summerfield et al., 1980).

Conclusion

Human language is characterized by a structure-dependent organization at all levels of the grammar, including phonology, syntax, morphology, and lexical semantics. This structural organization may have originated from the constraints imposed on error-free communication by the physical linear vectors of language production, but it is independent of the specific modality employed, be it speech or sign language. The fact that hierarchical structure dependencies are not manifest at the language surface level poses intriguing questions about the mechanisms underlying language acquisition in young children, which have only recently begun to be addressed experimentally. Children may exploit a combination of innate neurobiological factors and statistical (probabilistic and distributional) learning abilities. The development of full grammatical competence in children appears to be tied to the anatomo-functional maturation of left perisylvian cortical areas, including the left IFG and the superior temporal lobe, and of the white matter fiber tracts that interconnect these brain areas. A wide host of neuroimaging studies has demonstrated that the same anatomical brain structures, and notably the pars opercularis of Broca's area, play a crucial role in the processing and in the acquisition of hierarchical syntactic dependencies in adult subjects. This computational capacity is among the salient distinctive traits that differentiate the brains of humans from those of nonhuman primates and other vertebrates, and may thus be at the core of what makes us a linguistic species.

References

Aslin, R., Saffran, J., & Newport, E. (1998). Computation of conditional probability statistics by 8-month-old infants. *Psychological Science, 9,* 321–324.

Bahlmann, J., Schubotz, R. I., & Friederici, A. (2008). Hierarchical artificial grammar processing engages Broca's area. *Neuroimage, 42*(2), 525–534.

Bahlmann, J., Schubotz, R. I., Mueller, J. L., Koester, D., & Friederici, A. (2009). Neural circuits of hierarchical visuo-spatial sequence processing. *Brain Research, 1298,* 161–170.

Bates, E., & Dick, F. (2002). Language, gesture, and the developing brain. *Developmental Psychobiology, 40*(3), 293–310.

Bavelier, D., Corina, D., & Neville, H. (1998). Brain and language: A perspective from sign language. *Neuron, 21,* 275–278.

Bertoncini, J., Morais, J., Bijeljac-Babic, R., McAdams, S., Peretz, I., & Mehler, J. (1989). Dichotic perception and laterality in neonates. *Brain and Language, 37*(4), 591–605.

Bickerton, D. (1990). *Language and species.* Chicago: University of Chicago Press.

Bookheimer, S. (2002). Functional MRI of language: New approaches to understanding the cortical organization of semantic processing. *Annual Review of Neuroscience, 25*(1), 151–188.

Byrne, R., & Russon, A. (1998). Learning by imitation: A hierarchical approach. *Behavioral and Brain Sciences, 21*(5BR98), 667–721.

Capek, C. M., Grossi, G., Newman, A., McBurney, S. L., Corina, D., Roeder, B., et al. (2009). Brain systems mediating semantic and syntactic processing in deaf native signers: Biological invariance and modality specificity. *Proceedings of the National Academy of Sciences, USA, 106*(21), 8784–8789.

Capirci, O., Iverson, J., Pizzuto, E., & Volterra, V. (1996). Gestures and words during the transition to two-word speech. *Journal of Child Language, 23,* 645–673.

Caplan, D., Alpert, N., & Waters, G. (1998). Effects of syntactic structure and propositional number on patterns of regional cerebral blood flow. *Journal of Cognitive Neuroscience, 10*(4), 541–552.

Cartwright, T., & Brent, M. (1997). Early acquisition of syntactic categories: A formal model. *Cognition, 63,* 121–170.

Cheour, M., Ceponiene, R., Lehtokoski, A., Luuk, A., Allik, J., Alho, K., et al. (1998). Development of language-specific phoneme representations in the infant brain. *Nature Neuroscience, 1*(5), 351–353.

Chomsky, N. (1957). *Syntactic Structures*. The Hague: Mouton.

Conway, C., & Christiansen, M. (2001). Sequential learning in non-human primates. *Trends in Cognitive Sciences, 5*(12), 539–546.

Corina, D. (1998). Aphasia in users of signed languages. In P. Coppens, Y. Lebrun, & A. Basso (Eds.), *Aphasia in atypical populations* (pp. 261–309). Hillsdale, NJ: Erlbaum.

Dehaene-Lambertz, G., & Dehaene, S. (1994). Speed and cerebral correlates of syllable discrimination in infants. *Nature, 370*(6487), 292–295.

Dehaene-Lambertz, G., Dehaene, S., & Hertz-Pannier, L. (2002). Functional neuroimaging of speech perception in infants. *Science, 298*, 2013–1015.

Dehaene-Lambertz, G., & Houston, D. (1998). Faster orientation latency toward native language in two-month-old infants. *Language and Speech, 41*(1), 21–43.

Demonet, J., Thierry, G., & Cardebat, D. (2005). Renewal of the neurophysiology of language: Functional neuroimaging. *Physiological Review, 85*(1DTC05), 49–95.

Ejiri, K., & Masataka, N. (2001). Co-occurrence of preverbal vocal behavior and motor action in early infancy. *Developmental Science, 4*(1), 40–48.

Embick, D., Marantz, A., Miyashita, Y., O'Neil, W., & Sakai, K. (2000). A syntactic specialization for Broca's area. *Proceedings of the National Academy of Sciences, USA, 97*(11), 6150–6154.

Emmorey, K., Damasio, H., McCullough, S., Grabowski, T., Ponto, L., Hichwa, R., et al. (2002). Neural systems underlying spatial language in American Sign Language. *Neuroimage, 17*, 812–824.

Fitch, W., & Hauser, M. (2004). Computational constraints on syntactic processing in a nonhuman primate. *Science, 303*(5656FH04), 377–380.

Fletcher, P., Buchel, C., Josephs, O., Friston, K., & Dolan, R. (1999). Learning-related neuronal responses in prefrontal cortex studied with functional neuroimaging. *Cerebral Cortex, 9*(2), 168–178.

Fletcher, P., Zafiris, O., Frith, C. D., Honey, R. A. E., Corlett, P. R., Zilles, K., et al. (2005). On the benefits of not trying: Brain activity and connectivity reflecting the interactions of explicit and implicit sequence learning. *Cerebral Cortex, 15*(7), 1002–1015.

Fonteneau, E., & van der Lely, H. K. (2008). Electrical brain responses in language-impaired children reveal grammar-specific deficits. *PLoS ONE, 3*(3), 1–6.

Friederici, A. (2002). Towards a neural basis of auditory sentence processing. *Trends in Cognitive Sciences, 6*(2), 78–84.

Friederici, A. (2006). The neural basis of language development and its impairment. *Neuron, 52*(6), 941–952.

Friederici, A. (2009). Pathways to language: Fiber tracts in the human brain. *Trends in Cognitive Sciences, 13*(4), 175–181.

Friederici, A., Bahlmann, J., Heim, S., Schubotz, R. I., & Anwander, A. (2006). The brain differentiates human and non-human grammars: Functional localization and structural connectivity. *Proceedings of the National Academy of Sciences, USA, 103*(7), 2458–2463.

Gentner, T. Q., Fenn, K. M., Margoliash, D., & Nusbaum, H. C. (2006). Recursive syntactic pattern learning by songbirds. *Nature, 440*(7088), 1204–1207.

Gervain, J., Macagno, F., Cogoi, S., Peña, M., & Mehler, J. (2008). The neonate brain detects speech structure. *Proceedings of the National Academy of Sciences, USA, 105*(37), 14222–14227.

Gervain, J., Nespor, M., Mazuka, R., Horie, R., & Mehler, J. (2008). Bootstrapping word order in prelexical infants: A Japanese–Italian cross-linguistic study. *Cognitive Psychology*, *57*(1), 56–74.

Goldin-Meadow, S., & Mylander, C. (1998). Spontaneous sign systems created by deaf children in two cultures. *Nature*, *391*, 279–281.

Greenfield, P. (1991). Language, tools and brain: The ontogeny and phylogeny of hierarchically organized sequential behavior. *Behavioral and Brain Sciences*, *14*, 531–595.

Hampshire, A., Chamberlain, S. R., Monti, M. M., Duncan, J., & Owen, A. M. (2010). The role of the right inferior frontal gyrus: Inhibition and attentional control. *Neuroimage*, *50*(3), 1313–1319.

Hauser, M., Chomsky, N., & Fitch, W. (2002). The faculty of language: What is it, who has it, and how did it evolve? *Science*, *298*, 1569–1579.

Hirsh-Pasek, K., Kemler Nelson, D., Jusczyk, P., Cassidy, K., Druss, B., & Kennedy, L. (1987). Clauses are perceptual units for young infants. *Cognition*, *26*, 269–286.

Hoen, M., & Dominey, P. (2000). ERP analysis of cognitive sequencing: A left anterior negativity related to structural transformation processing. *Neuroreport*, *11*(14), 3187–3191.

Hoen, M., Pachot-Clouard, M., Segebarth, C., & Dominey, P. (2006). When Broca experiences the Janus syndrome: An ER-fMRI study comparing sentence comprehension and cognitive sequence processing. *Cortex*, *42*(4), 605–623.

Jackendoff, R. (1999). Possible stages in the evolution of the language capacity. *Trends in Cognitive Sciences*, *3*(7), 272–279.

Jackendoff, R. (2003). *Foundations of language*. Oxford: Oxford University Press.

Jusczyk, P. (1997). *The discovery of spoken language*. Cambridge, MA: MIT Press.

Jusczyk, P., Friederici, A., Wessels, J., Svenkerud, V., & Jusczyk, A. (1993). Infants' sensitivity to the sound patterns of native language words. *Journal of Memory and Language*, *32*(3), 402–420.

Keller, S. S., Crow, T., Foundas, A., Amunts, K., & Roberts, N. (2009). Broca's area: Nomenclature, anatomy, typology and asymmetry. *Brain and Language*, *109*(1), 29–48.

Klima, E., & Bellugi, U. (1979). *The signs of language*. Cambridge, MA: Harvard University Press.

Koechlin, E., & Jubault, T. (2006). Broca's area and the hierarchical organization of human behavior. *Neuron*, *50*(6), 963–974.

Kuhl, P. (2000). A new view of language acquisition. *Proceedings of the National Academy of Sciences, USA*, *97*(22), 11850–11857.

Lany, J., & Gómez, R. L. (2008). Twelve-month-old infants benefit from prior experience in statistical learning. *Psychological Science*, *19*(12), 1247–1252.

Lashley, K. (1951). The problem of serial order in behavior. In L. Jeffress (Ed.), *Cerebral mechanisms in behavior: The Hixon symposium* (pp. 112–146). New York: Wiley.

Lelekov-Boissard, T., & Dominey, P. (2002). Human brain potentials reveal similar processing of non-linguistic abstract structure and linguistic syntactic structure. *Neurophysiologie Clinique*, *32*, 72–84.

Liddell, S. (1980). *American Sign Language syntax*. New York: Mouton.

Lindenberg, R., Fangerau, H., & Seitz, R. J. (2007). "Broca's area" as a collective term? *Brain and Language*, *102*(1), 22–29.

Makuuchi, M., Bahlmann, J., Anwander, A., & Friederici, A. (2009). Segregating the core computational faculty of human language from working memory. *Proceedings of the National Academy of Sciences, USA*, *106*(20), 8362–8367.

Marcus, G., Vijayan, S., Bandi Rao, S., & Vishton, P. (1999). Rule learning by seven-month-old infants. *Science, 283*(5398), 77–80.

McClelland, J., & Plaut, D. (1999). Does generalization in infant learning implicate abstract algebra-like rules? *Trends in Cognitive Sciences, 3*(5), 166–168.

Mehler, J., Jusczyk, P., Lambertz, G., Halsted, N., Bertoncini, J., & Amiel-Tison, C. (1988). A precursor of language acquisition in young infants. *Cognition, 29*, 143–178.

Meyer, M., Friederici, A., & von Cramon, D. (2000). Neurocognition of auditory sentence comprehension: Event-related fMRI reveals sensitivity to syntactic violations and task demands. *Brain Research Cognitive Brain Research, 9*(1), 19–33.

Moro, A., Tettamanti, M., Perani, D., Donati, C., Cappa, S., & Fazio, F. (2001). Syntax and the brain: Disentangling grammar by selective anomalies. *Neuroimage, 13*(1), 110–118.

Musso, M., Moro, A., Glauche, V., Rijntjes, M., Reichenbach, J., Buchel, C., et al. (2003). Broca's area and the language instinct. *Nature Neuroscience, 6*(7MMG+03), 774–781.

Neville, H., Coffey, S., Holcomb, P., & Tallal, P. (1993). The neurobiology of sensory and language processing in language-impaired children. *Journal of Cognitive Neuroscience, 5*, 235–253.

Newman, A., Bavelier, D., Corina, D., Jezzard, P., & Neville, H. (2001). A critical period for right hemisphere recruitment in American Sign Language processing. *Nature Neuroscience, 5*(1), 76–80.

Ni, W., Constable, R., Mencl, W., Pugh, K., Fulbright, R., Shaywitz, S., et al. (2000). An event-related neuroimaging study distinguishing form and content in sentence processing. *Journal of Cognitive Neuroscience, 12*(1), 120–133.

Nowak, M., & Komarova, N. (2001). Towards an evolutionary theory of language. *Trends in Cognitive Sciences, 5*(7), 288–295.

Nowak, M., Plotkin, J., & Jansen, V. (2000). The evolution of syntactic communication. *Nature, 404*, 495–498.

Oberecker, R., & Friederici, A. (2006). Syntactic event-related potential components in 24-month-olds' sentence comprehension. *Neuroreport, 17*(10), 1017–1021.

Oberecker, R., Friedrich, M., & Friederici, A. (2005). Neural correlates of syntactic processing in two-year-olds. *Journal of Cognitive Neuroscience, 17*(10), 1667–1678.

Opitz, B., & Friederici, A. (2003). Interactions of the hippocampal system and the prefrontal cortex in learning language-like rules. *Neuroimage, 19*(4), 1730–1737.

Opitz, B., & Friederici, A. (2007). Neural basis of processing sequential and hierarchical syntactic structures. *Human Brain Mapping, 28*(7), 585–592.

Patel, A. (2003). Language, music, syntax and the brain. *Nature Neuroscience, 6*(7Pat03b), 674–681.

Peña, M., Bonatti, L., Nespor, M., & Mehler, J. (2002). Signal-driven computations in speech processing. *Science, 298*, 604–607.

Perruchet, P., & Rey, A. (2005). Does the mastery of center-embedded linguistic structures distinguish humans from nonhuman primates? *Psychonomic Bulletin and Review, 12*(2), 307–313.

Petitto, L. (1987). On the autonomy of language and gesture: Evidence from the acquisition of personal pronouns in American Sign Language. *Cognition, 27*(1), 1–52.

Petitto, L., Holowka, S., Sergio, L., & Ostry, D. (2001). Language rhythms in baby hand movements. *Nature, 413*, 35–36.

Petitto, L., Katerelos, M., Levy, B., Gauna, K., Tétreault, K., & Ferraro, V. (2001). Bilingual signed and spoken language acquisition from birth: Implications for the mechanisms underlying early bilingual language acquisition. *Journal of Child Language, 28,* 453–496.

Petitto, L., & Marentette, P. (1991). Babbling in the manual mode: Evidence for the ontogeny of language. *Science, 25,* 1493–1496.

Petitto, L., Zatorre, R., Gauna, K., Nikelski, J., Dostie, D., & Evans, A. (2000). Speech-like cerebral activity in profoundly deaf people processing signed languages: Implications for the neural basis of human language. *Proceedings of the National Academy of Sciences, USA, 97*(25), 13961–13966.

Poizner, H., Klima, E., & Bellugi, U. (1987). *What the hands reveal about the brain.* Cambridge, MA: MIT Press.

Pollard, C., & Sag, I. (1994). *Head-driven phrase structure grammar.* Chicago: University of Chicago Press.

Premack, D. (2004). Psychology. Is language the key to human intelligence? *Science, 303*(5656Pre04), 318–320.

Saffran, J. (2001). The use of predictive dependencies in language learning. *Journal of Memory and Language, 44,* 493–515.

Saffran, J., Aslin, R., & Newport, E. (1996). Statistical learning by 8-month-old infants. *Science, 274*(5294), 1926–1928.

Saffran, J., Pollak, S. D., Seibel, R. L., & Shkolnik, A. (2007). Dog is a dog is a dog: Infant rule learning is not specific to language. *Cognition, 105*(3), 669–680.

Saffran, J., Senghas, A., & Trueswell, J. (2001). The acquisition of language by children. *Proceedings of the National Academy of Sciences, USA, 98*(23), 12874–12875.

Senghas, A., & Coppola, M. (2001). Children creating language: How Nicaraguan Sign Language acquired a spatial grammar. *Psychological Science, 12*(4), 323–328.

Shannon, C. E., & Weaver, W. (1949). *The mathematical theory of communication.* Chicago: University of Illinois Press.

Shi, R., Werker, J., & Morgan, J. (1999). Newborn infants' sensitivity to perceptual cues to lexical and grammatical words. *Cognition, 72,* B11–B21.

Shore, C., Bates, E., Bretherton, I., Beeghly, M., & O'Connell, B. (1990). Vocal and gestural symbols: Similarities and differences from 13 to 28 months. In V. Volterra & C. Erting (Eds.), *From gesture to language in hearing and deaf children* (pp. 79–91). Berlin: Springer.

Silva-Pereyra, J., Rivera-Gaxiola, M., & Kuhl, P. (2005). An event-related brain potential study of sentence comprehension in preschoolers: Semantic and morphosyntactic processing. *Brain Research. Cognitive Brain Research, 23*(2–3), 247–258.

Silva-Pereyra, J. F., Klarman, L., Lin, L. J., & Kuhl, P. (2005). Sentence processing in 30-month-old children: An event-related potential study. *Neuroreport, 16*(6), 645–648.

Stromswold, K., Caplan, D., Alpert, N., & Rauch, S. (1996). Localization of syntactic comprehension by positron emission tomography. *Brain and Language, 52*(3), 452–473.

Studdert-Kennedy, M., & Lane, H. (1980). Clues from the differences between signed and spoken language. In U. Bellugi & M. Studdert-Kennedy (Eds.), *Signed and spoken language: Biological constraints on linguistic form – Dahlem Konferenzen* (pp. 29–40). Weinheim: Verlag Chemie GmbH.

Summerfield, A., Cutting, J., Frishberg, N., Lane, H., Lindblom, B., Runeson, J., et al. (1980). The structuring of language by the requirements of motor control and perception. In U. Bellugi & M. Studdert-Kennedy (Eds.), *Signed and spoken language: Biological constraints on linguistic form – Dahlem Konferenzen* (pp. 89–114). Weinheim: Verlag Chemie GmbH.

Terrace, H. S., Petitto, L., Sanders, R. J., & Bever, T. G. (1979). Can an ape create a sentence? *Science, 206*(4421), 891–902.

Tettamanti, M., Alkadhi, H., Moro, A., Perani, D., Kollias, S., & Weniger, D. (2002). Neural correlates for the acquisition of natural language syntax. *Neuroimage, 17*, 700–709.

Tettamanti, M., Rotondi, I., Perani, D., Scotti, G., Fazio, F., Cappa, S. F., et al. (2009). Syntax without language: Neurobiological evidence for cross-domain syntactic computations. *Cortex, 45*(7), 825–838.

Tettamanti, M., & Weniger, D. (2006). Broca's area: A supramodal hierarchical processor? *Cortex, 42*(4), 491–494.

13

How Does the Brain Establish Novel Meanings in Language? Abstract Symbol Theories Versus Embodied Theories of Meaning

Dorothee Chwilla

An Overview

The central topic of this chapter is how the mind/brain creates meaning. The high speed at which we comprehend language forms a major challenge for research on language. Here, we use event-related potentials (ERPs) to track semantic processing in real time. A further advantage of this approach is that there exists one ERP component, the N400, which is generally accepted to be highly sensitive to semantic factors (Kutas & Hillyard, 1980; see also Kutas, Kiang, & Sweeney, Volume 2, Chapter 26). The focus in this chapter will be on this component. We will first explore how the mind/brain creates familiar meanings, in particular abstract forms of world knowledge. Then we will proceed to the exciting question of how the mind/brain constructs novel meanings, not stored in semantic memory. I will present recent ERP results from our laboratory that reveal that familiar meanings, and, crucially, novel meanings too, are immediately accessed/integrated into the ongoing context. I will argue that the electrophysiological findings support embodied views of language and challenge abstract symbol theories of meaning.

General Background

In cognitive psychology and in the field of language there has been a shift from modular to interactive processing models. A good example are embodied theories of cognition that are of central importance for this chapter. According to embodied

The Handbook of the Neuropsychology of Language, First Edition. Edited by Miriam Faust.
© 2012 Blackwell Publishing Ltd. Published 2012 by Blackwell Publishing Ltd.

theories, mental *simulation* forms the basis of cognitive representation (e.g., Barsalou, 1999). These theories have in common that they are perceptual theories of cognition. A key assumption is that mental processes such as thinking or language understanding are based on the physical interactions that people have with their environment. In the same way that the body can be viewed as a support system for the mind, the mind can be viewed as a support system for the body. By shifting the basis of mental behaviour towards the body, the assumption is that mental processes are supported by the same processes that are used for physical interactions, that is, for perception and action.

According to the classical approach to meaning – that dominated linguistics and psycholinguistics for the past 40 years – meaning arises from the combination of *abstract symbols* into a representational structure. These theories are called *abstract symbol theories* of meaning (e.g., Collins & Loftus, 1975; Masson, 1995). This conception gave rise to different types of representation, such as feature lists, schemata, semantic nets, and connectionism. On this view, words have fixed meanings. The meaning of a word can be captured by defining a set of necessary and jointly sufficient features. High-dimensional models of meaning (latent semantic analysis, LSA, of Landauer & Dumais, 1997, and hyperspace analogue to language, HAL, of Burgess & Lund, 2000) have been presented as a variant of the classical abstract symbol theories. According to these high-dimensional models the meaning of a word is its vector representation in a high-dimensional space, and these vectors are similar to the abstract symbols used in classical theories of meaning. A major strength of the symbolic approach is that it allows representation of several kinds of knowledge (i.e., types and tokens, propositions and abstract concepts), as well as linguistic productivity by combining symbols. A fundamental critique of these theories is how meaning can arise from abstract symbols not grounded in perception or action (i.e., the grounding problem; Searle, 1980).

Embodied theories have challenged *abstract symbol theories* of meaning (e.g., Glenberg, 1997; MacWhinney, 1999). Embodied theories claim that meaning is based on our current interactions or previous experiences of interactions with objects in different environments. Current or past body–environment interactions guide people in how to think about, that is, *simulate* the perceptual and action details required by a situation. This view has been applied to the field of language comprehension. Relevant here is that several studies have provided clear evidence for interactions between language and action (e.g., Zwaan & Taylor, 2006).

Another challenge for abstract symbol theories comes from cognitive neuroscience. While the cortical systems for language and action traditionally were thought to be prime examples of independent and autonomous functional systems, strong evidence for brain mechanisms linking language and action has been provided.

A striking example is the work from Pulvermüller (2005). He investigated the processing of verbs involving actions with different parts of the body (leg, hand, and face). Pulvermüller showed that when participants read words for an action the motor system becomes active to represent its meaning. More specifically, verbs for head, arm, and leg actions produce head, arm, and leg activations in the respective areas of the motor cortex. These activations, as revealed by magnetoencephalogram, took place very fast – that is, within just a few hundreds of milliseconds. These results seem inconsistent with one of the main tenets of abstract symbol theories, that knowledge in the form of abstract symbols is stored in a semantic network, separate from the brain's modal systems for action, perception, and emotion.

Goals of This Chapter

The common goal of the ERP studies presented here was to test the different theories on the representation of word meaning (i.e., abstract symbol theories and embodied theories). The experimental results are organized in two parts. In Part 1 abstract symbol theories are tested in the context of the semantic priming paradigm. In two combined reaction-time ERP (RT/ERP) studies we explored the scope of semantic priming by testing for facilitation for word triplets that are exclusively related via world knowledge (e.g., PIANO – MOVE – BACKPAIN). Abstract symbol theories (like spreading activation models and distributed memory models) predict facilitation only for associative and semantic relations and cannot account for facilitation for abstract world knowledge relations.

The goal of the ERP studies presented in Part 2 was to test abstract symbol theories against embodied theories of meaning. This was accomplished by exploring how the mind/brain establishes novel meanings not stored in semantic memory (e.g., "to paddle with Frisbees"). Abstract symbol theories can only discover meaningfulness by consulting *stored* symbolic knowledge and therefore cannot explain facilitation for novel sensible situations. This constraint does not hold for embodied theories according to which meaningfulness resides in our knowledge of the possibilities and limitations of our body. The experimental parts are followed by a general discussion in which the implications of the ERP results – on the creation of novel meanings – for current theories of meaning will be discussed.

Throughout the chapter, I will focus on N400 which has been shown to be exquisitely sensitive to semantic factors. In the literature there is a debate about whether N400 reflects processes of lexical access (i.e., the ease with which a word can be activated from semantic memory; e.g., Kutas & Federmeier, 2000; Lau, Phillips, & Poeppel, 2008) or processes of integration (i.e., the ease with which a word can be fit into context; e.g., Chwilla, Brown, & Hagoort, 1995; Chwilla, Kolk, & Mulder, 2000; Friederici, 1995). It is noteworthy in this context to point out that the main result of the present chapter, that is, the immediate creation of novel meanings, supports the integration view and cannot be explained by the lexical access view. A discussion of the functional significance of N400, however, is outside of the scope of this chapter. Here N400 is used as a temporal landmark to track semantic processes in real time.

Part 1: How Does the Mind/Brain Create Familiar World Knowledge?

What makes a rose more similar to a lily than to a cactus? Why do we consider a rose a suitable present for a lover but not a cactus? These examples tap different kinds of knowledge. The first example taps differences in relatedness in terms of the organization of *semantic knowledge* (category membership). Answering the second question taps *world knowledge* – that is, general knowledge about objects and events that make up the world. Based on our experiences with the external world we have a huge storehouse containing all kinds of knowledge about the objects and events that surround us. While the organization of semantic knowledge is a central topic in cognitive (neuro)science, little is known about the representation of more abstract kinds of knowledge, like world knowledge. However, there is a growing consensus that a definition of semantic relatedness in terms of category membership is too limited to capture the multitude of factors that may contribute to word meaning. Other types of information that have been proposed to tap semantics are perceptual relations (e.g., PIZZA – COIN), functional relations, particularly instrument relations (e.g., BROOM – FLOOR), synonyms (e.g., STREET – ROAD) and antonyms (e.g., ORDER – CHAOS; for a review see Hutchison, 2003).

An effective tool to investigate the functional organization of semantic knowledge is the *semantic priming paradigm* (for a review see McNamara, 2005). Semantic priming refers to one of the best-documented findings in cognitive psychology, namely that a word (target) is processed faster and/or more accurately when it is preceded by a related word (prime). Semantic priming provides a window into the structure of semantic memory because facilitation of target processing can only occur on the basis of the particular type of information delivered by the prime. Of critical importance for models of representation and processing is the time course of the priming effect. If the knowledge becomes available very early to the reader/listener, this indicates that this aspect of information is central to word meaning.

Here, I will zoom in on more abstract world knowledge relations. World knowledge as illustrated by the example "we offer a red rose to our lover to declare a true love" refers to our notions of what kinds of objects and events occur in the world around us. How and when world knowledge is processed is of theoretical importance, because abstract symbol theories, like the popular spreading activation model (Collins & Loftus, 1975), distributed memory models (e.g., Masson, 1995), as well as all other priming models, predict facilitation only for concepts that share an associative relation or a semantic relation. Hence, they cannot account for facilitation for world knowledge relations.

Little is known about the accessibility of world knowledge relations. This is surprising because the use of world knowledge is essential for normal language understanding. Normal conversation is not so much about associative, semantic, or perceptual properties of words (e.g., that apples are fruit, are round, can be green or red) but about *events* or places that trigger schemata closely connected to our experiences. For instance, that in summer we can pick apples from trees, that we can buy apples on the market or in a grocery shop, that apples are tasteful in a pie, that apples lesson our thirst, and that eating an apple fits well with a diet. These examples illustrate that there is a multitude of more general types of knowledge that from the standpoint of the language user are retrieved without any effort but that have fallen outside the scope of psycholinguistic research and research in lexical semantics by linguists.

To my knowledge, there is one single study that tested for reaction time (RT) priming for world knowledge relations. This is the study of Moss, Ostrin, Tyler, and Marslen-Wilson (1995). They tested for priming for script knowledge in both the auditory and the visual modality. Scripts, also known as schemata, refer to knowledge structures or sets of expectations built on past experience that have been conceived as the building blocks of cognition (Rumelhart, 1980). Schemata are mental representations of stereotypical situations. A famous example is the restaurant script of Schank and Abelson (1977). A script for a restaurant involves the actors, props, entry and exit conditions, and action sequences like sitting at a table, ordering food from a menu, and drinking wine. Moss and colleagues built scripts by selecting a prime word like restaurant that referred to an event or place and so could evoke a script or schema. The targets referred to *typical elements* in the prime's script (e.g., RESTAURANT – WINE). Using a lexical decision task, in which participants had to make a word/nonword decision on the target, Moss et al. (1995) found RT priming for script knowledge in the auditory but not in the visual modality. Based on this finding, they concluded that script knowledge may be less central to word meaning than other kinds of semantic knowledge, like functional knowledge, for which they observed priming across modalities.

The absence of priming for script relations in the visual modality seems to support abstract symbol theories, according to which facilitation should only be observed for concepts that are associatively or semantically related. On the other hand, the results are not conclusive, because script priming did occur in the auditory modality. Nevertheless, the absence of visual script priming calls into question that world knowledge forms a central aspect of word meaning. If even typical elements of stereotypical scripts fail to elicit priming, then the evidence for the early availability of script knowledge is weak. This result is at odds with discourse studies (e.g., Cook & Myers, 2004) that have shown immediate facilitation for different kinds of world knowledge. Of direct relevance is a sentential ERP study of Hagoort, Hald, Bastiaansen, and Petersson (2004) in which the sensitivity of N400 to postlexical integration was exploited to compare the time course at which well-known facts and semantic knowledge are integrated into context. They compared sentences that were true based on general world knowledge like "Dutch trains are *yellow*" with false sentences "Dutch trains are *white*." These world knowledge violations were contrasted with a semantic selection restriction violation (e.g., "Dutch trains are *sour*"). The major result was that world knowledge was integrated in the same time-frame as semantic knowledge. However, the fact that Hagoort et al. observed similar N400 effects for semantic relations and world knowledge relations may critically depend on the presence of a lexical-sentential context.

In light of the theoretical importance of script priming for semantic priming models, we decided to test again for script priming in the visual modality (Chwilla & Kolk, 2005). To this end we constructed scripts consisting of triplets of words that presented a plausible scenario based on world knowledge (e.g., DIRECTOR – BRIBE – DISMISSAL). Importantly, the scripts as indicated by free association norms and other pretests were not associatively and/or semantically related in terms of feature overlap. Script-unrelated word triplets were built by pairing the target word with two unrelated prime words (e.g., VACATION – TRIAL – DISMISSAL). Our study differed from that of Moss et al. (1995) in two aspects. First, we used a shorter prime–target interval of 400 ms (as opposed to 1 s) to prevent fast decay of the visual primes. The occurrence of script priming in the auditory modality could be due to the fact that auditory primes leave a longer echoic trace that persists after target presentation. In our study, the two primes were presented simultaneously at central vision and immediately followed by the target. In the first study, participants had to indicate whether all three items were real Dutch words or not. Previous work from our laboratory has shown that this lexical decision variant is a sensitive measure of semantic priming (Chwilla & Kolk, 2002). Second, we used a two-word context and not a single-word context. The rational was that this enabled us to build more specific and in that sense more constrained short stories that may be more effective to represent script knowledge.

The prediction was that if script knowledge – in the absence of a sentential or pragmatic context – is immediately accessed/integrated into context, then a priming effect on RT and/or N400 should be obtained in lexical decision. The demonstration of script priming would have theoretical implications for abstract symbol theories (like spreading activation models and distributed memory models), because these models predict priming only for words that are either associatively and/or semantically related.

The main result was that we were successful in demonstrating a priming effect for words that were exclusively related via world knowledge. For RT significant priming was observed; lexical decision latencies were on average 25 ms faster for script-related than for script-unrelated scenarios. The RT effect was accompanied by an N400 effect (see Figure 13.1a). In particular, within the typical N400 window (400–500 ms post-target), a script priming effect was found for the frontal midline site and the left hemisphere. No N400 script priming effect was found for the right hemisphere. While the timing of the N400 effect fell well in the N400 window, the scalp distribution did not completely match that of the standard N400 effect for associative or semantic relations, which typically shows a bilateral central/posterior maximum. Therefore, it was not yet clear how the N400-like script priming effect relates to the standard N400 effect.

A second experiment was conducted to further determine the locus of script priming by increasing the contribution of meaning integration processes. In Experiment 2, we directed the attention of the participants to script knowledge. The

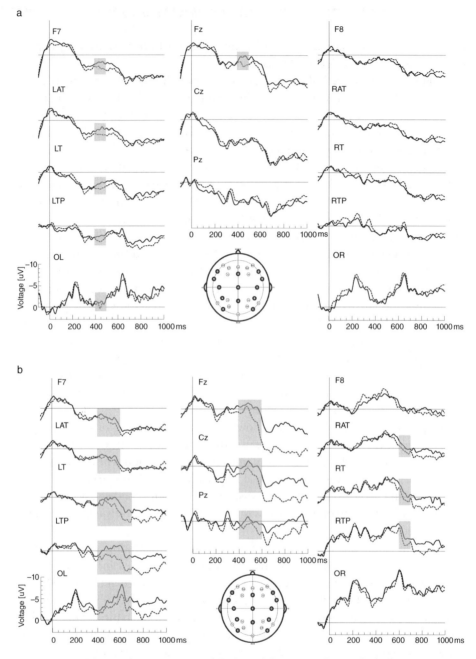

Figure 13.1 (a) Grand ERP averages of the lexical decision task time-locked to target onset (zero ms) for script-related targets (dotted line) and unrelated targets (solid line). Negativity is plotted upwards. The shaded areas indicate the time periods in which significant N400 effects were present. The electrode configuration is displayed by the bold circles. From Chwilla and Kolk (2005), with permission from Elsevier Science. (b) Grand ERP averages of the plausibility judgment task time-locked to target onset (zero ms) for script-related targets (dotted line) and unrelated targets (solid line) for a representative subset of sites. Negativity is plotted upwards. The shaded areas indicate the time periods in which significant N400 effects were present. From Chwilla and Kolk (2005), with permission from Elsevier Science.

basic idea was that the lexical decision task might not be optimal to investigate the processing of script information. The frequent occurrence of nonwords likely enhances the impact of lexical information at the cost of semantic or script information. The high emphasis on lexical information may disrupt normal language comprehension that outside of the laboratory is directed at the meaning level. In Experiment 2, we approximated normal language comprehension by using a task requiring exploitation of world knowledge. The same materials were presented as in Experiment 1, but all nonwords were removed. Participants had to judge if the three words together formed a plausible scenario based on world knowledge. This plausibility judgment task requires participants to integrate the three words and determine whether the word combination yields a familiar script. We assume that participants in everyday life search for the highest level of coherence that the material permits (Hess, Foss, & Carroll, 1995) and thus should be able to distinguish plausible from implausible scenarios. If the hypothesis that a higher-order meaning integration process gives rise to the script priming effects is correct, then increasing these integration processes of script information should enhance the N400 effect.

The change in task led to a strong increase in N400 script priming effect. Increasing the impact of meaning integration processes for script knowledge elicited a full-blown N400 effect. In contrast, with the lexical decision study, the N400 script priming effect showed a longer duration and was widely distributed across the scalp. The N400 effect in the plausibility judgment task resembled the standard N400 effect in terms of its morphology, time course, and bilateral central/parietal scalp distribution (see Figure 13.1b). The only difference with the standard N400 effect was that it was larger over the left hemisphere. A left-hemisphere advantage for script knowledge has also been reported in visual half-field studies, which supports the notion that the left hemisphere is more efficient in exploiting world knowledge (Faust & Babkoff, 1997).

Relation between script knowledge and semantic knowledge

The prevalent view among linguists and psycholinguists in the area of sentence and discourse processing is that there is no clear cut-off point between semantic knowledge and world knowledge (e.g., Clark, 1996). On the other hand, semantic priming theories make a distinction between semantic knowledge and world knowledge (e.g., Collins & Loftus, 1975; Masson, 1995) and predict priming only for semantic and not for world knowledge.

An argument in favor of a distinction between the two kinds of knowledge is that scripts represent more abstract relations that describe typical events in the real world, while semantic relations, like functional relations, are closely tied to the core meaning of the word. For semantic relations the integration process is based on more linguistic properties and involves determining the overlap of a finite set of semantic features. Integrating on the basis of script relations, on the other hand, likely involves the retrieval of – sometimes complex – scenarios as well as the determination of how well the various words "fit" this scenario. Therefore one might expect differences in the integration processes for the two kinds of knowledge.

What would be needed to clarify this issue is a direct comparison of the N400 priming effects elicited by these two kinds of relations. This was possible because the participants of the plausibility judgment task had also been tested in a semantic condition. Apart from the use of different materials (semantic vs. script relations), the procedure was the same. In the semantic condition, homographs were presented as target. In the critical semantic condition, Primes 1 and 2 were related to distinct meaning representations of the homograph (e.g., HAND – TREE – PALM) while the primes were unrelated to each other. In the unrelated condition the same target-word was preceded by two unrelated primes. Participants had to indicate whether one or both primes were semantically related to the target. A comparison of the time course of the N400 effects when based on semantic knowledge versus script knowledge did not reveal any differences in the onset of the N400 effects. The first reliable N400 effect for semantic relations was obtained in the 400–500 ms window. As for the script relations, there were no indications for an N400 effect in the preceding 300–400 ms window. These analyses show that the time course of the N400 effect for semantic relations and script relations was very similar (see Figure 13.2; for a comparison of the size and the scalp

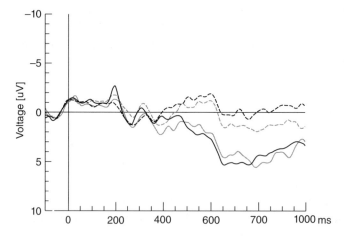

Figure 13.2 The grand average at electrode LTP (Wernicke's area) displaying the N400 semantic priming effect (the ERPs for the semantically related targets are indicated by the black line and those for the unrelated control targets are indicated by the black dashed line), and the N400 script priming effect (the ERPs for the script-related targets are indicated by the gray line and those for the script unrelated control targets are indicated by the gray dashed line) for the participants of Experiment 2. The ERPs are time-locked to target onset (zero ms). From Chwilla and Kolk (2005), with permission from Elsevier Science.

distribution of the effects see Chwilla and Kolk, 2005). Crucially for testing abstract symbol theories, these additional analyses reveal that script knowledge is immediately accessed/integrated.

So far, I have proposed that our scripts tap world knowledge. Are there objective measures that support the suggestion that our scripts are related via world knowledge? McKoon and Ratcliff (1992) proposed local co-occurrence frequency as a measure of familiarity. We have shown that a global measure of co-occurrence, namely, LSA of Landauer and Dumais (1997), is a sensitive measure for detecting subtle differences in semantic relatedness between items when alternative methods like free association and lexical co-occurrence suggested that the items were unrelated (Chwilla & Kolk, 2002). Therefore, we submitted our stimuli to LSA. These analyses indicated that the mean semantic similarity value was significantly larger for the script-related items (0.15) than for the unrelated items (0.07). The LSA analyses thus confirmed that our scripts present familiar and in that sense old contexts and therefore are readily available based on our notions of what kinds of objects and events make up the world.

Discussion

We have presented the first evidence of script priming in the visual domain. Across tasks script priming occurred for both RT and N400. For the auditory domain, script priming has already been reported (Moss et al., 1995). As in the present experiments, the primes were chosen such that they could evoke a script, but in contrast with the present experiments, the targets referred to typical elements in the prime's script. Given that Moss and colleagues used typical elements of the script as target it is unlikely that the absence of visual script priming was due to a weaker relatedness of the materials. Two factors in particular, the use of faster presentation conditions and the use of a two-word context, could account for the differences in results. Future studies are needed to determine which factor(s) are decisive for the elicitation of visual script priming effects.

Crucially, our RT and N400 data show that script priming can be obtained in the visual modality. At a more general level, the demonstration of script priming in the visual and in the auditory domain supports the view that facilitation for script information is a general finding. What do the results of the different tasks reveal about the accessibility of script knowledge? The occurrence of N400 effects in lexical decision bolsters the view that script knowledge forms a central aspect of word meaning that is immediately accessed when words are read. The plausibility judgment task revealed that directing attention to script relations enhanced the N400 script priming effects. Taken together, these results show that highlighting script knowledge by task can increase the priming effects for script relations but is not a necessary condition for N400 visual script priming to occur. The results on script priming are in line with the claim of Elman (2009) and of Hare, Jones, Thomson, Kelly, & McRae (2009) that event-based knowledge and relations play an important role in reading even when words are presented in isolation.

Locus of the script priming effect

The traditional account of automatic priming is that it is caused by spreading activation. The compound-cue model of Ratcliff and McKoon (1988) and the distributed memory model of Masson (1995) have been presented as competitors of spreading activation models. What all priming models, except for the compound-cue model, have in common is that they make a distinction between semantic knowledge and world knowledge. In particular, these models predict facilitation only for associative and semantic relations. The demonstration of RT and N400 priming for script relations, therefore, presents a challenge for current priming models. The only exception is the compound-cue model. According to this model, priming for semantic and associative relations occurs because the related words are more familiar in semantic memory than unrelated words. Latent semantic analysis revealed that this applied for our set of script relations. Thus, we conclude that the script priming effects can be explained by the automatic compound-cue integration model.

Important for our present purposes, the immediate integration of world knowledge is problematic for spreading activation models (e.g., Collins & Loftus, 1975) and distributed memory models (e.g., Masson, 1995). This is the case because these models can only account for priming for words that are associatively and/or semantically related. Abstract symbol models, therefore, lack the flexibility that is required to account for facilitation of world knowledge like the present script relations. In a similar vein, these models lack the flexibility to account for the facilitation occurring for different kinds of event-based relations reported by Hare and colleagues (2009). As pointed out by these authors, to account for the priming of event-based relations any spreading activation network model would need to include specific types of relations rather than simply undifferentiated association.

Part 2: How Does the Mind/Brain Create Novel Meanings?

World knowledge represents familiar knowledge based on our experiences with the external world. While the representation and processing of familiar knowledge is a heavily investigated research arena, little is known about how the mind/brain constructs novel meanings not stored in memory. Let me be clear about what I mean here by novel meaning. Imagine you are in Amsterdam sitting on a terrace overlooking one of the canals. It is a sunny afternoon and you enjoy watching boats passing by. Amongst them, you see a canoe with two boys paddling with Frisbees. "Paddling with Frisbees", as intense pretests of our materials have shown (Chwilla, Kolk, &

Vissers, 2007), represents a novel meaning that people have not encountered before. What we learn from daily life is that people can distinguish between novel sensible meanings (e.g., "to paddle with Frisbees") and novel insensible meanings (e.g., "to paddle with pullovers"). But how are we able to do this? Novel meanings are ubiquitous in language use. Novel words (often compounds) are constantly added to the vocabulary. Despite the novelty of the information, the sense of understanding is seldom lost. Therefore, an important question is how the mind/brain creates novel meanings, not stored in semantic memory?

The ERP studies that I will present were conducted to investigate how the mind/brain creates novel meanings in real time (Chwilla et al., 2007). Before presenting the goals and design of the studies I will describe in more detail the two approaches to the representation of word meaning in language comprehension.

Abstract symbol models versus embodied models of word meaning

According to the traditional cognitive (neuro)science approach the mind/brain is conceived of as an organ for building internal representations of the external world. The mind/brain essentially is a modular system largely unaffected by other modules (Fodor, 1975). A main assumption of the traditional cognitive science approach is that knowledge resides in a semantic memory system separate from the brain's modal systems for perception (vision, audition), action (movement, proprioception), and introspection (internal states including affect, motivations, intentions, metacognition; see Barsalou, 2009). Meaning arises from the syntactic combination of abstract, amodal symbols that are arbitrarily related to entities in the real world. For instance, according to the popular spreading activation model of Collins and Loftus (1975) meaning automatically arises from the pattern of relations among nodes in a network.

A very different approach is provided by perceptual theories of meaning, which gained popularity in the form of *embodied theories* of cognition (e.g., Barsalou, 1999; Glenberg, 1997; Lakoff, 1987; MacWhinney, 1999). Here, the brain's primary purpose is not to represent the external world but to regulate behavior. On this view, the brain is an equal player, next to the organism's body and the world. These three factors together form part of the physical substrate that causes behavior and cognition. A key question for embodied theories is how the brain, the body, and the world contribute to the creation and maintenance of real world behavior. A central assumption is that mental processes such as thinking or language comprehension are based on the physical interactions that people have with their environment.

The embodied framework has been applied to the field of language (e.g., Glenberg & Robertson, 1999, 2000; MacWhinney, 1999). The starting point is that the structure of the body is very important in that it determines the range of effective actions. The term *affordances* plays a crucial role. Following Gibson (1979), affordances are defined as the actions suggested by a particular object. For example, the affordances of a knife include cutting several kinds of objects, or defending oneself or somebody else, or attacking somebody, but they do not include watering flowers. Meaning arises from our current interactions, previous experiences of interactions, or imaged interactions with objects in different kinds of environments. Current or past body–environment interactions guide us in how to think about, that is, *simulate* the perceptual and action details required by a situation. Meaningfulness resides in our knowledge of the possibilities versus limitations of our body.

The most fully developed embodied view of language comprehension comes from Glenberg and colleagues. According to their "indexical hypothesis," understanding a sentence, such as "Jareb stood on the chair to change a light bulb," involves three steps. The first step is to index phrases to actual objects or to analogical perceptual symbols representing the objects. Thus, the noun phrase "the chair" may be taken to refer to an actual chair in the perceiver's environment or indexed to a prototypical representation of a chair that retains perceptual information; that is, a perceptual symbol. The second step is to use the indexed object or perceptual symbol to derive affordances. For example, a chair is typically used to sit on by an adult, but can also be used to stand on to reach for an object. The third step is to *mesh* the affordances guided by the syntax of the sentence. The language user combines the actions suggested by the chair and the actor, so that Jareb is on the chair rather than, say, under the chair. A sentence is meaningful to the extent that a reader/listener can mesh the objects and activities as directed by the sentence. A main advantage of the embodied approach is that because the model is based on perception, it brings us closer to a solution of the grounding problem.

Tracking the time course of novel meaning creation in real time

We conducted two ERP studies (Chwilla et al., 2007) with the aim of testing abstract symbol theories against embodied theories of meaning. This was accomplished by exploring how the mind/brain constructs novel meanings. In particular, we presented sentences that described a novel sensible context or a novel insensible context. For example, a context-setting sentence like "The scouts wanted to make music at the campfire" could be followed by a novel sensible sentence (e.g., "The boys searched for *branches* with which they went *drumming* and had a lot of fun"), or by a novel but senseless sentence (e.g., "The boys searched for *bushes* with which they went *drumming* and had a lot of fun"). Different pretests of the material verified that the novel contexts were indeed new. Critically, we demonstrated by using LSA that in more than 37,000 texts (selected from texts, novels, newspaper articles etc.), a central concept of each sentence (e.g., "drumming") appears in contexts that are orthogonal to the contexts in which the distinguishing concepts (e.g., "branches" and "bushes") appear.

Novel meaning creation is of theoretical importance, because embodied and disembodied theories make different predictions about the processing of novel meanings. Abstract symbol theories of meaning cannot explain how people can make sense out of novel sensible situations. The reason why these theories cannot explain superior performance for novel sensible versus novel insensible situations is that the only way they can discover meaningfulness is by consulting stored symbolic knowledge. However, this possibility was precluded by controlling the LSA values. In contrast, embodied theories of meaning can explain human ability to make sense out of new information not stored in long-term memory. On this view, people conceptualize specific situations, including those in which language is involved, by simulating themselves as full-bodied beings in these events. According to the indexical hypothesis, meaning for both familiar situations and novel situations evolves from meshing the affordances of the objects and activities as described by a sentence or discourse. What is meaningful and what is not depends on our knowledge about the possibilities and limitations of the human body and our experiences.

We used N400 to track the time course of novel meaning creation. Because nobody had yet probed for N400 effects to novel meanings, the aim of the first study was to investigate whether novel sensible meanings compared to novel insensible meanings elicit an N400 effect. Glenberg and Robertson (2000) have shown that participants judged new sensible sentences as more meaningful than new senseless sentences. To facilitate a comparison of the ERP results with the behavioral results, the procedure and task that we used was similar to that of Glenberg and Robertson (2000). That is, participants read the critical sentence, to which their brain activity was recorded, and then indicated how meaningful the sentence was given the context.

As predicted, participants judged novel sensible contexts as more meaningful than novel insensible contexts. The crucial question was whether novel sensible contexts not stored in semantic memory produced an N400 effect or not. The answer was yes. The main finding of Experiment 1 was that novel sensible contexts that were matched in terms of familiarity/semantic similarity by LSA to novel senseless contexts, elicited an N400 effect. The N400 effect to novel sensible contexts occurred in the same time-frame as the typical N400 effect to associative or semantic relations. It showed an onset at about 300 ms and peaked around 400 ms. The N400 effect to novel sensible contexts also resembled the classical N400 effect in terms of the wave shape and scalp distribution: it was maximal at central/posterior midline and bilateral posterior sites (see Figure 13.3a). Note that in a speeded RT version of this study no facilitation for novel sensible contexts was observed.

The exciting news of Experiment 1 was that we succeeded in constructing novel sensible stories, which according to LSA were *similar* in terms of association strength and semantic relatedness to the control stories, but nevertheless yielded an N400 effect. The occurrence of an N400 effect to novel sensible meanings compared to novel insensible ones cannot be explained by abstract symbol theories of meaning (e.g., Collins & Loftus, 1975; Masson, 1995; Ratcliff & McKoon, 1988). Because the critical words in the sentences were neither associatively nor semantically related, no facilitation should have been observed for novel sensible contexts according to these models. The results show that participants can establish new meanings not

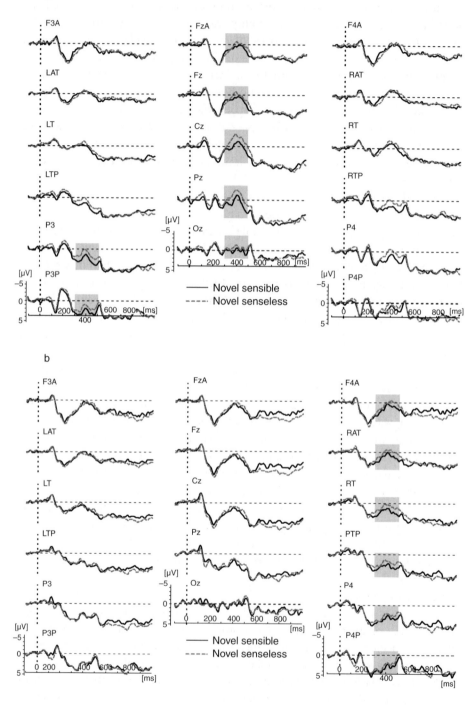

a

F3A

LAT

LT

LTP

P3

[μV]
−5
0
5

P3P

[μV]
−5
0
5
0 200 400 600 800 [ms]

FzA

Fz

Cz

Pz

[μV]
−5
0
5

Oz

0 200 400 600 800 [ms]

——— Novel sensible
- - - - Novel senseless

F4A

RAT

RT

RTP

P4

[μV]
−5
0
5

P4P

0 200 400 600 800 [ms]

b

F3A

LAT

LT

LTP

P3

[μV]
−5
0
5

P3P

0 200 400 600 800
[ms]

FzA

Fz

Cz

Pz

[μV]
−5
0
5

Oz

0 200 400 600 800
[ms]

——— Novel sensible
- - - - Novel senseless

F4A

RAT

RT

PTP

P4

[μV]
−5
0
5

P4P

0 200 400 600 800
[ms]

Figure 13.3   (a) Experiment 1. The grand mean ERP waveforms for the sensibility judgment task for a representative set of sites, time-locked to the onset of the critical word (time
point zero), relative to a 100 ms pre-critical word baseline. Negativity is plotted upward.
Shaded areas indicate the time periods and the set of electrodes that showed significant N400
effects. From Chwilla, Kolk, and Vissers (2007), with permission from Elsevier Science. (b)
Experiment 2. The grand mean ERP waveforms during reading for a representative set of
sites, time-locked to the onset of the critical word (time point zero), relative to a 100 ms
pre-critical word baseline. Negativity is plotted upward. Shaded areas indicate the time
periods and the set of electrodes that showed significant N400 effects. From Chwilla, Kolk,
and Vissers (2007), with permission from Elsevier Science.

←

stored in memory, and that the N400 is sensitive to such new meanings. The N400
effect to novel sensible contexts can be accounted for by the embodied theory of
language comprehension of Glenberg and Robertson (1999, 2000). Therefore, the
ERP data support embodied theories and call into question abstract symbol theories
of meaning.

A possible critique on the ERP study and some other behavioral studies that have
been presented as evidence supporting the embodied framework is that these studies
exploited artificial judgment tasks. In the ERP study, the task directed the participant's attention to the sensibility of the test sentence. It is clear that this task does
not comprise part of the reading process. Therefore, it can be argued that the N400
sensibility effect reflects task-induced strategies and not reading processes. On this
view, immediate integration of novel meanings may only occur when processing of
this information is in the focus of attention or overtly requested. In the latter case,
the facilitation for novel meanings would not inform us about the architecture of
the language comprehension system but instead would reflect an additional
function.

A second ERP study was conducted to clarify this issue. The aim of this study
was to test whether the N400 effect to novel sensible contexts reflects reading processes or task-specific strategies. In the second study, the same critical materials were
presented, but no additional task was given. All the participants were asked to do
was to read the context-setting paragraph and the test sentence while their EEG was
recorded. The predictions were straightforward: if the N400 effect to novel sensible
contexts observed in Experiment 1 reflects strategies induced by the judgment task,
then the N400 effect should disappear during reading. In contrast, if the N400 effect
to novel meanings reflects reading processes, then the effect should also show up in
Experiment 2.

The major result of Experiment 2 was that reading novel sensible contexts gave
rise to an N400 effect. As in the first study, the N400 sensibility effect resembled the
standard N400 effect in terms of the waveform and the timing of the effect (300–
500 ms window). The N400 effect started around 300 ms and peaked at 400 ms. The
only difference between studies was that the N400 sensibility effect in the reading
study was limited to the right hemisphere (see Figure 13.3b). Between-experiment
analyses confirmed that the N400 effect in Experiment 1 showed a bilateral central/

posterior maximum, whereas the N400 effect during reading was restricted to the right hemisphere. What could the difference in scalp distribution between the N400 effects reflect? At face value, the lateralization of the N400 sensibility effect in the reading study fits well with the idea that creative processes are mainly subserved by the right hemisphere. Such a specialization is consistent with a growing number of studies that point to a special involvement of the right hemisphere in comprehending more complex language, such as discourse processing (St George, Kutas, Martinez, & Serano, 1999), comprehending metaphors (e.g., Mashal, Faust, & Hendler, 2005), and getting jokes (e.g., Coulson & Wu, 2005). The fact that the N400 effect for lexical decision was maximal at centroparietal midline sites could reflect strategic processes.

Discussion

The important insight gained from Experiment 2 is that the N400 effect in relation to novel meanings generalized to normal reading. Based on the presence of an *immediate* N400 sensibility effect in Experiment 2, we reject the hypothesis that the N400 effect in relation to novel meanings was caused by strategic processes. The fact that the N400 effect to novel meanings occurs independent of task reveals that this effect is a general finding. This result has important implications for current theories of meaning.

Implications for abstract symbol versus embodied theories of meaning

We have demonstrated that novel sensible meanings compared to novel senseless meanings reliably elicit an N400 effect. To our knowledge, this is the first report of an N400 effect for new meanings that have to be created on the spot. The theoretical importance lies in the fact that the N400 effect to novel sensible contexts cannot be explained by high-dimensional models of meaning like LSA of Landauer and Dumais (1997) or by other abstract symbol theories of meaning (e.g., Collins & Loftus, 1975; Masson, 1995). According to abstract symbol theories, concepts can only be meaningfully related if they are associatively or semantically related by virtue of common experience. This does not apply to the novel sensible contexts presented in these ERP studies. Current measures of associative strength or semantic similarity (i.e., free association, category membership, local or global co-occurrence measures like LSA), therefore, cannot account for the N400 sensibility effect. Hence, theories that employ these methods as measures of semantic memory, in particular, spreading activation models, compound-cue models, distributed memory models, and high-dimensional theories of meaning, fail to explain the N400 effects to novel sensible contexts.

A fundamental problem that abstract symbol theories of meaning face is how meaningless symbols come to take on meaning. As pointed out by Searle in his famous Chinese Room example (1980) manipulation of abstract amodal symbols produces more abstract symbols, not meaning. Glenberg and Robertson (2000) claim that they have solved this grounding problem in their embodied approach to language. The starting point is that language is grounded in perception and action. Meaning arises from our current physical interactions with the environment or previous encounters with objects in different kinds of environments. Present or past body–environment interactions guide us in how to think about, that is, to simulate the perceptual and action details required by a situation. Meaningfulness resides in our knowledge about the possibilities and limitations of the human body. Therefore, the finding of an N400 effect to novel sensible situations can be accounted for by the embodied theory of language, in particular by the indexical hypothesis of Glenberg and Robertson (1999, 2000). This theory naturally explains why humans can make sense out of novel sensible situations but high-dimensional theories of meaning or abstract symbol theories cannot. Our N400 results, therefore, support an embodied approach to meaning.

The nature of the mental simulation process

The time course of the N400 sensibility effect – relative to the standard N400 effect – provides insight into the speed at which new meanings are constructed. Critically, the N400 effect in the case of novel meanings occurred in the same time frame (300–500 ms) as the standard N400 effect for associative or semantic relations. The N400 results demonstrate that immediate integration is not restricted to familiar meanings that based on learning history are stored in semantic memory. Immediate integration also occurs for novel meanings, although the latter relations have never been encountered. Crucial for the present goals, the immediacy of novel meaning creation as revealed by the present N400 effects has important repercussions for the nature of the mental simulation process.

The mental simulation process lies at the heart of embodied approaches to cognition and language comprehension. It could be argued that this mental simulation process represents some kind of strategy, in contrast to symbolic processing which proceeds in a strict bottom-up fashion and is automatic. The present ERP data speak to this issue. First, the immediate N400 effect to novel meanings during reading shows that the mental simulation process reflects normal reading processes rather than strategic processing. Second, the N400 results reveal that affordances are immediately generated even for novel, that is, for unfamiliar, situations, that have never been experienced before. Apparently, deriving affordances, that is, simulating new actions like "to paddle with Frisbees" or "to drum with branches," occurs with the same ease as deriving affordances for familiar actions like to "paddle with paddles" or "to drum with sticks." On the one hand, this ability seems astounding. On the other hand, if, as proposed by Hess and colleagues (1995), participants can't help but search for coherence and meaning whenever encountering words, then the speed at which new meanings are established becomes understandable. Humans are experts in extracting meaning.

Work from developmental psychology supports the idea that affordances are generated automatically. Gibson (1979), in his ecological theory of perception, proposed an innate mechanism for extracting important *visual* information from available stimulation. According to this nativist theory, any perceptually equipped animal can apprehend properties of the world that are relevant to action. They describe affordances as those action-related properties of the physical environment that afford, elicit, or suggest certain behavioural action. The organism's needs, motivations, and intentions in combination with the ecological context in which an element appears, indicate what the element affords. So, any organism will grasp what the environment affords in ecologically valid, natural terrains. Consistent with this, Borghi (2005) proposed that for simple actions visual input and object knowledge help subjects to extract affordances automatically. Language-acquisition studies further strengthen the link between language and action. Smith (2005) showed that action alters the shape categories formed by only 2-year-old children. In sum, the present N400 results, work from developmental psychology, and studies on language acquisition all bolster the claim that the mental simulation process reflects an automatic process.

General Discussion

The central topic of this chapter is how the mind/brain creates meaning in language. The ERP method was exploited to shed light on this issue by tracking the time course at which familiar and novel meanings are established.

With respect to familiar knowledge, people have certain expectancy patterns based on their experiences that are useful to interpret behaviour. In cognitive psychology, these expectancy patterns, called scripts or schemata, have been proposed to be the building blocks of cognition. From early childhood on, we build a large repertoire of scripts for all kinds of daily events, from climbing a staircase, biking, visiting a doctor versus visiting friends, to eating out at a restaurant. Daily life for the most part consists of scripts that help organize the world. Although pre-existing knowledge can lead to inaccuracies and illusions (for example, readers make inferences that are not present in the input which can lead to false recall; e.g., Bransford, Barclay, & Franks, 1972), in large majority of our interactions with the external world scripts are extremely helpful. The ERP data presented in Part 1 show that script knowledge forms a central aspect of word meaning that becomes available *immediately* when words are read.

An exciting question first posed by Plato is how the mind/brain constructs novel meanings. How can we make sense out of novel meanings like "to paddle with Frisbees," or "to use a comb to scratch icy car windows"? The ERP results, presented in Part 2, lead to the striking conclusion that novel meanings, although people never encountered them, become available immediately, that is within the same time frame as simple associative or semantic relations. Immediate access/integration occurs even though we have no experience or script for performing these novel actions. How come constructing novel meanings is not more (computationally) demanding than constructing familiar meanings?

To try to understand this, let us have a look at what a novel meaning, like "to paddle with Frisbees" is composed of. The words that the novel meaning consists of are familiar; what is new is the combination. Based on our world knowledge, we have a script for paddling, depicting an action typically performed with paddles, which consists of a series of actions like sitting in a canoe and moving paddles smoothly through the water by the respective arm, trunk, and leg movements to move the canoe forwards. Proper coordination of these bodily actions yields paddling. We also have semantic knowledge about Frisbees. We know that flying discs are called Frisbees. Frisbees are disc-shaped objects, which are generally plastic and roughly 20–25 cm in diameter with a lip. Dependent on our experience with Frisbees, we may also know that the shape of the disc, an airfoil in cross-section, allows it to fly by generating lift as it moves through the air while rotating. More generally known is that flying discs are thrown and caught for recreation. Likewise, we know that pullovers belong to the category of clothing, are a relatively heavy garment intended to cover the torso and arms of the human body and usually worn over a blouse, T-shirt, or other top. Pullovers can consist of wool, cotton, synthetic fibers, or some combination thereof. In brief, the concepts of a "Frisbee" and "pullover" are familiar chunks in semantic memory. But how can we grasp the meaning of the novel combination "to paddle with Frisbees"?

As should be clear, the symbolic approach fails to account for superior performance for novel sensible contexts. Immediate access/integration of completely unfamiliar contexts, therefore, forces us to accept explanations in terms of embodied actions. According to embodied approaches of language, in order to make sense out of novel meanings, these meanings have to be *grounded* in action or perception. To access and retrieve embodied knowledge, we project ourselves into a situation and simulate the perceptual and action details required by that situation. Scientists in the field of second-language acquisition have also often pointed out the importance of action for the grounding of novel meanings (Asher, 1977).

I propose that the process of analogy, which has been the focus of extensive research in cognitive science (Gentner, Holyoak, & Kokinov, 2001) provides an alternative for the symbolic approach. An analogy is a mapping between two represented situations, in which common relational structure is aligned. Analogical mapping refers to the process of establishing a structural alignment between two represented situations and then projecting inferences. Crucial for the present argument, Gentner and colleagues propose that through analogy, novel situations and problems can be understood in terms of familiar ones. Applying this idea to the present example, I propose that based on our analogical ability – the ability to perceive and use relational similarity – we combine (align) the paddling script with what we know about Frisbees. This combination (alignment) reveals that Frisbees, based on their physical properties (their size, form, stiffness, and light weight), make them a suitable object for paddling. In contrast, combining by way of analogy the script of paddling with our knowledge about pullovers (their lack of stiffness, and heavy weight when wet) conveys that paddling with pullovers will not work. As illustrated by the example, analogy can readily account for creative behavior. I would like to highlight the close relationship between analogies and metaphors (Lakoff, 1987). In fact, the majority of metaphors studied in the literature are analogies in that they convey chiefly relational commonalities (e.g., "These architects fight like lions"; "My job is a jail").

Our N400 results on novel meaning creation support the proposal of Gentner and Colhoun (2010) that analogical processes are at the core of relational thinking, which they suggest is key to human cognitive process and separates us from other intelligent creatures. Citing the authors, "The capacity for analogy ensures that every new encounter offers not only its own kernel of knowledge, but a potentially vast set of insights resulting from parallels past and future."

Conclusion

The goal of the present research was to test abstract symbol versus embodied approaches to meaning. In Part 1, we examined how abstract world knowledge is accessed/integrated into lexical semantic context. Immediate access/integration of world knowledge is problematic for abstract symbol theories and supports more flexible integration models, like the automatic compound-cue integration model. In Part 2, we tested abstract symbol theories and embodied theories of word meaning against each other by exploring how novel meanings are created. The immediate integration of novel meanings challenges abstract symbol theories and supports embodied approaches to language comprehension. Importantly, the immediate onset of the N400 effect to novel meanings and its task-independence support an automatic nature of the simulation process that lies at the heart of embodied approaches to cognition.

The ERP results presented here are at odds with the view that word meaning is performed by a central cognitive module. Our results add to the growing literature in language and nonlanguage domains that calls into question any clear dividing line between language and the brain's modal system for action. Overall, the results accord well with the view that a distributed cortical network is involved in meaning construction. I hope that I have made it clear that cognitive scientists should acknowledge the importance of embodiment for language use and meaning. For abstract symbol theories, it remains complicated to explain how we can talk about what we see (Jackendoff, 1987). The advantage of embodied approaches, in which language is grounded in perception and action, is that they naturally account for interactions of language with perception, action, and even emotion.

The question is whether the embodied versus symbolic approach should be viewed as competitors or as complementary approaches to the representation of meaning. Which approach to choose likely depends on the kind of concept. While perceptual symbols are very useful to represent concrete or highly imageable concepts, amodal abstract symbols may be needed to represent abstract concepts. Representational pluralism as proposed by Dove (2009) may be a prerequisite to cover the enormous spectrum of what we can do with language, from describing the foundations of logic to trying to describe a musical purely by means of abstract language – that is, without body language.

Note

Part of this chapter was written during a visit to the Centre for Language Science at Penn State University. I am grateful to Judith Kroll for insightful discussions and for being a wonderful host. I would like to thank Herman Kolk for fruitful collaboration over the years. I am grateful to Rob Schreuder for valuable comments on a previous version of this chapter. This chapter is dedicated to my dear friend, companion in science, music investigator, and foremost music-lover Dr Wout Croonen, who left us too soon.

References

Asher, J. (1977). Children learning another language: A developmental hypothesis. *Child Development, 48*, 1040–1048.

Barsalou, L. W. (1999). Perceptual symbol systems. *Behavioral and Brain Sciences, 22*, 577–660.

Barsalou, L. W. (2009). Simulation, situated conceptualization, and prediction. *Philosophical Transactions of the Royal Society B: Biological Sciences, 364*, 1281–1289.

Borghi, A. M. (2005). Object concepts and action. In D. Pecher & R. A. Zwaan (Eds.), *Grounding cognition: The role of perception and action in memory, language, and thinking* (pp. 8–34). Cambridge: Cambridge University Press.

Bransford, J. D., Barclay, J. R., & Franks, J. L. (1972). Sentence memory: A constructive versus interpretive approach. *Cognitive Psychology, 3*, 193–209.

Burgess, C., & Lund, K. (2000). The dynamics of meaning in memory. In E. Dietrich & A. Markman (Eds.), *Cognitive dynamics: Conceptual and representational change in humans and machines* (pp. 117–156). Hillsdale, NJ: Erlbaum.

Chwilla, D. J., Brown, C. M., & Hagoort, P. (1995). The N400 as a function of the level of processing. *Psychophysiology, 32*, 274–285.

Chwilla, D. J., & Kolk, H. H. J. (2002).Three-step priming in lexical decision. *Memory and Cognition, 30*, 217–225.

Chwilla, D. J., & Kolk, H. H. J. (2005). Accessing world knowledge: Evidence from N400 and reaction time priming. *Cognitive Brain Research, 25*, 589–606.

Chwilla, D. J., Kolk, H. H. J., & Mulder, G. (2000). Mediated priming in the lexical decision task: Evidence from event-related potentials and reaction time. *Journal of Memory and Language, 42*, 314–341.

Chwilla, D. J., Kolk, H. H. J., & Vissers, Th. W. M. (2007). Immediate integration of novel meanings: N400 support for an embodied view of language comprehension. *Brain Research, 1183*, 109–123.

Clark, H. H. (1996). *Using language*. Cambridge: Cambridge University Press.

Collins, A. M., & Loftus, E. F. (1975). A spreading-activation theory of semantic processing. *Psychological Review, 82*, 407–428.

Cook, A. E., & Myers, J. L. (2004). Processing discourse roles in scripted narratives: The influence of context and world knowledge. *Journal of Memory and Language, 50*, 268–288.

Coulson, S., & Wu, Y. C. (2005). Right hemisphere activation of joke-related information: An event-related brain potential study. *Journal of Cognitive Neuroscience, 17*, 494–506.

Dove, G. (2009). Beyond perceptual symbols: A call for representational pluralism. *Cognition, 110*, 412–431.

Elman, J. L. (2009). On the meaning of words and dinosaur bones: Lexical knowledge without a lexicon. *Cognitive Science, 33*, 547–582.

Faust, M., & Babkoff, H. (1997). Script as a priming stimulus for lexical decisions and with visual hemifield stimulation. *Brain and Language, 57*, 423–437.

Fodor, J. A. (1975). The language of thought. *New York*: Crowell Press.

Friederici, A. D. (1995). The time-course of syntactic activation during language processing: A model based on neuropsychological and neurophysiological data. *Brain and Language, 50*, 259–281.

Gentner, D., & Colhoun, J. (2010). Analogical processes in human thinking and learning. In A. von Müller & E. Pöppel (Series Eds.) & B. Glatzeder, V. Goel, & A. von Müller (Vol. Eds.), *On thinking* (vol. 2, *Towards a theory of thinking*, pp. 35–48). Springer-Verlag Berlin Heidelberg.

Gentner, D., Holyoak, K. J., & Kokinov, B. K. (Eds.). (2001). *The analogical mind*. Cambridge, MA: MIT Press.

Gibson J. J. (1979). *The ecological approach to visual perception. Boston*: Houghton. Mifflin.

Glenberg, A. M. (1997). What memory is for. *Behavioral and Brain Sciences, 20*, 1–55.

Glenberg, A. M., & Robertson, D. A. (1999). Indexical understanding of instructions. *Discourse Processes, 28*, 1–26.

Glenberg, A. M., & Robertson, D. A. (2000). Symbol grounding and meaning: A comparison of high-dimensional and embodied theories of meaning. *Journal of Memory and Language, 43*, 379–401.

Hagoort, P., Hald, L., Bastiaansen, M., & Petersson, K. M. (2004). Integration of word meaning and world knowledge in language comprehension. *Science, 304*, 438–441.

Hare, M., Jones, M., Thomson, C., Kelly, S., & McRae, K. (2009). Activating event knowledge. *Cognition, 111*, 151–167.

Hess, D. J., Foss, D. J., & Carroll, P. (1995). Effects of global and local context on lexical processing during language comprehension. *Journal of Experimental Psychology: General, 124*, 62–82.

Hutchison, K. (2003). Is semantic priming due to association strength or featural overlap? A "Micro-Analytic" review. *Psychonomic Bulletin and Review, 10*, 785–813.

Jackendoff, R. (1987). On beyond zebra: The relation of linguistic and visual information, *Cognition, 26*, 89–114.

Kutas, M., & Federmeier K. D. (2000). Electrophysiology reveals semantic memory use in language comprehension. *Trends in Cognitive Science, 4*, 463–470.

Kutas, M., & Hillyard, S. A. (1980). Reading senseless sentences: Brain potentials reflect semantic incongruity. *Science, 207*, 203–205.

Lakoff, G. (1987). *Women, Fire, and Dangerous Things*. Chicago: University of Chicago Press.

Landauer, T. K., & Dumais, S. T. (1997). A solution to Plato's problem: The latent semantic analysis theory of acquisition, induction, and representation of knowledge. *Psychological Review, 104,* 211–240.

Lau, E. F., Phillips, C., & Poeppel, D. (2008). A cortical network for semantics: (De)constructing the N400. *Nature Reviews Neuroscience, 9,* 920–933.

MacWhinney, B. (1999). The emergence of language from embodiment. In B. MacWhinney (Ed.), *The emergence of language* (pp. 213–256). Mahwah, NJ: Erlbaum.

Mashal, N., Faust, M., & Hendler, T. (2005). The role of the right hemisphere in processing nonsalient metaphorical meanings: Application of principal components analysis to fMRI data. *Neuropsychologia, 43,* 2084–2100.

Masson, M. E. J. (1995). A distributed memory model of semantic priming. *Journal of Experimental Psychology: Learning, Memory, and Cognition, 21,* 3–23.

McKoon, G., & Ratcliff, R. (1992). Spreading activation versus compound cue accounts of priming; mediated priming revisited. *Journal of Experimental Psychology: Learning, Memory, and Cognition, 18,* 1155–1172.

McNamara, T. P. (2005). *Semantic priming: Perspectives from memory and word recognition. Essays in cognitive psychology.* New York and Hove: Psychology Press.

Moss, H. E., Ostrin, R. K., Tyler, L. K., & Marslen-Wilson, W. D. (1995). Accessing different types of lexical semantic information: Evidence from priming. *Journal of Experimental Psychology: Learning, Memory, and Cognition, 21,* 863–883.

Pulvermüller F. (2005). Brain mechanisms linking language and action. *Nature Reviews Neuroscience, 6,* 576–582

Ratcliff, R., & McKoon, G. (1988). A retrieval theory of priming in memory. *Psychological Review, 95,* 385–408.

Rumelhart, D. E. (1980). Schemata. The building blocks of cognition. In R. J. Spiro, B. C. Bruce, & W. F. Brewer (Eds.), *Theoretical issues in reading comprehension* (pp. 33–58). Hillsdale, NJ: Erlbaum.

Schank, R. C., & Abelson, R. P. (1977). *Scripts, plans, goals and understanding.* Hillsdale, NJ: Erlbaum.

Searle, J. R. (1980). Minds, brains, and programs. *Behavioral and Brain Sciences, 3,* 417–457.

Smith, L. B. (2005). Action alters shape categories. *Cognitive Science, 29,* 665–679.

St George, M., Kutas, M., Martinez, A., & Sereno, M. I. (1999). Semantic integration in reading: Engagement of the right hemisphere during discourse processing. *Brain, 122,* 1317–1325.

Zwaan, R. A., & Taylor, L. J. (2006). Seeing, acting, understanding: Motor resonance in language comprehension. *Journal of Experimental Psychology: General, 135,* 1–11.

14

Motor and Nonmotor Language Representations in the Brain

Nira Mashal, Michael Andric, and Steven Small

Introduction

Typical face-to-face conversation involves an elaborate arrangement of movements. Both a speaker and his or her conversational partner exchange information about articulated speech via perception of mouth and lip movements. Virtually all face-to-face speech is also accompanied by spontaneously produced hand gestures. The brain coordinates all of these movements in various networks of regions, including some typically associated with language processing and others sometimes referred to as the "motor system." An important question is to what extent this motor system, beyond its role in producing actions, is also involved in perceiving them. The presence of motor system involvement in both producing and perceiving actions leads to a further line of inquiry seeking to discern the extent of its role in coding actions for comprehension. That is, might the motor system, via its regular responsibility in helping to produce and perceive actions, provide a basis for how the brain represents meaning more generally?

In this chapter, we discuss the motor regions of the cerebral cortex and their participation in a number of functions related to human language, i.e., producing and perceiving speech and language and representing the meaning of words and sentences. We first elaborate on motor system involvement in articulate speech, continue to characterize its involvement in manual gesture, and, lastly, discuss its more general role in interpreting a message's content.

Recent anatomical and physiological findings in the nonhuman primate brain have profoundly impacted our understanding of how actions are processed and

The Handbook of the Neuropsychology of Language, First Edition. Edited by Miriam Faust.
© 2012 Blackwell Publishing Ltd. Published 2012 by Blackwell Publishing Ltd.

understood neurobiologically. The cortical motor system of the primate is a collage of many anatomically and functionally distinguishable areas (Rizzolatti & Luppino, 2001). Single neuron recording studies have shown that in one of these areas of the macaque monkey, area F5 in the rostral part of the ventral premotor cortex, there exist neurons that code specific actions, possibly providing a "vocabulary" of motor action representations (Rizzolatti et al., 1988). Some of the neurons in F5 are active either when the monkey performs a specific mouth or hand action, or when it observes another monkey (or human) performing the same or a similar action. Such identified "mirror neurons" have also subsequently been found in the inferior parietal area PF (Fogassi, Gallese, Fadiga, & Rizzolatti, 1998). Mirror neurons have been proposed as the basis for a mechanism that transforms specific sensory information into a motor format, giving an immediate understanding of an observed motor act (Fabbri-Destro & Rizzolatti, 2008). A mirror mechanism is proposed to exist in humans as well, and similarly to mediate our understanding of actions (Fabbri-Destro & Rizzolatti, 2008; Rizzolatti & Arbib, 1998; Rizzolatti & Fabbri-Destro, 2008; Skipper, van Wassenhove, Nusbaum, & Small, 2007).

Does such a mechanism play a role in language comprehension via an observer's visual perceptions of a speaker's mouth and hand actions? Indeed, accumulating evidence suggests that areas of our own cortical motor system become active when we interpret spoken language (e.g., Meister, Wilson, Deblieck, Wu, & Iacoboni, 2007; Skipper et al., 2007; Wilson, Saygin, Sereno, & Iacoboni, 2004). The specific function of this motor activity, however, is still under considerable debate. Some have suggested that perceiving speech may incorporate a mechanism of simulating its production (Halle & Stevens, 1962; Liberman & Whalen, 2000). Existing data also admit alternate plausible theories emphasizing integration of motor and sensory information in perception (Hickok & Poeppel, 2004, 2007; Skipper, Nusbaum, & Small, 2006). Similarly, emerging data suggest that activity in motor regions is also present when we observe the hand gestures that accompany spoken language ("co-speech gestures"; e.g., Green et al., 2009; Skipper, Goldin-Meadow, Nusbaum, & Small, 2009; Willems, Ozyurek, & Hagoort, 2007), as well as the salient gestures that convey propositional meaning independent of speech ("emblems"; e.g., Villarreal et al., 2008). Moreover, cortical motor activity in language settings does not appear to be present just when perceiving the actions of its expression.

The question about the role of the motor system in language comprehension leads naturally to the more specific question about whether neurally instantiated motor programs are used in representing meaning more generally. Several studies of word and sentence processing have postulated that brain activity in primary and premotor cortices is used to represent the meaning of words and sentences. These studies have generally described such activity during the processing of action-related language, and not during processing of linguistic content unrelated to actions. Examples include activity in motor regions for processing action-related words (e.g., Hauk, Johnsrude, & Pulvermüller, 2004) and for sentences that describe oral, manual, and foot actions (e.g., Tettamanti et al., 2005). Thus, while we still lack a complete, systematic explanation of the role of the motor system in language, its involvement appears indisputable.

Speech Perception

When we observe someone speaking to us, we integrate auditory information from the speech stream with visual information from (especially) the lips and mouth to come up with the intended message. Evidence obtained from transcranial magnetic stimulation (TMS) and functional magnetic resonance imaging (fMRI) studies have suggested that a hearer might perceive speech in part (e.g., Skipper et al., 2006) or entirely (e.g., Liberman & Whalen, 2000) by simulating the articulatory gestures of the talker. This implies that some sort of motor mechanism – and by inference some motor regions of the brain – plays an important role in speech perception (e.g., Halle & Stevens, 1962; Massaro & Cohen, 1995; for review see Galantucci, Fowler, & Turvey, 2006). Thus, to find support for the notion that motor regions are involved in speech perception, a growing number of studies have used advanced brain imaging techniques to show similar brain regions activated during both speech perception and speech production tasks.

A large body of evidence obtained from fMRI has shown that audiovisual perception of monosyllables activates brain areas dedicated to speech production. A recent fMRI study showed that passive listening to meaningless monosyllables activates the ventral premotor cortex (PMv), an area also activated during production of the same syllables (Wilson et al., 2004). In a theoretical paper (Skipper et al., 2006), we have postulated that PMv integrates visual information from the face of the speaker with auditory information from the speech stream using motor commands that could have generated those movements. In this model, the flow of sensory information (backward model) maps and integrates the sensory information onto articulatory motor representations in the frontal lobe (forward model).

Subsequent work has been conducted with "illusory" audiovisual syllables, artificial audiovisual stimuli in which visual and auditory information are inconsistent, leading to a percept that is neither the auditory nor the visual component (McGurk & McDonald, 1976). These studies showed that observation and production overlap in multiple brain areas including premotor cortices and primary motor cortex (Skipper et al., 2007). When participants perceived an "illusory" incongruent /ta/ consisting of a visual image of the mouth producing /ka/ while hearing the audio /pa/, the activity in the motor area resembled the activity patterns evoked by the congruent audiovisual /ta/ more than /ka/ or /pa/. Interestingly, activity patterns in the visual cortex resembled the activity evoked by audiovisual /ka/, particularly early in the process, and activity patterns in auditory areas resembled the activity evoked by audiovisual /pa/, with similarly evolving time course.

A recent TMS study demonstrated neural activity in speech motor regions during passive speech perception, suggesting that activity in motor areas is causally linked to the perception of speech (Meister et al., 2007). That study used both fMRI and

TMS, first to localize premotor regions activated during both speech production and speech perception and then to apply slow (inhibitory) repetitive TMS (rTMS) over one of the previously identified premotor sites while participants heard a consonant–vowel syllable in noise. The subject had to identify it as pa, ta, or ka by pressing one of three keys. The results showed a decrease in the rate of correct responses for the speech perception task after applying TMS over the left premotor cortex as compared to baseline (no TMS). The authors concluded that the premotor area plays an essential role in speech perception, and that sensory regions are not in themselves sufficient for human perception. This suggests that a mechanism such as simulation, that couples action and perception, is critical for speech perception.

If motor brain regions are associated with speech perception, then listening to speech should lead to excitability of certain muscles, measured by motor-evoked potentials. Watkins et al. (2003) applied TMS over the face area of primary motor cortex to elicit motor-evoked potentials (MEPs) in the lip muscles. The MEPs were measured while participants listened to speech (continuous prose), listened to non-verbal sounds (e.g., glass breaking, bells ringing), viewed speech-related lip movements, and viewed eye and brow movements. The results indicated that either listening to speech or viewing speech-related actions enhanced the amplitude of motor-evoked potentials in the lip muscles compared to baseline. This effect was seen in response to stimulation of the left hemisphere but not the right hemisphere. This result provides evidence that speech perception of both auditory and visual information increases the excitability of the motor system involved in speech production.

Thus, neural systems for speech perception and speech production, traditionally localized in a dissociated way to the left posterior temporal and inferior frontal areas, respectively, seem to interact functionally during language comprehension (at least). Of course, it is well known since the nineteenth century that these systems are anatomically interconnected. Since Déjérine (1891, 1892), Broca's area, classically considered a motor speech production area, (e.g., Bookheimer, 2002; Broca, 1861) has been thought to be connected to Wernicke's area (Wernicke, 1874) by the arcuate fasciculus, although the original data on this connectivity came from gross anatomical inspection without physiological support. Neuroanatomical studies in monkeys (Yeterian & Pandya, 1985) support this connectivity in a homologous situation, and diffusion tensor imaging data from humans (Catani & Mesulam, 2008) have further elaborated the veracity of the original anatomical postulate (Déjérine, 1891). Geschwind (1966) built on these original concepts, and articulated a connectionist approach, summarizing what is now considered the classic Broca-Wernicke-Geschwind model of brain language relationships. According to his model, Broca's area is the center of expressive language, Wernicke's area is the center of receptive language, and the arcuate fasciculus serves as the connecting pathway between the two. The model predicts that lesions to Broca's area would cause Broca's aphasia, lesions to Wernicke's area would cause Wernicke's aphasia, and lesions to the arcuate fasciculus would cause conduction aphasia (Geschwind, 1971).

Since Geschwind, considerable research using the lesion analysis method, as well as research using newer technologies for studying brain–behavior relationships, are proving problematic for Geschwind's model. For example, it has become clear that the behavioral syndrome of Broca's aphasia is not caused by a lesion restricted to Broca's area, and can be caused by many other types of lesions (Feinberg & Farah, 1997). The same is true for Wernicke's aphasia (Ojemann, Ojemann, Lettich, & Berger, 1989). Conduction aphasia is more likely caused by a lesion to Wernicke's area than to the arcuate fasciculus (Anderson et al., 1999; Damasio & Damasio, 1980). Direct cortical stimulation of perisylvian areas that are associated with specific aphasic symptoms does not cause these symptoms as predicated by the model (Ojemann et al., 1989). Finally, a host of imaging studies, such as those reviewed here, suggest considerable integration of the neural mechanisms for production and perception of language.

The most recent connectionist model incorporates a connection between the rostral part of the inferior parietal lobule and the ventral premotor cortex and pars opercularis of the inferior frontal gyrus (IFGOp) via the superior longitudinal fasciculus, subcomponent III, and not through the arcuate fasciculus (Schmahmann et al., 2007). Spoken language areas, including auditory areas of the superior temporal gyrus, are also connected to frontal-motor areas through cortico-cortical connections (Makris et al., 1999; Rizzolatti & Luppino, 2001). These connections suggest that different cortical systems may interact functionally during language performance.

In summary, during the period since the original proposal of the connectionist model of Geschwind, particularly in the recent period of research with physiological and imaging techniques, researchers have greatly advanced their understanding of how speech production and perception are processed in the brain. Instead of referring to speech production and speech perception as two dissociated processes located in segregated yet connected brain "centers," its now known that speech perception and speech production interact during language performance and that speech perception integrally includes access to the speech motor system. After discussing the role of speech-associated gesture in language comprehension, which also involves direct involvement of the motor system, we will discuss the evidence that motor areas active during language comprehension in fact contribute to both comprehension and the representation of meaning.

Gesture Perception: Gestures Accompanying Speech

Co-speech gestures are those hand and arm movements that unknowingly accompany most spoken language (Kendon, 1994; McNeill, 1992, 2005). While a gesture is simply a "motion that embodies a meaning reliable to the accompanying speech" (McNeill, 2005), these actions vary in the types of information they contribute. For example, whereas *beat* gestures provide rhythmic "temporal highlighting" (McNeill, 1992) to their accompanying speech (e.g., using the hand like a baton and matching down motions with spoken intonations), representational *iconic* gestures depict semantic content in the context of accompanying speech (e.g., using downward directed wiggling fingers while describing someone walking). Such iconic gestures are thought to contribute to a message's meaning and interpretation (Goldin-Meadow, 2006; Kendon, 1994; McNeill, 2005). In pursuing a stronger appreciation for how the brain represents meaning, researchers are increasingly investigating the biology associated with processing these motor acts.

At a basic visual level, co-speech gestures are one class (among many) of biological movements. Thus, brain areas responsive to visually presented biological motion, e.g., portions of the superior temporal sulcus (STS) and adjoining middle occipital gyrus and anterior occipital sulcus (approximating V5/MT+), respond when observing such gestures (Dick, Goldin-Meadow, Hasson, Skipper, & Small, 2009; Kircher et al., 2009; Willems et al., 2007; Wilson, Molnar-Szakacs, & Iacoboni, 2008). More interesting, however, is that motor regions also appear to play a prominent role in interpreting these actions. As we just discussed in the context of mouth actions, neurophysiological data from monkeys suggest that understanding purposeful actions appears to be mediated by premotor and parietal responses similar to those involved in performing the actions (for reviews see Fabbri-Destro & Rizzolatti, 2008; Rizzolatti & Craighero, 2004). Brain imaging studies suggest similar mechanisms might operate in humans (Buccino et al., 2001). Does this include interpreting co-speech gestures? Although an entirely systematic profile of responses is not yet evident, generally, the research so far suggests yes.

Premotor and parietal activity when observing co-speech gestures

Significant neural responses in premotor and parietal cortices appear to be involved in the biology of observing co-speech gestures. For example, reliable premotor cortex activity is found when people view iconic co-speech gestures, either when compared to simple grooming movements (Holle, Gunter, Ruschemeyer, Hennenlotter, & Iacoboni, 2008), or when they are mismatched with a verb in a sentence (e.g., seeing someone say "hit" while performing a "writing" gesture; Willems et al., 2007). Premotor sensitivity is also evident in discourse settings when meaningful gestures (e.g., iconic, metaphoric, deictic) accompany continuous audiovisual story presentation (Skipper et al., 2009). In contrast, movements such as adjusting the collar and touching the cuff ("self-adaptive" movements) do *not* result in differential hemodynamic signal fluctuation (Skipper et al., 2009). Suggesting such responses extend to viewing co-speech gestures more generally, other studies also indicate premotor activity when people observe beat (Hubbard, Wilson, Callan, & Dapretto, 2009) and metaphoric (Kircher et al., 2009) gestures.

Further supporting the notion that premotor-parietal responses mediate action understanding is the finding that inferior parietal lobe activity occurs when people observe co-speech gestures (Dick et al., 2009; Green et al., 2009; Holle et al., 2008; Kircher et al., 2009; Skipper et al., 2009). The supramarginal gyrus (SMG), particularly, appears to play an important role. Differential hemodynamic signal fluctuation occurs in the SMG during story comprehension when meaningful co-speech gestures are presented compared to when they are not (Skipper et al., 2009). There is also strong effective connectivity between SMG and premotor cortices during co-speech gesture observation (Skipper et al., 2007, 2009). Interestingly, while Skipper et al. (2007, 2009) did not delineate right and left SMG, other work indicates functional differences between the two; for example, finding significant right SMG responses when gestures conveyed information unrelated to accompanying speech (Green et al., 2009).

Co-speech gesture processing also leads to differential functional activity across left and right intraparietal (IP) regions. For example, left IP activity dominates when a co-speech gesture is mismatched with a spoken verb in context (Willems et al., 2007), whereas right IP activity is prominent when observing co-speech gestures compared to grooming movements (Holle et al., 2008). Right IP activity is also found for observing beat gestures, but only when they are not accompanied by speech (Hubbard et al., 2009). It appears then that these IP responses reflect its involvement in action recognition, more generally, rather than reactivity to the message content per se.

Overall, co-speech gesture processing includes patterns of premotor and parietal activity similar to observing other purposeful actions such as grasping. However, co-speech gestures notably differ from grasping, often contributing semantic information pertinent to a speaker's message. Beyond extensive behavioral research (see McNeill, 1992, 2005), this idea is supported by results from event-related potential (ERP) studies documenting N400 effects – believed to reflect difficult integration of semantic information in context – pertaining to incongruence between words and gestures (Kelly, Kravitz, & Hopkins, 2004). Other studies dealing with the semantic relation between speech and gesture also find an N400 effect (Holle & Gunter, 2007; Kelly, Ward, Creigh, & Bartolotti, 2007; Ozyurek, Willems, Kita, & Hagoort, 2007; Wu & Coulson, 2005). Further, activity during co-speech gesture processing is often found in brain areas that are classically considered as integral to language interpretation, but, as with premotor and parietal responses, a wholly consistent pattern is still lacking.

Inferior frontal and temporal lobe activity when observing co-speech gestures

Co-speech gestures often add supplementary semantic information to a verbal message, and brain regions associated with processing such information respond when people perceive these gestures. For example, significant activity in the anterior left IFG, particularly the pars triangularis (IFGTr), is found when observing mismatches between an iconic gesture and a verb during sentence processing (Willems et al., 2007). Thus, left IFGTr may be particularly involved in interpreting meaning regardless of its expression in motor (e.g., as gesture) or verbal form. Similar findings in this region are apparent when people observe speech with gestures compared to speech alone (Dick et al., 2009; Kircher et al., 2009). Diverging from Willems et al. (2007), though, Dick et al. (2009) find this activation to be independent of the informativeness of the manual gesture, as the right IFGTr demonstrates stronger activity during observation of "self-adaptive" movements compared to meaningful co-speech gestures, and Green et al. (2009) find stronger bilateral IFGTr responses during observation of unrelated co-speech gestures compared to related ones Furthermore, IFGTr connectivity in a network including inferior parietal, temporal, and frontal motor regions appears to be strongest when observing "self-adaptive" movements and weakest when observing relevant gestures (Skipper et al., 2007). Perhaps when information from co-speech gestures appears to reduplicate that in speech, IFGTr involvement in interpretation is lower than when it does not. By this analysis, since self-adaptive movements do not contribute meaningful information, they would increase semantic retrieval and/or selection demands. Such an account fits with the Willems et al. (2007) finding of differential IFGTr activity when the gesture was "mismatched" to the verb since the hand information was no longer germane to the message, leaving relatively higher need for semantic retrieval.

Besides the frontal lobe, the temporal lobe has also been associated with processing meaning in language studies (Hickok & Poeppel, 2004; Martin & Chao, 2001; Wise et al., 2001), and temporal lobe activity does appear to be prominent during observation of co-speech gestures, as well. When gestures correspond to the semantics in a speaker's message, the anterior superior temporal region has strong connectivity with premotor regions (Skipper et al., 2007). Activity in this area also occurs when observing metaphoric gestures in isolation (Kircher et al., 2009). In the left posterior middle temporal gyrus (MTG), activity is greater for observing metaphoric (Kircher et al., 2009) or iconic (Green et al., 2009) gestures accompanying speech than for observing either speech or gesture alone. Existing theories associate anterior temporal lobe activity with the incorporation of semantic and syntactic structures into propositional representations of meaning, e.g., in sentence processing (Humphries, Binder, Medler, & Liebenthal, 2006; Noppeney & Price, 2004), and posterior activity with recognizing word meanings (Binder et al., 1997; Chao, Haxby, & Martin, 1999; Gold et al., 2006). These regions may be functioning in similar capacities in co-speech gesture processing, although it remains to be elaborated if their primary role in semantics is to interface sensory and conceptual representations (Hickok & Poeppel, 2004), to perform semantic recognition (Martin & Chao, 2001), and/or something else entirely.

Gesture Perception: Symbolic Hand Gestures (Emblems)

Another class of hand gestures, emblematic gestures or *emblems*, convey meaning independent of speech (Goldin-Meadow, 1999). Emblems are conventionalized manual actions that communicate symbolic meaning and can substitute for speech (e.g., giving a "thumbs up" to express "It's good"). With emblems, the hand action itself delivers an intended message. Unlike conventional sign languages, however, they are not combinatorial and lack the linguistic structures found in human language (McNeill, 2005). Rather, using a single hand position and movement, such gestures convey semantic, propositional information. Emblems thus have a unique combination of properties as both a single purposeful hand action and symbolic expression.

Premotor and parietal activity when observing symbolic gestures

Similar to co-speech gestures, perception of emblems leads to activation both in brain areas that are sensitive to biological movements (e.g., V5/MT and STSp) and in areas of the premotor and parietal cortex. Specifically, left ventral premotor cortex is regularly active during emblem observation (Lotze et al., 2006; Villarreal et al., 2008). Additionally, the intraparietal sulcus and inferior parietal lobule (SMG in particular) are also consistently active (Lotze et al., 2006; Nakamura et al., 2004; Villarreal et al., 2008). While localization of these parietal responses using fMRI has been either left-lateralized (Lotze et al., 2006) or bilateral (Nakamura et al., 2004; Villarreal et al., 2008), regional electrophysiological recordings during recognition of static pictures of emblems suggest right laterality (Nakamura et al., 2004). This lack of overall systematic lateralization suggests that emblem recognition may be associated with diffuse neural activity patterns across premotor and parietal cortices.

Inferior frontal and temporal lobe activity when observing symbolic gestures

Unlike co-speech gestures, emblems are typically used without accompanying speech, yet activation during emblem interpretation includes regions commonly associated with language interpretation. For example, left IFGOp, proximally marking the posterior part of Broca's area, is functionally responsive when observing emblems. This effect has been shown comparing activity for observing emblems versus rest (Lotze et al., 2006; Villarreal et al., 2008) and versus observing object-directed hand actions (Villarreal et al., 2008). Pars triangularis of the IFG is also responsive during emblem observation, whether on the right (Lotze et al., 2006; Nakamura et al., 2004) or bilaterally (Villarreal et al., 2008), and both IFGTr activity (Lotze et al., 2006; Villarreal et al., 2008) and activity of the pars orbitalis of the left IFG (Lotze et al., 2006) are greater for emblems than for pantomimed transitive hand actions.

In the temporal lobes, activity in the posterior portion of the MTG, associated previously with recognizing word meaning (Binder et al., 1997; Gold et al., 2006), is also present during emblem observation, and this activity is greater than for observing hand actions that do not directly convey meaning (Villarreal et al., 2008).

Significant activity when observing emblems is also present in the anterior temporal lobes (Lotze et al., 2006), in regions previously associated with semantic integration (Nopenney & Price, 2004; Stowe, Haverkort, & Zwarts, 2005), and sentence processing (Friederici, Opitz, & von Cramon, 2000; Humphries, Love, Swinney, & Hickok, 2005; Nopenney & Price, 2004).

Recall that unlike co-speech gestures or sign language, emblems are single expressions of meaning communicated in the absence of speech, and thus activation of these regions classically associated with language are responding to nonspeech expressions of meaning. Overall, it appears that emblem processing involves coordination of visual, premotor, and parietal activity with inferior frontal and temporal activity. One interpretation of these data is that the two inherent properties of emblems – as purposeful hand actions and expressions of semantic meaning – lead to integrated processing by two related neural networks in the brain. More generally, this pattern of responses suggests that the brain may be organized at one level by perceptual recognition (e.g., of a visually presented hand action), but at another level by the type of relevant information (e.g., semantic meaning) required for orchestrating functional response patterns.

Action Language

Thus far, we have discussed the role of the motor system in speech perception and language comprehension. Specifically, we have reviewed work on perception of the lips and mouth and how this might enhance speech perception, and perception of manual gestures – both those that accompany speech (co-speech gestures) and those that communicate meaning independent of speech (emblems) – and how they relate to language understanding. At this juncture, we will address the research on the more general role of the motor system in representing meaning related to action. What role might the motor system play in the processing of words or sentences describing actions, apart from their role during direct observation of such actions? One hypothesis that has been explored is that the motor system of the brain becomes active when processing language about actions, even when no related actions can be explicitly seen. A further hypothesis has been that not only does such activity exist, but it forms the basis of the neural representation of meaning, for language but also more generally. These hypotheses stand in direct contrast to the notion that words and sentences are understood through amodal mental representations (e.g., Fodor, 2001).

Reading, Listening, and the Motor System

Based on convergent findings from a number of neuroimaging studies, there is strong evidence that motor areas of the human brain are active during language comprehension, and good reason to believe that such motor activation does indeed contribute to comprehension (Aziz-Zadeh, Wilson, Rizzolatti, & Iacoboni, 2006; Hauk et al., 2004; Pulvermüller, Hauk, Nikulin, & Ilmoniemi, 2005; Tettamanti et al., 2005). For example, in one fMRI study subjects were asked to read words referring to arm, leg, or face actions (e.g., to pick, kick, lick, respectively) or to actually perform those movements by the fingers, leg, or tongue (Hauk et al., 2004). Since primary motor and premotor cortices both have a degree of somatotopic organization, it was possible to test whether areas in the motor cortex activated while reading action words were also active when actually performing the actions. Indeed, motor cortical activation elicited by an action word overlapped with the cortical representation of the action to which it referred. (Left inferior temporal and left inferior frontal activation were also present on word reading, as expected.) More specifically, activation for finger movements overlapped with activation produced by arm words in left precentral gyrus and in right middle frontal gyrus, and for foot movements and leg words in dorsal premotor areas and left dorsal pre- and post-central gyri. This study remarkably suggests that processing action words, like performing the actions themselves, activates motor and premotor cortices in a somatotopic fashion.

These data have been corroborated by a study using TMS. If the motor system is involved in understanding action-related sentences, then their presentation should modulate the listener's motor cortex activity. To test the hypothesis, motor evoked potentials (MEPs) were recorded from the hand and foot muscles while subjects listened to hand-action-related sentences (e.g., "He turned the key"), foot-action-related sentences (e.g., "He kicked the ball"), and sentences with abstract content (e.g., "He loved his country") serving as the control condition (Buccino et al., 2005). The MEPs of the hand and the foot muscles were recorded during single-pulse TMS of the subjects' hand and foot motor areas, respectively. The results revealed a decrease in the MEP amplitude recorded from the hand muscles during listening to hand-action-related sentences as compared to listening to both foot-related and abstract sentences. Also, a decrease in the MEP amplitude recorded from the foot muscles during listening to foot-action-related sentences was found as compared to listening to both hand-related and abstract sentences. These results support the view that motor areas are involved in understanding action-related sentences.

Using fMRI, Tettamanti et al. (2005) tested the hypothesis that the homologous human regions of the macaque mirror neuron system would be active when listening to descriptions of actions. Previous fMRI research suggested that observation of mouth actions induces activation in IFGOp, extending to the rostral-most sector of the ventral premotor cortex; that observation of hand actions induces activation in the ventral premotor cortex; and that observation of foot actions induces activation in the dorsal premotor cortex (Buccino et al., 2001; Buccino, Binkofski, & Riggio, 2004; Grezes, Armony, Rowe, & Passingham, 2003; Nishitani & Hari, 2002; Rizzolatti et al., 1996). Tettamanti et al. (2005) investigated the possibility that comprehension of actions relies on the observation–execution matching system not only when a person observes an action but also when the actions are verbally described by sentences. Subjects passively listened to sentences describing actions performed with the mouth (e.g., "I bite an apple"), the hand (e.g., "I grasp a knife"), and the leg (e.g., "I kick the ball"), and control sentences with abstract content (e.g., "I appreciate sincerity"). The results indicated that listening to mouth-related sentences, hand-related sentences, and foot-related sentences induces activation of different sectors of the left premotor cortex, depending on the effector used in the heard action-related sentence. Interestingly, IFGOp was the only brain region activated by action language but not abstract language, independent of body part. This suggests that during listening to action-related sentences, the IFGOp of Broca's area plays some more general role in processing action language. However, it should be noted that only partially overlapping activations were found for sentences describing mouth, hand, and leg actions in the left inferior parietal lobe, a region that is engaged in observing actions (e.g., Buccino et al., 2001). The authors concluded that listening to action-related sentences involving different effectors activates a left-lateralized fronto-parieto-temporal system that largely overlaps with the network activated during action execution and action observation.

Some evidence suggests that not only reading action words or listening to action-related sentences activates motor areas, but so does listening to sounds associated with actions. In a TMS study (Aziz-Zadeh, Iacoboni, Zaidel, Wilson, & Mazziotta, 2004), participants listened to sounds associated with bimanual actions (e.g., typing or tearing a paper), actions related to leg movement (e.g., walking), or control sounds (e.g., thunder). The results showed that during stimulation of the left hemisphere M1, sounds associated with bimanual actions produced greater motor corticospinal excitability than sounds of leg movements or control sounds. During stimulation of the right hemisphere M1, however, there was no difference in MEPs between manual and leg action sounds, suggesting a possible left hemisphere dominance in recognizing actions presented in the auditory modality. Thus, the available evidence reviewed so far is favorable to the account that a mirror mechanism plays a role in understanding the meaning of actions during reading word-actions (Hauk et al., 2004), action-related sentences (Tettamanti et al., 2005), and listening to action sounds (Aziz-Zadeh et al., 2004).

Nonetheless, one gap in our knowledge at present is the demonstration of a causal link between motor cortical activations and comprehension, i.e., the degree to which motor cortical activation during action language processing is necessary for comprehension. Certainly, the motor cortex plays a role in representing the meaning of action-related words and sentences. Nevertheless, although we have demonstration that understanding these words and sentences modulates the motor system (e.g., Buccino et al., 2005), we do not yet have demonstration that the motor system modulates the understanding of these words and sentences. Thus, while we can conclude with confidence that the motor cortex plays a role in representing the meaning of action-related language, we cannot yet absolutely characterize this role nor quantify its importance.

Motor imagery and the motor system

The accumulated data thus suggest that the motor regions involved in executing an action are active when a reader or hearer processes language about that action. Some researchers who believe that this motor cortex activity plays an integral role in comprehension propose a simulation account of the mechanism. One possible way of simulating action is to perform motor imagery, and there are several types of such imagery involving different brain networks (Solodkin, Hlustik, Chen, & Small, 2004). According to Gallese and Lakoff (2005), imagining the performance of an action and understanding the meaning of an action verb should be associated with the same neural activation. Willems, Toni, Hagoort, and Casasanto (2010) used fMRI to investigate this hypothesis with respect to action verbs. Neural activity was measured while subjects performed kinetic motor imagery of specific actions and an action-verb understanding task. In the imagery task, subjects had to explicitly imagine themselves performing the action verbs, which were either manual (e.g., "to throw") or nonmanual (e.g., "to kneel"). In the understanding task, subjects had to perform a lexical decision task to the written verbs. For each task, analysis was performed of areas more active for manual actions compared to nonmanual actions. There were no brain areas showing activity for both the imagery comparison and the language comparison. These results indicate that imagery may be a process distinct from understanding action verbs: whereas mental imagery is an effortful and explicit process, language understanding is fast and effortless. Furthermore, these results point to a double dissociation in motor areas between motor imagery and understanding of action verbs.

Summary

Speech, co-speech hand gestures, and emblems are all different ways to communicate and convey meaning: speech syllables are basic units from which words are composed, co-speech hand gestures are meaningful hand movements, contributing to the message the speaker wants to convey, and emblems are used to convey meaning independently of speech. Syllables and manual gestures require mouth and hand movements, respectively, and their use in communication involves an interaction between the "sender" (the speaker) of a message and its "receiver" (the hearer). The present chapter reviewed studies suggesting that the motor system may enhance language understanding when observing mouth and hand movements by representing the intended gesture within the motor system.

Furthermore, the motor system appears to play an important role in the understanding of action words, independently of the presence of observable lip and mouth movements. We have reviewed findings that may indicate a specific functional connection between motor and language networks of the human cerebral cortex. The macaque mirror neuron system has been suggested as a possible neural substrate in humans to account for the common brain regions that are activated not only during the perception of syllables, co-speech hand gestures, and emblems, but also in the motor aspects of performing the same communication acts. It is also possible that a human mirror mechanism plays a role in understanding the meaning of action words during reading and listening to action sounds. In other words, the involvement of motor regions in both perception and production of communicative actions could be based on activity in the mirror neurons of the frontal and parietal lobes, which play a role in both action execution and action observation. Future studies should unravel the more precise relation between action perception and action execution in humans and the mechanisms underlying their interaction in processing language.

References

Anderson, J. M., Gilmore, R., Roper, S., Crosson, B., Bauer, R. M., Nadeau, S., et al. (1999). Conduction aphasia and the arcuate fasciculus: A re-examination of the Wernicke-Geschwind model. *Brain Language, 70*(1), 1–12.

Aziz-Zadeh, L., Iacoboni, M., Zaidel, E., Wilson, S., & Mazziotta, J. (2004). Left hemisphere motor facilitation in response to manual action sounds. *European Journal of Neuroscience, 19*(9), 2609–2612.

Aziz-Zadeh, L., Wilson, S. M., Rizzolatti, G., & Iacoboni, M. (2006). Congruent embodied representations for visually presented actions and linguistic phrases describing actions. *Current Biology, 16*(18), 1818–1823.

Binder, J. R., Frost, J. A., Hammeke, T. A., Cox, R. W., Rao, S. M., & Prieto, T. (1997). Human brain language areas identified by functional magnetic resonance imaging. *Journal of Neuroscience, 17*, 353–362.

Blakemore, S. J., & Decety, J. (2001). From the perception of action to the understanding of intention. *Nature Reviews Neuroscience, 2*, 561–567.

Boatman, D. (2004). Cortical bases of speech perception: Evidence from functional lesion studies. *Cognition, 92*, 47–65.

Bookheimer, S. (2002). Functional MRI of language: New approaches to understanding the cortical organization of semantic processing. *Annual Review of Neuroscience, 25*, 151–188.

Buccino, G., Binkofski, F., Fink, G. R., Fadiga, L., Fogasi, L., Gallese, V., et al. (2001). Action observation activates premotor and parietal areas in a somatotopic manner: An fMRI study. *European Journal of Neuroscience, 13*, 400–404.

Buccino, G., Binkofski, F., Riggio, L. (2004). The mirror neuron system and action recognition. *Brain and Language, 89*(2), 370–376.

Buccino, G., Riggio, L., Melli, G., Binkofski, F., Gallese, V., & Rizzolatti, G. (2005). Listening to action-related sentences modulates the activity of the motor system: A combined TMS and behavioral study. *Brain Research. Cognitive Brain Research, 24*(3), 355–363.

Buccino, G., Vogt, S., Ritzi, A., Fink, G. R., Zilles, K., Freund, H.-J. et al. (2004). Neural circuits underlying imitation learning of hand actions: An event- related fMRI study. *Neuron, 42*, 323–334.

Catani, M., & Mesulam, M. (2008). The arcuate fasciculus and the disconnection theme in language and aphasia: History and current state. *Cortex, 44*(8), 953–961.

Chao, L. L., Haxby, J. V., & Martin, A. (1999). Attribute-based neural substrates in temporal cortex for perceiving and knowing about objects. *Nature Neuroscience, 2,* 913–919.

Damasio, H., & Damasio, A. R. (1980). The anatomical basis of conduction aphasia. *Brain, 103,* 337–350.

Déjerine, J. J. (1891). Sur un cas de cécité verbale avec agraphie suivi d'autopsie. *Mémoires de la Société de Biologie, 3,* 197–201.

Déjerine, J. J. (1892). Contribution a l'étude anatomo-pathologique et clinique des différentes variétés de cécité verbale. *Comptes Rendus Hebdomadaires des Sances et Mémoires de la Société de Biologie, 4,* 61–90.

Dick, A. S., Goldin-Meadow, S., Hasson, U., Skipper, J. I., & Small, S. L. (2009). Co-speech gestures influence neural activity in brain regions associated with processing semantic information. *Human Brain Mapping, 30,* 3509–3526.

Duffau, H., Capelle, L., Sichez, N., Denvil, D., Lopes, M., Sichez, J. P., et al. (2002). Intraoperative mapping of the subcortical language pathways using direct stimulations: An anatomofunctional study. *Brain, 125,* 199–214.

Fabbri-Destro, M., & Rizzolatti, G. (2008). Mirror neurons and mirror systems in monkeys and humans. *Physiology, 23,* 171–179.

Feinberg, T. E., & Farah, M. J. (Eds.). (1997). *Behavioral neurology and neuropsychology.* New York: McGraw-Hill.

Fodor, J. (2001). *The mind doesn't work that way.* Cambridge, MA: MIT Press.

Fogassi, L., Gallese, V., Fadiga, L., & Rizzolatti, G. (1998). Neurons responding to the sight of goal-directed hand/arm actions in the parietal area PF (7b) of the macaque monkey. Paper presented at the Annual Meeting of the Society of Neuroscience, Los Angeles, California.

Friederici, A. D., Opitz, B., & von Cramon, D. Y. (2000). Segregating semantic and syntactic aspects of processing in the human brain: An fMRI investigation of different word types. *Cerebral Cortex, 10,* 698–705.

Galantucci, B., Fowler, C. A., & Turvey, M. T. (2006). The motor theory of speech perception reviewed. *Psychonomic Bulletin and Review, 13*(3), 361–377.

Gallese, V., & Lakoff, G. (2005). The brain's concepts: The role of the sensory-motor system in conceptual knowledge. *Cognitive Neuropsychology, 22,* 455–479.

Geschwind, N. (1966). The organization of language and the brain. *Science, 170,* 940–944.

Geschwind, N. (1971). Current concepts: Aphasia. *New England Journal of Medicine, 284*(12), 654–656.

Gold, B. T., Balota, D. A., Jones, S. J., Powell, D. K., Smith, C. D., & Andersen, A. H. (2006). Dissociation of automatic and strategic lexical-semantics: Functional magnetic resonance imaging evidence for differing roles of multiple frontotemporal regions. *Journal of Neuroscience, 26,* 6523–6532.

Goldin-Meadow, S. (1999). The role of gesture in communication and thinking. *Trends in Cognitive Sciences, 3,* 419–429.

Goldin-Meadow, S. (2006). Talking and thinking with our hands. *Current Directions in Psychological Science, 15,* 34–39.

Green, A., Straube, B., Weis, S., Jansen, A., Willmes, K., Konrad, K., Kircher, T. (2009). Neural integration of iconic and unrelated coverbal gestures: A functional MRI study. *Human Brain Mapping, 30,* 3309–3324.

Grezes, J., Armony, J., Rowe, J., & Passingham, R. (2003). Activations related to "mirror" and "canonical" neurones in the human brain: An fMRI study. *Neuroimage, 18,* 928–937.

Halle, M., Stevens, K. N. (1962). Speech recognition: A model and a program for research. *IRE Transactions on Information Theory, IT-8,* 155–9.

Hauk, O., Johnsrude, I., & Pulvermüller, F. (2004). Somatotopic representation of action words in human motor and premotor cortex. *Neuron, 41,* 301–307.

Hickok, G., & Poeppel, D. (2004). Dorsal and ventral streams: A framework for understanding aspects of the functional anatomy of language. *Cognition, 92,* 67–99.

Hickok, G., & Poeppel, D. (2007). The cortical organization of speech processing. *Nature Reviews Neuroscience, 8,* 393–402.

Holle, H., & Gunter, T. C. (2007). The role of iconic gestures in speech disambiguation: ERP evidence. *Journal of Cognitive Neuroscience, 19,* 175–1192.

Holle, H., Gunter, T. C., Ruschemeyer, S.-A., Hennenlotter, A., & Iacoboni, M. (2008). Neural correlates of the processing of co-speech gestures. *Neuroimage, 39,* 2010–2024.

Holle, H., Obleser, J., Ruschemeyer, S.-A., & Gunter, T. C. (2010). Integration of iconic gestures and speech in left superior temporal areas boosts speech comprehension under adverse listening conditions. *Neuroimage, 49,* 875–884.

Hubbard, A. L., Wilson, S. M., Callan, D. E., & Dapretto, M. (2009). Giving speech a hand: Gesture modulates activity in auditory cortex during speech perception. *Human Brain Mapping, 30,* 1028–1037.

Humphries, C., Binder, J. R., Medler, D. A., & Liebenthal, E. (2006). Syntactic and semantic modulation of neural activity during auditory sentence comprehension. *Journal of Cognitive Neuroscience, 18,* 665–679.

Humphries, C., Love, T., Swinney, D., & Hickok, G. (2005). Response of anterior temporal cortex to syntactic and prosodic manipulations during sentence processing. *Human Brain Mapping, 26,* 128–138.

Iacoboni, M., Woods, R. P., Brass, M., Bekkering, H., Mazziotta, J. C., & Rizzolatti, G. (1999). Cortical mechanisms of human imitation. *Science, 286,* 2526–2528.

Kelly, S. D., Kravitz, C., & Hopkins, M. (2004). Neural correlates of bimodal speech and gesture comprehension. *Brain and Language, 89,* 253–260.

Kelly, S. D., Ward, S., Creigh, P., & Bartolotti, J. (2007). An intentional stance modulates the integration of gesture and speech during comprehension. *Brain and Language, 101,* 222–233.

Kemmerer, D., Gonzalez Castillo, J., Talavage, T., Patterson, S., & Wiley, C. (2008). Neuroanatomical distribution of five semantic components of verbs: Evidence from fMRI. *Brain and Language, 107,* 16–43.

Kendon, A. (1994). Do gestures communicate? A review. *Research on Language and Social Interactions, 27,* 175–200.

Kircher, T., Straube, B., Leube, D., Weis, S., Sachs, O., Willmes, K., et al. (2009). Neural interaction of speech and gesture: Differential activations of metaphoric co-verbal gestures. *Neuropsychologia, 47,* 169–179.

Liberman, A. M., & Whalen, D. H. (2000). On the relation of speech to language. *Trends in cognitive sciences, 4*(5), 187–196.

Lotze, M., Heymans, U., Birbaumer, N., Veit, R., Erb, M., Flor, H., et al. (2006). Differential cerebral activation during observation of expressive gestures and motor acts. *Neuropsychologia, 44,* 1787–1795.

Makris, N., Meyer, J. W., Batesa, J. F., Yeterian, E. H., Kennedy, D. N., & Caviness, V. S. (1999). MRI-based topographic parcellation of human cerebral white matter and nuclei: II. Rationale and applications with systematics of cerebral connectivity. *Neuroimage, 9*(1), 18–45.

Martin, A., & Chao, L. L. (2001). Semantic memory and the brain: Structure and processes. *Current Opinion in Neurobiology, 11*, 194–201.

Massaro, D. W. & Cohen, M. M. (1995). Perceiving talking faces. *Current Directions in Psychological Science, 4* (4), 104–109.

McGurk, H., & MacDonald, J. (1976). Hearing lips and seeing voices. *Nature, 264*, (5588), 746–748.

McNeill, D. (1992). *Hand and mind: What gestures reveal about thought.* Chicago: University of Chicago Press.

McNeill, D. (2005). *Gesture and thought.* Chicago: University of Chicago Press.

Meister, I. G., Wilson, S. M., Deblieck, C., Wu, A. D., & Iacoboni, M. (2007). The essential role of premotor cortex in speech perception. *Current Biology, 17*, 1692–1696.

Nakamura, A., Maess, B., Knosche, T. R., Gunter, T. C., Bach, P., & Friederici, A. D. (2004). Cooperation of different neuronal systems during hand sign recognition. *Neuroimage, 23*, 25–34.

Nishitani, N., & Hari, R. (2002). Viewing lip forms: Cortical dynamics. *Neuron, 36*, 1211–1220.

Noppeney, U., & Price, C. J. (2004). Retrieval of abstract semantics. *Neuroimage, 22*, 164–170.

Ojemann, G., Ojemann, J., Lettich, E., & Berger, M. (1989). Cortical language localization in left, dominant hemisphere: An electrical simulation mapping investigation in 117 patients. *Journal of Neurosurgery, 71*, 316–326.

Ozyurek, A., Willems, R. M., Kita, S., & Hagoort, P. (2007). On-line integration of semantic information from speech and gesture: Insights from event-related brain potentials. *Journal of Cognitive Neuroscience, 19*, 605–616.

Perani, D., Fazio, F., Borghese, N. A., Tettamanti, M., Ferrari, S., Decety, J., et al. (2001). Different brain correlates for watching real and virtual hand actions. *Neuroimage, 14*, 749–758.

Pulvermüller, F., Hauk, O., Nikulin, V. V., & Ilmoniemi, R. J. (2005). Functional links between motor and language systems. *European Journal of Neuroscience, 21*(3), 793–797.

Rizzolatti, G., & Arbib, M. A. (1998). Language within our grasp. *Trends in Neurosciences, 21*, 188–194.

Rizzolatti, G., Camarda, R., Fogassi, L., Gentilucci, M., Luppino, G., & Matelli, M. (1988). Functional organization of inferior area 6 in the macaque monkey: II. Area F5 and the control of distal movements. *Experimental Brain Research, 71*, 491–507.

Rizzolatti, G., & Craighero, L. (2004). The mirror-neuron system. *Annual Review of Neuroscience, 27*, 169–192.

Rizzolatti, G., & Fabbri-Destro, M. (2008). The mirror system and its role in social cognition. *Current Opinion in Neurobiology, 18*, 179–184.

Rizzolatti, G., Fadiga, L., Matelli, M., Bettinardi, V., Paulesu, E., Perani, D., et al. (1996). Localization of grasp representations in humans by PET: Observation versus execution. *Experimental Brain Research, 111*, 246–252.

Rizzolatti, G., & Luppino, G. (2001). The cortical motor system. *Neuron, 31*, 889–901.

Schmahmann, J. D., Pandya, D. N., Wang, R., Dai, G., D'Arceuil, H. E., de Crespigny, A. J., et al. (2007). Association fibre pathways of the brain: Parallel observations from diffusion spectrum imaging and autoradiography. *Brain, 130*(3), 630–653.

Shmuelof, L., & Zohary, E. (2005). Dissociation between ventral and dorsal fMRI activation during object and action recognition. *Neuron, 47*, 457–470.

Shmuelof, L., & Zohary, E. (2006). A mirror representation of others' actions in the human anterior parietal cortex. *Journal of Neuroscience, 26*, 9736–9742.

Skipper, J. I., Goldin-Meadow, S., Nusbaum, H. C., & Small, S. L. (2009). Gestures orchestrate brain networks for language understanding. *Current Biology, 19*, 661–667.

Skipper, J. I., Nusbaum, H. C., & Small, S. L. (2006). Lending a helping hand to hearing: A motor theory of speech perception. In M. A. Arbib (Ed.), *Action to language via the mirror neuron system* (pp. 250–286). Cambridge: Cambridge University Press.

Skipper, J. I., van Wassenhove, V., Nusbaum, H. C., & Small, S. L. (2007). Hearing lips and seeing voices: How cortical areas supporting speech production mediate audiovisual speech perception. *Cerebral Cortex, 17*, 2387–2399.

Solodkin, A., Hlustik, P., Chen, E. E., & Small, S. L. (2004). Fine modulation in network activation during motor execution and motor imagery. *Cerebral Cortex, 14*(11), 1246–1255.

Stowe, L. A., Haverkort, M., & Zwarts, F. (2005). Rethinking the neurological basis of language. *Lingua, 115*, 997–1042.

Tettamanti, M., Buccino, G., Saccuman, M. C., Gallese, V., Danna, M., Scifo, P., et al. (2005). Listening to action-related sentences activates fronto-parietal motor circuits. *Journal of cognitive neuroscience, 17*(2), 273–281.

Villarreal, M., Fridman, E. A., Amengual, A., Falasco, G., Gerscovich, E. R., Ulloa, E. R., et al. (2008). The neural substrate of gesture recognition. *Neuropsychologia, 46*, 2371–2382.

Watkins, K. E., Strafella, A. P., & Paus, T. (2003). Seeing and hearing speech excites the motor system involved in speech production. *Neuropsychologia, 41*, 989–994.

Wernicke, C. (1874). Der aphasischer Symptomenkomplex: Eine psychologische Studie auf anatomischer Basis. Breslau: Cohnand Weigert. Trans. G. H. Eggert (1977) in *Wernicke's works on aphasia: A sourcebook and review*. The Hague: Mouton, pp. 91–145.

Willems, R. M., Ozyurek, A., & Hagoort, P. (2007). When language meets action: The neural integration of gesture and speech. *Cerebral Cortex, 17*, 2322–2333.

Willems, R. E., Toni, I., Hagoort, P., & Casasanto, D. (2010). Neural dissociations between action verb understanding and motor imagery. *Journal of Cognitive neuroscience, 22*(10), 2387–2400.

Wilson, S. M., Molnar-Szakacs, I., & Iacoboni, M. (2008). Beyond superior temporal cortex: Intersubject correlations in narrative speech comprehension. *Cerebral Cortex, 18*, 230–242.

Wilson, S. M., Saygin, A. P., Sereno, M. I., & Iacoboni, M. (2004). Listening to speech activates motor areas involved in speech production. *Nature Neuroscience, 7*(7), 701–702.

Wise, R. J. S., Scott, S. K., Blank, S. C., Mummery, C. J., Murphy, K., & Warburton, E. A. (2001). Separate neural subsystems within "Wernicke's area." *Brain, 124*, 83–95.

Wu, Y. C., & Coulson, S. (2005). Meaningful gestures: Electrophysiological indices of iconic gesture comprehension. *Psychophysiology, 42*, 654–667.

Yeterian, E. H., & Pandya, D. N. (1985). Corticothalamic connections of the posterior parietal cortex in the rhesus monkey. *Journal of Comparative Neurology, 237*, 408–426.

15

What Role Does the Cerebellum Play in Language Processing?

Kristina A. Kellett, Jennifer L. Stevenson, and Morton Ann Gernsbacher

Beginning with Rolando and Flourens' early nineteenth-century documentation of the role of cerebellar lesions in disturbances of gait, posture, and voluntary coordination of movement, the cerebellum has been considered a primary player in motor behavior (Schmahmann, 1997). In 1922, Holmes was the first to document that focal cerebellar lesions produce speech motor deficits, suggesting a role for the cerebellum in speech production (Holmes, 1922). However, only recently has interest arisen in exploring the nonmotor roles the cerebellum might play in cognition, including language processing (Schmahmann, 1997).

Neuroanatomically, it is plausible that the cerebellum plays a role in language processing, given the reciprocal loops that link the cerebellum directly to or near the vicinity of language association regions in prefrontal cortex and temporal cortex. Output from the ventral dentate nucleus of the cerebellum projects to the ventrolateral nucleus of the thalamus and continues upward toward prefrontal regions (Leiner, Leiner, & Dow, 1986, 1991). Conversely, input to the cerebellum originates from the prefrontal cortex, as well as the upper bank of the temporal lobe's superior temporal sulcus, and traverses down through the pons and on to the lateral cerebellar hemispheres (Schmahmann, 1991; Schmahmann & Pandya, 1997). These cerebro-cerebellar loops may allow the cerebellum to act as an "adjunct of the cerebral cortex" (Leiner et al., 1986, p. 1006).

In the late 1980s, Petersen, Fox, Posner, Mintun, and Raichle (1989) conducted a pioneering study using positron emission tomography (PET). Not only was their collection of PET data a technological advance, but also their use of a high-level baseline condition, to control for the cerebellum's participation in speech motor execution, was an important innovation. Healthy adult participants mentally generated and spoke aloud verbs that were semantically related to visually presented nouns. The high-level baseline condition required participants to repeat target nouns aloud, therefore controlling for the factors involved in merely producing speech. Because the "repeating nouns aloud" baseline condition was subtracted from the "generating verbs aloud" condition, the remaining right cerebellar hemisphere activation provided a significant estimate of the nonmotor contributions of the cerebellum to language processing.

This chapter builds from Petersen et al.'s (1989) seminal experiment by reviewing the subsequent two decades of brain imaging studies of healthy adults performing phonological, lexical, semantic, syntactic, and discourse-level processes. To examine the cerebellum's role in language processing, our review follows the lead of Petersen et al. (1989) and includes only experiments that employed a high-level baseline that controls for motor processes. Our review also reports cerebellar lobular regions across studies to identify similar areas of activations for language tasks.

This chapter also confronts the problem of task difficulty. A common problem in experiments examining cerebellar activation is that most of the tasks used in the experimental conditions (e.g., mentally generating verbs) are more difficult than tasks used in the control conditions – even those control conditions considered high-level baseline (e.g., repeating nouns). More difficult tasks, in and of themselves, lead to greater levels of cerebellar activation (Ivry, 1997). This confound is not unique to language studies; it also complicates the interpretation of motor sequence learning (Jenkins, Brooks, Nixon, Fracowiak, & Passingham, 1994) and problem solving (Kim, Ugurbil, & Strick, 1994). For each of the studies reviewed, we discuss the implications of confounding by task difficulty.

In the final section of the chapter, we discuss theories of cerebellar function in relation to language processing, including the "timing hypothesis" (Keele & Ivry, 1991) and the notion of adaptive learning via error detection (Wolpert, Mialll, & Kawato, 1998). We conclude by suggesting that the cerebellum aids in more effortful linguistic processing, and we adopt the perspective that the cerebellum is a modulator rather than a generator of cognitive activity (Schmahmann, 1996).

Studies Reviewed

The studies reviewed in this chapter were identified in PubMed using various combinations of the following search terms: "fMRI," "PET," "cerebell*," "lexical," "semantic," "phonolo*," "syntax," "discourse," and "language." All studies chosen (1) reported cerebellar activity during a phonological, lexical semantic, syntactic, or higher-level discourse task; (2) scanned the whole brain; (3) did not use a priori regions of interest; (4) examined healthy adults; (5) presented linguistic stimuli (or stimuli approximating linguistic stimuli, e.g., false fonts) for both the experimental and baseline condition; (6) used similar input modality (auditory or visual) for both the experimental and baseline condition; and (7) equated across experimental and baseline conditions for response modality (e.g., pressing a button, speaking covertly, or speaking aloud). The search was not exhaustive but rather representative. A total of 38 experiments reported in 25 studies were reviewed.

To consolidate cerebellar anatomical localization across studies, coordinates reported in Talairach space were converted to Montreal Neurological Institute (MNI) space using the Lancaster transform (icbm2tal; Lancaster et al., 2007; Talairach & Tourneux, 1988). Talairach coordinates generated from a Brett transform were converted back to MNI space using a reverse Brett transform (Brett, Christoff, Cusack, & Lancaster, 2001). The Diedrichsen probabilistic atlas (created from 20 participants aligned to MNI space and labeled based on the Schmahmann cerebellar atlas) was used to anatomically localize cerebellar regions in FSLview (Diedrichsen, Balster, Flavell, Cussans, & Ramnani, 2009; Schmahmann, Doyon, Toga, Petrides, & Evans, 2000). Region labels (e.g., lobule VI, Crus I) were assigned based on the highest probability provided by the atlas. Studies that failed to report coordinates but did report lobules, were included in the review; however, studies reporting coordinates that localized out of bounds according to the Diedrichsen atlas were not included.

Areas of Inquiry

The following sections review phonological, lexical semantic, semantic, syntactic and discourse-level tasks respectively. The task comparison contrasts and corresponding neuroanatomical findings discussed in the sections below can be found in Table 15.1.

Phonology

Phonological processing requires decoding a spoken word or pseudoword (i.e., a nonword with a plausible sequence of sounds) into its respective phonemes (sounds). Phonological processes are also linked to orthographic processing (i.e., the processing of visual word parts, such as graphemes). A nonlexical route of orthographic processing is believed to support decoding a written word into its constituent graphemes and mapping those graphemes onto their phonological representations, which are assembled into the word's whole phonological representation. A lexical route is believed to involve mapping the entire word's phonology from its orthography, without assembling individual phonemes from graphemes (Coltheart, Rastle, Perry, Langdon, & Ziegler, 2001; Xu et al. 2001; Coltheart & Kohnen, Volume 2, Chapter 43).

Studies examining phonological processing have employed phonological fluency tasks (Gauthier, Duyme, Zanca, & Capron, 2009; Gourovitch et al., 2000; Schlosser et al., 1998), rhyming decision tasks (Xu et al., 2001), a vowel exchange task (Seki, Okada, Koeda, & Sadato, 2004), and the covert and overt articulation of

Table 15.1 Task comparison contrasts.

Reference	Category	Participants	Method	Contrast description	LH	Vermis	RH
Carreiras et al., 2007	Phonology	n = 36	fMRI	overt articulation of words/ pseudowords > overt and repeated articulation of "falso" to false fonts	VI	vermal VI/crus I/crus II, vermal VI	VI
Gauthier et al., 2009	Phonology	n = 11	fMRI	covert phonological fluency > counting; high fluency females	I-IV		crus II, I-IV
				covert phonological fluency > counting; low fluency females		vermal VIIIA, VI	
				covert phonological fluency > counting; high fluency males	crus I		crus II
				covert phonological fluency > counting; low fluency males	crus I		crus II, I-IV
Gourovitch et al., 2000	Phonology	n = 18	PET	overt letter fluency > overt production of over-learned sequence	crus I, VI		crus I
Herbster et al., 1997	Phonology	n = 10	PET	overt articulation of pseudowords > overt and repeated articulation of "hiya" to consonant strings	VI		crus I, VI
				overt articulation of regular and irregular words > overt and repeated articulation of "hiya" to consonant strings	VI		crus I

(continued)

Table 15.1 (continued)

Reference	Category	Participants	Method	Contrast description	LH	Vermis	RH
Joubert et al., 2004	Phonology	n = 10	fMRI	covert pronunciation of pseudowords > consonant strings			crus II, vermal VI/ lobule VI, I-IV
Moore & Price, 1999	Phonology	n = 8	PET	covert pronunciation of words > covert production of "ok" to false fonts	VI		
Schlösser et al., 1998	Phonology	n = 6	fMRI	covert phonological fluency > counting; females	VI		
				covert phonological fluency > counting; males			crus I
Seki et al., 2004	Phonology	n = 19	fMRI	vowel exchange > repetition; words	VI		
				vowel exchange > repetition; pseudowords	VIIIA		
Xu et al., 2001	Phonology	n = 12	PET	pseudowords rhyming > color matching with letters			VI
				word rhyming > color matching with letters			crus II
				alternate case rhyming > color matching with letters			crus II
Desmond et al., 1998	Lexical	n = 6	fMRI	word stem completion; words with many completions > few completions	IV/V		

						vermis VI, VII, VIII	VI, VIIA
				word stem completion; words with few completions > many completions			
Perani et al., 1999	Lexical	n = 14	PET	lexical decision > feature search			IX
Chee et al., 1999	Semantic	n = 8	fMRI	semantic > case categorization; visual domain			VIIB
Gourovitch et al., 2000	Semantic	n = 18	PET	semantic > case categorization; auditory domain	crus I/lobule VI, VI		crus II
Gurd et al., 2002	Semantic	n = 11	fMRI	overt semantic fluency > overt production of over-learned sequence			crus I
				covert semantic fluency > covert production of over-learned sequence			crus II
McDermott et al., 2003	Semantic	n = 20	fMRI	study semantically > phonologically related words	crus II		crus II
Miceli et al., 2002	Semantic	n = 9	fMRI	semantic > phonological categorization	V		I-IV
Petersen et al., 1989	Semantic	n = 7	PET	overt verb generation > overt word repetition; visual domain	crus I/VI, I-VI		VI
				overt verb generation > overt word repetition; auditory domain	I-V		VI
Roskies et al., 2001	Semantic	n = 20	PET	synonym > rhyming decision			crus I/VI, crus II

(continued)

Table 15.1 (*continued*)

Reference	Category	Participants	Method	Contrast description	LH	Vermis	RH
Seger et al., 2000	Semantic	n = 7	fMRI	covert verb generation; novel > repeated nouns	crus I		crus II, IV-VI
				covert verb generation; repeated > novel nouns	crus I, crus II		crus I, crus II, VIIB
				covert verb generation; unusual > first verb–noun pair	crus I, crus II		crus I, crus II
Tieleman et al., 2005	Semantic	n = 22	fMRI	semantic > case categorization	crus I, crus II		crus I, crus II
Tyler et al., 2004	Semantic	n = 12	fMRI	semantic decision > letter string matching			vermal VI/ lobule VI, crus II
Dogil et al., 2002	Syntax	n = 10	fMRI	overt manipulation of sentence word order > overt manipulation of list order	Not specified	Not specified	Not specified
Friederici et al., 2006	Syntax	n = 13	fMRI	covert reading of ungrammatical sentences > covert reading of grammatical sentences	crus I/lobule VI		
Stowe et al., 2004	Syntax	n = 16	PET	read syntactically ambiguous sentences > read syntactically unambiguous sentences			crus I
Giraud et al., 2000	Discourse	n = 6	PET	listened to story > listened to unrelated sentences	crus I		

pronounceable nonwords and words (Carreiras, Mechelli, Estevez, & Price, 2007; Herbster, Mintun, Nebes, & Becker, 1997; Joubert et al., 2004; Moore & Price, 1999).

Phonological fluency tasks require a participant to generate words beginning with a visually or aurally presented letter (e.g., given the letter *F*, the participant might generate *flower, forest, fortune,* etc.). Participants typically have a set amount of time to generate as many words per letter cue as they can without repeating a response. Therefore, participants must hear or read the target letter and hold that letter in memory while searching for suitable word completions, also while inhibiting previously given responses (Gourovitch et al., 2000).

Two studies, which aurally cued participants to covertly generate words and employed a high-level baseline of covert counting, reported unilateral right cerebellar activation (lobule VI, crus I, crus II; Schlosser et al., 1998) and more widespread bilateral cerebellar activation (left crus I, right crus I; Gauthier et al., 2009). A study that visually cued participants to generate words aloud relative to a high-level baseline of overtly reciting an over-learned sequence (e.g., months of the year) also produced bilateral cerebellar activation (bilateral crus I, left lobule VI; Gourovitch et al., 2000). Although accuracy was not reported in these studies, covert counting or reciting a well-practiced sequence is no doubt easier to perform than generating words in response to a cued letter. Therefore, the cerebellar activation reported in these studies could reflect any number of processes (e.g., more effortful search and retrieval of words as well as inhibition of previously provided responses.)

Rhyming decisions, which require participants to decide whether one word (e.g., *couch*) rhymes with another (e.g., *touch*), are believed to require decoding at a sublexical level of syllables and phonemes. In one study, participants made rhyming decisions on visually presented words, legal pseudowords (e.g., *louch*), and words presented in alternating upper and lower case (e.g., *cOucH*); for the baseline condition, participants made color-matching decisions on unpronounceable letter strings (Xu et al., 2001). Rhyming decisions on words (both the regular orthography and the alternate case conditions) produced right crus II activation, whereas rhyming decisions on pseudowords produced lobule VI activation, which also showed the strongest activation. However, because the baseline task, color matching, was significantly easier than the experimental task (as reflected in participants' faster latency and higher accuracy), the cerebellar activation might have been a function of task difficulty, and because rhyme matching requires the use of internal speech, whereas color matching does not, the cerebellar activation could reflect greater subarticulatory demands.

Vowel exchange tasks require participants to listen to or read a word, decode its phonological structure, and replace one of the vowels in the word with a vowel specified by the experimenter (e.g., replace the second vowel in *apartment* with the vowel /o/). One study reported that replacing a word or nonword's middle vowel with another vowel, compared with a baseline condition that required only repeating the word or nonword, elicited activation in the cerebellar vermis (VIIIa, VI; Seki et al., 2004). Vermal activation is unusual given the prevalence of cerebellar hemispheric activation found with other language tasks. The authors suggested that a higher level of sustained attention demanded by the vowel exchange task, compared with the word/nonword repetition task, was responsible for the vermal activation, given that sustained attention is believed to activate the cerebellar vermis (Lawrence, Ross, Hoffman, Garavan, & Stein, 2003; Seki et al., 2004; however, a review by Haarmeier & Thier, 2007, suggests a different interpretation of cerebellar activation in attention tasks, namely that working memory, oculomotor, or manual motor demands account for cerebellar activation rather than attention per se).

Finally, in one study (Herbster et al., 1997), participants pronounced aloud pseudowords and, as a control, viewed consonant letter strings while repeatedly articulating "hiya." The task comparison illustrated bilateral VI activity and right crus I activity; pronouncing aloud pseudowords arguably requires greater articulatory control relative to repeatedly articulating "hiya" while viewing letters strings. In another study (Joubert et al., 2004), participants silently pronounced pseudowords relative to silently pronouncing bolded letters within consonant letter strings (e.g., "bp" for "xt**bp**n"). The task comparison produced right crus II, paravermal VI, and anterior I-IV activation (Joubert et al., 2004). This study controlled for pre-articulatory demands by equating the number of phonemes to be pronounced in the experimental versus control task, suggesting that the observed cerebellar activation reflects mechanisms involved in the graphemic conversion of letters to phonological (or syllabic) representations.

Bilateral lobule VI was also activated alongside vermal VI when whispering words and nonwords was contrasted with whispering "falso" while viewing false fonts (Carreiras et al., 2007), and left lobule VI was activated when silently mouthing words was contrasted with mouthing "ok" while viewing false fonts (Moore & Price, 1999). Left lobule VI and right crus I of the cerebellum were activated when both regular words (i.e., consistent orthographic to phonological mapping) and irregular words (i.e., inconsistent orthographic to phonological mapping, "debt") were articulated, relative to "hiya" being repeated articulated to consonant letter strings (Herbster et al., 1997). Lobule VI has been implicated in articulatory planning processes (Ackermann, 2008), and the baseline comparison tasks of repeatedly saying "hiya," "falso," or "ok" most likely requires less articulatory planning than pronouncing aloud, whispering, or mouthing silently a varied set of real words or pseudowords.

In summary, whether requiring participants to generate words or make a decision based on phonological information, or whether requiring participants to read or speak aloud pseudowords, sublexical tasks seem to most commonly activate lobule VI, crus I and crus II of the cerebellum.

Lexical semantics

Word-level processing of a basic lexical semantic nature, such as passively viewing words relative to viewing consonant letter strings, can be considered to activate lexical knowledge, concomitantly drawing upon orthographic, phonological, and lexical semantic knowledge. Tasks that tap this type of lexical knowledge include lexical decision (Perani et al., 1999) and word stem completion (Desmond, Gabrieli, & Glover, 1998).

In a lexical decision task, participants decide whether a string of letters form a word, a task which is believed to engage lexical retrieval. In Perani et al. (1999), both the experimental task ("Is the stimulus a word?") and the baseline task ("Is an 'X' present in the letter string?") required making a yes/no decision with a button press. These two tasks appear to be well equated given that participants' responses latencies were equivalent in the two tasks. The contrast showed lobule IX activation; however, because few other language tasks have reported lobule IX activation, this finding merits further investigation for better understanding.

In a word stem completion task, participants either covertly or overtly identify the word for which only a stem, e.g., STE_, is provided. One study, in which participants pressed a button after covertly completing each word stem, manipulated whether there were many or few possible options for each stem (Desmond et al., 1998). Relative to the few-possible-completions condition, the many-possible-completions condition elicited left anterior quadrangular lobe (lobules IV/V) activation; in comparison, the few-possible-completions condition contrasted with many-possible-completions elicited widespread right cerebellar hemispheric activation (lobules VI and crus I/crus II) and vermal activation (vermal VI, VII, VIII). However, there is evidence from the behavioral results that the few-possible-completions condition was demonstrably more difficult than the many-possible-completions condition; the few-possible-completions condition led to lower completion rates and slower completion performance for those stems that participants could complete. The authors concluded that the right cerebellum plays a role in lexical search, given that the few-possible-completions condition relative to the many-possible-completions condition requires a more extensive lexical search to find viable word stem completions (Desmond et al., 1998). Taken together, the data from this word stem completion study and the lexical decision study reviewed above suggest that lexical semantic processing appears to most typically activate cerebellar lobules VI and crus I.

Semantics

Higher-level semantic processing calls upon semantic knowledge (i.e., meaning-based knowledge such as category exemplars or the semantic associations between words). Semantic tasks reviewed include semantic fluency (Gourovitch et al., 2000; Gurd et al., 2002), verb generation (Seger, Desmond, Glove, & Gabrieli, 2000), semantic categorization (Chee, O'Craven, Bergida, Rosen, & Savoy, 1999; Tieleman et al., 2005; Miceli et al., 2002), semantic decision (Roskies, Fiez, Balota, Raichle, & Petersen, 2001; Tyler, Bright, Fletcher, & Stamatakis, 2004), as well as a task of semantic-relatedness (McDermott, Petersen, Watson, & Ojemann, 2003).

Semantic fluency tasks involve accessing semantic knowledge of a given category to produce an exemplar from that category. Similar to phonological fluency tasks, semantic fluency tasks typically require participants to generate as many category exemplars as possible within a set amount of time without repeating a response. Participants listen to or read the name of a target category, hold that category name in memory while searching for suitable exemplars, and inhibit any previously given responses (for further details on semantic and phonological fluency tasks, see Pekkala, Volume 2, Chapter 30). In two studies, participants generated exemplars from cued categories (e.g., fruits, sports, cars), relative to generating an over-learned sequence (e.g., months of the year); participants were either visually cued and responded overtly (Gourovitch et al., 2000) or were aurally cued and responded covertly (Gurd et al., 2002). The task contrast elicited cerebellar activity respectively in right crus I (Gourovitch et al., 2000) or right crus II (Gurd et al., 2002).

However, in a practice session prior to the brain imaging component of the study (Gurd et al., 2002), participants made significantly more errors generating category exemplars than generating over-learned sequences, suggesting that the experimental task of category fluency was more difficult than the control task of generating over-learned sequences such as the months of the year. Thus, like phonological fluency tasks, cerebellar activation in semantic fluency tasks could reflect any number of cognitive processes involved in generating category exemplars relative to reciting a well-practiced sequence (e.g., more effortful search and retrieval, as well as inhibition of past responses). Error signals could be generated in relation to inhibiting previous responses; internal speech could be involved in searching for and retrieving viable answers.

Verb generation tasks entail producing a semantically associated verb to a presented noun. Participants are required to read or listen to a verb, hold that verb in memory while searching for and selecting a semantically related noun, and produce a response. In one study, widespread bilateral cerebellar activity was seen for covertly generating verbs to novel nouns compared with previously viewed nouns (left crus I and right crus II, VI, and V); the reverse contrast, covertly generating verbs for previously viewed nouns compared to novel nouns, elicited left crus I and crus II activity (Seger et al., 2000). However, because participants produced faster response times in the previously-viewed-nouns condition compared to the novel-nouns condition, an explanation based on task difficulty cannot be ruled out. In a direct manipulation of task difficulty, participants covertly generated verbs that formed an unusual relationship with the target noun (e.g., generating "throw" in response to "dish"). Relative to covertly generating the first verb that came to mind after viewing a noun, covertly generating unusual verbs led to bilateral cerebellar activity in crus I and crus II; participants also generated verbs more slowly in the "unusual verb" condition compared to the "first verb" condition (Seger et al., 2000).

Thus, greater cerebellar activation in these verb generation tasks could reflect error detection in the novel condition relative to the previously viewed condition as well as in the "unusual verb" condition relative to the "first verb" condition. In the previously viewed condition, participants already have experience generating verbs to the cue nouns; generating verbs to novel nouns would produce more error signals for retrieving a correct response and inhibiting incorrect responses. Likewise, generating unusual verb–noun relationships would entail rejecting more obvious, incorrect verb–noun relationships relative to generating the first verb that came to mind.

A task of semantic relatedness entails semantic retrieval operations to call upon semantic associations between words. In McDermott et al. (2003), participants viewed one word at a time and studied the semantic relatedness between the stimuli while covertly articulating words; the comparison task required participants to study the phonological relatedness between presented stimuli, also while covertly articulating words. The task contrast elicited bilateral crus II activation. Cerebellar activation could reflect semantic analysis, or control processes (e.g., strategic retrieval) beyond semantic analysis (Gold, Balota, Kirchoff, & Buckner, 2005). Because words can often be interpreted different ways depending on context (i.e., words can have multiple semantic representations), there are relatively more associations that can be made between words and semantic representations; in contrast, the number of associations between words and phonological structures tends to be limited by orthographic neighborhood because of somewhat regular spelling-to-sound relationships (Plaut, McClelland, Siedenberg, & Patterson, 1996). The greater number of associations between words and semantic representations relative to words and phonological structures would put greater demands on retrieval for the semantic-relatedness condition relative to the phonological-related condition (Gold et al., 2005). Greater retrieval demands (i.e., retrieving more information) may mean greater use of internal speech or articulatory planning processes; likewise, a higher number of associations in the semantic-relatedness condition relative to the phonological-relatedness condition could relate to greater selection demands and error signal generation (i.e., selecting correct associations and rejecting incorrect associations).

Semantic categorization tasks involve placing a stimulus word in one of two superordinate categories, requiring participants to retrieve the word's semantic properties and the categories' semantic properties, and to match the word to the correctly associated semantic category. In two studies, participants pressed a button to categorize visually presented nouns as either abstract or concrete (Chee et al., 1999), or as animal or object (Tieleman et al., 2005); the visual orthographic comparison task entailed pressing a button to categorize nouns as upper or lower case. The comparison contrast led to right lobule VIIB activity (Chee et al. 1999), or right crus I and crus II activity (Tieleman et al., 2005). Participants also pressed a button to categorize aurally presented nouns as abstract or concrete; when contrasted with an auditory syllable categorization task of categorizing nouns as having one or more syllables, left lobule VI, crus I as well as right crus II showed activation (Chee et al., 1999). A significant difference in response time between comparison conditions also existed, leading to a difference in performance difficulty (Chee et al., 1999; Tieleman et al., 2005); the semantic categorization task would entail greater processing effort associated with strategic retrieval, as opposed to identifying syllable count or case. In a separate study, participants semantically categorized visually presented nouns as animal or artifact relative to phonologically categorizing nouns as having a "k" or "tch" sound (Miceli et al., 2002). No significant difference in response time was seen between comparison tasks, and the corresponding cerebellar activity (left lobule V and right lobule I-IV) differed from the previously mentioned task comparisons eliciting lobule VI, crus I and crus II activity; other semantic and phonological comparison contrasts controlled for performance difficulty should be conducted to see if this differing task-related activation can be further substantiated.

For semantic decision tasks, participants answer yes or no regarding whether two words are semantically related. In Roskies et al. (2001), participants were visually presented with two words and indicated via button press if the two words were synonyms, relative to a phonological rhyming decision task in which participants indicated if two words rhymed; the contrast produced right crus II and medial right lobule VI/crus I activity. Participants were very slightly, but still significantly, slower and less accurate in the semantic decision task compared with the rhyming decision task. Additionally, participants performed the synonym task separately for hard-to-categorize synonyms and for easy-to-categorize synonyms. Right crus II was significantly more active for the hard categorization condition compared to the easy categorization condition; participants also performed more slowly and less accurately in the hard categorization condition relative to the easy condition.

In a different semantic decision paradigm, participants read two cue words, either nouns or verbs, followed by a probe word, after which participants pressed a button if the probe word was semantically related to one of the two cue words; for the baseline condition, participants indicated via button press if a probe letter string matched one of the first two presented letter strings (Tyler et al., 2004). Similar to Roskies et al. (2001), right crus II and crus I were activated in the semantic decision task relative to a letter-string-matching decision task (Tyler et al., 2004). Like other semantic tasks, cerebellar activation may reflect effortful involvement in control processes (e.g., retrieval).

In summary, semantic paradigms tend to activate crus I and crus II most often for tasks of semantic fluency, verb generation, semantic decision, semantic categorization, or a task of general semantic relatedness.

Syntax

Syntactic processing concerns the grammatical ordering of words and phrases at the sentence level. Because the cerebellum's involvement in syntax has not been a thoroughly researched topic, this review only provides three examples from the literature: tasks involving manipulating word order (Dogil et al., 2002), reading ungrammatical sentences (Friederici, Fiebach, Schlesewsky, Bornkessel, & Yves von

Cramon, 2006), and reading syntactically ambiguous sentences (Stowe, Paans, Wijers, & Zwarts, 2004).

In one study employing a word order manipulation task, participants actively arranged syntactic constituents to make a different, but equally grammatical sentence (Dogil et al., 2002). The German language allows syntactic constituents around a finite verb to be switched (e.g., "A customer has complained about the manager" can be rearranged to "About the manager has complained a customer"). In Dogil et al. (2002), participants covertly read a sentence, internally switched syntactic constituents, and overtly produced their response. The baseline task involved a "list reordering" task, in which participants covertly read a list of unrelated words, internally replaced the second item with the first, and overtly produced their response. The word order manipulation task relative to the list reordering task elicited bilateral cerebellar activation (although no coordinates or cerebellar regions were reported). Because stimuli in both tasks were controlled for their number of syllables (i.e., articulatory demand was equivalent), the cerebellar activation most likely does not reflect speech motor control processes (Dogil et al., 2002).

In another study (Friederici et al., 2006), participants covertly read ungrammatical sentences with an incorrect word order, and for a baseline condition participants covertly read grammatical sentences with a typical word order. Ungrammatical sentences relative to grammatical sentences produced activity in left crus I/lobule VI. There can be little doubt that reading ungrammatical sentences is not only more difficult but more fodder for any error detection mechanism; therefore, the greater reported cerebellar activation for reading ungrammatical sentences relative to grammatical sentences could reflect error detection.

When reading a syntactically ambiguous sentence, the ambiguity may not be resolved until later in the sentence, but the reader adopts a "best guess" interpretation based on highest syntactic frequency or simplicity until proven incorrect (e.g., Spivey & Tanenhaus, 1998). For example, "The red drops" can be followed by "fell onto the floor," or "onto the floor." Until the first word of the second phrase is read ("fell" or "onto"), the reader does not know whether "red" is an adjective or noun. However, because "red" is more frequently used as an adjective, the reader might assume that to be the case until suggested otherwise (Stowe et al., 2004). Participants in Stowe et al. (2004) read syntactically ambiguous sentences that by the end of each sentence resolved to the less frequent possibility; for a baseline condition, participants read syntactically unambiguous sentences. Reading ambiguous sentences led to greater right crus I activity, which could reflect an error detection process (i.e., when syntactically ambiguous sentences resolved to the less likely possibility, an error signal would be generated; Stowe et al., 2004).

Although additional research is needed to verify whether similar cerebellar regions are activated across syntactic tasks, the crus I/lobule VI activation of Friederici et al. (2006) and crus I activation of Stowe et al. (2004) is reminiscent of crus I and lobule VI activations found in aforementioned phonological, lexical-semantic, and semantic tasks.

Discourse

Discourse processing involves making connections between sentences to gain comprehension beyond the sentence level. Given the dearth of literature on cerebellar involvement in discourse processing, only one experiment will be discussed (Giraud et al., 2000).

Comparing related sentences with unrelated sentences assesses general discourse processing; participants listen or read related sentences and must recognize reoccurring concepts to build a coherent mental representation (Gernsbacher, Varner, & Faust, 1990; Robertson et al., 2000). In Giraud et al. (2000), participants passively listened to stories and unrelated sentences; listening to stories relative to unrelated sentences activated left crus I. Perhaps cerebellar activation corresponds to the greater effort needed to construct relationships between related sentences as opposed to unrelated. Considering crus I activation elicited in previously mentioned tasks, the difference in task effort between conditions could reflect similar task demands as found in lower-level phonological, lexical semantic, semantic, and syntactic tasks.

Functional Topography

Across phonological, lexical semantic, semantic, syntactic, and discourse tasks, cerebellar lobules VI, crus I and crus II appear to be predominantly activated for language processing; no one lobular region appears to be specialized for a given level of language processing, perhaps reflecting a common operation for the cerebellum across language tasks. As illustrated in Table 15.1, many of these findings seem to be right lateralized, likely reflecting the crossed relationship between the right cerebellum and left cerebral cortex language regions. A previous meta-analysis of experiments reporting task-related cerebellar activation in various language paradigms showed similar cerebellar lobular convergence: Stoodley and Schmahmann (2009) performed an activation likelihood estimation meta-analysis of 11 imaging studies employing language tasks, and reported significant concordance of foci within the cerebellar right lobule VI, crus I and crus II, as well as medial lobule VIIA and left lobule VI.

Additionally, lexical semantic tasks have been more "passive" in general (i.e., only requiring the reading of words) and generally activated lobule VI and crus I, whereas phonological, semantic, and syntactic tasks, which have, for the most part, required participants to perform an "active" manipulation of linguistic information (e.g., a rhyming decision), appeared to more often elicit crus II activation alongside crus I and lobule VI activation. The seemingly more widespread extent of "active" tasks could reflect increased task difficulty for "active" relative to "passive" types of tasks.

Task Difficulty: Coda and Theory

It is reasonable to think cerebellar activity in a language tasks could generally reflect task difficulty. A recent meta-analysis of 120 studies of lexical semantic task comparisons and semantic task comparisons was performed (Binder, Desai, Graves, & Conant, 2009). Not only did the stringent inclusion criteria require a selected study to employ a high-level baseline (to cancel out motor-related activity between task and baseline conditions), this meta-analysis also required task and baseline conditions to be equated on difficulty (i.e., either report a nonsignificant difference between task and baseline conditions for reaction time and accuracy, or pass the authors' assessment of difficulty equivalence). Interestingly, of the 1145 gathered foci across 120 studies, only 15 foci were of cerebellar activation. This may possibly reflect studies only imaging the supratentorial brain, or the role of the cerebellum in language processing could indeed be to aid more effortful language processing.

If the cerebellum shows activation when one task is more difficult than its comparison task, and if areas of activation appear to be more or less similar in lobular localization across different levels of language processing, then perhaps the cerebellum could assist effortful language processing through a more general mechanism. Theories of cerebellar function could be applied to language processing, including the "timing hypothesis" – particularly in relation to the temporal sequencing of syllables at the pre-articulatory level – as well as the cerebellum as an "internal model" that learns through error detection.

The "timing hypothesis" suggests the cerebellum is involved in tasks requiring the precise representation of temporal information (Ivry & Spencer, 2004). The neural architecture of the cerebellum supports representation of temporal information; for example, a signal propagated along one parallel fiber reaches successive Purkinje cells at incremental delays, allowing for the timing of discrete events (Braitenberg, 1967). Neuropsychological literature implicates the cerebellum in timing; cerebellar patients are impaired relative to controls in discriminating and producing timed intervals (Ivry & Keele, 1989). A review of neuroimaging studies on time measurement reported right lateral cerebellum activity for short-range or "automatic" timing tasks and left lateral cerebellum activity for long-range or "cognitive" timing tasks that, unlike automatic timing tasks, engage cognitive control mechanisms including working memory (Lewis & Miall, 2003). Timing is considered a general computational process of the cerebellum to which different cerebellar regions may contribute (Ivry & Spencer, 2004).

The timing hypothesis in relation to language processing proposes that the cerebellum is not directly involved in language processing but rather modulates language processing by timing linguistic functions represented at the level of the cerebral cortex (Keele & Ivry, 1991; Silveri, Leggio, & Molinari, 1994). Temporal modulation can conceivably be required for different linguistic processes, including sentence construction and comprehension (i.e., integrating phonological, semantic, and syntactic elements). A case study of a right cerebellar patient with agrammatic speech (the deficit morphological in nature) also showed reduced blood flow of the left cerebral hemisphere according to single-photon emission computerized tomography scans (Silveri et al., 1994). The phenomenon of crossed cerebro-cerebellar diaschisis presents when a lesion in a cerebellar hemisphere reduces input to anatomically connected regions in the contralateral cerebral hemisphere, as displayed by hypoperfusion or reduced blood flow in cerebral regions (Marien, Engelborghs, Fabbro, & De Deyn, 2001). At a 4-month follow-up, the patient's improvement of agrammatic symptoms paralleled increased left cerebral perfusion. Silveri et al. (1994) interpreted the patient's transient left cerebral hypoperfusion and agrammatic symptoms as evidence for the cerebellum modulating morphosyntactic processes, and suggested that the cerebellum provides correct timing for morphosyntactic operations in building sentences.

Cerebellar activation in language tasks may specifically reflect articulatory planning processes such as the temporal sequencing or parsing of an "inner speech code" (Ackermann, Mathiak, & Riecker, 2007). In a study where participants overtly repeated syllables at different rates relative to a passive listening condition, a functional connectivity analysis of task-related brain activity pointed to right superior cerebellar activation (lobule VI) within an articulatory planning network, and right inferior cerebellar activation within an articulatory execution network (Riecker et al., 2005). In a separate study, covertly repeating syllables relative to a resting baseline elicited bilateral superior cerebellar activation (lobules VI) for higher repetition frequencies (Wildgruber, Ackermann, & Grodd, 2001). From these results, internal speech can be considered a "pre-articulatory verbal code" related to articulatory planning processes, and is associated with lobule VI activation. Specifically, the cerebellum may modulate, based on linguistic constraints, the temporal structure of speech "motor programs" retrieved from a mental syllabary presumed to be stored in the left premotor cortex (Ackermann et al., 2007; Levelt, Roelofs, & Meyer, 1999). Articulatory planning processes in speech motor control could therefore conceivably assist cognitive behaviors requiring control of internal articulation, including language processes as well as language-related processes such as verbal working memory (Ackermann, 2008).

For example, it is often hypothesized that the superior cerebellum is engaged in subarticulatory rehearsal during the maintenance phase of verbal working memory tasks (e.g., Desmond et al., 1998). However, a recent review of cerebellar involvement in verbal working memory suggests the cerebellum participates in encoding and retrieval phases of verbal working memory tasks, rather than maintenance of verbal information through rehearsal (Ben-Yehudah, Guediche, & Fiez, 2007). Two event-related fMRI studies parsed apart encoding, maintenance, and retrieval phases in their verbal working memory tasks and only found superior cerebellar activity for encoding (Chen & Desmond, 2005), or encoding and retrieval phases (Chien & Fiez, 2001). Moreover, clinical data show that cerebellar lesions do not extinguish or reduce behavioral markers (e.g., word-length effect, articulatory suppression) of articulatory rehearsal (Ravizza et al., 2006), suggesting cerebellar activation from internal speech processing may reflect encoding and retrieval rather than rehearsal mechanisms per se.

Originating from earlier work on motor control, the cerebellum is thought of as a learning device (Gilbert & Thach, 1977; Marr, 1969). Theories of motor learning and control posit the cerebellum as internally modeling the motor system with the purpose of executing fast and accurate motion. Two basic forms of internal models generally exist: forward models predict the sensory outcomes of motor commands and inverse models predict the motor command that will cause a desired change in sensory outcomes (Ito, 2005; Wolpert et al., 1998). Error signals are generated by comparing predicted versus actual outcomes and can be used to adjust further predictions of the internal model, allowing the internal model to learn in an adaptive fashion. The concept of internal models in the motor system can be extended to cognition (Wolpert et al., 1998); imaging studies have examined cerebellar activity in relation to practice effects in language tasks. In Seger et al. (2000), verb generation to novel nouns produced more widespread cerebellar activation relative to previously viewed nouns. Similarly, in an earlier study, less activity in a right cerebellar region of interest along with diminished response time latencies were seen for generating verbs to previously viewed nouns relative to novel nouns (Raichle et al., 1994). However, not all evidence is in support of cerebellar involvement in practice effects for language tasks: cerebellar patients showed a decrease in response time across practice blocks in a verb generation task and did not differ in their performance from controls, demonstrating evidence of learning in spite of cerebellar lesions (Helmuth, Ivry, & Shimizu, 1997).

In imaging studies, the direction of activation for practice effects is also inconsistent; it is unclear whether learning increases or decreases activation (Kirschen, Chen, Schraedley-Desmond, & Desmond, 2005). While studies have shown decreased cerebellar activation in tasks for previously viewed stimuli relative to novel stimuli (e.g., Raichle et al., 1994; Seger et al., 2000), the effect of practice may increase cerebellar activation. For a verbal working memory task, participants displayed right lobule VI and right lobule VIIB/crus II after having practiced but not before practicing. Interpretation-wise, the increased cerebellar activity after practice may reflect consolidation of the cerebellum's internal model for automating the verbal working memory task (Kirschen et al., 2005); conversely, decreased cerebellar activity could reflect increased neural efficiency at accomplishing the task.

The aforementioned theories of cerebellar function are somewhat interrelated (Strick, Dum, & Fiez, 2009). For example, the precise representation of temporal information is needed to generate error signals when comparing predicted and actual outcomes (Ben-Yehudah et al., 2007). The temporal pre-articulatory representation of sounds, i.e., "internal speech," could in effect be present at all levels of language processing, whether phonological, lexical semantic, semantic, syntactic, or discourse.

In summary,

- Cerebellar modulation of language processing reflects differences in task difficulty across conditions in language tasks, as operationally defined by a difference in performance (e.g., reaction time and accuracy measurements) or general differences in task effort (e.g., processing fewer possible options vs. more possible options); cerebellar activity may reflect differential involvement from language-related processes such as verbal working memory, rather than linguistic processing per se.
- Across phonological, lexical semantic, semantic, syntactic, and discourse levels of language tasks, bilateral lobule VI, crus I and crus II largely seem to activate, with a preponderance toward right cerebellar hemisphere activity. A meta-analysis could more firmly substantiate the functional topography of language processing in the cerebellum. Cerebellar functional topography likely reflects anatomical connections to areas in the prefrontal and temporal cortices.
- The precise underlying mechanism for the cerebellum's modulation of language processing is unclear (i.e., whether related to learning mechanisms, pre-articulatory or "internal" speech, timing mechanisms, or some combination therein). These mechanisms could potentially assist language-related frontal cognitive control mechanisms (e.g., retrieval).

References

Ackermann, H. (2008). Cerebellar contributions to speech production and speech perception: Psycholinguistic and neurobiographical perspectives. *Trends in Neuroscience, 31*, 265–272.

Ackermann, H., Mathiak, K., & Riecker, A. (2007). The contribution of the cerebellum to speech production and speech perception: Clinical and functional imaging data. *The Cerebellum, 6*, 202–213.

Ben-Yehudah, G., Guediche, S., & Fiez, J. A. (2007). Cerebellar contributions to verbal working memory: Beyond cognitive theory. *The Cerebellum, 6*, 193–201.

Binder, J. R., Desai, R. H., Graves, W. W., & Conant, L. I. (2009). Where is the semantic system? A critical review and meta-analysis of 120 functional neuroimaging studies. *Cerebral Cortex, 19*, 2767–2796.

Braitenberg, V. (1967). Is the cerebellar cortex a biological clock in the millisecond range? *Progress in Brain Research, 25*, 334–346.

Brett, M., Christoff, R., Cusack, J., & Lancaster, J. (2001). Using the Talairach atlas with the MNI template. *Neuroimage, 13*, S85.

Carreiras, M., Mechelli, A., Estevez, A., & Price, C. J. (2007). Brain activation for lexical decision and reading aloud: Two sides of the same coin? *Journal of Cognitive Neuroscience, 19*, 433–444.

Chee, M. W. L., O'Craven, K. M., Bergida, R., Rosen, B. R., & Savoy, R. L. (1999). Auditory and visual word processing studied with fMRI. *Human Brain Mapping, 7*, 15–28.

Chein, J. M., & Fiez, J. A. (2001). Dissociation of verbal working memory system components during a delayed serial recall task. *Cerebral Cortex, 11*, 1003–1014.

Chen, S. H. A., & Desmond, J. E. (2005). Temporal dynamics of cerebro-cerebellar network recruitment during a cognitive task. *Neuropsychologia, 43,* 1227–1237.

Coltheart, M., Rastle, K., Perry, C., Langdon, R., & Ziegler, J. (2001). DRC: A dual route cascaded model of visual word recognition and reading aloud. *Psychological Review, 108,* 204–256.

Desmond, J. E., Gabrieli, J. D. E., & Glover, G. H. (1998). Dissociation of frontal and cerebellar activity in cognitive task: Evidence for a distinction between selection and search. *Neuroimage, 7,* 368–376.

Diedrichsen, J., Balster, J. H., Flavell, J., Cussans, E., & Ramnani, N. (2009). A probabilistic MR atlas of the human cerebellum. *Neuroimage, 46,* 39–46.

Dogil, G., Ackermann, H., Grodd, W., Haider, H., Kamp, H., Mayer, J., et al. (2002). The speaking brain: A tutorial introduction to fMRI experiments in the production of speech, prosody and syntax. *Journal of Neurolinguistics, 15,* 59–90.

Friederici, A. D., Fiebach, C. J, Schlesewsky, M., Bornkessel, I. D., & Yves von Cramon, D. (2006). Processing linguistic complexity and grammaticality in the left frontal cortex. *Cerebral Cortex, 16,* 1709–1717.

Gauthier, C. T., Duyme, M., Zanca, M., & Capron, C. (2009). Sex and performance level effects on brain activation during a verbal fluency task: A functional magnetic resonance imaging study. *Cortex, 45,* 164–176.

Gernsbacher, M. A., Varner, K. R., & Faust, M. (1990). Investigating differences in general comprehension skill. *Journal of Experimental Psychology, 16,* 430–445.

Gilbert, P. F. C., & Thach, W. T. (1977). Purkinje-cell activity during motor learning. *Brain Research, 128,* 309–328.

Giraud, A., Truy, E., Frackowiak, R. S. J., Gregoire, M., Pujol, J., & Collet, L. (2000). Differential recruitment of the speech processing system in healthy subjects and rehabilitated cochlear implant patients. *Brain, 123,* 1391–1402.

Gold, B. T., Balota, D. A., Kirchoff, B. A., & Buckner, R. L. (2005). Common and dissociable activation patterns associated with controlled semantic and phonological processing: Evidence from fMRI adaption. *Cerebral Cortex, 15,* 1438–1450.

Gourovitch, M. L., Kirkby, B. S., Goldberg, T. E., Weinberger, D. R., Gold, J. M., Esposito, G., et al. (2000). A comparison of rCBF patterns during letter and semantic fluency. *Neuropsychology, 14,* 353–360.

Gurd, J. M., Amunts, K., Weiss, P. H., Zafiris, O., Zilles, K., Marshall, J. C., et al. (2002). Posterior parietal cortex is implicated in continuous switching between verbal fluency tasks: An fMRI study with clinical implications. *Brain, 125,* 1024–1038.

Haarmeier, T., & Thier, P. (2007). The attentive cerebellum – myth or reality? *The Cerebellum, 6,* 177–183.

Helmuth, L. L., Ivry, R. B., & Shimizu, N. (1997). Preserved performance by cerebellar patients on tests of word generation, discrimination learning, and attention. *Learning and Memory, 3,* 456–474.

Herbster, A. N., Mintun, M. A., Nebes, R. D., & Becker, J. T. (1997). Regional cerebral blood flow during word and nonword reading. *Human Brain Mapping, 5,* 84–92.

Holmes, G. (1922). Clinical symptoms of cerebellar disease and their interpretation. *Lancet, 2,* 59–65.

Ito, M. (2005). Bases and implications of learning in the cerebellum – Adaptive control and internal model mechanism. *Progress in Brain Research, 148,* 95–108.

Ivry, R. (1997). Cerebellar timing systems. *International Review of Neurobiology, 41,* 555–573.

Ivry, R. B. & Keele, S.W. (1989). Timing functions of the cerebellum. *Journal of Cognitive Neuroscience, 1*, 136–152.

Ivry, R. B., & Spencer, R. M. C. (2004). The neural representation of time. *Current Opinion in Neurobiology, 14*, 225–232.

Jenkins, I. H., Brooks, D. J., Nixon, P. D., Fracowiak, R. S. J., & Passingham, R. E. (1994). Motor sequence learning: A study with positron emission tomography. *Journal of Neuroscience,14*, 3775–3790.

Joubert, S., Beauregard, M., Walter, N., Bourgouin, P., Beaudoin, G., Leroux, J., et al. (2004). Neural correlates of lexical and sublexical processes in reading. *Brain and Language, 89*, 9–20.

Keele, S. W., & Ivry, R. I. (1991). Does the cerebellum provide a common computation for diverse tasks? A Timing Hypothesis. *Annals of the New York Academy of Sciences, 608*, 179–211.

Kim, S. G., Ugurbil, K., & Strick, P. L. (1994). Activation of a cerebellar output nucleus during cognitive processing. *Science, 265*, 949–951.

Kirschen, M. P., Chen, S. H. A., Schraedley-Desmond, P., & Desmond, J. E. (2005). Load- and practice-dependent increases in cerebro-cerebellar activation in verbal working memory: An fMRI study. *Neuroimage, 24*, 462–472.

Lancaster J. L., Tordesillas-Gutierrez D., Martinez, M., Salinas F., Evans A. C., Zilles K., et al. (2007). Bias between MNI and Talairach coordinates analyzed using the ICBM-152 brain template. *Human Brain Mapping, 28*, 1194–1205.

Lawrence, N. S., Ross, T. J., Hoffman, R., Garavan, H., & Stein, E. A. (2003). Multiple neuronal networks mediate sustained attention. *Journal of Cognitive Neuroscience, 15*, 1028–1038.

Leiner, H. C., Leiner, A. L., & Dow, R. S. (1986). Does the cerebellum contribute to mental skills? *Behavioral Neuroscience, 100*, 443–454.

Leiner, H. C., Leiner, A. L., & Dow, R. S. (1991). The human cerebro-cerebellar system: Its computing, cognitive, and language skills. *Behavioral Brain Research, 44*, 113–128.

Levelt, W. J. M., Roelofs, A., & Meyer, A. S. (1999). A theory of lexical access in speech productions. *Behavioral and Brain Sciences, 22*, 1–38.

Lewis, P. A. & Miall, R. C. (2003). Distinct systems for automatic and cognitively controlled time measurement: Evidence from neuroimaging. *Current Opinion in Neurobiology, 13*, 250–255.

Marien, P., Engelborghs, S., Fabbro, F., & De Deyn, P. P. (2001). The lateralized linguistic cerebellum: A review and a new hypothesis. *Brain and Language, 79*, 580–600.

Marr, D. (1969). A theory of cerebellar cortex. *Journal of Physiology, 202*, 437–470.

McDermott, K. B., Petersen, S. E., Watson, J. M., & Ojemann, J. G. (2003). A procedure for identifying regions preferentially activated by attention to semantic and phonological relations using functional magnetic resonance imaging. *Neuropsychologia, 41*, 293–303.

Miceli, G., Turriziani, P., Caltagirone, C., Capasso, R., Tomaiuolo, F., & Caramazza, A. (2002). The neural correlates of grammatical gender: An fMRI investigation. *Journal of Cognitive Neuroscience, 14*, 618–628.

Moore, C.J., & Price, C. J. (1999). Three distinct ventral occipitotemporal regions for reading and object naming. *Neuroimage, 10*, 181–192.

Perani, D., Cappa, S. F., Schnur, T., Tettamanti, M., Collina, S., Rosa, M. M., et al. (1999). The neural correlates of verb and noun processing: A PET study. *Brain, 122*, 2337–2344.

Petersen, S. E., Fox, P. T., Posner, M. I., Mintun, M., & Raichle, M. E. (1989). Positron emission tomographic studies of the processing of single words. *Journal of Cognitive Neuroscience, 1*, 153–170.

Plaut, D. C., McClelland, J. L., Siedenberg, M. S., & Patterson, K. (1996). Understanding normal and impaired word reading: Computational principles in quasi-regular domains. *Psychological Review, 103*, 56–115.

Raichle, M. E., Fiez, J. A., Videen, T. O., MacLeod, A. K., Pardo, J. V., Fox, P. T., et al. (1994). Practice-related changes in human brain functional anatomy during nonmotor learning. *Cerebral Cortex, 4*, 1047–3211.

Ravizza, S. M., McCormick, C. A., Schlerf, J. E., Justus, T., Ivry, R. B., & Fiez, J. A. (2006). Cerebellar damage produces selective deficits in verbal working memory. *Brain, 129*, 306–320.

Riecker, A., Mathiak, K., Wildgruber, D., Erb, M., Hertrich, I., Grodd, W., & Ackermann, H. (2005). fMRI reavls two distinct cerebral networks subserving speech motor control. *Neurology, 64*, 700–706.

Robertson, D. A., Gernsbacher, M. A., Guidotti, S. J., Robertson, R. R. W., Irwin, W., Mock, B. J., et al. (2000). Functional neuroanatomy of the cognitive process of mapping during discourse comprehension. *Psychological Science, 11*, 255–260.

Roskies, A. L., Fiez, J. A., Balota, D. A., Raichle, M. E., & Petersen, S. E. (2001). Task-dependent modulation of regions in the left inferior frontal cortex during semantic processing. *Journal of Cognitive Neuroscience, 13*, 829–843.

Schlosser, R., Hutchinson, M., Joseffer, S., Rusinek, H., Saarimaki, A., Stevenson, J., et al. (1998). Functional magnetic resonance imaging of human brain activity in a verbal fluency task. *Journal of Neurology, Neurosurgery, and Psychiatry, 64*, 492–498.

Schmahmann, J. D. (1991). An emerging concept: The cerebellar contribution to higher function. *Archives of Neurology, 48*, 1178–1187.

Schmahmann, J. D. (1996). From movement to thought: Anatomic substrates of the cerebellar contribution to cognitive processing. *Human Brain Mapping, 4*, 174–198.

Schmahmann, J. D. (1997). Rediscovery of an early concept. In J.D. Schmahmann (Ed.), *The cerebellum and cognition* (pp. 4–20). San Diego, CA: Academic Press.

Schmahmann, J. D., Doyon, J., Toga, A., Petrides, M., & Evans, A. (2000). *MRI atlas of the human cerebellum.* San Diego, CA: Academic Press.

Schmahmann, J. D., & Pandya, D. N. (1997). The cerebrocerebellar system. *International Review of Neurobiology, 41*, 31–60.

Seger, C. A., Desmond, J. E., Glover, G. H., & Gabrieli, J. D. E. (2000). Functional magnetic resonance imaging evidence for right-hemisphere involvement in processing unusual semantic relationships. *Neuropsychology, 14*, 361–369.

Seki, A., Okada, T., Koeda, T., & Sadato, N. (2004). Phonemic manipulation in Japanese: An FMRI study. *Cognitive Brain Research, 20*, 261–272.

Silveri, M. C., Leggio, M. G., & Molinari, M. (1994). The cerebellum contributes to linguistic production: A case of agrammatic speech following a right cerebellar lesion. *Neurology, 44*, 2047–2050.

Spivey, M. J., & Tanenhaus, M. K. (1998). Syntactic ambiguity resolution in discourse: Modeling the effects of referential context and lexical frequency. *Journal of Experimental Psychology: Learning, Memory, Cognition, 24*, 1521–1543.

Stoodley, C. J., & Schmahmann, J. D. (2009). Functional topography in the human cerebellum: A meta-analysis of neuroimaging studies. *Neuroimage, 44*, 489–501.

Stowe, L. A., Paans, A. M. J., Wijers, A. A., & Zwarts, F. (2004). Activations of "motor" and other nonlanguage structures during sentence comprehension. *Brain and Language, 89,* 290–299.

Strick, P. L., Dum, R. O., & Fiez, J. A. (2009). Cerebellum and nonmotor function. *Annual Reviews of Neuroscience, 32,* 413–434.

Talairach, J., & Tournoux, P. (1988). *Co-planar stereotaxic atlas of the human brain.* New York: Thieme.

Tieleman, A., Seurinck, R., Deblaere, K., Vandemaele, P., Vingerhoets, G., & Achten, E. (2005). Stimulus pacing affects the activation of the medial temporal lobe during a semantic classification task: An fMRI study. *Neuroimage, 26,* 565–572.

Tyler, L. K., Bright, P., Fletcher, P., & Stamatakis, E. A. (2004). Neural processing of nouns and verbs: The role of inflectional morphology. *Neuropsychologia, 42,* 512–523.

Wildgruber, D., Ackermann, H., & Grodd, W. (2001). Differential contributions of motor cortex, basal ganglia, and cerebellum to speech motor control: Effects of syllable repetition rate evaluated by fMRI. *Neuroimage, 13,* 101–109.

Wolpert, D. M., Mialll, R. C., & Kawato, M. (1998). Internal models in the cerebellum. *Trends in Cognitive Science, 2,* 338–347.

Xu, B., Grafman, J., Gaillard, W. D., Ishii, K., Vega-Bermudez, F., Peitrini, P., et al. (2001). Conjoint and extended neural networks for the computation of speech codes: The neural basis of selective impairment in reading words and pseudowords. *Cerebral Cortex, 11,* 267–277.

Part IV

Coping with Higher-Level Processing: The Brain Behind Figurative and Creative Language

16

Bilateral Processing and Affect in Creative Language Comprehension

Heather J. Mirous and Mark Beeman

Language is creative. One of the hallmarks of human language is that it is endlessly generative. People use a small set of syntactic rules and a large, but finite, set of words to create and comprehend a seemingly infinite variety of sentences. Beyond that, people regularly use language even more creatively to further enrich their message, add nuance and emotion, to entertain, and to creatively solve problems.

Before we begin, a couple of disclaimers: first, this chapter describes the cognitive and neural bases of *some* aspects of verbal creativity, but does not purport to comprehensively explain the brain bases of creativity. Second, we will argue that the right hemisphere (RH) plays a relatively stronger role in verbal creativity than in other verbal processes, but we are not suggesting that creativity resides in the RH, is solely dependent on it, or any other simplistic pop psychology notions of the "creative hemisphere." However, there is now indisputable evidence that the RH does play a role in many aspects of verbal creativity, and it's not our fault if others see that as somehow similar to simplistic pop psychology (Dietrich, 2007). After all, in choosing hemispheres, pop psychology had a coin toss chance of success. More importantly, verbal creativity can be seen as the orchestration of myriad cognitive and brain processes, which we are only now beginning to delineate.

Creativity has been challenging to define over the years, but most researchers agree that it involves production or creation of something new that is useful, appreciated, or appropriate to the context (e.g., Amabile, 1983). Language that is novel and well understood is creative, particularly if it creates some new meaning. Some language behavior happens with the explicit goal of being creative. Some readers may recall (perhaps with mixed emotions) high-school writing classes devoted to "creative writing." Thus, other aspects of writing would seem to be, by default,

The Handbook of the Neuropsychology of Language, First Edition. Edited by Miriam Faust.
© 2012 Blackwell Publishing Ltd. Published 2012 by Blackwell Publishing Ltd.

uncreative. Writing poetry and creative fiction, using (and comprehending) novel metaphors, and other word play are clearly creative.

However, viewing creativity in language as a rare commodity, used only for special purposes, severely under-represents a critical aspect of language that contributes to daily comprehension and expression every day of our lives. Whether consciously aware of it or not, people frequently draw on aspects of creativity in order to understand and express language in ordinary, everyday activities and conversations. Speakers and listeners imply and understand meanings that "go beyond the words," and readers "read between the lines." People use metaphors, sarcasm, and irony, devise riddles, get jokes, and draw inferences about information not explicitly given in language input. Creative language use is critical to complete understanding in all media. From understanding movies, TV shows, advertisements, musical lyrics, reading stories, and even holding everyday conversation, all of these behaviors in language comprehension and production rely on our ability to understand and use creativity in language.

In this chapter, we will describe some of the cognitive processes and neural substrates that underlie a few categories of creative language use, highlighting similarities (and a few differences). We discuss how each hemisphere contributes to processing jokes, drawing inferences, and creatively solving problems (metaphor comprehension is covered in Volume 1, Chapters 19, 20, and 21) and outline a theoretical mechanism for these hemispheric differences. Finally, we will examine how positive mood facilitates and anxiety impedes the ability to make the semantic connections necessary for particularly creative language.

Bilateral Activation, Integration, and Selection (BAIS), with Relatively Coarser Semantic Coding in the Right Hemisphere

Before discussing particular types of creative language, we provide a framework (more fully described in Jung-Beeman, 2005) for understanding how both hemispheres contribute to multiple semantic processes necessary for creative language use. One general dimension on which creative language varies from more straightforward, prosaic language is the degree to which distant semantic relations – creativity researchers might say divergent thinking – are necessary. Much creative language requires the comprehender to make use of semantic information that seems less central to a word's definition, and of relatively distant associations rather than close, dominant associations. One way to describe such semantic processing is that it relies on *relatively coarser semantic coding*.

A great deal of evidence, including some to be discussed below, indicates that the RH codes semantic information more coarsely than the left hemisphere (LH; for review, see Jung-Beeman, 2005). When readers or listeners encounter a word, they activate (essentially, think about) a subset of concepts, properties, and associations (collectively referred to as *semantic fields*) related to that word. Evidence from a variety of sources suggests that the LH strongly activates a relatively smaller semantic field, or set of semantic features, those features most closely related to the current (apparent) context, or if context is impoverished, the dominant semantic features and interpretations. In contrast, the RH weakly activates a relatively larger semantic field, including features that are distantly related to the word or context, and secondary word interpretations; not *everything* potentially related to the word, but a broader set of related features than is activated in the LH (Chiarello, 1988; Chiarello, Burgess, Gage, & Pollock, 1990). Despite some obvious drawbacks, coarser semantic coding has one big advantage: the less sharply each word's meaning is specified, the more likely it is to connect in some distant way to other words in the context. These types of semantic connections appear central to creative language use.

The term "coarser semantic coding" provides a useful description of many language behaviors, but a further implication and goal is to link asymmetric semantic processing to asymmetric brain microcircuitry – specifically, to asymmetries in various features of neurons that influence the integration of inputs. As previously stated (Jung-Beeman, 2005), this is a huge leap, and there are many processing links between neuronal connections and understanding language. However, given that asymmetries exist in neuronal microcircuitries (for review, see Hutsler & Galuske, 2003) these are likely to have consequences in information processing; and, there must be some neuroanatomical basis for the asymmetries that indisputably exist in language processing.

Although the two hemispheres are roughly symmetrical, there are several established asymmetries. Some gross morphological asymmetries seem potentially related to language asymmetries, such as the LH having a relatively larger planum temporale (roughly speaking, the temporal plane just behind auditory cortex) and possibly Broca's area. While these asymmetries seem to favor stronger LH processing in language-related skills, the association is weak at best (perhaps absent in women, e.g., Chiarello et al., 2009). The LH also has a relatively higher ratio of gray to white matter; conversely, the RH has relatively more white matter, and a higher degree of functional interconnectivity (Semmes, 1968; Tucker, Roth, & Blair, 1986).

Asymmetries in coarseness of coding may be attributable to asymmetries at the microanatomic level. In brief, pyramidal neurons collect inputs through their dendrites, and, as such, differences in synaptic distributions along dendrites influence the type of inputs that cause these pyramidal neurons to fire. The range of cortical area over which neurons collect input could be termed their *input fields*. In association cortex (i.e., not primary sensory or motor areas) in or near language-critical areas such as Wernicke's area, Broca's area, and anterior temporal cortex, RH neurons have larger input fields than LH neurons (e.g., Jacob, Schall, & Scheibel, 1993; Scheibel et al., 1985; Seldon, 1981; for review, see Hutsler & Galuske, 2003). Specifically, they have more synapses overall and especially far from the soma (i.e., well dispersed). The LH pyramidal neurons have more synapses close to the soma. Because cortical connections are topographical, the spatial layout of the input fields have informational consequences – more dispersed input fields (in the RH) collect more differentiated inputs, perhaps requiring a variety of inputs to fire. More tightly distributed input fields (in the LH) collect highly similar inputs, perhaps causing the neuron to respond best to somewhat redundant inputs, and yielding relatively discrete processing units across cortical columns (Hutsler & Galuske, 2003). Similarly, outputs from neurons in superior temporal cortex are longer in the RH than in the LH, favoring more integrative processing in the RH (Tardif & Clarke, 2001).

These relative asymmetries in microcircuitry may allow each hemisphere to activate different fields of neurons in response to input. In terms of verbal processing, each hemisphere activates different semantic networks. Language areas of the LH, with neurons that have closely branching dendrites, are more adept at strongly activating smaller, more discrete semantic fields, i.e., engaging in relatively finer semantic coding (still coarse, but finer than in the RH). In contrast, language areas of the RH, with neurons that have broadly branching dendrites, are more adept at weakly activating larger, fuzzier semantic fields, i.e., engaging in relatively coarser semantic coding.

The BAIS framework (Jung-Beeman, 2005) further specifies that this general hemispheric asymmetry occurs in at least three distinct semantic processes that contribute to higher-level language comprehension: activation, integration, and selection. Each process is suited for different components of creative language processing and is supported by a distinct cortical region. The three processes are posited to be highly interactive, both within and across the hemispheres.

Semantic activation, depending mostly on bilateral Wernicke's area (broadly construed, including posterior superior temporal gyrus or STG) provides initial access to semantic features and associations (semantic representations that are highly distributed), activating features and first-order associations of the input word. Related processes may be supported by angular and supramarginal gyri (Booth et al., 2003), and perhaps inferior temporal lobe (Sharp, Scott, & Wise, 2004), with distinct areas important for different modalities of input and characteristics of information. As noted above, each input word elicits a semantic field in each hemisphere, a strongly focused one in the LH and a diffuse one in the RH. The two hemispheres likely store similar representations, but differ in dynamically accessing information, with the ultimate shape and size of the semantic fields modulated by context, memory load, and possibly mood.

Semantic integration is the process by which activated semantic concepts are connected to form a meaningful semantic relationship. Integration, seeming to depend on anterior temporal areas (middle and superior temporal gyri, perhaps temporal pole), computes the degree of semantic overlap in chunks of input, and allows for the elaboration of potentially useful connections. It may best be illustrated by an early neuroimaging study in which people showed stronger positron emission tomography (PET) signal in anterior temporal lobe of the RH when they had to comprehend ambiguous stories without a theme compared to when the theme was given, in the form of a title, before the story (St George, Kutas, Martinez, & Sereno, 1999).

Semantic selection allows competing activated concepts to be sorted out, inhibiting some concepts while selecting others for action (including but not limited to response production, for elaboration, or for consciousness). Selection modulates word-level semantic activation and message-level semantic integration. There is strong evidence that semantic selection depends on the inferior frontal gyrus (IFG). Indeed, it has been proposed that the IFG performs selection more generally, with semantic selection being just one aspect (e.g., Thompson-Schill, D'Esposito, Aguirre, & Farah, 1997; Zhang, Feng, Fox, Gao, & Tan, 2004). It is posited to interact with the other components: the more activated a concept (or integrative connection) is, the easier it is to select; the more selection is engaged, the narrower the scope of activation of concepts. Selection allows comprehenders to select concepts – given by the text or derived through integration – for output or to build their mental representation of the language they are comprehending.

Summary of coarser semantic coding

By itself, coarse semantic coding (of the RH) would be inadequate for comprehending language – if one couldn't even decide which meaning of a word was intended by a speaker (or writer), one would quickly get lost in almost any discourse. However, in many situations, semantic features that seemed initially irrelevant may add color or nuance to an interpretation, allow for the accommodation of unexpected subsequent input, or contribute to a wholesale reinterpretation of the initial input (for review, see Beeman, et al., 1994; Beeman, 1998; Jung-Beeman, 2005). These are the types of linguistic behaviors that are often critical to verbal creativity.

Jokes and Humor

A thoughtful wife has pork chops ready when her husband comes home from . . . fishing.

One inherently creative use of language is telling or understanding jokes and humor. Understanding jokes often relies on our ability to comprehend alternate, nonliteral, or "creative" word or phrase meanings as opposed to literal, dominant, straightforward meanings. After reading the example premise (from Coulson & Wu, 2005), *A thoughtful wife has pork chops ready when her husband comes home from . . .* most people would expect the word *work* (or similar phrases) to occur next. However, when they instead see *fishing*, a less-expected completion, people can easily integrate it with the prior context and (if they sense it is a joke), reinterpret that prior context in a new and interesting way. In short, they stop thinking of a stereotypical scenario of a dutiful wife making dinner for her husband, and reinterpret the phrase as depicting a comical scenario: a sarcastic wife making dinner in anticipation of her husband's failure (Coulson & Wu, 2005).

Patients with RH brain damage had long been observed to have difficulties understanding and/or responding to humor (e.g., Eisenson, 1962). Several decades ago,

Brownell and colleagues investigated this clinical observation in groups of patients with damage to the RH. These patients were not overtly aphasic, and seemed to understand simple straightforward sentences. However, they had a variety of more subtle difficulties understanding longer, more natural language while reading, listening to, or watching stories (for review, see Molloy, Brownell, & Gardner, 1988; also Beeman, 1993; 1998). Among their difficulties was understanding humor.

Historically, RH-damaged patients' difficulties with humor were sometimes assumed to be a function of impaired emotionality. However, another possibility is that the difficulty lay in making the unusual connections upon which humor (and inference, as discussed later) often turns. Brownell, Michel, Powelson, & Gardner (1983) postulated that jokes provide both coherence and surprise. The punchline fits the premise of the joke, but not in the expected way. Rather, understanding the punchline requires reinterpreting the prior context, in order to accommodate the new input, as we've seen above when readers encounter *fishing*.

In one study, nonaphasic patients with RH brain damage had difficulty understanding jokes, but they made systematic errors. After hearing and reading a premise, patients were asked to choose a "funny ending" from among several alternatives. When they erred, patients with RH damage chose surprising, but noncoherent endings (for the example above, they could choose *ballet*; Brownell et al., 1983). In contrast, patients with LH damage (the ones who could perform the task) also erred systematically, most often choosing coherent but nonsurprising endings (*work*, in above example; Bihrle, Brownell, Powelson, & Gardner, 1986). So it's not that RH-damaged patients had no sense of humor, but they didn't recognize the ways that a proper joke ending should fit with the premise.

Neuroimaging studies also suggest that joke comprehension makes particular demands on semantic processing of the RH. One functional magnetic resonance imaging (fMRI) study demonstrated increased fMRI signal in the middle temporal gyrus of the RH specifically related to "getting" semantic jokes (Goel & Dolan, 2001). Different brain areas seemed more sensitive to the affective component of the jokes, and to phonological processing related to jokes; but understanding jokes that turn on twists of meaning increased processing in the RH temporal lobe.

More recently, the process of reanalyzing and reorganizing prior context in light of new input has been termed *frame-shifting*, and is thought to be central to understanding many jokes and forms of humor (Coulson, 2001; see also Coulson & Davenport, Volume 1, Chapter 19). A series of event-related brain potential (ERP) experiments demonstrated differential sensitivity of the LH and RH to joke-related information (Coulson & Williams, 2005; Coulson & Wu, 2005).

In one study, jokes were one-liners such as the *fishing* joke above, with the joke being clinched in the final word, a *punch-word* so to speak (Coulson & Williams, 2005). The stem of the joke (everything up to *fishing*) was presented, one word at a time, in the center of the screen. ERPs were measured for the punch-word and a similarly unexpected but coherent straight ending. ERPs to these two target endings were contrasted with those elicited by a highly predictable ending. It is well established that predictability of a word inversely correlates with the N400 component of ERP signals: the more surprising and difficult to integrate a word is, given the preceding context, the bigger the N400. Thus, the N400 is often used as an index of priming, or how easily understood a word is, in context.

Because the researchers wished to examine hemispheric differences in joke comprehension and the source generators of ERP effects cannot be easily localized, the punch-words were briefly presented laterally, i.e., to the left or right of fixation. Thus, the critical word was presented to either the left visual field (LVF) or right visual field (RVF), thereby being directed initially to the RH or LH, respectively. Naturally, the highly expected endings elicited the smallest N400, regardless of which hemifield-hemisphere it was presented to. Critically, although the joke endings elicited a bigger N400 than the straight endings when viewed in the RVF/LH, the N400s to LVF/RH target words did not differ. In other words, the joke ending was just as well understood as the straight ending, when presented to the LVF/RH (Coulson & Williams, 2005).

But were those joke endings presented to the LVF/RH understood, or were the straight endings simply equally misunderstood? Although the N400 to both joke and straight endings presented to the LVF/RH appeared smaller than the joke N400 in the RVF/LH, a direct contrast of N400 effects across the hemifield conditions could be misleading. So, in another study, words related to joke understanding were contrasted with unrelated words. People viewed jokes that could be summarized with a single word, (such as *failure* for the fishing joke above, although the jokes were two-liners for the second study). After each joke, either the summarizing word or an unrelated word was presented as a target word. When presented to the LVF/RH, unrelated words elicited larger N400s than joke words; in contrast, no such difference was observed for RVF/LH target words (Coulson & Wu, 2005).

Other brain processes are also involved in comprehending jokes. Both the above ERP studies also observed later effects at the frontal scalp electrodes, likely related to working memory, retrieval, and selection processes that take advantage of RH semantic processing to further integrate and understand the joke (e.g., Coulson & Williams, 2005). Several different asymmetries could account for the increased role of RH semantic processing in joke comprehension, including coarser semantic coding (e.g., Beeman et al., 1994; Jung-Beeman, 2005), or more integrative (RH), rather than predictive (LH) processing (e.g., Federmeier & Kutas, 1999). In any case, the semantic information produced more strongly by the RH than by the LH allows people to see the distant connections between the punchline and the premise that allow them to reinterpret, or shift the frame, to see how a surprising ending may cohere after all.

As people encounter language, they expect it to make sense. If something initially doesn't make sense, people generally work harder to understand it. Fortunately, very often semantic processing prepares us to, if not expect particular input, at least be prepared for it. New input is often primed, because it fits so well with the context. In fact, the brain seems almost to predict what words will come next (one interpretation of the N400 is that it occurs to the extent these predictions are violated). When new input is surprising, comprehenders try to make sense of it. They could assume the topic has been completely changed, that they missed some input, or they could try to reread the context or use echoic memory and working memory to "replay" auditory input. Or, they could search internally for semantic overlap, however small, despite the surprise evoked by the more recent input. Coarser semantic coding, especially if it rises and falls over a slower timescale, is more likely to detect weak activation related to overlap of distant semantic relations. So, when people unexpectedly hear *the husband comes home from* . . . fishing, they may be surprised; but there may already be weak semantic activation somewhere in the brain – more likely as a result of RH than LH semantic processing – indicating potential connections between the new input and *thoughtful wife* and *pork chops ready*. That weak activation does not suffice to completely comprehend the utterance immediately, but it points the way to shifting the frame of the premise, which can then lead to fuller comprehension – and hopefully a small chuckle.

Story Theme and Inferences

There are other, more subtle ways that coarse semantic coding aids comprehension, sometimes in creative fashion. During comprehension, readers and listeners build mental representations of what they are hearing or reading (for review, see Zwaan & Rapp, 2006). In doing so, they try to maintain coherence between consecutive words and sentences (local coherence) as well as maintain overall coherence, or the big picture of the passage (global coherence). People are able to get the gist, or understand the theme of discourse, even when it is not explicitly stated. Patients with RH damage seem to have some difficulty doing so (Hough, 1990), and having to derive the gist of a long passage increases metabolism in the RH anterior temporal lobe, compared to when the theme was presented prior to the passage (St George et al., 1999).

Sometimes, maintaining coherence and getting the gist of a story requires people to "read between the lines," i.e., to draw connective inferences that bridge gaps in explicit input. In other words, comprehenders create meaning where none was explicitly given. Consider the following excerpt from a story:

> Although Barney had been planning his wife's fortieth birthday for weeks, he'd only managed to make one cake, and he wasn't quite finished with it. So he grabbed a spatula and took out the plain brown cake, setting it on the counter. After a few minutes, he put the colorful cake in the refrigerator.

In order to comprehend this passage, you needed to draw the inference that Barney frosted or decorated the cake. At the point that Barney grabbed a spatula and took out the plain brown cake, setting it on the counter, you could, potentially, predict that he was going to frost the cake. Evidence is somewhat mixed about how strongly people make such predictions, or *predictive inferences*. Later, when he put the colorful cake in the refrigerator, the coherence of the passage would be broken if you hadn't inferred that he frosted the cake. Such a point is sometimes called a *coherence point* (or *break*), and this type of inference is referred to as *backward* or *bridging* inference. As readers and listeners of language, we are constantly required to fill in gaps that are not explicitly stated in order to maintain coherence between changing states or events in what we are reading or hearing. Drawing inferences is an essential process in building locally and globally coherent mental representations (Albrecht & O'Brien, 1993; for review, see Graesser, Singer, & Trabasso, 1994; Singer, 2007).

Like understanding jokes, drawing inferences requires making distal or unusual connections between concepts (cf. Long, Johns, Jonathan, & Baynes, Volume 1, Chapter 5). Frost is only distantly related to the words *plain, brown,* and *cake.* It is somewhat more related to the whole phrase *plain brown cake.* It is slightly more related in the context of an upcoming birthday party. It is distantly related to *colorful cake.* But if comprehenders assume that the *colorful cake* is the same one as the *plain brown cake,* semantic overlap on the concept *frost* greatly facilitates drawing an inference that makes sense of it all.

As with jokes, patients with RH damage have also long been observed to have difficulties drawing connective inferences (e.g., Beeman, 1993; Brownell, Potter, Bihrle, & Gardner, 1986; McDonald & Wales, 1986). For example, after listening to (and simultaneously reading) very short scenarios implying an event, patients with RH damage answered questions about explicitly stated facts just as accurately as healthy elderly participants, but they answered questions about inferences at chance accuracy (Brownell et al., 1986). One could argue that they simply encoded inferences less strongly than explicitly stated information, hence forgot inferences more easily. However, another study showed that not only did patients with RH damage have difficulty answering inference questions, they also failed to show inference-related facilitation on a lexical decision task that occurred during the stories. That is, while listening to the above episode (during a longer story), participants simultaneously made lexical decisions to target words – some of which described the events being implied (*frost*). Age- and education-matched controls responded to the inference-related words more quickly than unrelated words (inference words for the other stories they heard), but patients with RH damage did not (Beeman, 1993). This suggests that, even at the moment the event was implied, these patients lacked semantic activation that would make it easier to draw the correct inferences. Other interpretations of the inference deficit with RH brain damage have been offered. E.g., it is possible that patients with RH damage have difficulty with inferences because they activate multiple interpretations (Tompkins, Fassbinder, Blake, Baumgaertner, & Jayaram, 2004), and do not effectively select the appropriate one. We suggest that the difficulty in selection is due to insufficient semantic overlap due to disrupted coarse semantic coding.

This is not to say that it would be impossible for these patients to draw inferences – merely that they could not draw them in an optimal way. What is the optimal way to draw such inferences? We suggest that while people comprehend stories, weak activation of concepts distantly related to input words can sometimes overlap and summate. Either activation on these concepts builds until it is just as strong as that from explicitly stated input, or when comprehenders detect a gap in coherence, the summated activation points them to concepts and events that may fill the gap and forge stronger connections across the text.

Evidence that the RH contributes to drawing inferences in healthy young comprehenders comes from both behavioral and neuroimaging studies. For instance, summation priming from three distantly related words (*foot-glass-pain*) appears to facilitate naming of a briefly presented target word (*cut*) more strongly in the LVF/RH than in the RVF/LH (Beeman et al., 1994). Furthermore, while listening to narratives participants show priming (or facilitation) for inference-related target words (e.g., after hearing the above excerpt, *frost* is read faster than *rain* – the inference-related word from a different story). Inference-related priming was examined at an early, predictive point (after hearing *he grabbed a spatula and took out the plain brown cake, setting it on the counter*) or at a late, bridging point (after hearing that *he put the colorful cake in the refrigerator*). At the predictive point, participants showed inference-related priming only for target words presented to the LVF/RH, and priming for RVF/LH target words only kicked in at the bridging point (Jung-Beeman, Bowden, & Gernsbacher, 2000). As noted above, it seems that RH coarser semantic coding is more likely to detect potential semantic overlap, and detect it earlier, so that when people need to draw inferences, information to fill the gap is already primed.

Neuroimaging data has further elucidated the specific cortical areas that support the component processes of drawing inferences. People reading sentence pairs that are moderately related, and thus encourage inferences to connect them, show greater activation in the RH, especially in the temporal lobe, than when they read either highly connected pairs that don't require inferences, or unrelated pairs for which no connection can be inferred (Mason & Just, 2004). But perhaps these sentence pairs, with varying degrees of relatedness, encouraged participants to adopt specialized strategies to connect them.

In our lab, whether using patients or healthy controls, or behavioral or neuroimaging methods, we've always used longer, natural-sounding stories, usually with multiple paragraphs each implying causal events. The belief is that participants will be more engaged, and at the same time, unable to adopt specialized strategies. Participants naturally listening to longer narratives (with no overt response required during the stories), showed stronger fMRI signal during stories that implied events compared to nearly identical stories – varying by only a few words – that explicitly stated the same events (Virtue, Haberman, Clancy, Parrish, & Jung-Beeman, 2006; Virtue, Parrish, & Beeman, 2008). At the predictive point (at which time an event was implied or explicitly stated), stronger signal for the implied or inference condition occurred in the STG of the RH (Virtue et al., 2006). At the coherence point (e.g., *colorful cake*), stronger signal for the implied condition occurred in the LH or bilaterally, in both STG and IFG (Virtue et al., 2006, 2008). Interestingly, the set of participants with the highest reading span (verbal working memory), who are most adept at drawing inferences, showed stronger fMRI signal in RH STG and IFG compared to participants lower in reading span (Virtue et al., 2006, 2008). While speculative, based on prior studies, these results may indicate that high working memory participants (St George, Mannes, & Hoffman, 1997) may have been integrating (anterior STG) and selecting (IFG) the inference at the coherence break, while low working memory participants were still activating (posterior STG) the concepts necessary to draw the inference (Virtue et al., 2006).

Of course other areas, such as medial frontal gyrus, are also likely important in detecting gaps in coherence (Ferstl, Rinck, & von Cramon, 2005). When no inferable concept readily presents itself, it appears that the search for connections depends largely on the IFG of the LH. This area seems to be highly active in many tasks involving more strategic, directed semantic search. It remains an open question whether in cases where the inference concept is primed, the final selection of an inference depends more crucially on frontal areas in the LH or RH (e.g., Virtue et al., 2006, 2008).

Drawing inferences is a subtle form of verbal creativity – when people comprehend concepts that weren't explicitly stated, they are essentially creating meaning. Drawing inferences is especially useful when comprehending creative language, or input that has multiple layers of meaning. Now we move on to other, more transparently creative aspects of language processing.

Verbal Creativity

There are numerous ways in which creativity can be expressed, even within the verbal domain. Inventing and understanding novel metaphors, including poetic metaphors, are discussed elsewhere in this volume (see Volume 1, Chapters 19, 20, and 21). In this section, we briefly cover a few other instances of generating creative verbal output. Such studies are more difficult to control than studies of experimenter-generated linguistic stimuli, and thus not unexpectedly remain relatively rare.

One study examined brain activity as people generated creative stories under various conditions (Howard-Jones, Blakemore, Samuel, Summers, & Claxton, 2005). Participants were instructed to generate either creative or uncreative stories, based on sets of three stimulus words that were either related or unrelated. As predicted, outside the brain scanner, people generated more creative stories when instructed to do so, and when generating stories that encompassed the unrelated words.

Inside the brain scanner, when the same participants were given the same types of instructions and stimuli (but not allowed to vocalize responses), different patterns of brain activity were recorded across the conditions. fMRI signal was stronger in extensive bilateral frontal areas (lateral and medial) when people were instructed to be creative than when instructed to be uncreative. Differences due to the word relatedness manipulation were smaller, but still, the unrelated condition – which elicited more creative stories, also elicited more activity in frontal brain areas. The two "creative" manipulations jointly increased activity in prefrontal cortex of the

RH, particularly the right medial frontal gyrus (Howard-Jones et al., 2005). Thus, the creative conditions seemed to evoke more top-down cognitive processing, mediated by prefrontal cortex, particularly in the RH. In contrast, the "uncreative" instruction and related word stimuli both elicited stronger activity than the creative conditions in the occipital lobes – as if participants were processing the visual input more intensely, to engage in "bottom-up" cognitive processing.

Several recent studies have examined how individuals generate simpler creative ideas, rather than whole stories. One used near-infrared spectroscopy to examine brain activity as musicians and matched nonmusicians performed a version of the classic divergent thinking task: to generate as many and as original ways to use a brick as possible. The musicians outperformed the controls in generating creative uses (as scored by blind judges). Musicians also showed stronger bilateral signal on the forehead, indicative of brain activity in bilateral frontal poles, whereas the nonmusicians showed left-lateralized activity for the divergent thinking task compared to a perceptual control task (Gibson, Folley, & Park, 2009).

Another study presented people with unusual situations (e.g., "a light in the darkness") and asked them to provide as many and as original ideas as possible to account for the situations (Grabner, Fink, & Neubauer, 2007). In this case, participants themselves rated the originality of each idea produced, and patterns of brain activity measured by electroencephalography (EEG) were contrasted for the more original versus less original ideas. In two different measures of EEG power, stronger activity for more original over less original ideas was observed in electrodes over the RH, particularly over right frontal cortex (Grabner et al., 2007).

In all these tasks, people were encouraged to come up with creative or original responses that still made sense given the stimuli and task demands. In all cases, it was assumed that more divergent thinking was required to generate more creative ideas; it is easy to see how coarser semantic coding would be advantageous for divergent thinking. Thus, it is not surprising that these experiments all showed the production of more creative ideas was associated with increased activity in right prefrontal cortical areas.

Insight and Creative Problem Solving

Another form of verbal creativity is creative problem solving, of which insight solving is one example. As with other forms of creativity, divergent thinking is often thought to be important. However, it should be noted that after an initial phase of divergence, achieving solution requires convergence – all pieces of the puzzle must fit together. Of course, to meet the typical criteria for creativity, of generating something both original and useful or appreciated, even stories generally converge in order to make sense. Likewise, as described above, even the surprise endings of jokes must cohere with the earlier premise, just in an unexpected way.

Our laboratory has been studying how people solve problems with insight for over a decade. Much of this work has been reviewed elsewhere (e.g., Kounios &

Beeman, 2009), so we will be brief here. The original motivation for beginning these studies was that the processes involved in solving with insight seemed uncannily similar to higher-level language processes, including drawing inferences, for which the RH seemed to contribute. Indeed, solving by insight seemed even more strongly to rely on the type of semantic processing posited to result from the relatively coarse semantic coding of the RH. Specifically, achieving solution insight is believed to occur when, after initially reaching impasse because the predominant solution strategies or associations to problem elements failed to bring a person closer to solution, people mentally restructure the problem. That is, they see the problem in a new light, in which the elements of the problem are related in a different way than initially interpreted. Often, this new structure appears suddenly, and as a whole – rather than being pieced together, and the whole influences the perception or understanding of the parts.

A variety of evidence suggests that unconscious processing contributes to restructuring, and solution, in important ways. People are often unaware of when they will approach solution by insight (Metcalfe & Wiebe, 1987), yet they recognize when a problem is solvable long before they can solve it (e.g., Bolte, Goschke, & Kuhl, 2003). Time away from the problem, called an incubation period, has long been thought to help people later achieve solution (e.g., Wallas, 1926). Indeed, people respond to solution words to problems that they haven't solved faster than to unrelated words (solutions to other problems), and this solution priming is especially evident in the LVF/RH (Bowden & Jung-Beeman, 1998). In fact, this solution priming occurs only when people report that they recognized the solution with a feeling of insight – that it came to them suddenly, and instantly they recognized that the solution fit the whole problem – as opposed to recognizing the solution more analytically (Bowden & Jung-Beeman, 2003).

Neuroimaging studies reveal several key brain areas that are more active as people solve with insight compared to when they solve analytically. Given that insight solutions seem to come as a whole, we expected that semantic integration in anterior STG of the RH might contribute to solving by insight. Indeed, just prior to the moment people solve with insight, fMRI signal increases in the temporal lobe of the RH, in anterior cingulate cortex (ACC), and in hippocampal regions (Jung-Beeman et al., 2004; Subramaniam, Parrish, Kounios, & Jung-Beeman, 2009). EEG also reveals a sudden burst of gamma band activity over the right temporal cortex just prior to insight solutions (Jung-Beeman et al., 2004). Prior to that gamma band activity, alpha band activity increases – again prior to insight solutions – over the occipital cortex. This likely reflects sensory gating, i.e., attenuation of visual processing, that allows individuals close to solution to quiet the sensory input to allow further processing of an idea that is weakly developing. It also implies that some part of the brain senses this weakly active potential solution – or simply a new association that, in this case, leads to solution.

Other distinctive brain processes precede successful solution by insight, earlier in the solving process, including reduced beta band EEG activity observed at electrodes over parieto-occipital cortex, and increased gamma band activity in right frontal electrodes (Sheth, Sandkühler, & Bhattacharya, 2009). Moreover, in the preparation interval before problems are presented, distinct patterns of brain activity are observed in both fMRI and EEG that distinguish trials in which people go on to solve problems with insight from those in which people go on to solve problems analytically (Kounios et al., 2006; Subramaniam et al., 2009). Preparation for insight (conscious and intentional or otherwise) is associated with increased activity in bilateral temporal lobes, presumably signaling readiness to pursue close and distant associations, and ACC, presumably signaling readiness to detect and/or switch between competing solution paths. Prior to problems being solved analytically, people showed relatively stronger activity in the occipital lobes (Kounios et al., 2006; Subramaniam et al., 2009), as if they were ready to concentrate on the stimuli and engage strictly bottom-up stimulus driven processing – just like those who generated uncreative stories (Howard-Jones et al., 2005).

Interestingly, EEG-measured patterns of brain activity during a resting state, before participants even knew what kind of tasks they would be performing, differed in people who tended to solve anagrams by insight, compared to people who tended to solve more analytically (by self-reports obtained after each successful anagram solution). Insight solvers showed stronger activity in electrodes over right temporal cortex as well as activity over occipital cortex that suggested more diffuse activation of the visual system – at rest (Kounios et al., 2008).

These patterns during resting state could reflect either individuals' preferred mode of spontaneous thought, or relatively stable – possibly even hardwired – differences in default network brain activity. Even if these observed differences originate in relatively stable traits, that doesn't mean they cannot vary across time (Kounios et al., 2008). The next section examines one variable that does vary across time and has been shown to influence cognitive and neural processing during creative verbal behavior – an individual's mood.

Mood Modulation of Creative Comprehension

Why does it seem that creativity flows freely at times, while at other times we can work methodically, but not achieve any breakthrough? Do we have any control over our creativity? Among other possible factors, *mood* seems to influence how creatively people use and comprehend language. Specifically, positive mood appears to facilitate creative comprehension, whereas anxiety likely impedes it. The mechanisms by which mood influences creative comprehension, perhaps via working memory, attention, or semantic access, are not yet completely clear.

Negative affect

While negative affect, such as sadness, anxiety (state, trait, and test anxiety), frustration, and depression can be beneficial to some types of cognitive processing, in many cases it has been shown to impair complex cognitive processing, such as learning new information, solving problems, and understanding discourse. Previous research has shown that negative affect, especially anxiety, can restrict working memory capacity and/or attentional focus, which in turn influence cognitive performance, for better or worse – worse, in the case of higher-level language processes that contribute to verbal creativity.

Working memory, or the capacity to maintain and manipulate information in mind (Baddeley, 1992) is important for many types of cognition, such as understanding written and spoken discourse, and may be especially important for more creative uses of discourse. Elevated anxiety (especially the anxiety felt at that moment, or *state* anxiety) seems to restrict functional working memory capacity, which then inhibits cognitive performance (Eysenck & Calvo, 1992).

Anxiety seems to impair, among other behaviors, the ability to draw inferences. In one study, high and low test-anxiety participants read sentence pairs and verified whether a following sentence was true – which could be judged only on the basis of inference (Richards, French, Keogh, & Carter, 2000). Compared to low test-anxiety participants, high test-anxiety participants made slower and less accurate judgments about the potential inferences. Also, high test-anxiety participants were slower to verify the unnecessary inferences than the necessary inferences, whereas low test-anxiety participants responded equally quickly to both inference types. Both effects suggest that high anxiety impedes working memory, which is especially important for verifying the unnecessary, elaborative inferences. In further support of this interpretation, directly increasing memory load (by requiring participants to keep six digits in mind while reading, rather than two) similarly impaired the performance of both groups, suggesting that perhaps high test-anxious participants put forth extra effort that helped them maintain similar levels of task effectiveness compared to low test-anxious participants (in line with the processing efficiency theory, Eysenck & Calvo, 1992).

Negative affect also restricts attentional resources and impairs cognitive performance (though working memory and attention effects may be related). For example, compared to neutral-mood college students, depressed college students were less able to detect inconsistencies in stories, and their judgments of passage difficulty less reliably predicted performance (Ellis, Ottaway, Varner, Becker, & Moore, 1997). When participants were notified that contradictions were present (to increase motivation), depressed students incorrectly identified noncontradictory statements as contradictory more often than participants in a neutral mood. The authors attributed these differences to the resource allocation model (Ellis & Ashbrook, 1988), which posits that during a depressed mood state, irrelevant and intrusive thoughts compete and interfere with cognition, meaning that the attentional resources that would otherwise be devoted to the task at hand are not fully available.

Besides competition from intrusive thoughts, negative affect may actually restrict attentional focus, highlighting relatively detail-oriented and local information, rather than global information (Gasper & Clore, 2002). Under negative affect, focus of attention can be even more specifically biased toward *particular* details, such as threatening stimuli (Easterbrook, 1959). In the context of text comprehension, for example, trait anxiety is associated with a bias toward making predictive inferences about ambiguous events that could be interpreted as threatening, but not toward nonthreatening events (Calvo & Castillo, 2001a,b; for further discussion, Blanchette & Richards, 2003).

Given that negative affect (sadness or anxiety, in different studies) narrows visual attention, it may also narrow conceptual attention, at least in contrast with positive affect. Thus it is not surprising that negative affect impairs processes like drawing inferences (Mirous & Beeman, submitted) and creative problem solving (Rowe, Hirsh, & Anderson, 2007; Subramaniam et al., 2009). We shall discuss such effects below, because they were observed together with the converse effect: positive affect facilitated inference processing and creative problem solving.

Positive affect

Contrary to negative affect, a positive mood, independent of arousal, enhances performance on several types of cognitive tasks. For example, positive affect facilitates creative thinking, problem solving, verbal fluency, classification of items, strategies used to make decisions, learning of a specific task, and even performance on previously mastered material, such as recall of addition and subtraction facts (for review, see Ashby, Isen, & Turken, 1999; Ashby, Valentin, & Turken, 2002) in adults and adolescents (Yasutake & Bryan, 1995) and in young children (Bryan & Bryan, 1991; Masters, Barden, & Ford, 1979).

As will become clear below, it seems likely that positive mood facilitates cognitive processing through broadened attention or otherwise altered cognitive control. One important potential mechanism involves a link between positive affect and the release of dopamine (Ashby, Isen, & Turken, 1999). This dopaminergic theory of positive affect suggests that during positive affect, moderate levels of dopamine released into the ACC facilitates executive attention, while moderate levels of dopamine released into prefrontal cortex facilitates working memory, both of which benefit creative processing (for further discussion, see Ashby, Valentin, & Turken, 2002).

Enhanced positive mood, whether simply assessed in participants or induced by experimenters, has been shown to enhance creative problem solving by a long, gradually building corpus of studies. Various types of creative problem solving improve when people are in a positive mood: from classic insight problems and the Remote Associate Test (Isen, Daubman, & Nowicki, 1987), to medical diagnostic hypothesis testing (Estrada, Isen, & Young, 1997), to negotiations (Carnevale & Isen, 1986), to workplace creativity (Amabile, Barsade, Mueller, & Staw, 2005). Being in a positive mood also improves people's rapid and intuitive judgments about the solvability of remote associate problems (Bolte et al., 2003).

Possibly, positive mood directly facilitates the retrieval of semantic information in response to input (Isen & Daubman, 1984; Isen, Johnson, Mertz, & Robinson,

1985). Indeed, the N400 effect indexing semantic relatedness is modulated by mood, such that positive affect causes more distantly related target words to elicit relatively smaller N400, as if the words seem more related when people are in a positive mood (Federmeier, Kirson, Moreno, & Kutas, 2001).

Alternatively, just as anxiety (or negative affect) narrows attention, positive affect broadens it (e.g., Gasper & Clore, 2002), and both do so in the conceptual domain as well as in the visual perceptual domain. Indeed, following induction into a more positive mood (compared to neutral or sad moods), participants demonstrated broader visual attention on the flanker task (when identifying the central letter, people were more influenced by the flanking letters they were supposed to ignore) and also solved remote associate problems better (Rowe et al., 2007). Moreover, under the positive mood induction, the two tasks were correlated: the better people performed on the Remote Associate Test items, the broader their visual attention was, as indexed by interference from the flanker letters.

We have observed similar effects in our lab while brain activity was assessed with fMRI. The more positive participants feel, the more compound remote associate problems they solve, and the increase in solutions is entirely attributable to solutions reportedly achieved by insight, rather than by analysis. In contrast, the more anxious people were, the more they solved problems analytically, and the less they solved problems by insight (Subramaniam et al., 2009).

Participants' mood was associated with changes in brain activity. Specifically, during the preparation period prior to problem onset, positive mood was associated with increased activation in the ACC. Note that this same area increases in activation prior to problems subsequently solved by insight, and also increases at the moment of solution. ACC is associated with both emotional response (ventral areas) and cognitive control (dorsal areas), such as detecting competing responses and switching attention between them in order to select the correct response. Given this, plus connections to other cognitive control regions such as dorsolateral prefrontal cortex, dorsal ACC seems well placed to help emotion modulate cognition. In terms of insight solving, we believe positive affect increased the breadth of attention (Gasper & Clore, 2002; Rowe et al., 2007), or decreased inhibition of nondominant word associations, allowing participants to detect weakly activated competing ideas. Weakly activated concepts that integrate distantly related problem elements in a new way are most likely processed in right STG. Thus, positive mood did not "turn on" the RH, but altered attention to make people more sensitive to quiet, weakly activated, but useful, concepts.

Like solving problems with insight, drawing inferences relies on connecting distantly related information, so mood could analogously modulate inference processing. In one recent study (Mirous & Beeman, submitted), we predicted that positive affect would facilitate drawing inferences (relative to anxious and neutral moods), while anxiety would impair drawing inferences (relative to positive and neutral moods). In a series of three experiments (positive vs. anxious mood, positive vs. neutral mood, and anxious vs. neutral mood), participants listened to stories that implied causal events.

While they listened to stories, participants named target words that either described or were unrelated to the implied inferences. As predicted, participants showed inference-related priming, naming the inference-related words faster than the unrelated words, when they appeared at the coherence point, the point in the story when coherence is broken if the inference is not drawn. To maintain coherence, comprehenders should select the appropriate inference concept to be included in their story representation at, or shortly after, the coherence point. Prior studies show IFG to be active at this point, either in the LH (Virtue et al., 2006), or bilaterally in comprehenders with higher working memory capacity (Virtue et al., 2008).

Importantly, this inference-related priming was modulated by mood, which was experimentally induced. Prior to each set of stories, participants viewed comical film clips to induce positive affect, scary film clips to induce anxiety, or neutral (nature) film clips to induce a more neutral mood (self-reported mood ratings confirmed that intended moods were established). Neither the causal events themselves nor the target words were particularly emotional, although some of the events might lead to emotional responses (more often negative than positive) for the story characters. Yet, participants showed reliably more priming when they were in a positive mood than when in a neutral or anxious mood, and reliably less priming (in fact, no priming) when they were in an anxious mood than when in a neutral or positive mood (Mirous & Beeman, submitted). This demonstrates that when people are in positive mood, they have better access to semantic information that will help them draw inferences important for fully comprehending stories.

Conclusion

Whether comprehending or producing it, creative language places greater emphasis on some processes than does more straightforward language behavior. This is not to say there are creative and uncreative language processes. Rather, creative language tends to emphasize the generation or detection of unusual semantic relations. As such, the RH's coarser coding version of semantic integration and semantic selection (particularly in generating creative ideas) plays a greater role in creative than in less creative language. Ultimately, truly creative language necessitates the use of many processes, across both hemispheres – especially as there can be a fine line between creative and nonsensical language.

Mood influences creative comprehension, as well as creative problem solving. Negative affect, particularly anxiety, restricts working memory and attention, and impairs creative cognition. Negative affect also has been linked to a narrow, detail-oriented, local focus of attention, which could be helpful in some cognitive tasks and harmful in others. Positive affect, on the other hand, has been linked to a wider, more global focus of attention, as well as to cognitive flexibility, both of which have proved helpful in creative comprehension tasks, but may be disruptive when intense focus is necessary. It is also possible that affect more directly influences the activation, integration, and/or selection of concepts needed to complete cognitive tasks, such as understanding and producing everyday discourse, which often relies on some creativity.

References

Albrecht, J. E., & O'Brien, E. J. (1993). Updating a mental model: Maintaining both local and global coherence. *Journal of Experimental Psychology: Learning, Memory, and Cognition, 19*, 1061–1070.

Amabile, T. M. (1983). The social psychology of creativity: A componential definition. *Journal of Personality and Social Psychology, 45*, 356–357.

Amabile, T. M., Barsade, S. G., Mueller, J. S., & Staw, B. M. (2005). Affect and creativity at work. *Administrative Science Quarterly, 50*, 367–403.

Ashby, F. G., Isen, A. M., & Turken, A. U. (1999). A neuropsychological theory of positive affect and its influence on cognition. *Psychological Review, 106*, 529–550.

Ashby, F. G., Valentin, V. V., & Turken, A. U. (2002). The effects of positive affect and arousal on working memory and executive attention: Neurobiology and computational models. In S. Moore & M. Oaksford (Eds.), *Emotional cognition: From brain to behavior* (pp. 245–287). Amsterdam: John Benjamins.

Baddeley, A. (1992). Working memory. *Science, 225*, 556–559.

Beeman, M. (1993). Semantic processing in the right hemisphere may contribute to drawing inferences. *Brain and Language, 44*, 80–120.

Beeman, M. (1998). Coarse semantic coding and discourse comprehension. In M. Beeman & C. Chiarello (Eds.), *Right hemisphere language comprehension: Perspectives from cognitive neuroscience* (pp. 255–284). Mahwah, NJ: Erlbaum.

Beeman, M., Friedman, R. B., Grafman, J., Perez, E., Diamond, S., & Lindsay, M. B. (1994). Summation priming and coarse semantic coding in the right hemisphere. *Journal of Cognitive Neuroscience, 6*, 26–45.

Bihrle, A. M., Brownell, H. H., Powelson, J. A., & Gardner, H. (1986). Comprehension of humorous and nonhumorous materials by left and right brain-damaged patients. *Brain and Cognition, 5*, 399–411.

Blanchette, I., & Richards, A. (2003). Anxiety and the interpretation of ambiguous information: Beyond the emotion-congruent effect. *Journal of Experimental Psychology: General, 132*, 294–309.

Bolte, A., Goschke, T., & Kuhl, J. (2003). Emotion and intuition: Effects of positive and negative mood on implicit judgments of semantic coherence. *Psychological Science, 14*, 416–421.

Bowden, E. M., & Jung-Beeman, M. (2003). Aha! Insight experience correlates with solution activation in the right hemisphere. *Psychonomic Bulletin and Review, 10*, 730–737.

Bowden, E. M., & Jung-Beeman, M. (1998). Getting the right idea: Semantic activation in the right hemisphere may help solve insight problems. *Psychological Science, 9*, 435–440.

Booth, J. R., Burman, D. D., Meyer, J. R., Gitelman, D. R., Parrish, T. B., & Mesulam, M. M. (2003). Relation between brain activation and lexical performance. *Human Brain Mapping, 19,* 155–169.

Brownell, H. H., Michel, D., Powelson, J. A., & Gardner, H. (1983). Surprise but not coherence: Sensitivity to verbal humor in right hemisphere patients. *Brain and Language, 18,* 20–27.

Brownell, H. H., Potter, H. H., Bihrle, A. M., & Gardner, H. (1986). Inference deficits in right brain-damaged patients. *Brain and Language, 29,* 310–321.

Bryan, T., & Bryan, J. (1991). Positive mood and math performance. *Journal of Learning Disabilities, 24,* 490–494.

Calvo, M. G., & Castillo, M. D. (2001a). Bias in predictive inferences during reading. *Discourse Processes, 32,* 43–71.

Calvo, M. G., & Castillo, M. D. (2001b). Selective interpretation in anxiety: Uncertainty for threatening events. *Cognition and Emotion, 15,* 299–320.

Carnevale, P. J. D., & Isen, A. M. (1986). The influence of positive affect and visual access on the discovery of integrative solutions in bilateral negotiation. *Organizational Behavior and Human Decision Processes, 37,* 1–13.

Chiarello, C. (1988). Lateralization of lexical processes in the normal brain: A review of visual half-field research. In H. A. Whitaker (Ed.), *Contemporary reviews in neuropsychology* (pp. 36–76). New York: Springer-Verlag.

Chiarello, C., Burgess, C., Gage, L., & Pollock, A. (1990). Semantic and associative priming in the cerebral hemispheres: Some words do, some words don't, . . . sometimes, some places. *Brain and Language, 38,* 75–104.

Chiarello, C., Welcome, S. E., Halderman, L. K., Towler, S., Julagay, J., Otto, R., & Leonard, C. M. (2009). A large-scale investigation of lateralization in cortical anatomy and word reading: Are there sex differences? *Neuropsychology, 23,* 210–222.

Coulson, S. (2001). *Semantic leaps: Frame-shifting and conceptual blending in meaning construction.* Cambridge: Cambridge University Press.

Coulson, S., & Williams, R. F. (2005). Hemispheric differences and joke comprehension. *Neuropsychologia, 43,* 128–141.

Coulson, S., & Wu, Y. C. (2005). Right hemisphere activation of joke-related information: An event-related brain potential study. *Journal of Cognitive Neuroscience, 17,* 494–506.

Dietrich, A. (2007). Who's afraid of a cognitive neuroscience of creativity? *Methods, 42,* 22–27.

Easterbrook, J. A. (1959). The effect of emotion on cue utilization and the organization of behavior. *Psychological Review, 66,* 183–201.

Eisenson, J. (1962). Language and intellectual modifications associated with right cerebral damage. *Language and Speech, 5,* 49–53.

Ellis, H. C., & Ashbrook, P. W. (1988). Resource allocation model of the effects of depressed mood states on memory. In K. Fiedler & J. Forgas (Eds.), *Affect, cognition and social behavior* (pp. 25–43). Toronto: Hogrefe.

Ellis, H. C., Ottaway, S. A., Varner, L. J., Becker, A. S., & Moore, B. A. (1997). Emotion, motivation, and text comprehension: The detection of contradictions in passages. *Journal of Experimental Psychology: General, 126,* 131–146.

Estrada, C. A., Isen, A. M., & Young, M. (1997). Positive affect facilitates integration of information and decreases anchoring in reasoning among physicians. *Organizational and Human Decision Processes, 72,* 117–135.

Eysenck, M. W., & Calvo, M. G. (1992). Anxiety and performance: The processing efficiency theory. *Cognition and Emotion, 6*, 409–434.

Federmeier, K. D., & Kutas, M. (1999). Right words and left words: Electrophysiological evidence for hemispheric differences in meaning processing. *Cognitive Brain Research, 8*, 373–392.

Federmeier, K. D., Kirson, D. A., Moreno, E. M., & Kutas, M. (2001). Effects of transient, mild mood states on semantic memory organization and use: An event-related potential investigation in humans. *Neuroscience Letters, 305*, 149–152.

Ferstl, E. C., Rinck, M., & von Cramon, Y. (2005). Emotional and temporal aspects of situation model processing during text comprehension: An event-related fMRI study. *Journal of Cognitive Neuroscience, 17*, 724–739.

Gasper, K., & Clore, G. L. (2002). Attending to the big picture: Mood and global versus local processing of visual information. *Psychological Science, 13*, 34–40.

Gibson, C., Folley, B. S., & Park, S. (2009). Enhanced divergent thinking and creativity in musicians: A behavioral and near-infrared spectroscopy study. *Brain and Cognition, 69*, 162–169.

Goel, V., & Dolan, R. J. (2001). The functional anatomy of humor: Segregating cognitive and affective components. *Nature Neuroscience, 4*, 237–238.

Grabner, R. H., Fink, A., & Neubauer, A. C. (2007). Brain correlates of self-rated originality of ideas: Evidence from event-related power and phase-locking changes in the EEG. *Behavioral Neuroscience, 121*, 224–230.

Graesser, A. C., Singer, M., & Trabasso, T. (1994). Constructing inferences during narrative text comprehension. *Psychological Review, 101*, 371–395.

Hough, M. S. (1990). Narrative comprehension in adults with right and left hemisphere brain-damage: Theme organization. *Brain and Language, 38*, 253–277.

Howard-Jones, P. A., Blakemore, S.-J., Samuel, E. A., Summers, I. R., & Claxton, G. (2005). Semantic divergence and creative story generation: An fMRI investigation. *Cognitive Brain Research, 25*, 240–250.

Hutsler, J., & Galuske, R. A. W. (2003). Hemispheric asymmetries in cerebral cortical networks. *Trends in Neurosciences, 26*, 429–435.

Isen, A. M., & Daubman, K. A. (1984). The influence of affect on categorization. *Journal of Personality and Social Psychology, 47*, 1206–1217.

Isen, A. M., Daubman, K. A., & Nowicki, G. P. (1987). Positive affect facilitates creative problem solving. *Journal of Personality and Social Psychology, 52*, 1122–1131.

Isen, A. M., Johnson, M. M., Mertz, E., & Robinson, G. F. (1985). The influence of positive affect on the unusualness of word associations. *Journal of Personality and Social Psychology, 48*, 1413–1426.

Jacob, R., Schall, M., & Scheibel, A. B. (1993). A quantitative dendritic analysis of Wernicke's area in humans. II. Gender, hemispheric, and environmental factors. *The Journal of Comparative Neurology, 327*, 97–111.

Jung-Beeman, M. (2005). Bilateral brain processes for comprehending natural language. *Trends in Cognitive Science, 9*, 512–518.

Jung-Beeman, M., Bowden, E. M., & Gernsbacher, M. A. (2000). Right and left hemisphere cooperation for drawing predictive and coherence inferences during normal story comprehension. *Brain and Language, 71*, 310–336.

Jung-Beeman, M., Bowden, E. M., Haberman, J., Frymiare, J. L., Arambel-Liu, S., Greenblatt, R., et al. (2004). Neural activity when people solve verbal problems with insight. *Public Library of Science – Biology, 2*, 500–510.

Kounios, J., & Beeman, M. (2009). The Aha! moment: The cognitive neuroscience of insight. *Current Directions in Psychological Science, 18,* 210–216.

Kounios, J., Fleck, J. I., Green, D. L., Payne, L., Stevenson, J. L., Bowden, E. M., et al. (2008). The origins of insight in resting-state brain activity. *Neuropsychologia, 46,* 281–291.

Kounios, J., Frymiare, J. L., Bowden, E. M., Fleck, J. I., Subramaniam, K., Parrish, T. B., et al. (2006). The prepared mind: Neural activity prior to problem presentation predicts subsequent solution by sudden insight. *Psychological Science, 17,* 882–890.

McDonald, S., & Wales, R. (1986). An investigation of the ability to process inferences in language following right hemisphere brain damage. *Brain and Language, 29,* 68–80.

Mason, R., & Just, M. (2004). How the brain processes causal inferences in text. *Psychological Science, 15,* 1–7.

Masters, J. C., Barden, C., & Ford, M. E. (1979). Affective states, expressive behavior, and learning in children. *Journal of Personality and Social Psychology, 37,* 380–390.

Metcalfe, J., & Weibe, D. (1987). Intuition in insight and noninsight problem solving. *Memory and Cognition, 15,* 238–246.

Mirous, H. J., & Beeman, M. (submitted). Mood makes or breaks meaning? Mood modulation of inference priming during story comprehension.

Molloy, R., Brownell, H. H., & Gardner, H. (1988). Discourse comprehension by right hemisphere stroke patients: Deficits of prediction and revision. In Y. Joanette & H. H. Brownell (Eds.), *Discourse ability and brain damage: Theoretical and empirical perspectives* (pp. 113–130). New York: Springer.

Richards, A., French, C. C., Keogh, E., & Carter, C. (2000). Test-anxiety, inferential reasoning and working memory load. *Anxiety, Stress and Coping, 13,* 87–109.

Rowe, G., Hirsh, J. B., & Anderson, A. K. (2007). Positive affect increases the breadth of attentional selection. *Proceedings of the National Academy of Science of the United States of America (PNAS), 104,* 383–388.

St George, M., Kutas, M., Martinez, A., & Sereno, M. I. (1999). Semantic integration in reading: Engagement of the right hemisphere during discourse processing. *Brain, 122,* 1317–1325.

St George, M., Mannes, S., & Hoffman, J. E. (1997). Individual differences in inference generation: An ERP analysis. *Journal of Cognitive Neuroscience, 9,* 776–788.

Scheibel, A. B., Fried, I., Paul, L., Forsythe, A., Tomiyasu, U., Wechsler, A., et al. (1985). Differentiating characteristics of the human speech cortex: A quantitative Golgi study. In D. F. Benson & E. Zaidel (Eds.), *The dual brain: Hemispheric specialization in humans* (pp. 65–74). New York: Guilford Press.

Seldon, H. L. (1981). Structure of human auditory cortex. II. Cytoarchitectonics and dendritic distributions. *Brain Research, 229,* 277–294.

Semmes, J. (1968). Hemispheric specialization: A possible clue to mechanism. *Neuropsychologia, 6,* 11–26.

Sharp, D. J., Scott, S. K., & Wise, R. J. S. (2004). Retrieving meaning after temporal lobe infarction: The role of the basal language area. *Annals of Neurology, 56,* 836–846.

Sheth, B. R., Sandkühler, S., & Bhattacharya, J. (2009). Posterior beta and anterior gamma predict cognitive insight. *Journal of Cognitive Neuroscience, 21,* 1269–1279.

Singer, M. (2007). Inference processing in discourse comprehension. In G. Gaskell (Ed.), *Oxford handbook of psycholinguistics* (pp. 343–359). New York: Oxford University Press.

Subramaniam, K., Parrish, T., Kounios, J., & Jung-Beeman, M. (2009). A brain mechanism for facilitation of insight by positive affect. *Journal of Cognitive Neuroscience, 21,* 415–432.

Tardif, E., & Clarke, S. (2001). Intrinsic connectivity of human auditory areas: A tracing study with Dil. *European Journal of Neuroscience, 13*, 1045–1050.

Thompson-Schill, S. L., D'Esposito, M., Aguirre, G. K., & Farah, M. J. (1997). Role of left inferior prefrontal cortex in retrieval of semantic knowledge: A re-evaluation. *Proceedings of the National Academy of Science, 94*, 14792–14797.

Tompkins, C. A., Fassbinder, W., Blake, M. O., Baumgaertner, A., & Jayaram, N. (2004). Inference generation during text comprehension by adults with right hemisphere brain damage: Activation failure versus multiple activation. *Journal of Speech, Language, and Hearing Research, 47*, 1380–1395.

Tucker, D. M., Roth, D. L., & Blair, T. B. (1986). Functional connections among cortical regions: Topography of EEG coherence. *Electroencephalography Clinical Neurophysiology, 63*, 242–250.

Virtue, S., Haberman, J., Clancy, Z., Parrish, T., & Jung-Beeman, M. (2006). Neural activity of inferences during story comprehension. *Brain Research, 1084*, 104–114.

Virtue, S., Parrish, T., & Beeman, M. (2008). Inferences during story comprehension: Cortical recruitment affected by predictability of events and working memory capacity. *Journal of Cognitive Neuroscience, 20*, 2274–2284.

Wallas, G. (1926). *The art of thought.* New York: Franklin Watts.

Yasutake, D., & Bryan, T. (1995). The influence of affect on the achievement and behavior of students with learning disabilities. *Journal of Learning Disabilities, 28*, 329–334.

Zhang, J. X., Feng, C., Fox, P. T., Gao, J., & Tan, L. H. (2004). Is left inferior frontal gyrus a general mechanism for selection? *NeuroImage, 23*, 596–603.

Zwaan, R. A., & Rapp, D. N. (2006). Discourse Comprehension. In M. J. Traxler & M. A. Gernsbacher (Eds.), *Handbook of Psycholinguistics, Second Edition* (pp. 725–764). Amsterdam: Elsevier, Inc.

17

Two-Track Mind: Formulaic and Novel Language Support a Dual-Process Model

Diana Van Lancker Sidtis

This chapter presents a historical and critical survey of phraseology, the study of formulaic language, in the context of analytic, experimental, and biological approaches. It begins with Weinreich's (1969) early reluctance to explore the topic in a scholarly way and follows a circuitous path through linguistic, psychological, and neurological studies, culminating in current views of formulaic language as an integral component of speech performance and language competence (Fillmore, 1979; Locke & Bogin, 2006; Pawley & Syder, 1983). Linguistic and psychological studies have grappled with the question of whether idioms (as a prime example of a formulaic expression) are best described as compositional, i.e., composed of constituent parts, or unitary, i.e., processed as whole units. The preponderance of the evidence supports a *dual-process model of language*, whereby novel expressions and formulaic expressions differ essentially in how they are learned or acquired, stored, and processed (Kempler & Van Lancker, 1993; Kuiper, 2009; Van Lancker Sidtis, 1973, 2004, 2008; Wray & Perkins, 2000). Novel expressions are made up of lexical items assembled by grammatical rules; these communicate new information. In contrast, formulaic expressions, known in their unitary shape to the language user, are acquired and processed according to unique properties. Biological studies provide strong evidence for this distinction, as damage to different brain areas produces different effects on the two modes of language, novel (or propositional) and formulaic (Van Lancker Sidtis, Kempler, Ahn, & Yang, 2011). It is the purpose of this chapter to describe and clarify this distinction.

The Handbook of the Neuropsychology of Language, First Edition. Edited by Miriam Faust.
© 2012 Blackwell Publishing Ltd. Published 2012 by Blackwell Publishing Ltd.

Background

Before the advent of generative grammar, a little-known field study laboriously documented actual use of proverbs by citizens in a small German village over a period of three years (Hain, 1951). More recently, with the advent of computerized corpora of spoken and written language, more information about the presence of formulaic expressions in natural discourse has been gained (Aijmer, 1996; Altenberg, 1998; Fellbaum, 2002; Moon, 1998). However, serious scientific attention to formulaic expressions has evolved slowly. In a 1969 book chapter entitled "Problems in the analysis of idioms" (published two years after his demise in 1967), the linguist Uriel Weinreich apologized for taking up "so unfashionable a topic," that for many "would surely smack of the most outlandish romanticism" (p. 23). How the scholarly world has changed in 40 years! Since then, hundreds of serious articles touching on the structure and use of idioms have appeared. (Entering "idiom studies" as a Google search term in October 2009 yielded 1,720,000 links; entering "formulaic language" brings up 532,000.) Now, formulaic language, the broader rubric which encompasses idioms as well as an extremely large array of other fixed, familiar expressions, is a legitimate field of study (e.g., Coulmas, 1994; Sidtis, 2011; Van Lancker, 1988, 1994; Van Lancker Sidtis, 2008, 2010; Wray, 2002).

Description of Formulaic Expressions

Describing formulaic expressions is simple but not easy. Simply put, they differ from all other utterances in that they are not novel – not newly created. It is not so easy to provide a comprehensive description to such a heterogeneous set (Figure 17.1). The properties of formulaic expressions – stereotyped form, conventionalized meaning, and appropriate, contextual usage conditions – are known to the native speaker. Stereotyped form includes word order and specific lexical composition as well as phonetic, prosodic, and vocal features that typically appear with a given formulaic expression. Although the canonical version, or "formuleme," has its signature stereotyped form, in actual usage most formulaic expressions are modified. It can undergo word addition, morphemic alteration, and various kinds of constituent movement. A speaker utilizing a formuleme will take care that it remains recognizable. This is the constraint governing flexibility. (The many studies devoted to the question of formulaic expression flexibility will be summarized below.) Prosodic shape, including intonation, voice quality, and phonetic detail, is usually specified. The expression *I wouldn't want to be in his shoes* must have a sentence accent on the next to last word. The wildly popular *What-ever!* favored by younger speakers features an aspirated voiceless stop and hyperarticulated syllables. Often formulaic expressions must be spoken with specialized vocal material to make the grade: the American comedian Steve Martin's *Well, excuse me!* and, from a popular dialect in New York, *Fuggedaboudit* (*Forget about it*) come to mind.

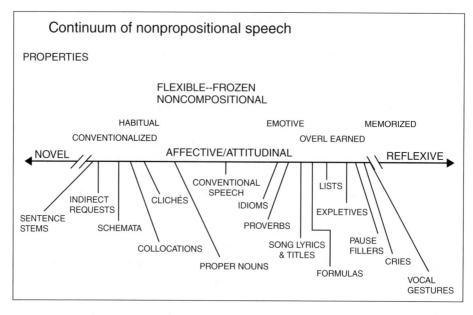

Figure 17.1　Schematic continuum of "nonpropositional speech," currently known as formulaic expressions, from most reflexive to most novel. Properties of expressions are listed above the line. It is proposed that as routinized motor gestures, formulaic expressions rely in large part on basal ganglia. Since they are holistic, affective, and context-bound, formulaic expressions require an intact right hemisphere for normal performance.

Conventionalized meaning in formulaic utterances refers to a range of nonstandard, nonliteral semantic relations. These expressions signal a complex meaning structure that reaches beyond the usual lexical meanings. Idioms – *Keep a stiff upper lip, Wears her fingers to the bone* – meet this criterion by definition. Most conversational speech formulas also fit this description: saying *Right* in a conversational turn does not necessarily mean that the previous utterance was deemed to be correct, but merely acknowledges the turn, or it may be a sarcastic comment. The meaning of saying *Have a nice day* is a primarily social one. *Can it be true?* uttered in conversation, is not literally or grammatically a question, but is an expression of surprise. Semantic ingredients that are nearly always present in the complex meaning structure of formulaic expressions, including idioms and speech formulas, are evaluative, attitudinal, and affective connotations. On the one hand, a novel utterance can be neutral. *The cat is lying on the couch* gives no clue about anyone's opinion, feeling, or judgment about the sentence content. Almost any idiom or speech formula, on the other hand, carries precisely these kinds of nuances: *Just in the nick of time* (tension, relief); *It's way over my head* (exasperation, confusion); *Where have you been all my life?* (affirmation, compliment), *I met someone* (intrigue, excitement) and so on.

The third property, the sociolinguistic or appropriate contextual usage conditions governing the use of formulaic expressions, is probably the most subtle. Circumstances surrounding the communication, in which the formula appears, must have specific characteristics to constitute native usage. Fine-grained and detailed contingencies of formality, register, and social context adhere to the utterances and cause them to stand out when these are violated. Sometimes it is difficult to say why a formulaic expression isn't "right" in that discourse unit. Often those that are not right in contextual terms are generated by second-language speakers. These contextual errors can be heard in international interviews and diplomatic presentations. (Second-language speakers are also apt to err in details of stereotyped form or conventionalized meaning, as is well understood in second-language learning studies; Weinert, 1995).

These three properties, stereotyped form, conventionalized meaning, and contextual conditions characterize the formulaic utterance and belong to it, as part of language competence, and are all known to the speaker/listener. This personal knowledge can be viewed as the fourth property. Familiarity in the form of memorial knowledge, which belongs to every formulaic expression, is the least discussed by speech scientists. Yet language users know these expressions along with their properties (Bell & Healey, 1992; Jackendoff, 1994). What is meant by saying that speakers *know* the expression? This fact is abundantly obvious in the world around us, for example, in newspaper advertisements and headlines. In a recent example in a home-town paper, advertising copy by a group called *careerbuilder.com* trumpets a headline: "We have over 600,000 jobs." Under this statement two lines appear: "One of them is right for you. Heck, dozens are right for you." The addition of "heck," a speech formula in the form of an expletive, indicates knowledge of normal usage by the advertisement's writer and expectation by the writer of like knowledge in the readership. Further, this stylistic turn appeals to a conversational, intimate level of discourse.

In many cases, humor is constructed around the play between literal and idiomatic meanings of ditropic expressions – sentences and phrases that allow for both a literal and an idiomatic interpretation, such as "The coast is clear." A high proportion of cartoon humor is made up of precisely this specialized kind of pun. In a cartoon by Barsotti, for example, a king, opening a present with a look of surprise at the contents of the box, says "Why, this is fit for me!" Again, this, like so many other efforts at humor, illustrates that the readership of the magazine in which the cartoon appeared (*The New Yorker*) is familiar with ditropic ambiguity, and that the readers will recognize the allusion to the formulaic expression *This is fit for a king*. It is only because of these two features – the ditropic pun and familiarity with the underlying formulaic expression – that the cartoon achieves humor.

There is evidence from many sources that speakers are familiar with a large array of formulaic expressions. Anecdotally, listeners smile and nod on hearing lists of these expressions. Native speakers explicitly endorse knowing them. In class at the university, for example, students quickly understand the notion of formulaic expressions and immediately begin contributing examples (Van Lancker Sidtis, 2011). This is a very natural, easy concept for language users. In addition, formal studies have shown that people identify formulaic expressions when presented with lists randomized with novel expressions (Van Lancker Sidtis & Rallon, 2006).

The four factors – form, meaning, context, and personal knowledge – distinguish formulaic expressions in principle and practice from novel ones, and lead to the proposal that formulaic and novel language are qualitatively different from the points of view of linguistic analysis and speaker performance. First to be reviewed in this chapter are linguistic studies, which consider formal, structural properties. As some of these questions are addressed by probing speakers' responses, linguistic studies morph into psycholinguistic approaches, which measure users' performance. Finally, the review proceeds to evidence from neurological disorders that show how formulaic and novel language are stored and processed according to disparate cerebral mechanisms.

Linguistic and Psycholinguistic Studies of Formulaic Expressions

A burning question in linguistic approaches has always been: What is a structural descriptive approach to formulaic expressions? Attempts to answer these questions have utilized analytic tools as well as psychological testing. Two camps have jousted back and forth between presenting analytic solutions and proposing that formulaic expressions are unitary, similar to lexical items (Titone & Connine, 1999). Weinreich's (1969) treatment of idioms proposed a structural-analytic solution which was not viable. Some scholars then classified the idiom as a fixed lexical item (Heringer, 1976; Swinney & Cutler, 1979), while others continued to consider idioms as a compositional (Burt, 1992; Gibbs, 1980, 1994), positing various degrees of "frozenness" in idioms (Gibbs, Nayak, & Cutting, 1989). Structural descriptions were presented about flexibility versus frozenness, compositionality and semantic transparency (Cacciari & Tabossi, 1988, 1993; Estill & Kemper, 1982; Gibbs & Gonzales, 1985; Nunberg, Sag, & Wasow, 1994). Fraser (1970) proposed that the alleged relative fixedness of idioms was related to which transformations they could undergo. Some time later, Cutler (1982) suggested that the proposed frozenness parameter reflected the age of the expression. Subsequent studies of aphasic speakers showed no effect of a frozenness parameter in performance on idiom recognition (Papagno & Genoni, 2004).

Comprehension studies: how do listeners process idioms?

Using idioms, speakers convey ideas and emotions using words that do not refer to their usual lexical meanings. *She's skating on thin ice* can be said without referring to skating or ice, but to convey the idea of risky behavior. Three models proposed to explain this are literal-first (serial) processing, literal and idiomatic (parallel) processing, and direct access of idiomatic meaning. Bobrow and Bell (1973) proposed that idioms are lexical items stored in memory and that upon encountering an idiom, the comprehension device first attempts a literal interpretation. After failing, the idiom retrieval mode kicks in and the idiom is selected from the look-up list. Thus, serial processing predicts greater response time latencies for idioms than for literal utterances because literal interpretation is the first step in any language task. However, studies revealed that visual classification was faster for idioms than for matched literal phrases (Swinney & Cutler, 1979), suggesting that idiomatic meaning is processed in parallel with literal meaning, and that idioms are stored and retrieved whole.

The question remains as to how fixed expressions can undergo syntactic modifications and maintain their pragmatic identity and conventionalized meaning. For example, one could say *For years, she had been totally skating on really the thinnest ice,* and listeners, depending on context, could assume the nonliteral meaning, as examined in indirect questions (Gibbs, 1981). Experimental approaches to these questions involve measuring production errors, response time, accuracy in recall and recognition memory tasks, and various kinds of rating surveys (Gibbs & Gonzales, 1985; Gibbs, Nayak, Bolton, & Keppel, 1989). The various findings of syntactic and lexical flexibility have led to hybrid psycholinguistic models (Cacciari & Tabossi, 1988; Smolka, Rabanus, & Rösler, 2007), which integrate both literal-first and idiomatic-only approaches. However, the heterogeneity of formulaic expressions and the variety of flexible variants have defied linguistic description in credible structural terms (Hillert & Swinney, 2001). This stalemate can be resolved by considering the notion of the *formuleme,* which is the canonical form of the expression known to the speaker and can be manipulated using grammatical rules.

Support for the psycholinguistic distinction between formulaic and novel expressions comes from the fact that native speakers distinguish idiomatic from literal expressions on the basis of the auditory signal alone in both production and perception. An early study by Lieberman (1963) revealed different articulatory patterns for words when produced in a formulaic or novel context. Van Lancker and Canter (1981) demonstrated that listeners could distinguish literal from idiomatic meanings of ditropic sentences (those with balanced ambiguity between literal and idiomatic meanings, such as "It broke the ice") produced by native speakers, without benefit of other context, and acoustic analyses indicated that pitch contours, pausing, and word length were significantly involved in distinguishing the meanings (Van Lancker, Canter, & Terbeek, 1981). Recently, similar studies were conducted on Korean ditropic sentences. When the sentences were auditorily presented singly or in pairs, native listeners of Korean were able to discriminate between idiomatic and literal meanings. In a second task, listeners provided goodness ratings for each utterance, indicating to what extent each item was a good idiomatic or literal exemplar. There was a significant correlation between recognition performance and goodness ratings, reflecting listeners' knowledge of these categories. Acoustic analysis indicated that literal sentences had significantly longer durations and duration variations, while idiomatic sentences were characterized by greater variation in intensity.

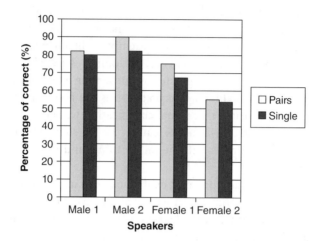

Figure 17.2 Performance results for Korean ditropic sentences in the listening study, in which utterances were heard singly and as randomized pairings. Listeners successfully recognized idiomatic and literal meanings by 3 of the 4 speakers. The first 3 speakers were born and raised in Korean. The fourth speaker (second female) had spent 3 years in early childhood in the US.

Another significant difference was seen in the last two syllables of sentences: idiomatic sentences featured rising fundamental frequency contour significantly more often, while literal sentences were produced with falling fundamental frequency contour (Figure 17.2).

These results indicate that literal and idiomatic utterances have a separate status and that acoustic cues serve to distinguish them. These findings more generally support the notion that propositional and formulaic language form different categories in grammatical competence. Further support for this view comes from studies showing that people remember idioms as chunks rather than composite forms (Horowitz & Manelis, 1973; Osgood & Hoosain, 1974; Pickens & Pollio, 1979; Simon, 1974), a result also obtained for Chinese idioms (Simon, Zhang, Zang, & Peng, 1989).

Production studies in normal speakers

Several creative approaches to studying the production of formulaic expressions have been designed. Speech-error elicitation experiments showed that idioms are not devoid of information about their syntactic and semantic structure (Cutting & Bock, 1997). Interference in the form of blending errors – *The way the cookie bounces; It's not rocket surgery! Well, that's all water over the bridge* – was more likely to occur between idioms sharing the same syntactic form, and the resultant word substitutions were in the same grammatical class. Indeed, during speech production, speakers can discern grammatical form and lexical meaning in these expressions, and hence syntactic and semantic operations can be performed on any formulaic expression. However, the properties of formulaic expressions reviewed above – stereotyped form, conventionalized meanings, conditions of use, and familiarity – must all be recognized in a veridical model of language competence. These facts about formulaic expressions are revealed in surveys, sentence completion studies, and word association studies (Clark, 1970; Van Lancker Sidtis & Rallon, 2004). A series of idiom production experiments by Sprenger (2003) using a priming paradigm addressed these questions. These studies yielded the notion of *superlemma*, which corresponds to the idea proposed in this article of canonical form or *formuleme*. Similarly, more extensive analysis of speech errors involving idioms derived from a very large database suggests that "idioms are both compositional and noncompositional at the same time, at different levels of processing" (Kuiper, van Egmond, Kempen, & Sprenger, 2007, p. 324). This super-lemma or formuleme is stored and processed as a whole, but because it contains syntactic and semantic information of various kinds (as does any linguistic entity in the speaker's repertory), it can link to other parts of the lexicon and grammar. These and other studies lead to the perspective that formulaic and novel language exist side by side.

Dual-process model of language competence

The dual-processing model states that formulaic expressions, which by definition have stereotyped form, conventionalized meanings, contextual constraints, and familiarity to a language community (Kitzinger, 2000), exist in harmony with the grammar, which consists of rules and a lexicon (Lounsbury, 1963). Inconsistencies arising from idiom studies can be explained by the normal interplay of formulaic and novel processing, such that formulaic expressions, depending on the intent and verbal creativity of the speaker, can be altered using standard grammatical processes. The interesting point is not that formulaic expressions can be semantically transparent and composed and are therefore alterable, but that there is a *known entity to analyze and to alter*.

Cerebral Processing: Comprehension Studies

Although the original observations on preserved automatic speech were made in the speech of persons with severe aphasia, most experimental studies of brain processing related to this topic address *comprehension* of *idioms*. Early such studies identified the right hemisphere as involved. Using frozen metaphors such as *heavy heart* in a picture matching task, Winner and Gardner (1977) found that persons with right hemisphere damage performed poorly. A similar result was obtained later using a similar picture matching task for recognition of idioms and speech formulas (Kempler & Van Lancker, 1996), called the Familiar and Novel Language Comprehension test (FANL-C). In this protocol, 20 formulaic expressions, such as *I'd like to give you a piece of my mind*, are matched with 20 novel expressions, each with four line drawings provided for a pointing response. Studies using this protocol indicate greater deficits in recognizing formulaic expressions than novel expressions following right hemisphere damage, with the converse observed in left hemisphere damage (Kempler & Van Lancker, 1993; Kempler, Van Lancker, Marchman & Bates, 1999; Van Lancker & Kempler, 1987). Broader research has suggested that appreciation of social and linguistic context is also diminished in right hemisphere damage (Brownell, Gardner, Prather, & Martino, 1995; Gardner, Brownell, Wapner, & Michelow, 1983; Joanette & Brownell, 1990); these qualities are called upon for successful processing of formulaic language. However, a few recent articles highlight a role of the left hemisphere in comprehension of idioms with less evidence attaching to a significant involvement of the right hemisphere (Papagno & Genoni, 2004; Papagno, Tabossi, Colombo, & Zampetti, 2004; see also Cacciari & Papagno, Volume 1, Chapter 18). Some of these discrepancies may be attributed to the different task demands in processing the material (Kacinek & Chiarello, 2007; Papagno & Caporali, 2007). Further, it has often been observed that both hemispheres participate in a given cognitive function but may do so using different strategies (Drews, 1987; Bogen, 1969). The finding that persons with right hemisphere damage performed better than the left-brain-damaged group on idiom recognition is difficult to interpret, given the weight of other findings about right and left hemisphere functions (Papagno, Curti, Rizzo, Crippa, & Colombo, 2006). Severity, location, and size of lesions may differ importantly in groups studied. Presence or absence of subcortical damage has been seen to influence cognitive performance, but only recently have contributions of subcortical structures been considered; these are reviewed in the production section below. In a creative comprehension study using functional brain imaging, passive listening to affective-prosodic interjections, a primitive version of formulaic expressions, elicited bilateral temporal as well as subcortical activation (Dietrich, Hertrich, Alter, Ischebeck, & Ackermann, 2008).

Production studies in neurological disorders

Whether there is an underlying language ability that equally supports comprehension and production of language remains a debated question in most realms of the language sciences (see review in Van Lancker Sidtis, 2006). Earlier theories utilized the notion of the ideal speaker–hearer, for whom general grammatical knowledge could be assumed and described. However, in performance, as is well known from studies of aphasia, striking differences in ability to produce novel utterances are observed in production compared to comprehension. This dissociation is also true for formulaic language. In some cases, production of formulaic language is preserved alongside impaired performance in comprehension, and the reverse is also seen. Formulaic language abilities are dissociated in comprehension and production modes.

Cerebral participation in novel and formulaic speech production   As is well known, production of novel utterances engages left-sided cortical areas of the brain including the inferior frontal gyrus (Broca's area), sensorimotor strip, and supplementary motor area via the neural pathways described above, aroused by the reticular formation and the aqueductal grey matter in the brainstem, exchanging commands via the pyramidal and extrapyramidal tracts to the peripheral nervous system (cranial and spinal nerves). Auditory monitoring is enabled by the superior temporal gyrus. Complex motor gestures are executed and monitored by the basal ganglia with participation by the limbic system, which modulates emotion. Integration of motor speech gestures is aided by the thalamus and the cerebellum, especially the right cerebellum. Integration of cortical and subcortical systems, coordinating cognitive and affective streams of information, characterizes all communicative performance (Panksepp, 2003). Damage to any of these structures may interfere with production of spontaneous, novel language.

Modern notions of formulaic language arise from earlier discussions surrounding the phenomenon of "automatic speech" as consistently observed in aphasia. The term "automatic speech" (Hughlings Jackson, 1874) indexed preserved vocalizations in severe neurogenic language deficit, including emotional outbursts, swearing, *yes*, and *no*, among many others. The terms "voluntary" and "propositional" were used to refer to contrasting novel or newly created utterances. The dichotomy has also been seen as corresponding to conscious versus nonconscious, routinized versus constructed, or holistic versus combinatorial. A closer look at the use of these expressions brings more confusion than clarity. "Low level" grammatical processes in spontaneous speech, such as subject–verb agreement, proceed automatically. On the other hand, emotional utterances may be voluntarily produced and human speech is imbued with affect (Panksepp, 2003). Recurrent, nonlinguistic aphasic utterances (such as *bi di bi di*) can be delivered "voluntarily." Comparisons with nonhuman communication are not enlightening. Research in nonhuman animals indicates that calls may be produced with referential and intentional content (Cheney & Seyfarth, 1980, 1990; Marler, 1998). In humans, reflexive and volitional control systems join to produce vocal sound, and volitional control of activity involves both cortical and subcortical systems (Ludlow, 2005). Therefore, while much of formulaic language derives from categories subsumed under the previous rubric "automatic speech," current use favors the newer, generic term.

Formulaic (formerly automatic) speech, comprising over-learned, recited, and/ or emotional utterances of various kinds, including counting, speech formulas (salutations and conversational fillers), swearing, nursery rhymes, familiar lyrics and familiar songs, and all other such expressions known by native speakers (see Figure 17.1; Code, 1994; Hughlings Jackson, 1874; Van Lancker, 1993; Van Lancker & Cummings, 1999; Wray, 2002; Wray & Perkins, 2000) depend on neurological mechanisms that differ from spontaneous speech. There is evidence for significant right hemisphere control modulation of production of formulaic expressions beyond the centuries-old observation of preserved automatic speech in aphasia following left hemisphere damage. (Some have insisted that intact left hemisphere structures are modulating any residual speech.) A dramatic demonstration comes from a postsurgical interview of a normally developing, right-handed adult who underwent left hemispherectomy for treatment of brain cancer (Van Lancker & Cummings, 1999). The subject was profoundly aphasic, but produced residual speech consisting of well-articulated expletives (*goddammit*), pause fillers (*well, uh*), and sentence stems (*I can't, that's a*), all classical examples of formulaic speech. He also performed pragmatically appropriate gestures, such as sighing, laughing, and *tsk*. Further support arises from mouth asymmetry studies, showing greater left-sided openings for counting and greater right-sided opening for word generation in aphasic subjects (Graves & Landis, 1985).

A controlled study indicated superior processing of formulaic compared to matched novel speech production tasks in aphasic subjects in all but the repetition tasks (Lum & Ellis, 1999). A similar, more extensive design examined performance of unilaterally brain-damaged subjects on repetition, sentence completion, and comprehension tasks (spoken and written) involving matched formulaic (idioms and speech formulas) and novel expressions (Van Lancker Sidtis et al., 2011). Significant differences for utterance types were found for sentence completion (Figure 17.3) and for comprehension using the FANL-C, replicating earlier findings

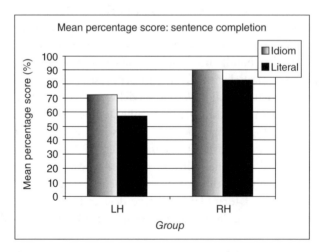

Figure 17.3 Mean percentage correct responses for the sentence completion task is seen on the vertical (Y) axis. Responses on idioms are compared with matched novel utterances using the Comprehension Nonliteral Language Protocol (Van Lancker Sidtis et al., 2010). Left hemisphere (LH) damaged subjects completed significantly more idioms than literal (novel) utterances; performance on the two tasks did not differ significantly for right hemisphere (RH) damaged subjects.

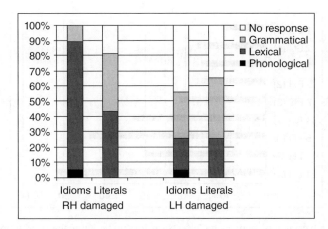

Figure 17.4 Right (RH) and left hemisphere (LH) damaged subjects show different error patterns on sentence completion for idiomatic and novel (literal) exemplars. The right hemisphere group made more lexical errors, suggesting deficient processing of formulaic language.

(Kempler & Van Lancker, 1996). Repetition accuracies for formulaic and novel utterances did not differ overall, but the left and right hemisphere damaged groups showed different error profiles, with the right hemisphere group committing more lexical errors on idiom repetition (Figure 17.4). These results support the claim for different cerebral representation of formulaic and novel language, but indicate that the contrast is best revealed not in repetition, but when tasks resemble spontaneous speech. (Recent studies have revealed significant differences in speech measures for spontaneous and repeated modes – Kempler, & Van Lancker, 2002; Sidtis, Rogers, Godier, Tagliati, & Sidtis, 2010 – further supporting the notion that meaningful differences between formulaic and novel speech are better sought in spontaneous than in repeated or read speech.) In a related study, left- and right-brain-damaged persons differed in producing the contrasts in ditropic sentences (those with either an idiomatic or literal meaning), in that contrastive timing cues were more successfully executed by the right hemisphere damaged group (Belánger, Baum, & Titone, 2009).

Other approaches have examined the incidence of formulaic expressions in the spontaneous speech of persons with neurogenic disease. Discourse studies using speech of persons who had suffered left or right hemisphere stroke revealed that, compared to normal speakers, the proportion of formulaic language was significantly lower following right hemisphere damage and significantly higher in patients with left hemisphere damage and aphasia (Van Lancker Sidtis & Postman, 2006; Speech samples A and B, Appendix I). In a later study, a left hemisphere damaged subject with transcortical sensory aphasia, whose semantic deficit was profound, yielded the highest proportion of formulaic expressions (Speech sample C, Appendix I), while proportions of formulaic language in two right hemisphere damaged

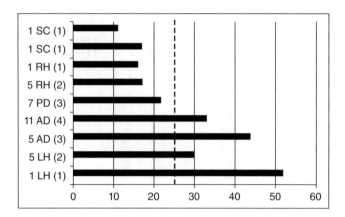

Figure 17.5 Overview of neurogenic effects on formulaic language production from four discourse studies, showing proportions of words in formulaic expressions on the horizontal axis and patients on the vertical axis (SC = subcortical damage; RH = right hemisphere damage; LH = left hemisphere damage). Results are taken from single case and group studies (first number indicates number of subjects in study). Number in parenthesis refers to publications: (1) Sidtis et al. (2009); (2) Van Lancker Sidtis and Postman (2006); (3) Rogers et al. (2010); (4) Bridges and Sidtis (2010). The dotted line represents an average from 24 age- and education-matched normal-control subjects. Here it can be seen that subcortical and right hemisphere damage results in a lower proportion of words in formulaic expressions, while Alzheimer's disease and left hemisphere damage is associated with a larger proportion of words in formulaic expressions.

subjects were low, in agreement with the group study above (Sidtis, Canterucci, & Katsnelson, 2009; Figure 17.5).

In functional brain imaging studies in humans, bilateral activation for both propositional and selected types of formulaic speech (counting, Pledge of Allegiance) has been reported (Blank, Scott, Murphy, Warburton, & Wise, 2002; Bookheimer, Zeffiro, Blaxton, Gaillard, & Theodore, 2000). These and similar inconsistencies between robust, often-replicated findings from the clinical lesion literature and imaging results indicate that functional imaging results must be interpreted with caution (see review by J. Sidtis, 2007). In contrast, in another brain imaging study, measures of cerebral blood flow for naming and counting differed. Using partial least squares analysis of PET (positron emission tomography) regional cerebral blood flow, Van Lancker, McIntosh, and Grafton (2003) identified three latent variables as naming-vocalization, naming, and counting. The first two latent variables were significantly associated with Broca's area and the third corresponded with diffuse representation and basal ganglia sites.

Subcortical contribution to formulaic language   Previous decades emphasized the human cortex as the mediator of the higher cognitive functions unique to humans, highlighting language as an exclusively human function with primarily cortical representation. Recently, significant functionality for human behavior is attributed to basal ganglia/limbic systems (Lieberman, 2002), the mediators of motoric and emotional behaviors (Marsden, 1982; Panksepp, 1998, 2003). Recent studies reveal an important contribution of the basal ganglia to initiation, execution, and monitoring of human speech and language (MacLean, 1990; Marsden, 1982). Unique kinds of learning are associated with the basal ganglia (Graybiel, 1998; Knowlton, Mangels, & Squire, 1996); these include acquisition and execution of gestures that are compatible with processing of formulaic expressions.

The limbic system, in integration with basal ganglia structures, modulates mood, emotion, attention, and arousal. Affective functions are held to have a status in human behaviors as valued as cognitive functions: "A proper neuronal conceptualization of affective processes may be essential for making sense out of many brain functions" (Panksepp & Burgdorf, 2003, p. 536). Emotional vocalizations in humans and in nonhuman animals are likely the result of coordinated activity in limbic-basal ganglia nuclei. As mentioned above, formulaic expressions typically incorporate affective and attitudinal nuances. As will be discussed below, some have associated formulaic expressions with emotional cries in human and nonhuman vocalization.

Clinical and experimental evidence suggests a role of subcortical nuclei in production of formulaic language (Van Lancker Sidtis, 2004). In three published cases, subcortical damage led to significantly reduced incidence of formulaic expressions (Sidtis et al., 2009; Speedie, Wertman, T'air, & Heilman, 1993; see Figure 17.5; Speech sample C in Appendix I). Other studies show impoverished production of formulaic expression in Parkinson's disease, an illness of the basal ganglia (Illes, Metter, Hanson, & Iritani, 1988; Rogers, Sidtis, & Sidtis, 2010). Conversely, dysfunction of the basal ganglia/limbic system in persons with Tourette's syndrome is associated with hyperstimulated incidence of expletives (coprolalia; see Van Lancker & Cummings, 1999). In humans, formulaic and emotional vocalizations occurred when subcortical sites were electrically stimulated during stereotaxic surgical techniques, usually for treatment of epilepsy (Petrovici, 1980; Schaltenbrand, 1965). During a functional magnetic resonance imaging (fMRI) study using a naming task, instead of correctly naming pictures depicting *drown*, *yelling*, *clapping*, and so on, some subjects emitted formulaic expression, such as *help*, *yay*, and *hey*. In this study, right sided and subcortical structures showed an activation response that was not present when the correct action names were produced (Postman-Caucheteux, 2007).

Formulaic utterances in an evolutionary perspective   Formulaic utterances bear a resemblance to animal calls, and thus may offer clues to the evolution of vocal control mechanisms (Code, 2005; Wray, 2000). Animal vocalization indicates warnings and facilitates social interactions. Similarly, some formulaic language in humans, such as swearing and other interjections, are likely mediated by limbic system structures and, presumably, were originally intended to perform the social functions of repulsing intruders and expressing anger and dissatisfaction. In humans, the older system may continue to perform, in ways only partially understood, in singing and in emotional and routinized vocal behaviors.

Thus it has been proposed that emotional and over-learned utterances foreshadowed human language (Code, 2005; Wray, 1998, 2000). Indeed, there is evidence of a hierarchical system that has evolved, consisting at an earlier period of emotional responses mediated by subcortical nuclei and modulated through right hemisphere cortical networks, and having an essential relationship to modern day formulaic expressions (Jaynes, 1976; Van Lancker, 1979). It has long been known that while human language is cortically represented, animal vocalizations can be elicited only by stimulation of subcortical nuclei (Jürgens, 2002; Ploog, 1975). Some scholars have proposed that subcortical structures, which are evolutionarily "old," have also (in addition to cortical lobes) been highly elaborated in the human (Lieberman, 2002). In this view, routinized vocal behaviors occur as species-specific vocalizations in nonhuman mammals, and survive in humans as emotional and formulaic vocalizations. Either alongside the emotional systems or arising out of them, depending on one's viewpoint, are combinatorial systems, seen only in humans and modulated by left hemisphere cortical mechanisms (Kreiman & Sidtis, 2011).

Language development and autism

Normal language acquisition involves two differentiated processes, whereby children acquire whole expressions and then later work out the compositional properties (Locke, 1993, 1995; Peters, 1977, 1983). These two modes of acquiring language appear to proceed in tandem throughout childhood and into adolescence, following different maturational schedules (Kempler, et al., 1999). In some developmental disorders, the holistic mode predominates; this is often seen in persons on the autistic spectrum.

Repetition appears to be an innate function in learning and is a normal occurrence in conversational speech (Wolf & Sidtis, 2010). In child language acquisition, the term *imitation* is used to refer to this ubiquitous phenomenon, and children are heard to imitate the speech around them. However, the role and requirement of frequency of exposure for successful acquisition of grammar has long been under debate. For acquisition of formulaic expressions, it is arguable that frequency of exposure is not a crucial factor. Elsewhere we have proposed that formulaic expressions, because of their special qualities of nonliteral meaning, affective nuances, and context dependency, are subject to rapid uptake in language development by children and adolescents (Reuterskiold & Sidtis, submitted). This learning process is comparable to other kinds of one-trial learning, as seen in imprinting or flashbulb memories (Brown & Kulik, 1977; Horn, 1985). It is supported by recent studies documenting incidental learning of phonetic and linguistic material following single or brief exposure to an utterance (Goldinger, 1996; Gurevich, Johnson & Goldberg, 2010). This copying of verbal material appears as an isolated functionality and is seen in its purist form in some autistic children.

The contrast between novel and formulaic language assumes extreme manifestation in autism, but little understanding of its meaning has emerged (Bogdashina, 2005). Here we also see an abrupt dissociation between production and comprehension. Echolalia, the copying of whole utterances spoken by self or others, is observed in many children diagnosed with autism; meaning comprehension of these expressions is minimal (Cohen & Volkmar, 1997). In addition to near exact repetition of the speech of others, some children show mitigated repetition, in which pronouns and grammatical endings are changed appropriately: *Are you happy today?* Is repeated as *Am I happy today?* and may further appear several times as *I am happy today*. Prosody is often altered and takes deviant shapes. In the language disorder of autism, grammatical and lexical competence is severely impoverished or nonexistent. The initiative to speak may also be only weakly present or not present at all. In these cases, the preserved formulaic mode, manifest in repetition and perseveration, is distorted and pathological, in that it does not function to acquire the very large number of socially appropriate and nonliteral expressions, as in normal language learning, but some communicative function is occasionally seen using these expressions (Dobbinson, Perkins, & Boucher, 2003; Prizant, 1983; Prizant & Duchan, 1981). In extreme cases, the formulaic mode is limited to mimicking advertisement jingles, sayings, and other salient expressions in the media, copying rhythmic as well as articulatory features (Paul, 2004).

Formulaic language in Alzheimer's disease

The dissociation between production and comprehension of formulaic language emerges clearly in Alzheimer speech. Anecdotally, persons with the moderate to severe cognitive deficits associated with probable Alzheimer's disease have been observed to produce an array of formulaic utterances (*Excuse me! Good-bye; See you later*) with normal expression, long after semantic abilities have been severely compromised. Preliminary findings in our laboratory reveal a proportion of formulaic expressions in Alzheimer spontaneous speech that is significantly higher than matched normal control subjects (Bridges & Sidtis, 2010; Rogers et al., 2010; see Figure 17.5). Formulaic expressions appear to constitute a portion of what has been previously referred to as "empty speech" in Alzheimer's disease (Speech Sample E, Appendix I). Despite retention of a repertory of formulaic expressions in production, comprehension of idioms and social speech formulas is impaired in Alzheimer's disease (Kempler, Van Lancker, & Read, 1988; Papagno, Lucchelli, Muggia, & Rizzo, 2003), reflecting the dissociation between production and comprehension mentioned above.

Interestingly, the form of the formulaic expression may be distorted in Alzheimer speech: *No but they come home every little while; It's way back in the head; Made up mind to; Not a very going out man*. These errors take a different shape from the formulaic speech errors observed in normal subjects (Cutting & Bock, 1997; Kuiper et al., 2007). In addition to these distortions of form, pragmatic constraints are also often violated, in that the social context is inappropriate. The Alzheimer patient may say *It's nice to see you again* to a stranger. While formulaic expressions are retained to a greater degree than abilities to produce novel utterances, the cognitive disorder does affect formulaic form, meaning, and pragmatic constraints. Preservation of formulaic language in Alzheimer's disease lends support to the thesis of subcortical involvement in formulaic language, as Alzheimer's disease afflicts cortical layers, leaving basal ganglia intact until late in the disease progression.

Conclusions: Dual-Process Processing of Novel and Formulaic Language

An overview of psychological and neurological observations leads to a model of normal language competence comprising two disparate modes. These processing modes differ primarily in the nature of the units, or building blocks, that are produced and comprehended. Formulaic expressions have been called giant lexical units or superlemmas. Although this perspective remains controversial, most findings have supported what has been called "the lexical hypothesis." The term "lexical" is less than useful because formulaic expressions have several properties that distinguish them crucially from words: wide-ranging intraphrase flexibility, mandatory affective and attitudinal nuances, and, in many cases, considerable length. More appropriate is the term "formuleme," referring to the canonical expression known to native speakers in terms of its form, meaning, and pragmatic contingencies. Formulemes are stored as a whole with a range of unique characteristics pertaining to phonetic, lexical, and prosodic form and conventionalized meaning encompassing an array of social and affective connotations. Pragmatic contingences constrain the social settings that are appropriate for the expression. In contrast, novel expressions are formed using grammatical rules to select and arrange lexical items into strings. Psychological and neurological evidence reviewed above indicates that formulaic and grammatical modes of competence are processed differently and that they are in continuous interplay with each other. Even more striking is the fact that native speakers know – by heart – the form, meaning, and pragmatics of hundreds of thousands of such expressions. Personal familiarity with the canonical shapes, or formulemes, overshadows other factors, such as whether or not idioms are transparent or compositional when manipulated by speakers.

Evidence from several subdisciplines in the language sciences supports the view that formulaic and novel expressions are stored and processed according to different principles. Speakers' performance in psychological experiments lends support to the notion of formulaic expressions as holistically stored and processed, in contrast to novel expressions, which are by definition composed by rules. Neurological evidence further reveals that these differences between novel and formulaic pattern differently for production and comprehension modes. Comprehension of idioms, as a subset of formulaic language, is impaired in damage to both cerebral hemispheres, but production of formulaic expressions is significantly higher in left hemisphere than right hemisphere damage. Autistic and Alzheimer subjects produce an overabundance of formulaic expressions but show deficient ability to comprehend them or to utilize them according to pragmatic principles; the basal ganglia are preserved in Alzheimer's disease until very late in the disease progression. Production of formulaic expressions is diminished in Parkinson's disease, in which basal ganglia are compromised from the beginning of the disease progression. Comprehension of formulaic expressions is undertaken by both hemispheres according to different strategies, while production of formulaic expressions relies more heavily on a right-hemisphere-subcortical circuit.

Implications for Evaluation and Treatment in Communicative Disorders

Evaluation techniques in neurogenic language disorders in current standard practice take only minimal notice, if any, of formulaic language. In aphasia, occasional elicitation of so-called "automatic speech," such as counting to 10 or 20 and recitation of nursery rhymes, is limited and reveals only the tip of the iceberg that constitutes formulaic language competence. During evaluation of spontaneous speech, clinicians seldom distinguish between formulaic expressions and novel speech as present in the speech sample. For initial intake as well as for assessment of recovered speech ability, this distinction is of prime importance in understanding the language profile of the patient. In Speech Sample F (Appendix I), an aphasic patient has recovered a quantity of speech in the fifth training period. Of 139 words, 64% appear in standard formulaic expressions, and 7% (*big, small*) are probably idiosyncratically processed formulaic expressions (words and phrases adapted into the formulaic mode). In right hemisphere damage, the paucity of formulaic language in conversation could impact the patient's communicative function. Such failures have been misread by family members and acquaintances as recalcitrance or mood disorder. When correct identification in type of recovered speech – formulaic or novel, is performed, more enlightened treatment can proceed. For example, in cases where the prevailing mode of disordered or recovered speech is formulaic, as in left hemisphere damage and autism, this kind of speech might be supported and molded toward the ends of improved functional socialization and communication. Where it is impoverished, in right or subcortical damage and Parkinsonism, treatment utilizing conversational formulas could be designed.

References

Aijmer, K. (1996). *Conversational routines in English*. London, New York: Longman.

Altenberg, B. (1998). On the phraseology of spoken English: The evidence of recurrent word-combinations. In A. P. Cowie (Ed.), *Phraseology: Theory, analysis and application* (pp. 101–124). Oxford: Clarendon Press.

Belánger, N., Baum, S., & Titone, D. (2009). Use of prosodic cues in the production of idiomatic and literal sentences by individuals with right- and left-hemisphere damage. *Brain and Language, 110*, 38–42.

Bell, R. A., & Healey, J. G. (1992). Idiomatic communication and interpersonal solidarity in friends' relational cultures. *Human Communication Research, 3*, 307–335.

Blank, S. C., Scott, S., Murphy, K., Warburton, E., & Wise, R. (2002). Speech production: Wernicke, Broca and beyond. *Brain, 125*, 1829–1838.

Bobrow, S., & Bell, S., (1973). On catching on to idiomatic expressions. *Memory and Cognition, 19*, 295–308.

Bogdashina, O. (2005). *Communication issues in autism and Aspergers syndrome. Do we speak the same language?* London: Jessica Kingsley Publishers.

Bogen, J. E. (1969). The other side of the brain II: An appositional mind. *Bulletin of the Los Angeles Neurological Societies, 324*, 191–219.

Bookheimer, S. Y., Zeffiro, T. A., Blaxton, T. A., Gaillard, P. W., & Theodore, W. H. (2000). Activation of language cortex with automatic speech tasks. *Neurology, 55*, 1151–7.

Bridges, K., & Sidtis, D. (2010). Language studies in early and late onset Alzheimer's disease. Paper presented at FLaRN Conference, Paderborn, Germany.

Brown, R., & Kulik, J. (1977). Flashbulb memories. *Cognition, 5*, 73–93.

Brownell, H. H., Gardner, H., Prather, P., & Martino, G. (1995). Language, communication, and the right hemisphere. In H. S. Kirshner (Ed.), *Handbook of neurological speech and language disorders* (vol. 33, pp. 325–349). London: Informa Healthcare.

Burt, J. S. (1992). Against the lexical representation of idioms. *Canadian Journal of Psychology, 46*(4), 582–605.

Cacciari C., & Tabossi P. (1988). The comprehension of idioms. *Journal of Memory and Language, 27*, 668–683.

Cheney, D. L., & Seyfarth, R. M. (1980). Vocal recognition in free-ranging vervet monkeys. *Animal Behavior, 28*, 362–367.

Cheney, D. L., & Seyfarth, R. M. (1990). *How monkeys see the world.* Chicago: University of Chicago Press.

Clark, H. H. (1970). Word associations and linguistic theory. In J. Lyons (Ed.), *New horizons in linguistics* (pp. 271–286). Baltimore: Penguin Books.

Code, C. (1994). Speech automatism production in aphasia. *Journal of Neurolinguistics, 8*(2), 135–148.

Code, C. (2005). First in, last out? The evolution of aphasic lexical speech automatisms to agrammatism and the evolution of human communication. *Interaction Studies, 6*, 311–334.

Cohen, D. J., & Volkmar, F. R. (Eds.). (1997). *Handbook of autism and pervasive developmental disorders.* New York: Wiley & Sons.

Coulmas, F. (1994). Formulaic language. In R.E. Asher (Ed.), *Encyclopedia of language and linguistics* (pp. 1292–1293). Oxford: Pergamon.

Cutler, A., (1982). Idioms: The colder the older. *Linguistic Inquiry, 13*, 3178–320.

Cutting, J. C., & Bock, K. (1997). That's the way the cookie bounces: Syntactic and semantic components of experimentally elicited idiom blends. *Memory-Cognition, 25*(1), 57–71.

Dietrich, S., Hertrich, I., Alter, K., Ischebeck, A., & Ackermann, H. (2008). Understanding the emotional expression of verbal interjections: A functional MRI study. *NeuroReport, 19*(18), 1751–1755.

Dobbinson, S., Perkins, M. R., & Boucher, J. (2003). The interactional significance of formulas in autistic language. *Clinical Linguistics and Phonetics, 17*(4), 299–307.

Drews, E. (1987). Quantitatively different organization structure of lexical knowledge in the left and right hemisphere. *Neuropsychologia, 25,* 419–427.

Estill, R. B., & Kemper, S., (1982). Interpreting idioms. *Journal of Psycholinguistic Research, 11,* 559–569.

Fellbaum, C. (Ed.). (2007). *Idioms and collocations: Corpus-based linguistic and lexicographic studies (corpus and discourse) research in corpus and discourse.* Birmingham, UK: Continuum Press.

Fillmore, C. (1979). On fluency. In C. J. Fillmore, D. Kempler & W. S.-Y. Wang (Eds.), *Individual differences in language ability and language behavior* (pp. 85–102). London: Academic Press.

Fraser, B. (1970). Idioms within a transformation grammar. *Foundations of Language, 6,* 22–42.

Gardner, H., Brownell, H. H., Wapner, W., & Michelow, D. (1983). Missing the point: The role of the right hemisphere in the processing of complex linguistic materials. In E. Perecman (Ed.), *Cognitive processing in the right hemisphere* (pp. 169–192). New York: Academic Press.

Gibbs, R. W. (1980). Spilling the beans on understanding and memory for idioms in conversation. *Memory and Cognition, 8*(2), 149–156.

Gibbs, R. W. (1981). Your wish is my command: Convention and context in interpreting indirect requests. *Journal of Verbal Learning and Verbal Behavior, 20,* 431–444.

Gibbs, R. W. (1994). *The poetics of mind: Figurative thought, language, and understanding.* New York: Cambridge University Press.

Gibbs, R. W., & Gonzales, G. P., (1985). Syntactic frozenness in processing and remembering idioms. *Cognition, 20,* 243–259.

Gibbs, R. W., Nayak, N. P., Bolton, J. L., & Keppel, M. E. (1989). Speaker's assumptions about the lexical flexibility of idioms. *Memory and Cognition, 17*(1), 58–68.

Gibbs, R. W., Nayak, N. P., & Cutting, C. (1989). How to kick the bucket and not decompose: analyzability and idiom processing. *Journal of Memory and Language, 28,* 576–593.

Goldinger, S. D. (1996). Words and voices: Episodic trace in spoken work identification and recognition memory. *Journal of Experimental Psychology: Learning, Memory, and Cognition, 22*(5), 1166–1183.

Graves, R., & Landis, T. (1985). Hemispheric control of speech expression in aphasia. *Archives of Neurology, 42,* 249–251.

Graybiel, A. M. (1998). The basal ganglia and chunking of action repertoires. *Neurobiology of Learning and Memory, 70,* 119–136.

Gurevich, O., Johnson, M. A., & Goldberg, A. E. (2010). Incidental verbatim memory for language. *Language and Cognition, 2*(1), 45–78.

Hain, M. (1951). *Sprichwort und Volkssprache.* Giessen: Wilhelm Schmitz Verlag. English trans., in D. Sidtis & S. Mohr (Eds.), *Formulaic language in the field*, Anja Tachler, translator. Copyright.

Heringer, J. T. (1976). Idioms and lexicalization in English. In Shibetani, M. (Ed.), *Syntax and semantics* (vol. 6). New York: Academic Press.

Hillert, D., & Swinney, D. (2001). The processing of fixed expressions during sentence comprehension. In A. Cienki, B. J. Luka, & M. B. Smith (Eds.), *Conceptual and discourse factors in linguistic structure* (pp. 107–1210). Stanford, CA: CSLI Publications.

Horn, G. (1985). *Memory, imprinting and the brain*. Oxford Psychology Series No. 10. Oxford: Clarendon Press.

Horowitz, L. M., & Manelis, L. (1973). Recognition and cued recall of idioms and phrases. *Journal of Experimental Psychology, 100*, 291–296.

Hughlings Jackson, J. (1874). On the nature of the duality of the brain. In J. Taylor (Ed.), *Selected writings of John Hughlings Jackson* (vol. 2, pp. 129–145). London: Hodder & Stoughton.

Illes, J., Metter, E. J., Hanson, W. R., & Iritani, S. (1988). Language production in Parkinson's disease: Acoustic and linguistic considerations. *Brain and Language, 33*, 146–160.

Jackendoff, R. (1995). The boundaries of the lexicon. In M. Everaert, E. van der Linden, A. Schenk & R. Schreuder (Eds.), *Idioms: Structural and psychological perspectives* (pp. 133–166). Hillsdale, NJ: Erlbaum.

Jaynes, J. (1976). *The origin of consciousness in the breakdown of the bicameral mind*. Boston MA: Houghton Mifflin.

Joanette, Y., & Brownell, H. (Eds.). (1990). *Discourse ability and brain damage: Theoretical and empirical perspectives*. New York: Springer-Verlag.

Jürgens, U. (2002). Neural pathways underlying vocal control. *Neuroscience and Biobehavioral Reviews, 26*(2), 235–258.

Kacinik, N. A., & Chiarello, C. (2007). Understanding metaphors: Is the right hemisphere uniquely involved? *Brain and Language, 100*(2), 188–207.

Kempler, D., & Van Lancker, D. (1993). Acquisition and loss of familiar language: Idiom and proverb comprehension. In F. R. Eckman (Ed.), *Language acquisition and language disorders* (vol. 4, *Confluence: Linguistics, L2 acquisition, speech pathology*, pp. 249–257). Amsterdam/Philadelphia: J. Benjamins.

Kempler, D., & Van Lancker, D. (1996). The Formulaic and Novel Language Comprehension Test (FANL-C). Copyright. (For complete test materials, see http://blog.emerson.edu/daniel_kempler/fanlc.html).

Kempler, D., & Van Lancker, D. (2002). The effect of speech task on intelligibility in dysarthria: Case study of Parkinson's disease. *Brain and Language, 80*, 449–464.

Kempler, D., Van Lancker, D., Marchman, V., & Bates, E. (1999). Idiom comprehension in children and adults with unilateral brain damage. *Developmental Neuropsychology, 15*(3), 327–349.

Kempler, D., Van Lancker, D., & Read, S. (1988). Comprehension of idioms and proverbs by Alzheimer patients. *Alzheimer Disease and Associated Disorders – An International Journal, 2*, 38–49.

Kitzinger, C., (2000). How to resist an idiom. *Research on Language and Social Interaction, 33*, 121–154.

Knowlton, B., Mangels, J., & Squire, L. (1996). A neostratal habit learning system in humans. *Science, 273*, 1399–1402.

Kreiman, J., & Sidtis, D. (2011). *Foundations of voice studies: Interdisciplinary approaches to the production and perception of voice*. Boston: Wiley-Blackwell.

Kuiper, K. (2009). *Formulaic genres*. UK: Palgrave Macmillan.

Kuiper, K., van Egmond, M., Kempen, G., & Sprenger, S. (2007). Slipping on superlemmas: Multi-word lexical items in speech production. *The Mental Lexicon, 2*(3), 313–357.

Lieberman, P. (1963). Some effects of semantic and grammatical context on the production and perception of speech. *Language and Speech, 6*, 172–187.

Lieberman, P. (2002). *Human language and our reptilian brain: The subcortical bases of speech, syntax, and thought*. Cambridge, MA: Harvard University Press.

Locke, J. L. (1993). *The child's path to spoken language*. Cambridge, MA: Harvard University Press.

Locke, J. L. (1995). Development of the capacity for spoken language. In P. Fletcher & B. MacWhinney (Eds.), *The handbook of child language* (pp. 278– 302). Oxford: Blackwell.

Locke, J. L., & Bogin, B. (2006). Language and life history: A new perspective on the development and evolution of human language. *Behavioral and Brain Sciences, 29*, 259–325.

Lounsbury, F.G. (1963). Linguistics and psychology. In S. Koch (Ed.), *Psychology: Study of a science* (pp. 553–582). New York: McGraw-Hill.

Ludlow C. L. (2005). Central nervous system control of the laryngeal muscles in humans. *Respiratory Physiology and Neurobiology, 147*, 205–222.

Lum, C. C., & Ellis, A. W. (1994). Is nonpropositional speech preserved in aphasia? *Brain and Language, 46*, 368–391.

MacLean, P. D. (1990). *The triune brain in evolution*. New York: Plenum.

Marler, P. (1998). Animal communication and human language. In G. Jablonski & L. C. Aiello (Eds.), *The origin and diversification of language*. Wattis Symposium Series in Anthropology. Memoirs of the California Academy of Sciences, No. 24 (pp. 1–19). San Francisco: California Academy of Sciences.

Marsden, C. D. (1982). The mysterious motor function of the basal ganglia: The Robert Wartenberg lecture. *Neurology, 32*, 514–539.

Moon, R. E. (1998). Fixed expressions and text: A study of the distribution and textual behaviour of fixed expressions in English. *Oxford Studies in Lexicology and Lexicography*. Oxford: Clarendon Press.

Nunberg, G., Sag, I. A., & Wasow, T. (1994). Idioms. *Language, 70*, 491–538.

Osgood, C., & Hoosain, R. (1974). Salience of the word as a unit in the perception of language. *Perception and Psychophysics, 15*, 168–192.

Panksepp, J. (1998). *Affective neuroscience: The foundations of human and animal emotions*. New York: Oxford University Press.

Panksepp, J. (2003). At the interface of affective, behavioral and cognitive neurosciences: Decoding the emotional feelings of the brain. *Brain and Cognition, 52*, 4–14.

Panksepp, J., & Burgdoff, J. (2003). "Laughing" rats and the evolutionary antecedents of human joy? *Physiology and Behavior, 79*, 533–547.

Papagno, C., & Caporali, A. (2007). Testing idiom comprehension in aphasic patients: The effects of task and idiom type. *Brain and Language, 100*(2), 208–220.

Papagno, C., Curti, R., Rizzo, S., Crippa, F., & Colombo, M. R. (2006). Is the right hemisphere involved in idiom comprehension? A neuropsychological study. *Neuropsychology, 20*(5), 598–606.

Papagno, C., & Genoni, A. (2004). The role of syntactic competence in idiom comprehension: A study on aphasic patients. *Journal of Neurolinguistics, 17*, 371–382.

Papagno, C., Lucchelli, F., Muggia, S., & Rizzo, S., (2003). Idiom comprehension in Alzheimer's disease: The role of the central executive. *Brain, 126*, 2419–2430.

Papagno, C., Tabossi, P., Colombo, M., & Zampetti, P. (2004). Idiom comprehension in aphasic patients. *Brain and Language, 89*(1), 226–234.

Paul, R. (2004). Autism. In R. D. Kent (Ed.), *The MIT handbook of communication disorders* (pp. 151–120). Cambridge, MA: MIT Press.

Pawley, A., & Syder, F. H. (1983). Two puzzles for linguistic theory: Nativelike selection and nativelike fluency. In J. C. Richards & R. Schmidt (Eds.), *Language and Communication* (pp. 191–225). London: Longman.

Peters, A. M. (1977). Language-learning strategies: Does the whole equal the sum of the parts? *Language, 53*, 560–573.

Peters, A. M. (1983). *The units of language acquisition.* Cambridge: Cambridge University Press.

Petrovici, J.-N. (1980). Speech disturbances following stereotaxic surgery in ventrolateral thalamus. *Neurosurgical Review, 3*(3), 189–195.

Pickens, J. D., & Pollio, H. R. (1979). Patterns of figurative language competence in adult speakers. *Psychological Research, 40*, 299–313.

Ploog, D. (1975). Vocal behavior and its "localization" as prerequisite for speech. In K. J. Zülch, O. Creutzfeldt, & G. C. Galbraith (Eds.), *Cerebral localization.* Berlin: Springer-Verlag.

Postman-Caucheteux, W. A., Hoffman, S., Picchioni, D., McArdle, J., Birn, R., & Braun, A. (2007). Distinct activation patterns for accurate vs. inaccurate naming of actions and objects: An fMRI study with stroke patients with chronic aphasia. *Brain and Language, 103*, 150–151.

Prizant, B. M. (1983). Language acquisition and communicative behavior in autism: Toward an understanding of the "whole" of it. *Journal of Speech and Hearing Disorders, 48*, 296–307.

Prizant, B. M., & Duchan, J. (1981). The functions of immediate echolalia in autistic children. *Journal of Speech and Hearing Disorders, 46*, 241–249.

Reuterskiold, K., & Sidtis, D. (submitted). Incidental learning of formulaic expressions.

Rogers, T., Sidtis, D., & Sidtis, J. (2010, March). Formulaic language production and comprehension in Alzheimer's and Parkinson's disease. Paper presented at FLaRN Conference, Paderborn, Germany.

Schaltenbrand, G. (1965). The effects of stereotactic electrical stimulation in the depth of the brain. *Brain, 88*, 835–840.

Sidtis, D. (2011). Teaching "Linguistic approaches to nonliteral language": We really knew how to have fun. In K. Kuiper (Ed.), *Teaching Linguistics* (pp. 110–136). England: Equinox.

Sidtis, D., Canterucci, G., & Katsnelson, D. (2009). Effects of neurological damage on production of formulaic language. *Clinical Linguistics and Phonetics, 23*(15), 270–284.

Sidtis, D., Rogers, T., Godier, V., Tagliati, M., & Sidtis, J. J. (2010). Voice and fluency changes as a function of speech task and deep brain stimulation. *Journal of Speech Language and Hearing Research, 53* 1167–1177.

Sidtis, J. J. (2007). Some problems for representation of brain organization based on activation in functional imaging. *Brain and Language, 102*, 130–140.

Simon, H. A. (1974). How big is a chunk? *Science, 183*, 482–448.

Simon, H. A., Zhang, W., Zang, W., & Peng, R. (1989). STM capacity for Chinese words and idioms with visual and auditory presentations. In H. A. Simon (Ed.), *Models of thought* (Vol. 2, pp. 68–75). New Haven and London: Yale University Press.

Smolka, E., Rabanus, S., & Rösler, F. (2007). Processing verbs in German idioms: Evidence against the configuration hypothesis. *Metaphor and Symbol, 22*(3), 213–231.

Speedie, L. J., Wertman, E., T'air, J., & Heilman, K. M. (1993). Disruption of automatic speech following a right basal ganglia lesion. *Neurology, 43*, 1768–1774.

Sprenger, S. A. (2003). *Fixed expressions and the production of idioms.* (Unpublished doctoral dissertation). University of Nijmegen.

Swinney, D. A., & Cutler, A. (1979). The access and processing of idiomatic expressions. *Journal of Verbal Learning and Verbal Behavior, 18*, 523–534.

Titone, D.A., & Connine, C. M. (1999). On the compositional and noncompositional nature of idiomatic expressions. *Journal of Pragmatics, 31,* 1655–1674.

Van Lancker, D. (1973). Language lateralization and grammars. In John Kimball (Ed.), *Studies in syntax and semantics* (vol. 2, pp. 197–204). New York: Academic Press.

Van Lancker, D. (1979). Review of the book *The origin of consciousness in the breakdown of the bicameral mind,* by Julian Jaynes. *Forum Linguisticum, 4,* 72–91.

Van Lancker, D. (1988). Nonpropositional speech: Neurolinguistic studies. In Andrew Ellis (Ed.), *Progress in the psychology of language* (pp. 49–118). Hillsdale, NJ: Erlbaum.

Van Lancker, D. (1994). Nonpropositional speech in aphasia. In G. Blanken, J. Dittmann, J. Grimm, J. C. Marshall, & C.-W. Wallesch (Eds.), *Linguistic disorders and pathologies: An international handbook* (pp. 215–225). Berlin: Walter de Gruyter.

Van Lancker, D., & Canter, G. J. (1981). Idiomatic versus literal interpretations of ditropically ambiguous sentences. *Journal of Speech and Hearing Research, 46,* 64–69.

Van Lancker, D., Canter, J., & Terbeek, D. (1981). Disambiguation of ditropic sentences: Acoustic and phonetic cues. *Journal of Speech and Hearing Research, 24,* 330–335.

Van Lancker, D., & Cummings, J. (1999). Expletives: Neurolinguistic and neurobehavioral perspectives on swearing. *Brain Research Reviews, 31,* 83–104.

Van Lancker, D., & Kempler, D. (1987). Comprehension of familiar phrases by left but not by right hemisphere damaged patients. *Brain and Language, 32,* 265–277.

Van Lancker, D., McIntosh, R., & Grafton, R. (2003). PET activation studies comparing two speech tasks widely used in surgical mapping. *Brain and Language, 85,* 245–261.

Van Lancker Sidtis, D. (2004). When novel sentences spoken or heard for the first time in the history of the universe are not enough: Toward a dual-process model of language. *International Journal of Language and Communication Disorders, 39*(1), 1–44.

Van Lancker Sidtis, D. (2006). Has neuroimaging solved the problems of neurolinguistics? *Brain and Language, 98,* 276–290.

Van Lancker Sidtis, D. (2008). Formulaic and novel language in a "dual process" model of language competence: Evidence from surveys, speech samples, and schemata. In R. L. Corrigan, E. A. Moravcsik, H. Ouali & K. M. Wheatley (Eds.), *Formulaic language* (vol. 2, *Acquisition, loss, psychological reality, functional applications,* pp. 151–176). Amsterdam: Benjamins Publishing Co.

Van Lancker Sidtis, D. (2010). Formulaic and novel expressions in mind and brain: Empirical studies and a dual process model of language competence. In J. Guendouzi, F. Loncke, & M. Williams (Eds.), *The handbook of psycholinguistic and cognitive processes: Perspectives in communication disorders.* London: Taylor & Francis.

Van Lancker Sidtis, D., & Postman, W. A. (2006). Formulaic expressions in spontaneous speech of left- and right-hemisphere damaged subjects. *Aphasiology, 20*(5), 411–426.

Van Lancker Sidtis, D., & Rallon, G. (2004). Tracking the incidence of formulaic expressions in everyday speech: Methods for classification and verification. *Language and Communication, 24,* 207–240.

Van Lancker Sidtis, D., Kempler, D., Ahn, J.-S., & Yang, S.-Y. (2011). Results of the Comprehensive Nonliteral Language Protocol on left- and right-hemisphere damaged subjects. Manuscript in preparation.

Weinert, R. (1995). The role of formulaic language in second language acquisition: A review. *Applied Linguistics, 16*(2),180–205.

Weinreich, V. (1969). Problems in the analysis of idioms. In J. Puhvel (Ed.), *Substance and structure of language* (pp. 23–82). Los Angeles: University of California Press.

Winner, E., & Gardner, H. (1977). The comprehension of metaphor in brain-damaged patients. *Brain, 100,* 717–729.

Wolf, R., & Sidtis, D. (2010). Examination in the relationship between formulaic language and pragmatic repetition in conversational discourse. Paper presented at FLaRN Conference, Paderborn, Germany.

Wray, A. (1998). Protolanguage as a holistic system for social interaction. *Language and Communication, 18,* 47–67.

Wray, A. (2000). Holistic utterances in protolanguage: The link from primates to humans. In C. Knight, J. R. Hurford & M. Studdert-Kennedy (Eds.), *The evolutionary emergence of language: Social function and the origins of linguistic form* (pp. 285–302). Cambridge: Cambridge University Press.

Wray, A. (2002). *Formulaic language and the lexicon.* Cambridge: Cambridge University Press.

Wray, A., & Perkins, M. (2000). The functions of formulaic language: An integrated model. *Language and Communication, 20,* 1–28.

Appendix I. Speech Samples

(Formulaic expressions are <u>underlined</u>)

A   Subject with left hemisphere damage and aphasia (from a group study of 5 subjects; Van Lancker Sidtis & Postman, 2006)
Do I work?
<u>Christ</u> I work <u>every damn day and half night</u>
'cause it's '<u>cause what else you going to do?</u>
<u>Go crazy?</u> Doing . . .
<u>Well</u> 'tis <u>long story but</u> . . .
That property that we built . . .
<u>There's a long story</u>.

B   Subject with right hemisphere damage (from a group study of 5 subjects; Van Lancker Sidtis & Postman, 2006)
I worked at General Electric for forty something years.
<u>And I</u> ran a big machine . . . about as big as this room.
<u>And I</u> worked in jet engines . . . all my life . . . <u>ever since</u>
<u>well</u> I worked on superchargers
before before jets came into being
in 1941 I worked on superchargers till I went in . . .
I enlisted in the Air Force . . . or the army.

C   Subject with transcortical sensory aphasia (single-case studies; Sidtis, Canterucci, & Katsnelson, 2009)
Patient: <u>I came, I saw, I conquered.</u>
Clinician: *What else did you use to do? . . . Were you an engineer?*
Patient: Yes, I was an engineer. <u>It's more important.</u>
<u>It's that I</u> . . . <u>I said good morning. I said good morning.</u>

And . . . or . . . I didn't even say good morning.
I just said Hi, how are you? How are you? And we . . . we . . . Hi, good morning.
How are you. It was 9, 8:30, 9:00.
I decided to . . . I did very, very well, and then, all of a sudden.
It's a long story. But I think I know what I'm talking about. I hope so. I hope
so, too.

D   Speech of a subject with subcortical damage (the first SC [subcortical] case on
    Figure 17.5; Sidtis, Canterucci, & Katsnelson, 2009)
    I felt wonderful, it was a great day.
    Um, I didn't think I was gonna graduate and I made it through college.
    We had a party and my grandmother was there, my father's mother, and my
    friends were there, and it was just a great day.
    Well, I woke up and I was in unfamiliar surroundings,
    I was in the hospital and I didn't know what had happened,
    and I was depressed because I couldn't move my left side of my leg,
    and my arm was hurting and I had a sore in the palm of my hand,
    I guess where I had been pressing.

E   Speech of an Alzheimer subject (sample taken during group study; Rogers,
    Sidtis, & Sidtis, 2010)
    Honey. And I have other things to do for others.
    So I just (sighs)
    What do you need I- I nine (?) and n-
    and just uh a couple of things and-
    and then and please don't come to me
    when I could be there or there or there okay?

F   Recovery of fluent speech in an aphasic patient after five training sessions
    (sample from Dr Jacqueline Stark, Vienna, Austria)
    Test 1 Uh. TV? My Monday is uh . . . bank uh. TV . . . my . . . Monday uh
    bank. hm.
    Test 5 Uh . . . uh good morning . . . uh . . . um . . . me uh I want a . . . big big
    ter// uh terevision, all right? Um, big. All right? And uh . . . money? Yes.
    Fine . . . um . . . big   and.   uh . . . small   um . . . TV.   yes . . . uh   small
    um . . . Uh . . . sky and cricket ands . . . tennis and . . . uh soccer and movies
    and news and . . . all right? Um . . . right. Uh . . . where? Ah! All right! Boah!
    nice! Wow! Big! And small! Ho-ho, Jesus! Uh . . . price? What? two thou-
    sand . . . oh Jesus! hm . . . wait. um . . . hm hm hm. yes . . . alright . . . um . . .
    I. will uh . . . I will phone and uh . . . uh. woman, yes? And uh um . . . wife, yes.
    Um . . . maybe all right . . . maybe uh. two thousand? Oh, Jesus. All right. Uh
    phone and wait, all right? Uh . . . oh, Jesus! Hi! Jane um . . . phew . . . uh . . . w
    hat is the matter? Money? Oh, Jesus . . . all right . . . all right! thank you! see
    you! Uh salesman . . . uh . . . money, yes . . . fine . . .

18

Neuropsychological and Neurophysiological Correlates of Idiom Understanding: How Many Hemispheres Are Involved?

Cristina Cacciari and Costanza Papagno

Introduction

As the philosopher John Searle claimed, idiomatic expressions are so pervasive in everyday language that speakers seem to follow an implicit rule: *Speak idiomatically unless there is some special reason not to* (Searle, 1979, p. 50). Figurative language is extremely pervasive in everyday language: according to an estimate proposed by Jackendoff (1995), there are as many fixed expressions as there are words in American English, more or less 80,000 (Jackendoff, 1995). Some years ago, Pollio, Barlow, Fine, and Pollio (1977) estimated that people use about 6 nonliteral fixed expressions per minute of discourse, specifically 1.8 new metaphors and 4.08 *conventionalized* metaphors (as *John is an elephant* or *That lawyer is a shark*). Assuming that people engage in conversation on average 2 hours a day, a person utters 4.7 million novel metaphors and 21.4 million frozen ones over a 60-year average lifespan.

In this chapter, we review the literature concerning the neural architecture underlying idiom comprehension in language-unimpaired and language-impaired participants. Just some words on the limitation of this review chapter: we only consider studies on the neuropsychological and neurophysiological correlates of idiom comprehension and leave aside studies concerning other forms of figurative language (e.g., metaphor, proverbs; see Thoma & Daum, 2006). Since we are specifically interested in the brain areas recruited during idiom processing, we did not consider the (few) studies on idiom comprehension that employed event-related scalp-recorded brain potentials (for an overview, see Vespignani, Canal, Molinaro, Fonda,

The Handbook of the Neuropsychology of Language, First Edition. Edited by Miriam Faust.
© 2012 Blackwell Publishing Ltd. Published 2012 by Blackwell Publishing Ltd.

& Cacciari, 2010). This technique in fact provides fine-grained information on the timing with which cognitive processes occur but it does not provide reliable information on the specific brain regions recruited.

The organization of the chapter is as follows: we start from defining the identity of the linguistic strings considered in this chapter, namely idiomatic expressions, and how these differ from other members of the huge family that goes under the name of *figurative language*. Then we examine the neuropsychological literature following a chronological criterion: first we consider the studies on idiom comprehension from the 1970s to the 1990s, and then the more recent studies. We move to the studies that directly assessed the neural architecture underlying idiom comprehension by employing transcranial magnetic stimulation (TMS), a technique that can be used to disrupt, reversibly and transiently, the normal activity of a brain region), and functional magnetic resonance imaging (fMRI). Finally we draw some conclusions about possible answers to the basic question that motivated this chapter, *How many hemispheres are involved?*

What an Idiom Is and Is Not

When a speaker/reader encounters a sentence, s/he is generally able to judge whether it is intended literally or not. The ease with which people deal with this distinction in everyday discourse belies the complexity of the distinction between literal and figurative language. Many researchers have expressed serious doubts as to whether a sharp distinction can (or should) be drawn between these two varieties of language. A partial and maybe more promising alternative is to use the notion of *level of conventionalization* that is generally considered to be based on a continuum that goes from *not conventional at all* to *fully conventional*. The position of idioms along this continuum can be conceived as closest to the *fully conventional* pole. Idiomatization in fact is a process: to reach the status of idiom, an expression must become conventionalized for a linguistic community (Cacciari, 1993).

Defining what an idiom is and the difference between an idiom and other types of figurative expression (e.g., metaphor, proverb, cliché, and collocation) might seem at a first glance a useless task. In contrast, as we will see in this chapter, there is an underestimation of the role played by the linguistic characteristics of the experimental stimuli employed in experimental and clinical studies, and very often researchers mistake an idiom for a proverb or a metaphor. Since, as we explain below, these expressions indeed differ from a semantic and syntactic point of view, this confusion might be problematic. Therefore, it is necessary to point out not only what an idiom is but also what an idiom *is not*.

Operationally, *an idiomatic expression is a string of constituents whose meaning is not necessarily derived from that of the constituent parts*. The idiomatic meaning is stored in semantic memory together with word meanings, concepts, and many other types of multiword strings (e.g., lines of poetry, advertisings, and song titles). In general the relationship between lexical items and phrasal meaning is to a large extent arbitrary and learned.

Idioms differ from metaphors (even though many idioms diachronically derive from metaphors) since metaphors (either the more frozen or conventionalized ones) do not have a unique standardized meaning and can convey more than one meaning (even a rather conventionalized metaphor as *John is an elephant* conveys different meanings, for instance that he is clumsy, extremely big, a blunderer, etc.). Idioms do have a unique meaning that can be specialized but not changed by context. We cannot retrieve and productively combine words online to create an idiomatic expression (Konopka & Bock, 2009). Some idioms allow semantic variations within a more or less fixed template, but this should not be confounded with true metaphorical language. In contrast, we can create a metaphor on the fly, albeit not necessarily a good one. Metaphors have to do with categorization processes (Cacciari & Glucksberg, 1994; Glucksberg, 2001) while idioms with meaning have to do with retrieval from semantic memory. Idioms also differ from proverbs (e.g., *You can't get blood from a stone*; *A point in time saves nine*) since the latter are full sentences, temporarily undefined, signaled by specific grammatical, phonetic and/ or rhetorical patterns or by a binary structure (theme/comment). Proverbs are often used as general comments to shared communicative situations, and are generally true statements, both literally and figuratively (Ferretti, Schwint, & Katz, 2007; Turner & Katz, 1997).

The First Neuropsychological Studies on Idiom Comprehension: The Rise of the RH Hypothesis

The psycholinguistic models on idiom processing are generally based on language-unimpaired participants (for overviews, see Cacciari, Padovani, & Corradini, 2007; Cacciari & Tabossi, 1993; Vespignani et al., 2010) and assume that in order to understand an idiom, lexical integrity is required. Therefore, injuries to the left hemisphere (LH), typically resulting in aphasic impairments, ought to damage, along with other linguistic skills, patients' ability to comprehend idiomatic expressions. However, at odds with this prediction, a widely accepted view in the neuropsychological literature assumes that damage to the LH may have no major consequences on idiom comprehension, and it is the nondominant right hemisphere (RH) that is important for the processing of idiomatic expressions (Van Lancker Sidtis & Postman, 2006).

The idea that the comprehension of idiomatic expressions is predominantly subserved by the RH (henceforth referred to as *the RH hypothesis*) originates from a misinterpretation of the results of the first classical lesion study on metaphor comprehension (Winner & Gardner, 1977). Winner and Gardner found that aphasic left-brain-damaged (LBD) patients were correct when they had to associate a metaphoric expression with the matching picture, whereas right-brain-damaged (RBD) patients, despite being able to verbally explain the correct meaning of metaphors, chose the pictures corresponding to the literal meaning. On the contrary, the five LBD patients who could be tested in the oral modality gave literal explanations despite choosing metaphorical pictures.

Since then, Winner and Gardner's results have been taken to support the RH hypothesis for figurative language comprehension tout court. However, this study concerned the comprehension of a specific type of figurative language, namely, metaphors and not idioms. Although this finding has been taken as evidence that RBD patients are impaired in comprehending all figurative language, it may only indicate that RBD patients are defective in comprehending metaphors, not necessarily idioms, and/or in picture matching. And in fact a greater difficulty with pictorial material is constantly reported when RBD patients are tested (e.g., Papagno, Curti, Rizzo, Crippa, & Colombo, 2006).

Studies specifically focused on idiom comprehension in language-impaired patients did not provide conclusive evidence in support of the RH hypothesis. The first researchers testing idiomatic expressions were Stachowiak, Huber, Poeck, and Kerschensteiner (1977) who were almost ignored in the neuropsychological literature on figurative language comprehension. They investigated the semantic and pragmatic strategies used for comprehending auditorily presented short stories containing idioms by four subgroups of aphasic patients (Broca, Wernicke, amnestic, and global aphasics), RBD patients, and normal controls. Participants were required to choose the picture (out of five) appropriate to the story. Half of the stories were commented using semantically transparent idioms and half with semantically opaque idioms (i.e., idioms with a close vs. remote relationship between literal and figurative meaning, respectively). Overall, the performance was better with transparent than with opaque idioms. The comprehension of idioms in the aphasic groups was not poorer than that of the other groups: in fact the distribution of idiomatic choices was similar across groups, except for the Wernicke group which produced slightly more literal responses. Stachowiak et al. (1977) interpreted the lack of a significant difference between aphasics and controls as suggesting that aphasics heavily relied on the pictorial information provided by context. Whether or not aphasic patients had difficulty in comprehending idioms if presented out of a verbal or pictorial context was not investigated. However, it is possible that if a particular word or sentence was not understood, enough cues in the context were available to let them infer the misunderstood part. Thus verbal redundancy could have made up for the difficulties at word and sentence levels.

Some years later, Van Lancker and Kempler (1987; see also Van Lancker Sidtis, Volume 1, Chapter 17) and Kempler, Van Lancker, Marchman, and Bates (1999) reported a *double dissociation* between idiom comprehension and novel sentence comprehension in LBD and RBD patients tested with a sentence-to-picture matching task: while RBD participants had normal performance on novel (literal) sentences and performed poorly on familiar (figurative) sentences, aphasic patients had the opposite pattern. The test consisted of 40 test items, namely 20 familiar phrases, including proverbs, idioms, and contextually bound social interaction formulas (*I'll get back to you later*), and 20 novel sentences constructed to match the familiar ones in length, surface grammatical structure, and word frequency. The foils for familiar phrases were two concrete interpretations related to individual words in the stimulus sentence (the picture is described by a sentence including a content word of the familiar phrase); the third foil represented the opposite figurative meaning of the familiar phrase. In a first version there was a picture representing the literal interpretation, instead of a concrete interpretation. The target was a picture representing the figurative meaning of the sentence. However, several methodological flaws render the interpretations of these results somewhat difficult. For example, at a closer look one can see that even if literal and non-literal sentences were matched in structure, the linguistic expressions were rather heterogeneous and comprised idioms, proverbs, and collocations such as *I'll get back to you later*. Very few controls on the psycholinguistic properties of the stimuli were reported (e.g., familiarity, length, and syntactic structure). Moreover, clinical features such as the severity of aphasia and the presence of additional neuropsychological deficits (e.g., attentional, perceptual, or spatial deficits) were not reported. The time of testing with respect to the time of onset of aphasia was variable, and it was not specified whether patients underwent language rehabilitation. The possibility that language-impaired participants had additional neuropsychological deficits deserved more attention since when sensory or cognitive deficits associated with RH damage result in sub-optimal processing of critical elements, or deplete available resources for further analysis, patients might be particularly likely to resort to the less demanding choice (the literal alternative). In fact, the pictures representing literal sentences might be less demanding for visuo-perceptual and visuospatial skills. Indeed the picture complexity of literal sentences is generally lower than that of idiomatic sentences: literal sentences typically only have a single concrete interpretation, and limited visuospatial and attentional resources might suffice. This is not true for pictures depicting idiomatic meanings that are often abstract and therefore difficult to represent at a pictorial level. It could then be the case that patients' performance was influenced by pictorial complexity and/or ambiguity. This is confirmed by a recent study on aphasics that showed significant correlations between idiom comprehension (tested with a sentence-to-picture matching task) and star cancellation or line bisection tests (Papagno et al., 2006). Finally, in Van Lancker and Kempler's study the performance of aphasic patients on familiar phrases was considered close to normal even though their mean percentage of correct responses was 72% as compared to 97.3% of controls. This suggests that LBD patients' performance was at least mildly impaired.

Similar concerns on the clinical implications and interpretation of the study of Van Lancker and Kempler (1987) were raised some years later by Tompkins, Boada, and McGarry (1992). Indeed, Tompkins et al. correctly pointed out that defining the meaning of an idiom or choosing a picture in a matching task are the end-products of multiple computations, so the sources of failure on such tasks are hard to correctly spell out. In other words, offline tasks are distant in time (and correspondingly in terms of cognitive operations) and far from being able to detect the initial retrieval or computation of meaning. By contrast, online tasks require a response to some aspect of the input during, rather than after, comprehension processes. To investigate the extent to which online versus offline tasks might produce different results, Tompkins et al. tested 20 RBD patients (40% of them with neglect), 20 LBD (65% of them with aphasia), and 20 neurologically intact controls. Participants performed two idiom comprehension tasks: the primary task was an online word-monitoring task in which participants listened to a sentence and pressed a button as quickly as possible when they heard a specific target word. Target words (e.g., *rat*) were concrete nouns that were the final constituent of ambiguous familiar idioms (e.g. *smell a rat*). Target monitoring was measured in three experimental conditions: idiomatic contexts, literal contexts that biased toward a literal interpretation of ambiguous idioms, and control contexts in which the target did not occur in an idiom (e.g., *saw a rat*). Brain-damaged participants performed similarly to normal controls in that all responded faster to target nouns in idiomatic and literal contexts compared to control contexts. The secondary task was an offline task in which participants were asked to give a meaning definition of 12 highly familiar idiomatic strings. In this task, brain-damaged participants performed poorly and made more errors than controls, without any difference between RBD and LBD. Therefore, adults with unilateral brain damage were able to activate and retrieve the meaning of familiar idioms. Their idiom interpretation deficits most likely reflect impairment at some later stage of information processing. However, it should be noted that only 65% of LBD patients were aphasic and that the standard deviations in the word monitoring tasks were rather high suggesting a huge variability in the patients' performance. It is likely that if subgroups had been distinguished, the performance of aphasics would have been significantly worse than that of controls in the online task. In addition, as in previously mentioned studies, no information about the lesion site or size was given, but only a rough topological distribution in anterior, posterior, mixed, and subcortical lesions.

Recent Neuropsychological Studies on Idiom Comprehension: The Fall of the RH Hypothesis

The studies described above definitively showed that the hypothesis that the RH plays a major role in idiom comprehension has a number of important limitations. More recent neuropsychological studies provided direct evidence of the involvement of the LH, specifically of the temporal lobe, in idiom comprehension. It should be noted that the studies that appeared in this period of time differ in many methodological respects from the previous ones: for instance, many of the more recent studies provide detailed information about the criteria of selection of the participants, and on the anatomical assessment of the lesion sites; the experimental materials are more controlled as far as the psycholinguistic variables known to affect linguistic processing are concerned.

In a sentence-to-picture matching task, Papagno, Tabossi, Colombo, and Zampetti (2004) presented 10 aphasic patients and 10 healthy controls with highly familiar unambiguous idioms (the literal meaning of the string was implausible or the sentence ill-formed). Each idiom was paired with pictures representing the idiomatic interpretation, the literal interpretation, or an unrelated situation. Aphasic patients were severely impaired in that they chose the wrong picture in half of the trials. When the same patients were asked to orally define the meaning of the same set of idioms, their accuracy dramatically increased (although their performance was significantly worse than that of controls). This suggests that the picture matching paradigm may underestimate the patient's ability to comprehend idioms.

The analysis of the individual errors in the sentence-to-picture matching task showed that patients did not choose at random: in fact they selected the unrelated alternative only a few times (the number of unrelated choices was comparable to that of the healthy participants). A further analysis of the responses given by aphasic patients with semantic deficits indicated that they took advantage of syntactic information: when presented with syntactically ill-formed idioms or with idioms with infrequent syntactic structures, patients with good syntactic competence made fewer literal errors than with well-formed idioms. In sum, these patients retrieved the figurative interpretation only when the linguistic analysis of the string failed to yield acceptable results. This suggests that aphasic patients made use of spared language abilities in order to comprehend idiomatic expressions, for example, syntactic competence (Papagno et al., 2004) when lexical semantic knowledge was impaired. When semantic knowledge was defective, aphasic patients accepted the literal interpretation, even when semantically implausible, basically because their semantic deficits did not allow them to recognize sentence implausibility. On the contrary, semantic knowledge was used when syntactic analysis was defective.

Papagno and Genoni (2004) tested 11 aphasic patients with syntactic deficit but spared semantic knowledge (plus a corresponding number of healthy controls) with an auditory sentence presentation mode and two tasks: a sentence-to-picture matching task and a grammaticality judgment task. They showed that idiom comprehension was significantly impaired in patients as compared to controls. Moreover, the patients' ability to comprehend idioms inversely correlated with the plausibility of the literal interpretation of the idiom string: the more plausible the literal interpretation was, the greater was the probability that the patient selected the picture corresponding to the literal meaning. Interestingly, idiom comprehension correlated with grammaticality judgment and in particular with the patients' ability to recognize the correct grammatical form of an idiom. This is a further piece of evidence that the more language processing is preserved, the more idiom comprehension is preserved as well.

Papagno et al.'s study (2006) was explicitly designed to assess the comprehension of unambiguous idiom in RDB and LBD patients (15 and 12, respectively) by means of a string-to-picture matching task. While all LBD patients were aphasic, the RBD patients showed various degrees of visuospatial impairment. In fact, idiom comprehension significantly correlated with visuospatial tasks in RBD patients. Eight of the 12 LBD patients were impaired in idiom comprehension, and overall the performance of the LBD patients was significantly worse than that of their matched controls.

As Tompkins et al. (1992) noted, some of the deficits previously reported for RBD adults might be partly an artifact of the differential plausibility of the literal meanings, alone or in combination with patients' visuospatial deficits. The RBD patients, though impaired, performed significantly better than LBD patients; their performance was correlated with visuospatial abilities and was significantly affected by lesion site, being particularly impaired in patients with a cortical and/or subcortical frontal lesion.

The Effect of the Task and of the Type of Idiom

Idiomatic expressions do not form a homogeneous group: they might be semantically ambiguous or not, they might be more or less familiar, they might differ in terms of semantic transparency (i.e., the extent to which the idiomatic meaning is inferable from the literal meaning of the string). The possibility exists that different types of idiomatic expression could undergo different kinds of processing and that the comprehension of ambiguous versus unambiguous idioms might be selectively disrupted.

To test the effect of the ambiguity of the idiom string, Cacciari et al. (2006) investigated the comprehension of ambiguous idioms in 15 aphasic patients using a word-to-sentence matching task. Syntactically simple sentences containing an idiom were paired with four words: a word corresponding to the idiomatic interpretation of the string, a word semantically associated with the last constituent word of the idiom string, and two unrelated foils (one foil was either an abstract or concrete word depending on the semantic class of the idiom target, and the other a word that could literally complete the verb in the verb phrase). The task was to choose the target word with the best fit with the figurative meaning of the sentence. Aphasic patients were significantly more impaired than matched controls. Semantically associated errors were significantly more frequent than unrelated errors. This might depend either on a lack of recognition of the idiomatic nature of the string (Cacciari & Tabossi, 1988) that prevented aphasics from retrieving the idiom meaning from semantic memory or on deficient inhibition of the word meaning associated with the final constituent word of the idiom string. The retrieval of the figurative meaning might have been blocked by a sort of processing loop in which the patient was unable to get rid of the literal meaning of the string. Since the language resources of aphasics are damaged, a greater involvement of executive control was required thus depleting the attentional pool and preventing the appropriate suppression/inhibition of the literal meaning. However, this study was not designed to tease apart these two explanations.

However, the disproportionate choice of the literal answer may depend on the task. Therefore Papagno and Caporali's study (2007) investigated whether, and to what extent, idiom comprehension in aphasic patients was influenced by the task and by the ambiguous versus unambiguous nature of idioms. Fifteen aphasics (and 15 controls) were involved in two experiments: in the first experiment, they were tested with three different tasks (sentence-to-picture and sentence-to-word match-ing tasks, and oral definition task) using simple sentences containing unambiguous idioms. The results showed high variability among aphasic patients, with some severely impaired and others performing nearly as well as the control group. The patients' performance was influenced by the severity of the language deficit (for instance, the oral definition task could not be performed by some nonfluent patients), but also and even more so by the type of task. While in fact it had no influence on the performance of neurologically unimpaired participants, it did affect aphasic patients and for a variety of reasons: reduced expressive skills in the oral definition task, and dysexecutive problems in the sentence-to-picture matching task (but also in the sentence-to-word matching task with ambiguous idioms, see Experiment 2). Indeed, a comparison of the results in the three tasks showed that aphasic patients performed significantly better with the sentence-to-word matching task (see Cacciari et al.'s 2006 study for the details on the experiment design) than with the other two tasks. In the sentence-to-word matching task, one foil was semantically associated with the last constituent word of the idiom string; and two words were unrelated foils. Specifically, the first type of unrelated word was either an abstract or a concrete word depending on the nature of the idiomatic target. The second type of unrelated foil was a word that could plausibly complete the verb in the verb phrase. The target was a word corresponding to the idiomatic interpreta-tion of the sentence. The overt representation of the literal meaning in the sentence-to-picture matching task (i.e., a bizarre picture corresponding to the idiom's literal interpretation) had in fact a strong interference effect, similar to that observed in the Stroop test. When an explicit pictorial representation of the idiom's literal meaning was available, patients were unable to suppress it. This confirms that the literal interpretation somehow remained active while the sentence was processed, even when it had very low plausibility. In the sentence-to-word matching task none of the target words referred to the literal meaning of the idiom string, and this decreased the interference of the literal interpretation. Therefore the errors (very numerous as compared to controls) indeed indicate lack of knowledge of the idi-omatic meaning. Since literal errors especially appeared when the literal interpreta-tion was overtly *offered* to the patient, it could be the case that when the figurative meaning is lost (or not accessed) and the literal alternative (i.e., the word or picture corresponding to the literal interpretation of the idiom string) is absent, the patients chose the (wrong) answer that preserves the semantic class (abstract/concrete) of the correct choice. This further suggests some level of processing of the sentential meaning.

In the second experiment of Papagno and Caporali's study (2007), patients and controls were presented with simple sentences containing either ambiguous or unambiguous idioms in a sentence-to-word matching task. Again, patients per-formed significantly worse than controls, but with a different pattern of errors for unambiguous compared to ambiguous idioms (significantly more unrelated errors preserving the semantic class, and significantly more literal associate errors, respec-tively). This different pattern of errors, together with the absence of correlation with general language impairment for unambiguous idioms, suggests that the two types of idiom might have been processed differently by aphasics. In support of this hypothesis, in this same study two patients were found with a double dissociation. One patient was severely impaired on ambiguous idiom comprehension, but had a noticeably better performance on unambiguous idioms, while the other made no errors on ambiguous idioms and performed at chance on unambiguous idioms.

Further evidence for differential processing of ambiguous and unambiguous idioms came from a single case study (Papagno & Cacciari, 2010). Idiom comprehension was investigated in an Italian semantic dementia patient (M.C.) with conceptual damages affecting both naming and comprehension of concrete nouns, while abstract nouns, verbs, and adjectives (both abstract and concrete) were spared (Papagno, Capasso, & Miceli, 2009). Since idioms convey abstract figurative meanings, we assessed whether idiom comprehension was preserved in M.C. as it was for abstract literal meanings, and tested the extent to which the number of meanings associated to a linguistic unit affected M.C.'s comprehension processes. Therefore we employed ambiguous and unambiguous idioms (together with polysemous and nonpolysemous words). Only the comprehension of unambiguous idioms (and of nonpolysemous words) was impaired despite the fact that both types of idiom string conveyed abstract mental states.

In sum, there is consistent evidence suggesting a double dissociation: while there are patients severely impaired on ambiguous idiom who display a noticeably better performance on unambiguous idioms, other patients make no errors on ambiguous idioms but perform at chance on unambiguous idioms. Overall, aphasic patients unexpectedly showed better performances with ambiguous idioms, as if a plausible literal meaning helped in retrieving the idiomatic meaning.

The observation of this double dissociation in patients has interesting parallels in the psycholinguistic literature on word processing in healthy participants. It has been often reported that semantically ambiguous words are recognized faster than nonambiguous words (e.g., Rubinstein, Garfield, & Millikan, 1970) especially in lexical decision studies. Several interpretations of this *ambiguity advantage* have been provided that postulate a lexical architecture based on either inhibitory lexical networks (e.g., Kellas, Ferraro, & Simpson, 1988) or competition between patterns of activation of word meanings (e.g., Gaskell & Marslen-Wilson, 1997). Recently this *ambiguity advantage* has been put under scrutiny by several authors (for an overview, see Rodd, Gaskell, & Marslen-Wilson, 2002). The main result is that multiple related word senses, as in polysemous words, produce a processing advantage while multiple unrelated meanings, as in homonyms, delay recognition producing an ambiguity disadvantage (e.g., Rodd et al., 2002). Rodd et al. interpreted these results as suggesting competition to activate a distributed semantic representation: while the different meanings of a homonym (e.g., *bank*) compete for activation and produce interference that delays recognition times, the rich and intertwined semantic representation associated with polysemous words that have many related senses (e.g., *rose*) facilitate their recognition. The possibility exists that ambiguous idioms behave as polysemous words, especially when there is a close semantic relationship between the literal and figurative interpretation of the idiom string. Further evidence that, aside from ambiguity, not all idiomatic expressions are processed alike came from a case study of a Finnish deep dyslexic patient (Nenonen, Niemi, & Laine, 2002). The authors investigated the patient's comprehension of verb phrase and noun phrase idioms with a reading task. The authors found that the syntactic structure of the different types of Finnish idiom modulated the ability of the deep dyslexic to comprehend idioms. However, it is not clear to what extent these results were influenced by the nature of the task that might have been particularly problematic for a deep dyslexic.

Although we showed that there is ample evidence of impairment of idiomatic processing in aphasia, there are also aphasics with preserved idiom comprehension (Hillert, 2004). Hillert tested two German LBD patients (one with Wernicke's and the other with global aphasia), one RDB patient, and one healthy control using a cross-modal lexical decision paradigm. He found no difference between aphasics and the two controls. However, aside from the very scarce number of patients and controls, the results might have been influenced by the lower processing demand of the comprehension of the German noun compounds used in the study. Indeed, noun phrase idioms have proved to be easier to access than verb phrase idioms (Nenonen et al., 2002) that are the most frequent form of idiom in the literature on aphasic patients.

Transcranial Magnetic Stimulation and Brain Imaging Studies

Most of the neurophysiological studies on figurative language are devoted to metaphors and only a few investigated idiom comprehension. To our knowledge, there are only three studies that used the repetitive transcranial magnetic stimulation (rTMS) technique and three fMRI studies (we do not consider two fMRI studies, Boulenger, Hauk, & Pulvermüller, 2009, and Aziz-Zadeh & Damasio, 2008, on the relationship between language and motor system, that used idioms and metaphors as experimental materials). We start with rTMS studies.

The first study that used an *interference approach* by means of offline rTMS to investigate the neural substrates of idiom comprehension was that of Oliveri, Romero, and Papagno (2004). In this study familiar unambiguous idiom strings were paired with two pictures representing the idiomatic or the literal meaning of the string. Fifteen healthy participants were asked to decide which one of the pictures matched the string meaning. The scalp positions for stimulation were the posterior temporal site (corresponding to BA 22) and a frontal site (BA 44/45) both on the RH and LH (plus a baseline without stimulation). In general, the reaction times increased following LH rTMS while they were unaffected by RH rTMS. The distribution of reaction times and errors was mostly affected by stimulation of the left temporal site as compared to the other sites and to the baseline. Left frontal rTMS induced less prominent, nonsignificant, disruption whereas right temporal rTMS facilitated participants' performance.

A subsequent rTMS study by the same group (Fogliata et al., 2007) was devoted to testing the temporal dynamics of activation of left prefrontal and temporal cortices. If the prefrontal cortex is involved in activating the figurative interpretation of unambiguous idioms, its activation should appear early in idiom processing. On the other hand, the authors hypothesized that if a suppression mechanism is at work, the frontal activity might persist even when the temporal activity decreases. To this end, rTMS was applied over the left middle frontal gyrus (BA 9) and left superior/middle temporal cortex (BA 22) at four different time points (0, 40, 80, and 120 ms after picture presentation). Forty-three participants were presented with short sentences that could be literal or contain a familiar unambiguous idiom. Each sentence was paired with four pictures (for idioms they represented the correct idiomatic meaning, the literal meaning, a context containing the noun phrase of the idiom, or an unrelated situation). Again, a sentence-to-picture matching task was used. The rTMS interfered with the task when delivered 80 ms after picture presentation at both frontal and temporal sites. However, stimulation at 120 ms after picture representation had an effect on accuracy, which occurred only at the prefrontal site, supporting the idea that a mechanism of inhibition/suppression was at work. In contrast, literal sentence comprehension was unaffected by prefrontal stimulation at any times suggesting that the role of the prefrontal cortex was specific to idiom comprehension (see the study by Romero Lauro, Tettamanti, Cappa, & Papagno, 2008, presented below).

In another study (Rizzo, Sandrini, & Papagno, 2007) that used the same online stimulation paradigm and experimental materials, the scalp sites stimulated with the rTMS in 14 participants were the right and left dorsolateral prefrontal cortex (DLPFC). The study was designed to use the interference paradigm provided by rTMS for testing the hypothesis that lesions in these areas might be at the origin of the impairment in idiom comprehension found in RBD patients. Both left and right rTMS slowed down the reaction times of all sentences (consistently with the brain imaging literature on the involvement of the DLPFC in sentence processing) and decreased idiom's accuracy. In sum, both the left and right DLPFC were involved in the selection of the appropriate response in the case of idioms, presumably because of inhibition of the literal meanings.

We now turn to fMRI studies (Mashal, Faust, Hendler, & Jung-Beeman, 2008; Romero Lauro et al., 2008; Zempleni, Haverkort, Renken, & Stowe, 2007, see also Rapp, Volume 1, Chapter 20). In an event-related fMRI study, Zempleni et al. (2007) visually presented 17 participants with literally plausible idioms in sentences that biased the readers toward the figurative or literal interpretation of the idiom strings. These were contrasted with sentences containing unambiguous idioms and literal sentences. Participants read the sentences for comprehension and carried out a relatedness decision whenever a word printed in red appeared after a sentence (which happened only on filler sentences). The major finding of this study is that idiom comprehension (for both ambiguous and unambiguous idioms), as measured by contrasting figurative versus literal sentences, was supported by bilateral inferior frontal gyri and left middle temporal gyrus. The right middle temporal gyrus was also involved, but almost exclusively for ambiguous idioms.

Another event-related fMRI study was carried out by Romero Lauro et al. (2008). They asked 22 participants to decide whether the meaning of a sentence, that either was literal or contained an ambiguous or an unambiguous idiom, matched a picture. The results revealed that making judgments about literal and idiomatic sentences yielded a common network of cortical activity, involving language areas of the LH. However, the nonliteral task elicited overall greater activation, both in terms of magnitude and spatial extent. In particular, Romero Lauro et al. found a bilateral frontotemporal network of increased cortical activity for idiomatic compared with literal sentences. The idiomatic condition activated bilaterally the inferior frontal gyrus and the anterior middle temporal gyrus (BA 21). Specifically, the left superior frontal (approximately covering BA 9), as well as the left inferior frontal gyrus, were specifically involved in processing idiomatic sentences. As to the RH, activation was seen in the middle temporal gyrus and in the temporal pole. In contrast with Zempleni et al.'s study, Romero Lauro et al. did not find any difference between ambiguous and unambiguous idioms.

The last fMRI study on idiom comprehension was carried out by Mashal et al. (2008) who examined the role of the LH and RH in processing the dominant/ idiomatic and the subordinate/literal meaning of familiar ambiguous idioms (a behavioral divided visual field experiment was also carried out, but we concentrate on the fMRI experiment). The study is based on the *graded salience hypothesis* (Giora, 2003) that predicts that subordinate/literal interpretations are processed in the RH while dominant/idiomatic interpretations primarily engage the LH. This hypothesis is at odds with what was found by Romero Lauro et al. (2008) but is compatible with Zempleni et al.'s (2007) results. Fourteen participants were instructed to perform one of two different tasks: to think about the idiomatic meaning of the sentences or to think about the literal meaning of the idiom or of the literal sentence (a third of the sentences were literal and the remaining contained ambiguous idioms). Prior to each block, instructions on how to process the sentences, idiomatically or literally, were visualized to the participants. No control is reported on whether or not participants indeed identified the idiomatic meaning, or thought of the idiomatic versus literal meaning (note that 50 out of 75 experimental sentences contained idioms). This is a serious confound especially because of the interpretations assigned to the brain activity reported in this study. The brain activation obtained for the (*presumed*, in our view) idiomatic processing of idioms, compared to the literal processing of the literal sentences, showed that three areas of the LH had greater activation: the inferior frontal gyrus, the middle temporal gyrus and the thalamus, as in the previous studies. The comparison between the (again *presumed*) literal processing of idioms with the (*presumed*) idiomatic processing of idioms showed greater activation in the RH middle temporal gyrus (as in Zempleni et al., 2007, while in Romero Lauro et al., 2008, such activation concerned unambiguous idioms as well), in the anterior part of the right superior temporal gyrus and in the left and right anterior insula. The opposite contrast (idiomatic vs. literal processing of idioms) identified significant activation only in the left inferior frontal gyrus.

These fMRI results (together with the behavioral results obtained with the divided visual field paradigm) were interpreted by Mashal et al. (2008) as evidence of an RH advantage in processing subordinate/nonsalient literal meaning of familiar ambiguous idioms, and an LH advantage in processing the dominant/idiomatic meaning of the idiom strings. However, as we said, the most problematic aspect of this interesting study remains the fact that there is no overt task (either online or offline) that could to some extent guarantee that indeed participants entered into either a literal or an idiomatic mode of processing as instructed prior to the block beginning and remained *faithful* and stable to that processing mode for the entire block. It should be noted that these results in large part are inconsistent with the bilateral activation patterns found in both Zempleni et al. (2007) and Romero Lauro et al. (2008). In contrast, the left-sided brain activations observed by Mashal et al. (2008) are consistent with lesion data of aphasic patients where a left temporal lesion is associated with a literal interpretation of the sentence. In fact, when the LH *is* damaged and the RH is not, the idiom's literal interpretation is the first to be activated and produced by the patient.

Mashal et al. interpreted their results as evidence for the graded salience hypothesis (Giora, 2003). However it is not clear to what extent the notion of salience interacts or overlaps with that of meaning dominance: as has been shown by decades of studies on lexical ambiguity processing, when a word or a string of words has two meanings, one of them typically is dominant (and corresponds to the prepotent response). Idioms are no exception and the results can be reinterpreted as showing that dominant (often more frequent) meanings are elaborated mostly via the LH, regardless of their literal or figurative nature.

Conclusion

As we hope it is clear from this chapter, the identification of the neuropsychological and neurophysiological correlates of idiom understanding is still a fascinating challenge for models of language processing. The title contains a basic question that has animated the first phase of the studies on idiom comprehension in language-impaired participants and has continued to exert a role also in the second phase: How many hemispheres are involved in idiom comprehension?

A simple way to respond is that both hemispheres indeed play a role in idiom language, although not an equally dominant one (for an interesting hypothesis on the labor division of the LH and RH to be applied to figurative language comprehension, see Beeman, 1998, and Mirous & Beeman, Volume 1, Chapter 16). This should come as no surprise since after all idioms are linguistic units, and the prevalence of the LH in sentence processing is well established. The explicit comparison of RBD and LBD patients (as in Papagno et al., 2006) and the literature on each of these groups indicated that LBD patients were impaired in idiom comprehension. The impaired performance on idioms of RBD patients was related to: (1) visuospatial deficits that were particularly relevant when patients were tested with pictorial materials; (2) lesions localized in the prefrontal (cortical or subcortical) region. This was confirmed by the fact that, when these lesions were absent, RBD patients' performance on idioms was not different from that of controls. The evidence reported in many neuropsychological and neurophysiological studies on a role of the right (and not only the left) dorsolateral prefrontal cortex (but also of the subcortical white matter) could explain why figurative (and idiomatic in particular) language impairment has been considered a right-brain-damage consequence: since the exact lesion site was often not reported, it could well be the case that a number of patients had prefrontal lesions.

From an anatomical point of view, two sites are thought to be relevant for the patients' performance: a cortical and/or subcortical frontal area particularly involved in the comprehension of ambiguous idioms, and a cortical temporal region constantly involved when unambiguous idiom comprehension is impaired. These results were supported by rTMS studies on healthy participants using both offline (Oliveri et al., 2004) and online paradigms (Fogliata et al., 2007; Rizzo et al., 2007).

Prefrontal regions appear to be involved in: (1) the retrieval of the figurative meaning of idioms from semantic memory; (2) monitoring of the response; and (3) inhibition of an alternative interpretation (especially with the picture matching task). Once a sentence containing an idiom is linguistically processed and two possible interpretations are available, a response must be selected and the outcome monitored. Selection and monitoring of internally generated responses are likely to be performed by the central executive whose neural correlates are supposed to be in the prefrontal lobe. Indeed, as we saw, patients with prefrontal lesions produce a higher number of literal interpretations as compared to patients with lesions not involving the prefrontal lobe. The role of the prefrontal cortex in language control has been demonstrated in a number of studies with sentence processing tasks in which the listener/reader needs to maintain the information online for a certain period (Friederici, 2002).

In a nutshell, idiom comprehension seems to be subserved by a bilateral neural network as opposed to the exclusive participation of the RH. Specifically, converging evidence from lesion studies and rTMS and fMRI studies indicates that the neural network activated during idiom comprehension also involves: (1) in the LH, the temporal cortex and the superior medial frontal gyrus and the inferior frontal gyrus; (2) in the RH, the superior and middle temporal gyri, the temporal pole, and the inferior frontal gyrus.

References

Aziz-Zadeh, L., & Damasio, A. (2008). Embodied semantics for actions: Findings from functional brain imaging. *Journal of Physiology, 102,* 35–39.

Beeman, M. (1998). Coarse semantic coding and discourse comprehension. In M. Beeman & C. Chiarello (Eds.), *Right hemisphere language comprehension. Perspective from cognitive neuroscience* (pp. 255–284). Mahwah, NJ: Erlbaum.

Boulenger, V., Hauk, O., & Pulvermüller, F. (2009). Grasping ideas with the motor system: Semantic somatotopy in idiom comprehension. *Cerebral Cortex, 19*, 1905–1914.

Cacciari, C. (1993). The place of idioms in a literal and metaphorical world. In C. Cacciari & P. Tabossi (Eds.), *Idioms. Processing, structure, and interpretation* (pp. 27–55). Hillsdale, NJ: Erlbaum.

Cacciari, C., & Glucksberg, S. (1994). Understanding figurative language. In M. A. Gernsbacher (Ed.), *Handbook of psycholinguistics* (pp. 447–477). New York: Academic Press.

Cacciari, C., Padovani, R., & Corradini, P. (2007). Exploring the relationship between individuals' speed of processing and their comprehension of spoken idioms. *European Journal of Cognitive Psychology, 19*(3), 417–445

Cacciari, C., Reati, F., Colombo, M. R., Padovani, R., Rizzo, S., & Papagno, C. (2006). The comprehension of ambiguous idioms in aphasic patients. *Neuropsychologia, 44*, 1305–1314.

Cacciari, C., & Tabossi, P. (1988). The comprehension of idioms. *Journal of Memory and Language, 27*, 668–683.

Cacciari, C., & Tabossi, P. (Eds.). (1993). *Idioms. Processing, structure, and interpretation*. Hillsdale, NJ: Erlbaum.

Ferretti, T. R., Schwint, C. A., & Katz, A. (2007). Electrophysiological and behavioral measures of the influence of literal and figurative contextual constraint on proverb comprehension. *Brain and Language, 101*, 38–49.

Fogliata, A., Rizzo, S., Reati, F., Miniussi, C., Oliveri, M., & Papagno, C. (2007). The time course of idiom processing. *Neuropsychologia, 45*, 3215–3222.

Friederici, A. D. (2002). Towards a neural basis of auditory sentence processing. *Trends in Cognitive Sciences, 6*, 78–84.

Gaskell, M. G., & Marslen-Wilson, W. D. (1997). Integrating form and meaning: A distributed model of speech perception. *Language and Cognitive Processes, 12*, 613–656.

Giora, R. (2003). *On our minds. Salience, context and figurative language*. Oxford: Oxford University Press.

Glucksberg, S. (2001). *Understanding figurative language*. Oxford: Oxford University Press.

Hillert, D. (2004). Spared access to idiomatic and literal meanings: A single-case approach. *Brain and Language, 89*, 207–215.

Jackendoff, R. (1995). The boundaries of the lexicon. In M. Everaert, E. van den Linden, A. Schenk, & R. Schreuder (Eds.), *Idioms: structural and psychological perspectives* (pp. 133–166). Hillsdale, NJ: Erlbaum.

Kellas, G., Ferraro, F. R., & Simpson, G. B. (1988). Lexical ambiguity and the time course of attentional allocation in word recognition. *Journal of Experimental Psychology: Human Perception and Performance, 14*, 601–609.

Kempler, D., Van Lancker, D., Marchman, V., & Bates, E. (1999). Idiom comprehension in children and adults with unilateral brain damage. *Developmental Neuropsychology, 15*, 327–349.

Konopcka, A. E., & Bock, K. (2009). Lexical or syntactic control of sentence formulation? Structural generalizations from idiom production. *Cognitive Psychology, 58*, 68–101.

Mashal, N., Faust, M., Hendler, T., & Jung-Beeman, M. (2008). Hemispheric differences in processing the literal interpretation of idioms: Converging evidence from behavioral and fMRI studies. *Cortex, 44*, 848–860.

Nenonen, M., Niemi, J., & Laine, M. (2002). Representation and processing of idioms: Evidence from aphasia. *Journal of Neurolinguistics, 1,* 43–58.

Oliveri, M., Romero, L., & Papagno, C. (2004). Left but not right temporal lobe involvement in opaque idiom comprehension: A repetitive transcranial magnetic stimulation study. *Journal of Cognitive Neuroscience, 16,* 848–855.

Papagno, C., & Cacciari, C. (2010). The comprehension of idioms in a patient with a reversed concreteness effect. *Journal of Neurolinguistics.* doi:10.1016/j,jneuroling.2010.06.002

Papagno, C., Capasso, R., Miceli G. (2009). Reversed concreteness effect for nouns in a subject with semantic dementia. *Neuropsychologia, 47,* 1138–1148. doi:10.1016/j.neuropsychologia.2009.01.019

Papagno, C., Capasso, R., Zerboni, H., & Miceli, G. (2009). A reverse concreteness effect in a subject with semantic dementia. *Brain and Language, 103,* 90–91.

Papagno, C., & Caporali, A. (2007). Testing idiom comprehension in aphasic patients: The effects of task and idiom type. *Brain and Language, 100,* 208–220.

Papagno, C., Curti, R., Rizzo, S., Crippa, F., & Colombo, M. R. (2006). Is the right hemisphere involved in idiom comprehension? A neuropsychological study. *Neuropsychology, 20,* 598–606.

Papagno, C., & Genoni, A. (2004). The role of syntactic competence in idiom comprehension: A study on aphasic patients. *Journal of Neurolinguistics, 17,* 371–382.

Papagno, C., Lucchelli, F., Muggia, S., & Rizzo, S. (2003). Idiom comprehension in Alzheimer's disease: The role of the central executive. *Brain, 126,* 2419–2430.

Papagno, C., Tabossi, P., Colombo, M., & Zampetti, P. (2004). Idiom comprehension in aphasic patients. *Brain and Language, 89,* 226–234.

Pollio, H., Barlow, J., Fine, H., & Pollio, M. (1977). *Metaphor and the poetics of growth: Figurative language in psychology, psychotherapy and education.* Hillsdale, NJ: Erlbaum.

Rizzo, S., Sandrini, M., & Papagno, C. (2007). The dorsolateral prefrontal cortex in idiom interpretation: An rTMS study. *Brain Research Bulletin, 71,* 523–528.

Rodd, J., Gaskell, G., & Marslen-Wilson, W. (2002). Making sense of semantic ambiguity: Semantic competition in lexical access. *Journal of Memory and Language, 46,* 245–266.

Romero Lauro, L. J., Tettamanti, M., Cappa, S. F., & Papagno, C. (2008). Idiom comprehension: A prefrontal task? *Cerebral Cortex, 18,* 162–170.

Rubinstein, H., Garfield, L., & Millikan, J. A. (1970). Homographic entries in the internal lexicon. *Journal of Verbal Learning and Verbal Behavior, 9,* 487–494.

Searle, J. R. (1979). *Expression and meaning: Studies in the theory of speech acts.* Cambridge: Cambridge University Press.

Stachowiak, F., Huber, W., Poeck, K., & Kerschensteiner, M. (1977). Text comprehension in aphasia. *Brain and Language, 4,* 177–195.

Thoma, P., & Daum, I. (2006). Neurocognitive mechanisms of figurative language processing. Evidence from clinical dysfunctions. *Neuroscience and Behavioral Review, 30,* 1182–1205.

Tompkins, C. A., Boada, R., & McGarry, K. (1992). The access and processing of familiar idioms by brain-damaged and normally aging adults. *Journal of Speech and Hearing Research, 35,* 626–637.

Turner, N., & Katz, A. (1997). The availability of conventional and of literal meaning during the comprehension of proverbs. *Pragmatics and Cognition, 5,* 199–233.

Van Lancker, D., & Kempler, D. (1987). Comprehension of familiar phrases by left but not by right hemisphere damaged patients. *Brain and Language, 32,* 265–277.

Van Lancker Sidtis D., & Postman, W. A. (2006). Formulaic expressions in spontaneous speech of left and right hemisphere damaged subjects. *Aphasiology, 20*(5), 411–426.

Vespignani, F., Canal, P., Molinaro, N., Fonda, S., & Cacciari, C. (2010). Predictive mechanisms in idiom comprehension. *Journal of Cognitive Neuroscience, 22*(8), 1682–1700.

Zempleni, M. Z., Haverkort, M., Renken, R., & Stowe, L. A. (2007). Evidence for bilateral involvement in idiom comprehension: An fMRI study. *NeuroImage, 34*, 1280–1291

Winner, E., & Gardner, H. (1977). The comprehension of metaphor in brain-damaged patients. *Brain, 100*, 717–729.

19

Cognitive Neuroscience of Creative Language: The Poetic and the Prosaic

Seana Coulson and Tristan S. Davenport

Creativity in Language

In the comedy film *Office Space*, a depressed software technician named Peter shambles into his place of work and is greeted with the phrase, "Looks like someone has a case of the Mondays." Although readily understood by native speakers, creative language such as this has received scant attention from researchers in the cognitive neuroscience of language. Under the assumption that the essential feature of language is its compositionality (e.g., Dowty, Wall, & Peters, 1981), linguists have attempted to explain how the meanings of sentences can be derived from their syntactic structure and the meanings of their constituent words. Accordingly, researchers in psychology and neuropsychology have targeted knowledge of grammar and of word meaning, investigating their development in children, their breakdown in brain damage, and the way they operate in healthy adults.

However, there are a number of reasons for researchers in cognitive neuroscience to shift their focus from the most straightforward cases of literal meaning to more creative instances of language use such as the one cited above. First, while many people think of creative language as being confined to artistic venues, it is in fact far more common than many people realize (Gibbs, Wilson, & Bryant, in press). Second, the diversity of creative language highlights the range of different cognitive processes people bring to bear on language production and comprehension. Finally, the study of figurative language has led to an important locus of generativity in language, namely the human ability to interpret linguistic expressions in light of real-world knowledge and contextual factors (Coulson, 2001).

The Handbook of the Neuropsychology of Language, First Edition. Edited by Miriam Faust.
© 2012 Blackwell Publishing Ltd. Published 2012 by Blackwell Publishing Ltd.

The line of dialogue above highlights not only Peter's melancholy, but also two constructs from cognitive linguistics that help account both for creative uses of language, and for more straightforward instances of literal meaning (Fauconnier & Turner, 2002). The first such construct is *frames*, hierarchically structured representations of background knowledge activated by elements in a discourse (Fillmore, 1976). For example, this snippet of movie dialogue calls upon at least two frames. The phrase "a case of" activates a frame concerned with sickness and ailments. The mention of "Monday" activates cultural knowledge about the seven-day week and Monday's importance as the first obligatory day of work. In fact, without background knowledge about the work week, the statement is not readily interpretable. For example, an Israeli whose work week begins on Sunday might find the statement anomalous, in spite of knowing where Monday falls in the sequence of days.

In order to reach the desired interpretation, a second theoretical device is needed, namely an ability to activate *mappings*, or correspondences, between the appropriate elements in each of these conceptual domains. Features of the work-week frame pertaining to Monday are mapped onto features of the sickness frame that have compatible conceptual structure. Thus an illness, which is frequently unpleasant and beyond one's control, can be readily identified with Monday. In the integrated interpretation, Monday is the very ailment from which Peter suffers.

This chapter focuses on two well-defined examples of creative language that utilize frames and mappings: jokes and metaphors. We begin each section with a review of cognitive neuroscience research used to test and develop models of the comprehension of these phenomena, and follow with a review of evidence for the importance of the right hemisphere (RH) in each. We conclude with some speculations about the potential relevance of such research to general issues relevant to meaning in language.

Joke Comprehension

The study of joke comprehension addresses the importance of frames for language comprehension, since many jokes are funny because they invite the listener to use one frame to help interpret the information presented in the initial part of the joke, only to reveal frame-incompatible information at the punchline. For example, consider, "I let my accountant do my taxes because it saves time: last spring it saved me ten years." Initially, the listener activates a busy-professional frame. However, at the punchline "saved me ten years" it becomes apparent that a crooked-businessman frame is more appropriate. While lexical reinterpretation is important, to truly appreciate this joke it is necessary to recruit background knowledge about the particular sorts of relationships that can obtain between business people and their accountants so that the initial busy-professional interpretation can be mapped into the crooked-businessman frame. The semantic and pragmatic reanalysis necessary to understand narrative jokes such as this is known as *frame-shifting*, and the humor of a narrative joke is related in part to the contrast between the two frames (Coulson, 2001).

Patient studies of joke comprehension

Researchers in neuropsychology have long noted that joke comprehension is compromised in patients with RH lesions, especially when there is damage to the anterior portion of the frontal lobe (Brownell, Michel, Powelson, & Gardner, 1983; Shammi & Stuss, 1999). In one classic study, RH damaged (RHD) patients were given the set-up for a number of jokes and asked to pick the punchline from an array of three choices: straightforward endings, non sequitur endings, and the correct punchline. While age-matched controls had no trouble choosing the punchlines, RHD patients tended to choose the non sequitur endings, suggesting they understood that jokes involve a surprise ending, but were impaired on the frame-shifting process required to re-establish coherence.

Remarkably, the performance of RHD patients on joke comprehension tasks is slightly worse than that of left hemisphere damaged (LHD) patients whose communicative difficulties are seemingly more severe. To compare these groups, Bihrle and colleagues used nonverbal materials (cartoons) that required frame-shifting. Patients were shown the first 2 frames of the cartoon and asked to pick an ending that made it funny. On each trial, they were given two alternatives: the correct ending, and either a straightforward ending, a neutral non sequitur, or a humorous non sequitur. Though both patient groups were impaired on this task, the LHD patients were more likely to err by choosing straightforward endings, while RHD patients showed a consistent preference for non sequitur endings, especially the humorous non sequiturs, which tended to involve slapstick humor (Bihrle, Brownell & Gardner, 1986).

The latter finding suggests the deficits RHD patients experience in the comprehension and production of humor is not attributable to the emotional problems associated with some kinds of RHD, but rather from deficits in inferential processing. Moreover, subsequent research has demonstrated that RHD patients also have difficulty interpreting nonjoke materials that require semantic reanalysis (Brownell, Potter, Bihrle, & Gardner, 1986). Taken together, these observations indicate that the difficulty RHD patients experience understanding humorous materials is cognitive rather than emotional, and involves the inferential reanalysis in frame-shifting.

Cognitive electrophysiology of joke comprehension

The neurophysiology of joke comprehension has also been studied in healthy adults via the noninvasive recording of event-related brain potentials (ERPs). One virtue of this technique is that it allows the researcher to take advantage of reasonably well-understood ERP components associated with processing different sorts of linguistic information, such as the link between the N400 and semantic integration processes (for further details, see Kutas, Kiang, and Sweeney, Volume 2, Chapter 26). The N400 component of the ERPs was first noted in experiments contrasting sentences that ended sensibly and predictably with others that ended with an incongruous word. Congruous words elicited a late positive wave, while incongruous endings elicited a negative wave beginning about 200 ms after word onset and peaking at 400 ms (Kutas & Hillyard, 1980). Subsequent experiments have demonstrated a strong inverse correlation with the predictability of the eliciting word within a given sentence context (DeLong, Urbach, & Kutas, 2005; Kutas, Lindamood, & Hillyard, 1984). In general, experimental manipulations that make semantic integration more difficult result in larger amplitude N400, while those that facilitate it reduce N400 amplitude (van Berkum, Hagoort, & Brown, 1999).

Given the impact of frame-shifting on language interpretation, one might expect the underlying processes to be reflected in the brain's real-time response to jokes. Accordingly, Coulson and Kutas (2001) compared ERPs elicited by sentences that ended as jokes requiring frame-shifting with nonfunny "straight" endings consistent with the contextually evoked frame. Two types of jokes were tested, high constraint jokes such as (1) which elicited at least one response on a sentence completion task with a cloze probability of greater than 40%, and low constraint jokes such as (2) which elicited responses with cloze probabilities lower than 40%. Cloze probability is a measure of a word's predictability in a sentence context obtained via a sentence completion task. For example, when given the sentence fragment in (1), 81% of participants produced the word "face"; thus, the cloze probability of "face" in this context is 81%. For both (1) and (2) the word in parentheses was the most popular response on the cloze task.

1 I asked the woman at the party if she remembered me from last year and she said she never forgets a (face 81%).
2 My husband took all the money we were saving to buy a new car and blew it all at the (casino 18%).

To control for the fact that joke endings are (by definition) unexpected, the straight controls were chosen so that they matched the joke endings for cloze probability, but were consistent with the frame evoked by context. For example, the straight ending for (1) was "name" (the joke ending was "dress"), while the straight ending for (2) was "tables" (the joke ending was "movies"). The cloze probability of all four ending types (high and low constraint joke and straight endings) was equal, and ranged from 0–5%.

Coulson and Kutas (2001) found that ERPs to joke endings differed in several respects from those to the straight endings, depending on contextual constraint as well as participants' ability to get the jokes. In good joke comprehenders, high but not low constraint joke endings elicited a larger N400 than the straight endings, presumably because the activation of the relevant frame facilitated lexical integration of the high constraint straight endings relative to the jokes. Similar effects may have been absent from the low constraint stimuli, because those sentences led to the activation of a diverse set of frames that were less likely to be consistent with the straight endings.

However, both sorts of jokes (high and low constraint) elicited a late positivity in the ERP (500–900 ms post-onset), as well as a slow sustained negativity 300–900 ms post-onset, evident over left frontal sites. The sustained negativity at left frontal sites has been suggested to reflect the manipulation of information in working memory (Coulson & Kutas, 2001; Coulson & Lovett, 2004). The late positivity is an ERP effect often associated with the activation of information in memory (i.e., retrieval), consistent with the suggestion that joke comprehension requires the activation of a novel frame.

In poor joke comprehenders, jokes elicited a negativity between 300 and 700 ms after the onset of the sentence final word. The absence of the late positivity and the left frontal negativity in the poor joke comprehenders' ERPs suggests that these effects index cognitive operations important for actually getting the joke. The poor joke comprehenders apparently searched for a coherent interpretation of the joke endings, but because they were unable to retrieve the frame necessary to get the joke, they did not generate the ERP effects observed in good joke comprehenders.

These demonstrations of the brain's relatively early sensitivity to discourse level manipulations are consistent with the dynamic inferencing mechanisms assumed in many frame-based models of comprehension. For example, based on computational considerations, Shastri (1999) proposed that frame-based inferences necessary for language comprehension occur in a time-frame on the order of hundreds of milliseconds, in keeping with the observation that joke comprehension modulates the ERPs 300 ms after the onset of a critical word (Coulson & Kutas, 2001; Coulson & Lovett, 2004). In such models, comprehension is achieved by binding elements of the discourse representation to frames in long-term memory (Coulson, 2001; Lange, 1989). Such models help explain how speakers are able to rapidly and routinely compute predictions, explanations, and speaker intentions (Shastri & Ajjanagadde, 1993; van Berkum, 2008).

Hemispheric asymmetry and joke comprehension

Studies reviewed above have revealed a number of laterally asymmetric ERP effects suggestive of hemispheric asymmetry in joke comprehension, but do not directly speak to RH involvement due to limitations on the spatial resolution of the EEG signal. However, studies in neurologically intact individuals using the *hemi-field priming* paradigm also suggest differences in the contribution of the two cerebral hemispheres for the comprehension of creative language use such as that in jokes. The *priming* part of the hemi-field priming paradigm refers to a core phenomenon in psycholinguistics, the finding that people respond faster and more accurately to a word (e.g., "dog") when it is preceded by a semantically related (or otherwise associated) word (e.g., "cat"), than if it has been preceded by an unrelated word (e.g., "umbrella"). The *hemi-field* part of hemi-field priming refers to the fact that in this paradigm stimuli are presented to either the left or the right visual hemi-field (LVF/RVF).

Because stimuli presented outside the center of gaze are initially processed only by the opposite hemisphere, hemi-field presentation is thought to shift the balance of word processing, thus allowing the experimenter to probe each hemisphere's sensitivity to various semantic manipulations (Hellige, 1983; Zaidel, 1983). Although information presented in this way is rapidly transmitted to both hemispheres, the hemi-field technique is thought to reveal initial hemisphere-specific computations (Chiarello, 1991). Consequently, left visual field presentation is typically abbreviated as LVF/RH, while right visual field presentation is abbreviated RVF/LH.

Indeed, researchers who use the hemi-field priming paradigm report a number of results that suggest the two cerebral hemispheres differ in the way they establish the meaning of linguistic stimuli. Though these studies consistently find that RVF/LH presentation leads to shorter reaction times on priming tasks, presentation to the RVF/LH does not necessarily yield more robust *priming effects*, viz. the difference in reaction times between words preceded by lexical associates and words preceded by unrelated words (Chiarello, 1988). For example, though most single word priming studies using strongly associated words (such as "cat" and "dog") report equivalent priming with RVF/LH and LVF/RH presentation, nonassociated category members such as "goat" and "dog" yield greater priming effects with LVF/RH presentation (Chiarello, Burgess, Richards, & Pollock, 1990).

These observations have led some theorists to speculate that hemispheric differences in semantic activation might explain the disparate effect of LHD and RHD on the comprehension of language. One suggestion is that semantic activations in the LH are more specific than those in the RH, described as "fine" versus "coarse" semantic coding (Beeman et al., 1994; Chiarello et al., 1990; see also Mirous & Beeman, Volume 1, Chapter 16). Words in the RH are represented by means of wide semantic fields, while words in the LH are represented via a narrow range of features relevant to the immediate discourse context. Although coarse RH semantic activations would predictably include contextually irrelevant information, diffuse RH activation might provide additional information that makes joke processing easier. Similarly, reduced access to these semantic activations in RHD patients could result in joke comprehension deficits.

One chief source of evidence for the coarse coding hypothesis comes from an experiment in which centrally presented trios of words served as "summation primes" for a weakly related lateralized target (Beeman et al., 1994). For example, "cry, foot, glass" served as *summation primes* for the target "cut," and as *direct primes* for the target "laugh" which was semantically related to one of the prime words. Accuracies on a naming task indicated that, relative to unrelated items, both hemispheres benefited from both sorts of primes. However, there was an RVF/LH advantage for the direct primes and an LVF/RH advantage for summation primes. Beeman and colleagues argue that these findings suggest the RH benefits from the summed activation of shared features within a set of semantic fields.

Coulson and Wu (2005), however, note that the features of "foot" and "glass" do not, in fact, intersect. They suggest that summation priming results because these elements can be linked in a cognitive model in which glass can be construed as an instrument that induces a change of state in a patient, such as a foot. Rather than the sheer breadth of activation, hemispheric differences might thus be related to the type of semantic activations in each hemisphere. For example, the RH may preferentially activate stored knowledge about typical situations when glass, feet, and crying might co-occur, while the LH is more sensitive to linguistic cues that overtly specify the same types of complex relations.

Coulson and Wu (2005) argue that such hemispheric differences reflect RH coding of thematic and relational information. RHD patients have greater difficulty than those with LHD at recalling the theme of stories they have read (Hough, 1990). Further, neuroimaging research with healthy adults also suggests the importance of RH temporal lobe activity in processing thematic information. In a story comprehension task using materials modeled after the classic Bransford and Johnson study (1972), St George and colleagues report greater RH temporal lobe activation when thematic information was not provided for ambiguous paragraphs than when thematic information was provided by the inclusion of titles for the paragraphs (St George, Kutas, Martinez, & Sereno, 1999).

Hemispheric differences in semantic activation

Hemispheric differences in semantic activation might explain why RHD is associated with a detrimental effect on the comprehension of narrative jokes that require frame-shifting. Like Beeman's summation triads, jokes require the listener to access nonovertly encoded information to understand the connection between one's initial interpretation and the construal implied by the joke's punchline. For example, in the joke "The replacement player hit a home run with my girl," the reader must reinterpret information about a baseball game by accessing background information about romance.

Understanding one-line jokes Several hemi-field presentation studies in our laboratory have addressed whether hemispheric differences in semantic activation in healthy adults are relevant for joke comprehension. To do so, we used a variant of the hemi-field priming paradigm in which the measure of priming is the amplitude of the N400 component of the ERP. The use of an ERP measure of priming has a number of advantages over traditional behavioral measures, including the possibility of assessing the degree to which hemi-field presentation actually shifts the contribution of each hemisphere to stimulus processing. Further, whereas the response latencies in behavioral measures of priming are determined by a number of cognitive processes, including stimulus evaluation, response selection, and response execution, ERPs provide an ongoing record of the brain response from the onset of the stimulus until the execution of a response. Finally, ERPs can provide measures of the stimulus evaluation process in the absence of an overt response.

To assess whether hemispheric differences in semantic activation affect the difficulty of joke comprehension, we recorded ERPs as healthy adults read laterally presented "punch-words" to one-line jokes (Coulson & Williams, 2005). As noted above, the critical word in a joke often elicits a larger N400 than a similarly unexpected "straight" ending for the same sentence: the N400 joke effect (Coulson & Kutas, 2001). We reasoned that if hemispheric differences in semantic activation are relevant for joke comprehension, lateral presentation of joke ("girl") versus straight ("ball") endings for sentences such as "A replacement player hit a home run with my" would result in different N400 joke effects as a function of visual field of presentation. In this sentence comprehension paradigm, the difficulty of joke comprehension is indexed by the size of the N400 joke effect with larger effects pointing to relatively more processing difficulty. In fact, N400 joke effects were smaller when the critical words were presented to the LVF/RH than the RVF/LH, suggesting joke comprehension was easier with LVF/RH presentation (Coulson & Williams, 2005).

In a similarly motivated study, we measured ERPs elicited by laterally presented probe words that were preceded either by a joke, or by a nonfunny control (Coulson & Wu, 2005). Since all jokes turned on the last word of the sentence, control sentences were formed by replacing the sentence final word with a "straight" ending. For example, to construct a control for the following joke "Everyone has so much fun diving from the tree into the swimming pool, we decided to put in a little water," the word "water" was replaced by "platform". Probes (such as "crazy") were designed to be related to the meaning of the joke, but unrelated to the meaning of the straight control. In this sentence prime paradigm, the activation of information relevant to joke comprehension was signaled by differences in the size of the N400 elicited by related versus unrelated probes. The more active joke-related information was, the larger the N400 relatedness effect could be expected to be. Consistent with the hypothesis that the RH activates thematic and relational information important for joke comprehension, Coulson and Wu (2005) found larger N400 relatedness effects with LVF/RH presentation (see also Hull, Chen, Vaid, & Martinez, 2005, for comparable evidence using behavioral measures).

Understanding puns   It is, however, important not to construe jokes as a monolithic language phenomenon. The word play in puns, for example, is different from that in more semantically based jokes discussed above. While semantic jokes begin by suggesting one interpretation of the discourse situation only to replace it with another at the punchline, the point of puns is to promote multiple meanings. For example, in "Old programmers never die, they just lose their memory," the word "memory" can refer either to a human ability or to an electronic device, and both meanings are contextually appropriate. Indeed, the humorous nature of a pun derives from the listener's ability to simultaneously maintain two, possibly conflict-ing, meanings for the same word or phrase. In contrast to jokes that rely on frame-shifting, puns might be expected to rely more on LH mechanisms for the activation of conventional meanings.

Coulson and Severens (2007) addressed hemispheric sensitivity to the different meanings of a pun using a sentence priming paradigm with puns and pun-related probe words. ERPs were recorded as healthy adults listened to puns and read probe words presented in either participants' left or right visual hemi-fields. Probe words were either highly related to the pun that preceded them, moderately related to the pun that preceded them, or unrelated. For example, the highly related probe for "During branding cowboys have sore calves," was "cow" and the moderately related probe was "leg".

The activation of pun-related information was assessed by the presence of relat-edness effects on the N400 component of the ERP and on positive waveforms that frequently follow the N400 such as the late positive complex (LPC). Results sug-gested that initially both meanings of a pun were equally active in the LH while only the highly related probes were active in the RH; by 500 ms after the offset of the pun, however, both meanings were available in both hemispheres (Coulson & Severens, 2007).

Studies with puns thus differ from research reviewed above that suggest a RH advantage in understanding the critical word in a joke (Coulson & Williams, 2005), and in the activation of joke-related information (Coulson & Wu, 2005). While pun-related information is eventually available to both hemispheres, the LH showed an initial advantage that may reflect the importance of this hemisphere (especially the left frontal lobe) in coding the association between a word's phono-logical form and its conventional meaning. Consistent with this interpretation, a neuroimaging study that compared brain activity during the comprehension of semantic jokes with nonfunny controls revealed bilateral temporal lobe activa-tions, while an analogous comparison using puns revealed left frontal activations (Goel & Dolan, 2001). Whereas the RH and LH temporal lobe activation presum-ably reflects memory processes necessary for the inferential demands of jokes, the LH frontal activations to puns were consistent with the need to retrieve word meanings.

Neural substrate of joke comprehension

The involvement of the RH in humorous materials that involve frame-shifting is supported by an fMRI study in which neurologically intact participants viewed pairs of funny and nonfunny cartoons (Bartolo, Benuzzi, Nocetti, Baraldi, & Nichelli, 2006). As in the linguistic stimuli employed by Coulson and colleagues, the funny cartoon pairs employed by Bartolo et al. achieved their humorous effect by creating an expectation and confounding it. A key feature of Bartolo et al.'s stimuli, however, was that the expectation being manipulated depended on the intentions of the character depicted in the cartoon. Participants showed increased activation in right inferior frontal gyrus, as well as left middle and superior temporal gyri, while viewing the funny cartoon pairs.

Interestingly, the activations described by Bartolo et al. (2006) are markedly similar to those activated in a study of the attribution of intention (Brunet, Sarfati, Hardy-Baylé, & Decety, 2000). This result suggests that theory of mind may be crucial to understanding jokes, a connection also made by Winner, Brownell, Happé, Blum, and Pincus (1998) in a study of RHD patients' ability to distinguish between lies and jokes. Winner et al (1998) designed stories such that in order to distinguish lies from jokes, participants had to attribute a second-order belief (i.e., a belief about someone else's belief) to a character in the story. The RHD patients were significantly less adept at distinguishing lies from jokes than the neurologically intact controls. The difficulty RHD patients experienced distinguishing lies from jokes was thus argued to be derived from an inability to correctly attribute beliefs and intentions to others.

More generally, the recruitment of brain regions for understanding various sorts of creative language is best understood by relating these regions to the underlying cognitive processes. Because there are many different ways that linguistic utterances can diverge from literality, we should expect to observe a similar diversity in networks of brain areas recruited to comprehend them. Just as the brain areas activated in the comprehension of literal language differ as a function of the degree to which visual imagery or emotions are evoked (Ferstl, Rinck, & Cramon, 2005; Just, Newman, Keller, McEleny, & Carpenter, 2003), so too should we expect the comprehension of various kinds of nonliteral language to differ as a function of the cognitive processes they engender. In the following section, we provide a selective review of the literature on the cognitive neuroscience of metaphoric language, a creative use of language that differs from that in jokes in a number of important ways.

Metaphor

Relative to other sorts of figurative language (e.g. sarcasm, jokes, and so forth), metaphor has received the vast majority of the attention of researchers in cognitive neuroscience (see, e.g., the special issue of *Brain and Language* devoted to the neural correlates of nonliteral language; Giora, 2007). A speaker uses a metaphor whenever she refers to one domain with vocabulary more generally associated with another. For example, in "I made some good arguments, but in the end he crushed me with statistics," the speaker uses "crushed," a verb of physical action, to discuss the outcome of a verbal argument. In contrast to the traditional view of metaphor as a departure from normal language use, cognitive linguists have argued that metaphor is a pervasive phenomenon in everyday language (Lakoff & Johnson, 1980; Lakoff & Turner, 1989; Turner, 1991), and often explains the way that word meanings change over time (Sweetser, 1990).

Electrophysiological studies

Much research on the neural basis of metaphor has been motivated by classical accounts of metaphor comprehension that posit a two-stage model in which literal processing is followed by metaphorical processing (Grice, 1975; Searle, 1979). Although this model has been undermined by behavioral data (see Gibbs, 1994; Glucksberg, 1998, for review), the idea of a qualitatively distinct mode of metaphor processing is supported by influential work in the patient literature, which suggested RHD is particularly detrimental to the comprehension of metaphors (Winner & Gardner, 1977). Because the two-stage model involves predictions about the time course of processing, a number of investigators have exploited the temporal resolution available in the ERP signal to test when metaphoric meanings become available (e.g., Pynte, Besson, Robichon, & Poli, 1996).

For example, Kazmerski, Blasko, and Dessalegn (2003) and colleagues used an ERP study of the metaphor interference effect (MIE) to demonstrate that metaphorical meanings are activated early in the processing stream. This effect is elicited when participants are asked to evaluate the literal truth of sentences which are either literally true, literally false, or metaphorically true (but literally false). The MIE refers to the increased response times to reject metaphorically true sentences such as "The divorce is a nightmare," compared to literally false sentences such as "The divorce is a table" (Glucksberg, Gildea, & Bookin, 1982). Because the task demands that the participant attend only to the literal meaning of these sentences, the MIE is interpreted as reflecting the automatic activation of metaphoric meanings.

Kazmerski and colleagues observed an MIE in participants' reaction times, as it took participants longer to respond "no" to the metaphorical sentences than their literal counterparts (Kazmerski et al., 2003). Interestingly, the MIE was only 11 ms in participants with low IQ (<100), but was 35 ms in participants with high IQ (>115). The ERP correlates of the MIE included a smaller N400 for the metaphorically true sentences than the literally false sentences, suggesting participants found metaphorical words easier to process than the anomalous endings, as well as a larger late positivity for the metaphors, perhaps reflecting the greater difficulty in responding "no" to these items. Moreover, these ERP effects were marked and robust in the high IQ group, but largely absent in the low IQ group whose behavioral MIE was also negligible.

Research to date thus suggests that, contrary to the standard model of metaphor comprehension, metaphoric meanings are available quite early in processing, affecting the ERPs beginning 250–300 ms after the onset of a metaphorical word (Kazmerski et al., 2003; Pynte et al., 1996). Decontextualized metaphors such as "Those fighters are lions," elicit slightly larger N400s than plausible literal controls such as "Those animals are lions" (Pynte et al., 1996), suggesting they place more demands on semantic integration processes. However, metaphors elicit smaller N400s than implausible literal controls such as "The rumor is a lumberjack"

(Kazmerski et al., 2003), suggesting they are easier to process than incongruous sentence completions. This latter finding casts doubt on the suggestion that the enhanced N400 relative to plausible literal endings indexes their literal incongruity.

Coulson and Van Petten (2002) have suggested that N400 amplitude to metaphors is driven by the complexity of mapping and blending operations involved in the comprehension of metaphors, but also in the comprehension of literal language. In our model, metaphor comprehension involves coordinating various conceptual domains in a blend, a hybrid model that consists of structure from multiple conceptual domains, and that often develops emergent structure of its own. Metaphor comprehension involves the temporary construction of simple cognitive models along with the establishment of mappings, or, systematic correspondences among objects and relationships represented in various models. Mappings are based on relationships such as identity, similarity, or analogy. Consequently, metaphoric meanings – that use analogy to link objects in different conceptual domains – do not fundamentally differ from meanings that employ other sorts of mappings.

For instance, understanding the metaphor in "All the nurses at the hospital say that surgeon is a butcher," requires coordinating conceptual structure associated with surgery, butchery, and a blend of the two. To understand this metaphor, it is necessary to apprehend mappings between surgeon and butcher, patient and dead animal (e.g., cow), as well as scalpel and cleaver. However, it also involves the construction of a blended model that integrates some information from each of the two domains. In this example, the blend inherits the goals of the surgeon, and the means and manner of the butcher. The inference that the surgeon is incompetent arises when these structures are integrated to create a hypothetical agent with both characteristics.

Similar conceptual operations are involved in understanding literal language. For example, understanding butcher in "During the war, that surgeon had to work as a butcher," also requires the comprehender to establish mappings and integrate information about a surgeon's training and skill with general information about butchers, and other aspects of the context (Coulson & Matlock, 2001). One might, for instance, infer that the surgeon in question was overqualified for his job, or that he was forced to work as a butcher in a labor camp. Differences in the comprehensibility of these butcher sentences, then, might be less a matter of their figurativity than the extent to which they require the comprehender to activate additional information to establish mappings and elaborate the blend.

To test these ideas, Coulson and Van Petten (2002) compared ERPs elicited by words in three different contexts on a continuum from literal to figurative, as suggested by conceptual integration theory (Fauconnier & Turner, 1998). For the literal end of the continuum, they used sentences that prompted a literal reading of the last term, as in "He knows that whiskey is a strong intoxicant." At the metaphoric end of the continuum, they used sentences such as "He knows that power is a strong intoxicant." The literal mapping condition, hypothesized to fall somewhere between the literal and the metaphoric uses, involved sentences such as, "He has used cough syrup as an intoxicant." Literal mapping stimuli employed fully literal uses of words in ways that were hypothesized to include some of the same conceptual operations as in metaphor comprehension. These sentences described cases where one object was substituted for another, one object was mistaken for another, or one object was used to represent another – all contexts that require the comprehender to set up a mapping, that is, understand a correspondence, between the two objects in question and the domains in which they typically occur.

In the time window in which the N400 is observed (300–500 ms post-onset), ERPs in all three conditions were qualitatively similar, displaying similar wave shape and scalp topography, suggesting that processing was similar for all three sorts of contexts. Moreover, as predicted, N400 amplitude differed as a function of mapping complexity, with literals eliciting the least N400, literal mappings the next-most, and metaphors the most N400, suggesting a concomitant gradient of processing difficulty. The graded N400 difference argues against the literal/figurative dichotomy inherent in the standard model, and suggests processing difficulty associated with figurative language is related to the complexity of mapping and conceptual integration.

A similar result was obtained by Lai, Curran, and Menn (2009), who observed ERPs elicited by literal sentences ("Every soldier in the frontline was attacked"), metaphors employing conventional conceptual mappings ("Every point in my argument was attacked"), metaphors employing novel mappings ("Every second of our time was attacked"), and sentences employing anomalous, nonsensical mappings ("Every drop of rain was attacked"). They observed enlarged amplitudes early in the N400 window for all conditions except the literal. Later, beyond 440 ms post-stimulus, the novel metaphor and anomalous mapping conditions elicited continuing negativities while the literal and conventional metaphor conditions elicited more positive waveforms. Lai and colleagues interpreted the early N400 effect as evidence that both conventional and novel metaphors require real-time processing of conceptual mappings. The later effect was taken to show that the novel conceptual mapping required more time and/or processing resources, once again underscoring the importance of conceptual mapping complexity, rather than the literal/figurative distinction, per se.

Although the comprehension of metaphorical meanings poses a challenge that is greater than that associated with literal language of comparable syntactic complexity, there does not seem to be much evidence to support a view of metaphor comprehension as involving a qualitatively distinct processing mode. ERP studies of metaphor comprehension suggest metaphoric meanings are active during the same temporal interval as literal meanings (Kazmerski et al., 2003). As in the case of literal language, semantic integration difficulty of metaphoric language is largely a function of contextual support (Pynte et al., 1996), and may also be attributable to demands of conceptual mapping and blending operations (Coulson & Van Petten, 2002; Lai et al., 2009).

Hemispheric asymmetry in metaphor comprehension

Results reviewed above thus suggest that qualitatively similar processing mechanisms underlie the comprehension of literal and metaphorical meanings. By contrast, the study of patients with brain damage has suggested that the LH is the province of literal language, while the RH is the preferred substrate of metaphorical meanings (e.g., Winner & Gardner, 1977). However, the early theory that the comprehension abilities of the RH were especially suited for metaphor was based on sparse data, and may have suffered from the assumption that all forms of "nonstandard" language use – metaphor, jokes, sarcasm, and so forth – had the same neural bases. Indeed, the ability to understand figurative language is compromised not only by unilateral lesions in the RH, but also by lesions to the LH (Gagnon, Goulet, Giroux, & Joanette, 2003; Giora, 2000; Papagno, Tabossi, Colombo, & Zampetti, 2004; see also Cacciari & Papagno, Volume 1, Chapter 18), and by neurological conditions that compromise executive functions, such as Down's syndrome (Papagno & Vallar, 2001), and Alzheimer's disease (Papagno, 2001).

Similarly, whereas an early neuroimaging study of metaphor comprehension in neurologically intact adults revealed greater blood flow increase in the RH when participants read blocks of sentences containing metaphors than when they read literal control sentences (Bottini et al., 1994), more recent work has argued against the RH as the preferred substrate of metaphor comprehension (see Coulson, 2008, for a review; cf. Faust, Volume 1, Chapter 21). For example, an fMRI study in which task difficulty was well matched for literal and metaphorical sentences revealed additional LH activation for metaphors (Rapp, Leube, Erb, Grodd, & Kircher, 2004; see also Rapp, Volume 1, Chapter 20). Other studies in which investigators have made significant efforts to control for task difficulty have revealed LH activations in comparisons of literal versus metaphorical meanings (Lee & Dapretto, 2006; Rapp, Leube, Erb, Grodd, & Kircher, 2007). RH recruitment may thus depend on overall task difficulty, rather than the figurativity of the meanings (Coulson & Van Petten, 2002).

In general, RH activation is associated with complex sentences and discourse level processing (Bookheimer, 2002; Kircher, Brammer, Andreu, Williams, & McGuire, 2001; St George et al., 1999; Rehak, Kaplan, & Gardner, 1992), suggesting that it is semantic complexity that triggers the recruitment of RH areas. Functional MRI studies of literal language comprehension indicate that when sentence comprehension places increased demands on lexical and syntactic processes, increased activation both in classic LH language areas and in their RH homologues is observed (Keller, Carpenter, & Just, 2001). Finally, a systematic review of frontal hemodynamic activity revealed that additional RH activation was observed as a wide variety of tasks became more difficult (Duncan & Owen, 2000).

The bulk of the evidence from the hemi-field priming paradigm also argues against the portrait of the RH as the preferred substrate of metaphor comprehension. An early report by Anaki and colleagues suggested that while metaphoric meanings are initially activated in both hemispheres, they are only sustained in the RH (Anaki, Faust, & Kravets, 1998). However, subsequent attempts to replicate results reported by Anaki and colleagues have failed (Kacinik, 2003). Further, hemi-field priming studies using sentential stimuli have revealed priming for both literal and metaphorical meanings with presentation to both visual fields (Kacinik & Chiarello, 2007), and even shown more pronounced metaphor priming with presentation to the RVF/LH (Faust & Weisper, 2000).

Similarly, Coulson and Van Petten (2007) recorded ERPs as participants read sentence contexts that promoted either a literal or a metaphorical meaning of the sentence-final word presented in either the RVF/LH or the LVF/RH. Although the hemi-field presentation paradigm had measurable effects both on participants' behavior and their ERPs, it did not modulate the size of the N400 metaphoricity effect. These data suggest that both hemispheres are sensitive to the processing difficulty engendered by metaphorically used nouns in sentence contexts.

Results reviewed above are in keeping with the claim that the brain does not treat literal and metaphoric language as qualitatively distinct categories. Neural resources recruited for metaphor comprehension have been found to vary as a function of factors such as the novelty and complexity of the mapping that also impact the comprehension of literal language. Indeed, recent work in the hemi-field priming paradigm suggests both hemispheres have the capacity to comprehend metaphorical meanings. Given that metaphoric mapping is a basic mechanism of meaning extension, perhaps it is not surprising that both hemispheres are similarly sensitive to metaphoric meaning.

Conclusion

Language researchers have historically assumed that literal meanings were basic, and creative language phenomena such as metaphor involved fundamentally different processing mechanisms with a RH substrate. In an effort to concentrate on tractable problems, many researchers have focused on literal meanings, thereby avoiding the more difficult problem of figurative language. However, studies exploring the use of context in both literal and figurative language processing have pointed to common mechanisms which may underlie both. In brief, these proposed mechanisms include frames, the memory structures activated during language use (Fillmore, 1976), along with a means to activate correspondences between and within frames, permitting the conceptual mapping and integration that underlies much linguistic creativity (Coulson, 2001).

The neural mechanisms supporting these abilities may be distributed unevenly between the two cerebral hemispheres. Specifically, human lesion studies have suggested important roles for RH in comprehending two kinds of creative language, jokes (Birhle et al, 1986; Brownell et al., 1983) and metaphors (Winner & Gardner, 1977). Electrophysiological and imaging data largely support this contention in the case of jokes, showing a RH advantage for joke processing (e.g., Bartolo et al., 2006; Coulson & Wu, 2005). For metaphor, on the other hand, the data have argued against the hypothesized RH advantage (e.g., Rapp et al., 2004; Coulson & Van Petten, 2007). Although both metaphors and jokes rely extensively on the activation and integration of background knowledge, jokes also require the suppression of some aspects of the initial interpretation and the reintegration of others. As such, the study of creative language provides a valuable window into the real-time activation of semantic knowledge and its use in language processing.

References

Anaki, D., Faust, M., & Kravets, S. (1998). Cerebral hemispheric asymmetries in processing lexical metaphors. *Neuropsychologia, 36,* 353–362.

Bartolo, A., Benuzzi, F., Nocetti, L., Baraldi, P., & Nichelli, P. (2006). Humor comprehension and appreciation: An fMRI study. *Journal of Cognitive Neuroscience, 18*(11), 1789–1798.

Beeman, M. J., Friedman, R., Grafman, J., Perez, E., Diamond, S., & Lindsay, M. (1994). Summation priming and coarse coding in the right hemisphere. *Journal of Cognitive Neuroscience, 6,* 26–45.

Bihrle, A., Brownell, H., & Gardner, H. (1986). Comprehension of humorous and nonhumorous materials by left- and right-brain-damaged patients. *Brain and Cognition, 5,* 399–411.

Bookheimer, S. (2002). Functional MRI of language: New approaches to understanding the cortical organization of semantic processing. *Annual Review of Neuroscience, 25,* 151–188.

Bottini, G., Corcoran, R., Sterzi, R., Paulesu, E., Schenone, P., Scarpa, P., et al. (1994). The role of the right hemisphere in the interpretation of figurative aspects of language: A positron emission tomography activation study. *Brain, 117*(6), 1241–1253.

Bransford, J., & Johnson, M. (1972). Contextual prerequisites for understanding: Some investigations of comprehension and recall. *Journal of Verbal Learning and Verbal Behavior, 11,* 717–726.

Brownell, H., Michel, D., Powelson, J., & Gardner, H. (1983). Surprise but not coherence: Sensitivity to verbal humor in right-hemisphere patients. *Brain and Language, 18,* 20–27.

Brownell, H., Potter, H., Bihrle, A., & Gardner, H. (1986). Inference deficits in right brain-damaged patients. *Brain and Language, 27,* 310–321.

Brunet, E., Sarfati, Y., Hardy-Baylé, M., & Decety, J. (2000). A PET investigation of the attribution of intentions with a nonverbal task. *NeuroImage, 11*(2), 157–166.

Chiarello, C. (1988). Lateralization of lexical processes in the normal brain: A review of visual half-field research. In H. A. Whitaker (Ed.), *Contemporary reviews in neuropsychology* (pp. 36–76). New York: Springer.

Chiarello, C. (1991). Interpretations of word meanings by the cerebral hemispheres: One is not enough. In P. Schwanenflugel (Ed.), *The psychology of word meanings* (pp. 251–278). Hillsdale, NJ: Erlbaum.

Chiarello, C., Burgess, C., Richards, L., & Pollock, A. (1990). Semantic and associative priming in the cerebral hemispheres: Some words do, some words don't . . . sometimes, some places. *Brain and Language, 38,* 75–104.

Coulson, S. (2001). *Semantic leaps: Frame-shifting and conceptual blending in meaning construction.* Cambridge: Cambridge University Press.

Coulson, S. (2008). Metaphor comprehension and the brain. In R. Gibbs (Ed.), *The Cambridge Handbook of Metaphor and Thought* (pp. 177–194). Cambridge: Cambridge University Press.

Coulson, S., & Kutas, M. (2001). Getting it: Human event-related brain response in good and poor comprehenders. *Neuroscience Letters, 316,* 71–74.

Coulson, S., & Lewandowska-Tomaszczyk, B. (Eds.). (2005). *The literal and nonliteral in language and thought.* Frankfurt: Peter Lang.

Coulson, S., & Lovett, C. (2004). Handedness, hemispheric asymmetries, and joke comprehension. *Cognitive Brain Research, 19,* 275–288.

Coulson, S., & Matlock, T. (2001). Metaphor and the space structuring model. *Metaphor and Symbol, 16,* 295–316.

Coulson, S., & Severens, E. (2007). Hemispheric asymmetry and pun comprehension: When cowboys have sore calves. *Brain and Language, 100,* 172–187.

Coulson, S., & Van Petten, C. (2002). Conceptual integration and metaphor: An ERP study. *Memory and Cognition, 30*(6), 958–968.

Coulson, S., & Van Petten, C. (2007). A special role for the right hemisphere in metaphor comprehension? ERP evidence from hemifield presentation. *Brain Research, 1146,* 128–145.

Coulson, S., & Williams, R. W. (2005). Hemispheric asymmetries and joke comprehension. *Neuropsychologia, 43,* 128–141.

Coulson, S., & Wu, Y. C. (2005). Right hemisphere activation of joke-related information: An event-related potential study. *Journal of Cognitive Neuroscience, 17*(3), 494–506.

DeLong, K., Urbach, T., & Kutas, M. (2005). Probabilistic word pre-activation during language comprehension inferred from electrical brain activity. *Nature Neuroscience, 3,* 1117–1121.

Dowty, D., Wall, R., & Peters, S. (1981). *Introduction to Montague semantics.* Dordrecht, Netherlands: D. Reidel Publishing Company.

Duncan, J., & Owen, A. (2000). Common regions of the human frontal lobe recruited by diverse cognitive demands. *Trends in Neuroscience, 23,* 475–483.

Fauconnier, G., & Turner, M. (1998). Conceptual integration networks. *Cognitive Science, 22,* 133–187.

Fauconnier, G., & Turner, M. (2002). *The way we think.* New York: Basic Books.

Faust, M., & Weisper, S. (2000). Understanding metaphoric sentences in the two cerebral hemispheres. *Brain and Cognition, 43*(1–3), 186–191.

Ferstl, E., Rinck, M., & Cramon, D. (2005). Emotional and temporal aspects of situation model processing during text comprehension: An event-related fMRI study. *Journal of Cognitive Neuroscience, 17,* 724–739.

Fillmore, C. J. (1976). The need for frame semantics within linguistics. *Statistical methods in linguistics, 12*(5), 5–29.

Gagnon, L., Goulet, P., Giroux, F., & Joanette, Y. (2003). Processing of metaphoric and non-metaphoric alternative meanings of words after right- and left-hemispheric lesion. *Brain and Language, 87,* 217–226.

Gibbs, R. (1994). *The poetics of mind: Figurative thought, language, and understanding.* Cambridge: Cambridge University Press.

Gibbs, R., Wilson, N., & Bryant, G. (in press). Figurative language: Normal adult cognitive research. In M. Spivey, M. Joanisse, & K. McRae (Eds.), *The Cambridge Handbook of Psycholinguistics.* Cambridge: Cambridge University Press.

Giora, R. (1991). On the cognitive aspects of the joke. *Journal of Pragmatics, 16,* 465–485.

Giora R. (1992). Literal vs. figurative language: Different or equal? *Journal of Pragmatics, 34,* 487–506.

Giora, R. (2000). Differential effects of right-and left-hemisphere damage on understanding sarcasm and metaphor. *Metaphor and symbol, 15*(1), 63–83.

Giora, R. (2003). *On our mind: Salience, context, and figurative language.* New York: Oxford University Press.

Giora, R. (2007). Is metaphor special? *Brain and Language, 100*(2), 111–114.

Glucksberg, S. (1998). Understanding metaphors. *Current Directions in Psychological Science, 7*(2), pp 39–43.

Glucksberg, S., Gildea, P., & Bookin, H. B. (1982). On understanding nonliteral speech: Can people ignore metaphors? *Journal of Verbal Learning and Verbal Behavior, 21*(1), 85–98.

Goel, V., & Dolan, R. J. (2001). The functional anatomy of humor: Segregating cognitive and affective components. *Nature Neuroscience, 4,* 237–238.

Grice, H. (1975). Logic and conversation. In P. C. J. Morgan (Ed.), *Syntax and semantics* (vol. 3, *Speech Acts,* pp. 41–58). New York: Academic Press.

Hellige, J. (1983). *Cerebral hemisphere asymmetry: Method, theory, and application.* Santa Barbara, CA: Praeger Publishing, Inc.

Hough, M. (1990). Narrative comprehension in adults with right- and left-hemisphere brain damage: Theme organization. *Brain and Language, 38,* 253–277.

Hull, R., Chen, H.-C., Vaid, J., & Martinez, F. (2005). Great expectations: Humor comprehension across hemispheres. *Brain and Cognition, 57,* 281–282.

Just, M. A., Newman, S., Keller, T. A., McEleny, A., & Carpenter, P. A. (2003). Imagery in sentence comprehension: An fMRI study. *Neuroimage, 21,* 112–124.

Kacinik, N. A. (2003). *Hemispheric processing of literal and metaphoric language* (Unpublished doctoral dissertation). University of California, Riverside, Riverside.

Kacinik, N. A., & Chiarello, C. (2007). Understanding metaphors: Is the right hemisphere uniquely involved? *Brain and Language, 100,* 188–207.

Kazmerski, V., Blasko, D., & Dessalegn, B. (2003). ERP and behavioral evidence of individual differences in metaphor comprehension. *Memory and Cognition, 31*(5), 673–689.

Keller, T. A., Carpenter, P. A., & Just, M. A. (2001). The neural bases of sentence comprehension: A fMRI examination of syntactic and lexical processing. *Cereb Cortex, 11*(3), 223–237.

Kircher, T., Brammer, M. J., Andreu, N., Williams, S., & McGuire, P. K. (2001). Engagement of right temporal cortex during processing of linguistic context. *Neuropsychologia, 39,* 798–809.

Kutas, M., & Hillyard, S. A. (1980). Reading senseless sentences: Brain potentials reflect semantic incongruity. *Science, 207,* 203–205.

Kutas, M., Lindamood, T., & Hillyard, S. A. (1984). Word expectancy and event-related brain potentials during sentence processing. In S. Requin (Ed.), *Preparatory states and processes* (pp. 217–237). Hillsdale, NJ: Erlbaum.

Kutas, M., & Van Petten, C. (1994). Psycholinguistics electrified. In M. Gernsbacher (Ed.), *Handbook of psycholinguistics* (83–143). San Diego, CA: Academic Press.

Lai, V., Curran, T., & Menn, L. (2009). Comprehending conventional and novel metaphors: An ERP study. *Brain Research, 1284*, 145–155.

Lakoff, G. (1987). *Women, fire, and dangerous things: What categories reveal about the mind.* Chicago: University of Chicago Press.

Lakoff, G., & Johnson, M. (1980). *Metaphors we live by.* Chicago: University of Chicago Press.

Lakoff, G., & Turner, M. (1989). *More than cool reason: A field guide to poetic metaphor.* Chicago: University of Chicago Press.

Lange, T. E., & Dyer, M.G. (1989). High-level inferencing in a connectionist network. *Connection Science, 1*, 181–217.

Lee, S., & Dapretto, M. (2006). Metaphorical vs. literal word meanings: fMRI evidence against a selective role of the right hemisphere. *Neuroimage, 29*, 536–544.

Martin, A. (2001). Functional neuroimaging of semantic memory. In R. Cabeza & A. Kingstone (Eds.), *Handbook of functional neuroimaging of cognition* (pp. 153–186). Cambridge, MA: MIT Press.

Martin, A., & Chao, L. (2001). Semantic memory and the brain: Structure and processes. *Current Opinion in Neurobiology, 11*(2), 194–201.

Papagno, C. (2001). Comprehension of metaphors and idioms in patients with Alzheimer's disease: A longitudinal study. *Brain, 124*(7), 1450–1460.

Papagno, C., Tabossi, P., Colombo, M., & Zampetti, P. (2004). Idiom comprehension in aphasic patients. *Brain and Language, 89*, 226–234.

Papagno, C., & Vallar, G. (2001). Understanding metaphors and idioms: A single-case neuropsychological study in a person with Down syndrome. *Journal of the International Psychological Society, 7*(4), 516–527.

Pynte, J., Besson, M., Robichon, F., & Poli, J. (1996). The time-course of metaphor comprehension: An event-related potential study. *Brain and Language, 55*, 293–316.

Rapp, A., Leube, D., Erb, M., Grodd, W., & Kircher, T. (2004). Neural correlates of metaphor processing. *Cognitive Brain Research, 20*, 395–402.

Rapp, A., Leube, D., Erb, M., Grodd, W., & Kircher, T. (2007). Laterality in metaphor processing: Lack of evidence from functional magnetic resonance imaging for the right hemisphere theory. *Brain and Language 100*, 142–147.

Rehak, A., Kaplan, J., & Gardner, H. (1992). Sensitivity to conversational deviance in right-hemisphere damaged patients. *Brain and Language, 42*, 203–217.

Rugg, M. D., & Coles, M. (Eds.). (1995). *Electrophysiology of mind: Event-related brain potentials and cognition.* Oxford: Oxford University Press.

Searle, J. (1979). *Expression and meaning: Studies in the theory of speech acts.* Cambridge: Cambridge University Press.

Shammi, P., & Stuss, D. T. (1999). Humour appreciation: A role of the right frontal lobe. *Brain, 122*(4), 657–666.

Shastri, L. (1999). Advances in SHRUTI: A neurally motivated model of relational knowledge representation and inference using temporal synchrony. *Applied Intelligence, 11*, 79–108.

Shastri, L., & Ajjanagadde, V. (1993). From simple associations to systematic reasoning: A connectionist representation of rules, variables, and dynamic bindings using temporal asynchrony. *Behavioral and Brain Sciences, 16*(3), 417–494.

St George, M., Kutas, M., Martinez, A., & Sereno, M. I. (1999). Semantic integration in reading: engagement of the right hemisphere during discourse processing. *Brain, 122*(7), 1317–1325.

Sweetser, E. (1990). *From etymology to pragmatics: Metaphorical and cultural aspects of seman-tic structure*. Cambridge: Cambridge University Press.

Turner, M. (1991). *Reading minds: The study of English in the age of cognitive science*. Princeton, NJ: Princeton University Press.

Van Berkum, J. (2008). Understanding sentences in context: What brainwaves can tell us. *Current Directions in Psychological Science, 17*(6), 376–380.

Van Berkum, J., Hagoort, P., & Brown, C. (1999). Semantic integration in sentence and discourse: Evidence from the N400. *Journal of Cognitive Neuroscience, 11*(6), 657–671.

Winner, E., Brownell, H., Happé, F., Blum, A., & Pincus, D. (1998). Distinguishing lies from jokes: Theory of mind deficits and discourse interpretation in right hemisphere brain-damaged patients. *Brain and Language, 62*, 89–106.

Winner, E., & Gardner, H. (1977). The comprehension of metaphor in brain-damaged patients. *Brain, 100*, 719–727.

Zaidel, E. (1983). A response to Gazzaniga: Language in the right hemisphere, convergent perspectives. *American Psychologist, 38*(5), 542–546.

20

The Brain Behind Nonliteral Language: Insights From Brain Imaging

Alexander Michael Rapp

Nonliteral expressions constitute a challenge for comprehension as they go beyond the literal meaning of the words and require the ability to process more than the literal meaning of an utterance in order to grasp the speaker's intention in a given context. Several definitions exist for nonliteral ("figurative") language, however there is some consensus that metaphors, idioms, proverbs, and ironic expressions are among the most important types. This chapter will review the current functional brain imaging evidence on their comprehension.

A clearer picture of the functional neuroanatomy behind nonliteral language comprehension may be of interest for several reasons. First, nonliteral expressions constitute a challenging semantic phenomenon per se as they represent an integral part of our everyday language and thinking processes (Lakoff & Johnson, 1980) and are remarkably frequent in everyday speech (Gibbs, 1994, 2000; Markert & Hahn, 1997; Whalen, Pexman, & Alastair, 2009). Comprehension of figurative expressions optionally involves other processes like mapping of semantic domains (e.g., metaphor; Rapp, Leube, Erb, Grodd, & Kircher, 2004), integration of world knowledge (e.g., metonymy; Rapp, Erb, Grodd, Bartels, & Markert, in press), and theory of mind (TOM) processes (e.g., irony; Happe, 1996; Rapp et al., 2010). Beyond scientific, research on the functional neuroanatomy of nonliteral language is as well of clinical interest. For instance, much interest in the neuroanatomy of nonliteral language comes from psychiatry research. Patients with neurodevelopmental psychiatric disorders such as schizophrenia or autism show deficits in the comprehension of nonliteral expressions whereas other language skills are relatively preserved (Kircher, Leube, Erb, Grodd, & Rapp, 2007; Martin & McDonald, 2004; Rapp, 2009;

The Handbook of the Neuropsychology of Language, First Edition. Edited by Miriam Faust.
© 2012 Blackwell Publishing Ltd. Published 2012 by Blackwell Publishing Ltd.

Thoma & Daum, 2006). So far, more than 100 studies have investigated nonliteral language comprehension in schizophrenia (Rapp & Schmierer, 2010), and an increasing number of studies apply nonliteral language paradigms in patients with autism (Gold & Faust, 2010; Martin & McDonald, 2004) and Alzheimer's dementia (see Rapp & Wild, submitted).

Beyond psychiatric conditions, much interest on nonliteral language came from researchers interested in language impairment resulting from brain lesions in the left or right cerebral hemisphere. Although there is no question that the left hemisphere is the superior language processor, a growing body of research has demonstrated significant linguistic abilities in the "nonverbal" right hemisphere (Jung-Beeman, 2005; Lindell, 2006). Traditionally, especially the processing of nonliteral and figurative expressions is attributed to a greater or lesser extent to the right cerebral hemisphere (Bookheimer, 2002; Bottini et al., 1994; Burgess & Chiarello, 1996). For metaphors, this is sometimes named the "right hemisphere theory" of metaphor processing. One strong version of this theory predicts that metaphors are predominantly processed by the right hemisphere. Two other neurolinguistic theories strongly influenced research on the neuroanatomy of nonliteral language as well. Beeman's coarse semantic coding theory (Beeman et al., 1994; Beeman, 1998; Jung-Beeman, 2005; Mirous & Beeman, Volume 1, Chapter 16) proposes that the left hemisphere specializes in processing only fine (close) semantic relationships while the right hemisphere is adept at both fine (close) and coarse (distant) semantic relationships. According to this theory, mapping of distant semantic fields during metaphor comprehension would result in right hemisphere brain activity. Giora (Giora, 1997; Giora, Zaidel, Soroker, Batori, & Kasher, 2000) introduced the "graded salience hypothesis." According to this theory, only novel, nonsalient nonliteral stimuli are processed in the right hemisphere, whereas salient, "fossilized" expressions are processed in the left cerebral hemisphere.

Brain Lesion Studies on Metaphor

The last decade brought an enormous increase in our knowledge of the functional neuroanatomy of language. One reason is the widespread use of functional brain imaging techniques, i.e., functional magnetic resonance imaging. However, the first direct evidence on the functional neuroanatomy of nonliteral language came from patients with brain lesions (Benton, 1968; Van Lancker, 1990; Winner & Gardner, 1977) and several new brain lesion studies during the last decade improved our understanding. At least 16 studies investigated the comprehension of metaphoric expressions (Table 20.1), supplemented by additional studies on proverb (Benton, 1968; Brundage & Brookshire, 1995; Paul, Van Lancker Sidtis, Schieffer, Dietrich, & Brown, 2003; Ulatowska et al., 1995, 2001) and idiom comprehension (e.g., Cacciari et al., 2006; Kempler, Van Lancker, Marchman, & Bates, 1999; Papagno & Caporali 2007; Papagno, Curti, Rizzo, & Crippa, 2006; Papagno, Tabossi, Colombo, & Zampetti, 2004; Tompkins, Boada, & McGarry, 1992; Van Lancker, 2006; see also

Table 20.1 Brain lesion studies on metaphor comprehension.

Authors	Year	Stimuli (word vs. Sentence level)	Probands	Number of RHD probands	Number of metaphoric stimuli	Task
Winner & Gardner	1977	phrasal	RH LH AD HC	22	18	sentence-to-picture matching
Brownell et al.	1984	word	LH RH HC	10	4	word matching
Brownell et al.	1990	word	RH LH HC	15	16	word matching
Tompkins	1990	word	RH LH HC	25	18	word/nonword decision
Hillekamp et al.	1996	word	RH LH HC	18	30	word-to-picture matching
Mackenzie et al.	1997	phrasal	RH HC	17	?[1]	sentence-to-picture matching
Giora et al.	2000	phrasal	RH LH HC	27	4	verbal explanation
Zaidel et al.	2002	phrasal (aber kurz)	RH LH HC	27	2 mal 4	sentence-to-picture matching
Gagnon et al.	2003	word	RH LH HC	10	20	word matching
Rinaldi et al.	2004	phrasal	RH HC	50	20	sentence-to-picture matching, multiple choice
Champagne et al.	2004	phrasal	RH HC	10	2 mal 10	verbal explanation plus MC
Klepousniotou & Baum	2005	word	RH LH HC	8	18?	word/nonword decision
Klepousniotou & Baum	2005	phrasal	RH LH HC	8	18?	lexical decision
Brownell et al.	2007	phrasal	RH	3	3	verbal explanation
Champagne et al.	2007	phrasal	RH SCZ HC	15	?	?

? = not reported; HC = healthy control subjects; LH = left hemisphere damaged; RH = right hemisphere damaged; AD = Alzeimer's disease.
[1]Metaphor subtest of the right hemisphere language battery (Bryan, 1989).

Cacciari & Papagno, Volume 1, Chapter 18 and Van Lancker Sidtis, Volume 1, Chapter 17).

In a seminal study of the field, Winner and Gardner (1977) investigated the comprehension of conventional metaphoric expressions (like "A heavy heart can really make a difference") in probands with damage to either the left or the right cerebral hemisphere. The results showed an effect of both task and lesion lateralization on performance: patients with right hemisphere lesions had preserved ability to understand phrasal metaphors (Winner & Gardner, 1977), a finding that was later replicated with other studies (Giora et al., 2000; Rinaldi, Marangolo, & Baldassarri, 2004; Zaidel, Kasher, Soroker, & Batori, 2002). This preserved ability of right hemisphere lesioned patients to understand metaphors correctly suggests that the left hemisphere has the ability to process conventional phrasal metaphors correctly. However, in a different task of the same study, Winner and Gardner tested the ability to match the same metaphors with an appropriate picture. In this task, patients with right hemisphere lesioned probands were impaired, which could suggest an impairment to work with a metaphoric meaning, but could alternatively be confounded by impaired skills in picture matching (Zaidel et al., 2002). The methodological quality of lesion studies on metaphor is on average high (Table 20.1), however altogether lesion studies are heterogeneous in their results and cannot provide a definite picture on what modulates right hemisphere involvement in metaphor comprehension. For example, Rinaldi et al. (2004) replicate Winner's and Gardner's finding of right-hemisphere-damaged impairment in matching metaphors with an appropriate picture. However, the same group of patients was less impaired in matching metaphors with an appropriate verbal description. As well, language impairment in right hemisphere lesions may partially recover (Brownell et al., 2007; Lundgren, Brownell, Cayer-Meade, & Roy, 2006; Lundgren, Brownell, Roy, & Cayer-Meade, 2006) and some studies have considerable intervals between lesion onset and time of assessment.

Functional Magnetic Resonance Research

An alternative approach to investigating the functional neuroanatomy of nonliteral language is research with functional magnetic resonance imaging (fMRI). Compared to brain lesion studies, a *disadvantage* of fMRI is that a lack of activation indicates far less evidence that a brain region is *not* involved in a task (for further considerations related to interpretation of fMRI data, see Van Lancker Sidtis, Volume 1, Chapter 17). However, an advantage of this technique is that healthy individuals with selected properties can be investigated.

So far, at least 29 fMRI studies have been published on nonliteral language in healthy subjects (Table 20.2). The available research covers a variety of different tasks and nonliteral language types: 5 studies used idioms as stimuli, 7 ironic/sarcastic expressions, 18 investigated metaphors, and one metonymy. At least three additional studies were published as an abstract (Mason, Prat, & Just, 2008;

Table 20.2 fMRI studies on nonliteral language comprehension.

	Autoren	Year	NL Language type	Language	Number of subjects	Novel stimuli	Salient	Evidence for RH involvement	Included in metanalysis below
1	Rapp et al.	2004	metaphor	German	15	x		no	x
2	Mashal et al.	2005	metaphor	Hebrew	15	x	x	yes	
3	Uchiyama et al.	2006	irony	Japanese	20			no	x
4	Eviatar & Just	2006	irony metaphor	English	16		x	yes / no	
5	Wang et al.	2006	irony	English	(18) (+18)			yes	
6	Wang et al.	2006	irony	English	12 (+12)			yes	x
7	Lee & Dapretto	2006	metaphor	English	12		x	no	x
8	Stringaris et al.	2006	metaphor	English	12		x	yes	
9	Aziz-Zadeh et al.	2006	metaphor	English	12		?	–	
10	Wakusawa et al.	2007	irony, metaphor	Japanese	38		x	yes	x
11	Ahrens et al.	2007	metaphor	Chinese	8	x	x	yes	x
12	Stringaris et al.	2007	metaphor	English	11		x	no	x
13	Mashal et al.	2007	metaphor	Hebrew	15	x	x	yes	x
14	Rapp et al.	2007	metaphor	German	17	x		no	
15	Zempleni et al.	2007	idiom	Dutch	15		x	yes	x

No.	Study	Year	Trope	Language	N				
16	Shibata et al.	2007	metaphor	Japanese	13	x		x	no
17	Mashal et al.	2008	idiom	Hebrew	14	x	x		yes
18	Lauro et al.	2008	idiom	Italian	22	x	x		yes
19	Boulenger et al.	2008	idiom	English	18	x	x		yes
20	Chen et al.	2008	metaphor	English	14	x		x	no
21	Mashal et al.	2009	metaphor	Hebrew	15	x		x	yes
22	Hillert & Buracas	2009	idiom	English	10	x			yes
23	Yang et al.	2009	metaphor	English	18	x	x	x	yes
24	Schmidt & Seger	2009	metaphor	English	10	x	x	x	yes
25	Rapp et al.	2010	irony	German	15	x			yes
26	Yang et al.	2010	metaphor	English	18	x	x	x	yes
27	Mashal & Faust	2010	metaphor	Hebrew	10		x		–
28	Rapp et al.	2010	metonymy	German	14	x	x		yes
29	Shibata et al.	2010	irony	Japanese	13	x	x		yes

Mejía-Constaín, Arsenault, Monchi, Senhadji, & Joanette, 2008) or book-chapter (Yu, Kim, Kim, & Nam, 2009).

The first fMRI study on *metaphor* comprehension was published by Rapp et al. (2004). In their study, the comprehension of short, novel, syntactically simple metaphors (like "the lover's words are harp sounds") relative to literal control stimuli (like "the lover's words are lies") matched for tense and word frequency were investigated. Both hemispheres were involved in the contrasts for metaphoric and literal stimuli against baseline, but – contrary to the study hypothesis – no right hemisphere activation was detected in the direct comparison.

Metaphoric relative to matched literal stimuli activated a left frontotemporal network with maxima in the anterior-inferior part of the left inferior frontal gyrus (IFG; BA 45/47), anterior temporal (BA 20) and posterior middle/inferior temporal (BA 37) gyri. This result was divergent from a previous, often cited, positron emission tomography (PET) study by Bottini et al. (1994), in which right hemisphere activation was found for phrasal metaphoric expressions.

More evidence for a role of the left IFG in metaphor comprehension came from subsequent fMRI studies. For instance, Eviatar and Just (2006) used a ROI-analysis (region-of-interest analysis) in 16 subjects whilst reading brief three-sentence stories that concluded with either a literal, metaphoric, or ironic sentence. Metaphoric utterances resulted in significantly higher levels of activation in the left IFG and in bilateral inferior temporal cortex than the literal and ironic utterances.

Some evidence for right hemisphere theory of metaphor comes from fMRI research by Stringaris and colleagues (Stringaris, Medford, Giampetro, Brammer, & David, 2007). In their fMRI study, subjects read short English sentences with either metaphoric ("Some surgeons are butchers"), literal ("Some surgeons are fathers"), or nonmeaningful sentences ("Some surgeons are shelves"). Metaphoric relative to literal stimuli showed activation differences in both cerebral hemispheres: on the one hand, results further strengthened Rapp et al.'s finding (2004) of an important role for BA 47 in metaphor comprehension, on the other hand, right hemisphere contribution was found in the right middle temporal gyrus. In another study (Stringaris et al., 2006), 12 healthy subjects read metaphoric or literal stimuli, followed by a single word, which could be semantically related or not to the preceding sentence context. Judging unrelated words as contextually irrelevant was associated with increased fMRI signal in the right ventrolateral prefrontal cortex (BA 47) in the metaphoric, but not the literal, condition.

Using Chinese stimuli, Ahrens et al. (2007) found a small difference between conventional metaphors and literal sentences in the right inferior temporal gyrus, but the differences between anomalous metaphors and literal sentences were quite large and involved bilateral activation. However, a limitation of this study is the significantly reduced understandability of the novel metaphors and the relatively small number of study subjects (n = 8) which makes the results presumably more susceptible for interindividual differences. In another study, Aziz-Zadeh, Wilson, Rizzolatti, and Iacoboni (2006) investigated comprehension of metaphorical phrases describing actions. A severe limitation of this study is that only 5 metaphorical stimuli were used.

So far 5 studies directly compared novel and salient metaphoric expressions (Ahrens et al., 2007; Mashal, Faust, Hendler, & Jung-Beeman, 2005, 2007; Schmidt & Seger, 2009; Yang, Edens, Simpson, & Krawcyk, 2009). In all studies, novel metaphoric expressions induced stronger blood oxygen level dependent (BOLD) response than salient stimuli. However, in the latter 4 studies (with whole brain analysis) only 43% of the reported maxima for direct comparison data locate to the right cerebral hemisphere.

Three fMRI-studies investigated the comprehension of metaphoric word pairs (Lee & Dapretto, 2006; Mashal et al., 2005, 2007; see also Faust, Volume 1, Chapter 21). The distinction between word and sentence level could be of importance since metaphoric words might have different lateralization patterns (Faust & Weisper, 2000; Rapp, Leube, Erb, Grodd, & Kircher, 2007). However, the word-level fMRI studies are themselves heterogeneous in terms of hemispheric lateralization. Lee and Dapretto (2006) found no fMRI activation in the right cerebral hemisphere. In contrast, Mashal and colleagues (2005, 2007) found evidence for a significant RH contribution on word level. Mashal and colleagues (2007) investigated novel metaphors ("pearl tears") in comparison to conventional metaphors ("bright student). Novel metaphoric expressions activated more the right superior temporal sulcus and RH IFG as well as BA 46 of the left hemisphere. Recently, one study (Mashal & Faust, 2010) investigated text level (stanzas). Unexpectedly, this study did not find any activation maxima for metaphoric > literal stimuli.

Five studies from 5 different countries so far have investigated the comprehension of *idioms* (Boulenger, Hauk, & Pulvermüller, 2009; Hillert & Buracas, 2009; Lauro, Tettamanti, Cappa, & Papagno, 2008; Mashal, Faust, Hendler, & Jung-Beeman, 2008; Zempleni, Haverkort, Renken, & Stowe, 2007). Studies used four different languages (Table 20.2). Zempleni and colleagues investigated comprehension of familiar idioms in sentence context in 17 healthy subjects (Zempleni, 2006; Zempleni et al., 2007). Two types of idioms were used as stimuli: literally plausible, ambiguous idioms and literally implausible, unambiguous idioms. The idiomatic versus literal sentence contrast elicited activation in the bilateral inferior frontal gyri and in the bilateral middle temporal gyri. The right temporal lobe was particularly involved in the processing of ambiguous idioms. Whereas Zempleni et al. applied a word-relatedness task in Dutch language, in another study by Lauro et al. (2008) subjects had to decide whether Italian idioms matched in meaning with a picture. Idioms specifically activated the left frontal and temporal cortex. Activations were also seen in the right superior and middle temporal gyri, in the temporal pole, and in the right IFG. Mashal et al. (2008) investigated processing of idioms in a block design with Hebrew stimuli. Again, both hemispheres were involved in direct comparison contrasts. Two studies used English-language stimuli: Hillert and Buracas (2009) found a role of Broca's area during comprehension of idioms, a finding that was also found in a study by Boulenger and colleagues (2009). The study by Mashal and colleagues (2008) provided evidence for the graded salience hypothesis using

Hebrew idioms: whereas processing salient meanings (the idiomatic meaning of idioms and the literal interpretations of a literal sentence) involved left hemisphere regions, the processing of nonsalient meanings (the literal interpretation of idioms) was associated with increased activity in right brain regions (Mashal et al., 2008).

So far, only one study investigated the comprehension of *metonymies* using fMRI (Rapp et al., in press). In this study, short phrasal metonymies activated a predominantly left frontotemporal network with maxima in the left and right IFG and the left middle temporal gyrus relative to matched literal control stimuli.

In contrast to other types of nonliteral language, research on *ironic expressions* is less dominated by the question of hemispheric lateralization. Irony comprehension draws clinical interest mostly because it essentially involves perspective-taking and second-order theory of mind processes (Blasko & Kazmerski, 2006; Colston & Gibbs, 2002; Happé, 1996; Sprong, Schothorst, Vos, Hox, & van Engeland, 2007). Lesions studies on irony comprehension sometimes do not disentangle the role of the cerebral hemispheres. Consistently, they point towards an important role of the medial prefrontal cortex in irony comprehension (see Rapp et al., 2010, for overview on lesion studies). A role of the medial prefrontal regions is as well supported by the six fMRI studies that so far used ironic stimuli (Rapp et al., 2010; Shibata, Toyomura, Itoh, & Abe, 2010; Uchiyama et. al, 2006; Wakusawa et al., 2007; Wang, Lee, Sigman, & Dapretto, 2006a, 2006b).

An ALE Meta-Analysis

An additional approach to illustrate the current evidence of nonliteral language anatomy is the application of a coordinate-based meta-analysis technique, the so-called activation likelihood estimation (ALE) method (Eickhoff et al., 2009; Turkeltaub, Eden, Jones, & Zeffiro, 2002). This research tool identifies consistent regions of activation across a collection of fMRI studies. The calculation is based on the reported activation maxima in the study publications and their number of study subjects. Coordinates are then modeled with a Gaussian function to accommodate the spatial uncertainty associated with a reported coordinate and are analyzed for where they converge (Laird et al., 2009).

We (Rapp, Mutschler et al., submitted) recently applied this methodology to the available fMRI studies on nonliteral language. Not all studies reported in Table 20.2 could be included, since inclusion of studies reporting data only from "region of interest" analysis could bias the analysis towards these regions. Twenty-one studies were included (Table 20.2). In these studies, approx. 250 activation maxima for direct comparison of nonliteral > literal stimuli are reported, about 30% of them correspond to the right cerebral hemisphere. An important cautionary remark is, however, that the number of reported maxima in fMRI research strongly interdepends with the chosen significance level (the lower the significance level, the larger the number of reported maxima; see also Wilke & Lidzba, 2007, for lateralization effects). Results could therefore be biased in the direction of the chosen significance levels.

Results of the meta-analysis of all studies comparing nonliteral and literal stimuli directly are shown in Figure 20.1a. Overall, nonliteral stimuli induce stronger activation in bilateral, yet more left-lateralized frontotemporal network. The strongest cluster is located in the left IFG (BA 45/9/44). Sixteen out of the 21 studies contribute to this cluster. The right hemisphere homologue of this brain region represents the second strongest cluster (right IFG/BA 47).

The ALE meta-analysis thus strengthens evidence for *a* role of the right hemisphere in nonliteral language comprehension. However, there is no right hemisphere *dominance* as only two out of 14 significant clusters are located in the right cerebral hemisphere. Such a dominance would be predicted by a strong version of the right hemisphere theory. Other clusters locate in the middle temporal gyrus bilaterally and in the left hemisphere paracingulate gyrus and the left thalamus.

A similar, but not identical pattern of activation was seen when only the 10 studies on *metaphor* were included into another ALE analysis. Again, bilateral, left > right clusters were detected in the IFG. Other clusters were activated inter alia in the left middle frontal gyrus (BA 9), and bilaterally in the parahippocampal gyrus and middle temporal gyrus.

A subanalysis only for salient metaphoric stimuli (with the activation reported for salient stimuli in Ahrens et al., 2007; Chen, Widick, & Chatterjee, 2008; Lee & Dapretto, 2006; Mashal et al., 2007; Schmidt, Kranjex, Cardillo, & Chatterjee, 2009; Stringaris et al., 2007) showed only left hemisphere clusters (Figure 20.1a). In contrast, a subanalysis only for nonsalient stimuli (from Ahrens et al., 2007; Mashal et al., 2007; Mashal, Faust, Hendler, & Jung-Beeman, 2009; Rapp et al., 2004; Schmidt & Seger, 2009; Shibata, Abe, Terao, & Miyamoto, 2007, Yang et al., 2009) showed clusters of activation in both hemispheres (Figure 20.1a). Of note, however, still more clusters were located in the left cerebral hemisphere, so that the right cerebral hemisphere seems to be involved, but not dominant.

The 5 studies on *idiom* comprehension (Boulenger et al., 2009; Hillert & Buracas, 2009; Lauro et al., 2007; Mashal et al., 2008; Zempleni et al. 2007) were included into another ALE meta-analysis (Figure 20.1b). A cautionary remark is that 5 studies is presumably a low number for an ALE analysis. All studies reported activation maxima in both hemispheres (18 out of 48 reported maxima are in the right hemisphere). The ALE analysis showed four significant clusters (Rapp, Mutschler, et al., submitted). The strongest cluster was once more in the left IFG. Only one cluster in the medial frontal lobe showed small elongation into the right cerebral hemisphere. Altogether, the network for idioms is similar to the one for salient metaphors (Figure 20.1b).

Five studies were included into an ALE meta-analysis *of irony/sarcasm* (Rapp et al., 2010; Shibata et al., 2010; Uchiyama et al., 2006; Wakusawa et al., 2007; Wang et al., 2006b). Although this is a small number of studies for an ALE analysis, three clusters came out significant. The largest cluster was in the right superior/middle temporal gyrus (BA 22/21/41). The studies by Uchiyama et al., Wang et al., and

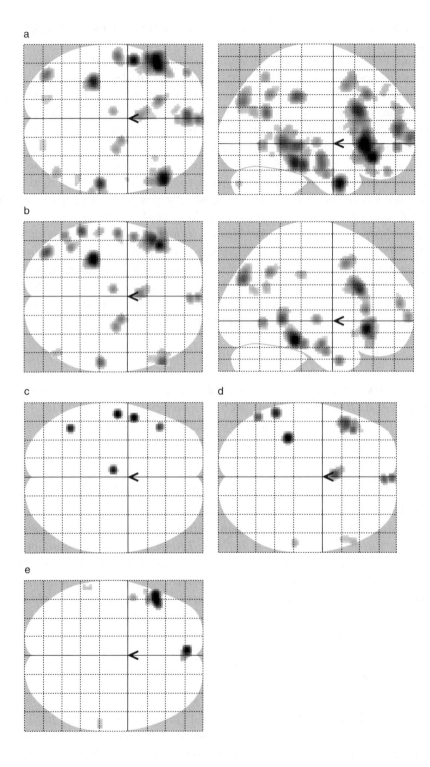

Figure 20.1 ALE meta-analysis of studies on nonliteral language (from Rapp, Mutschler, et al., submitted). Significance level p < 0.001, extent 5 vx in all analysis. (a) ALE meta-analysis of 21 fMRI studies on nonliteral language (marked with X in Table 20.2). (b) ALE meta-analysis of studies reporting contrasts for salient metaphoric > literal stimuli. Data included from studies no. 1, 7, 11, 12, 13, 16, 20, 21, 23, 24 in Table 20.2. (c) ALE meta-analysis of studies reporting contrasts for salient metaphoric > literal stimuli. Data included from studies no. 7, 11, 12, 13, 20, 24 in Table 20.2. (d) ALE meta-analysis of studies reporting contrasts for novel metaphoric > literal stimuli. Data included from studies no. 1, 11, 13, 16, 21, 23, 24 in Table 20.2. (e) ALE meta-analysis of studies reporting contrasts for idioms > literal stimuli. Data included from studies no. 15, 17, 18, 19, 22 in Table 20.2.

Shibata et al. contribute to this cluster. This finding is congruent with the fMRI studies by Eviatar and Just (2006) who found BOLD response induced by ironic stimuli in this region using a ROI-approach and the study by Wang et al. (2006a) indicating a role of the right temporal lobe for irony comprehension in children. Recently, Rapp et al. (2010) reported a correlation between right temporal lobe BOLD response during irony comprehension and psychometric schizotypy. Schizotypy is a personality trait that likewise is associated with hemispheric lateralization differences (Somers, Sommer, Boks, & Kahn, 2009) and has genetic and clinical similarities with schizophrenia (Raine, 2006). Findings from the brain lesion studies are compatible with the fMRI studies in respect to the right middle superior temporal gyrus in irony appreciation (Giora et al., 2000; Zaidel et al., 2002). Another cluster of activation was present in the medial frontal gyrus. Like in most brain lesion studies, this cluster was located in the right medial prefrontal lobe. In contrast, most fMRI studies on irony reported more left medial frontal contribution (see Rapp et al., 2010). Medial frontal brain activation could likewise be a correlate of second-order theory of mind processing, a mental operation that is essentially involved in irony comprehension (Blasko & Kazmerski, 2006; Colston & Gibbs 2002; Happé, 1996; Sprong et al. 2007). The two latest-published studies (Rapp et al., 2010; Shibata et al., 2010) contributed to a third cluster located in the right premotor cortex.

Conclusion

So far, it is evident that right hemisphere contribution is present in most studies of nonliteral language. However, it is less clear which factors contribute to the extent of the right hemisphere's involvement. Rather than "nonliterality" per se, other factors like salience (Giora, 2007) or figurativeness (Schmidt et al., 2010) could play an important role. The exact role of such influencing factors, however, is so far not yet clear. Overall, studies using salient stimuli reported less right hemisphere contribution than novel stimuli (Rapp, Mutschler, et al., submitted). However, some inconsistent findings are incompatible with a strong version of the graded salience hypothesis (e.g. Rapp et al. 2007). Many current findings point towards a central role of the left (and to a lesser extent the right) IFG in the comprehension of non-literal language. In their initial study, Rapp et al. (2004) claimed that especially the anterior-inferior part, corresponding to BA 45/47, plays a key role in nonliteral language comprehension. However, newer research indicates that not only the anterior-inferior, but additional other parts of the IFG (including Broca's area) are active during nonliteral language comprehension. The IFG plays a key role in semantic language comprehension on a sentence level (Bookheimer, 2002). Research on literal language indicates that this brain region plays a central role in integrating semantic meanings into a sentence context (e.g., Arcuri, 2003; Zhu et al., 2009). During metaphor comprehension, activation of this region could be a correlate of bringing together distant semantic meanings. As well, this region plays an important role in integrating world knowledge into a sentence context (Pylkkänen, Oliveri, & Smart, 2009). For example, Hagoort and colleagues (Hagoort, Hald, Bastiaansen, & Petersson, 2004; Hagoort, 2005) found an effect of integrating world knowledge on the BOLD reponse in the left IFG, especially in BA 45 and 47. Beyond this, the IFG of both hemispheres may contribute to unification of discourse information with previously stored knowledge in long-term memory during comprehension of literal and nonliteral sentences (Hagoort, 2005; Menenti, Petersson, Scheeringa, & Hagoort, 2009).

References

Ahrens, K., Liu, H., Lee, C., Gong, S., Fang, S., & Hsu, Y. Y. (2007). Functional MRI of conventional and anomalous metaphors in Mandarin Chinese. *Brain and Language, 100,* 163–171.

Arcuri, S. M. (2003). *Neural and cognitive studies of thought disorder in schizophrenia* (Unpublished doctoral dissertation). Kings College London Institute of Psychiatry, University of London.

Aziz-Zadeh, L., Wilson, S. M., Rizzolatti, G., & Iacoboni, M. (2006). Congruent embodied representations for visually presented actions and linguistic phrases describing actions. *Current Biology, 16,* 1818–1823.

Beeman, M. (1998). Coarse semantic coding and discourse comprehension. In M. Beeman & C. Chiarello (Eds.), *Right hemisphere language comprehension: Perspectives from cognitive neuroscience* (pp. 255–284). Mahwah, NJ: Erlbaum.

Beeman, M., Friedman, R. B., Grafman, J., Perez, E., Diamond, S., & Lindsay, M. B. (1994). Summation priming and coarse semantic coding in the right hemisphere. *Journal of Cognitive Neuroscience, 6,* 26–45.

Benton, A. L. (1968). Differential behavioral effects in frontal lobe disease. *Neuropsychologia, 6,* 53–60.

Blasko, D. G., & Kazmerski, V. A. (2006). Erp correlates of individual differences in the comprehension of nonliteral language. *Metaphor and Symbol, 21*(4), 267–284.

Bookheimer, S. (2002). Functional MRI of language: New approaches to understanding the cortical organization of semantic processing. *Annual Review of Neuroscience, 25,* 151–188.

Bottini, G., Corcoran, R., Sterzi, R., Paulesu, E., Schenone, P., Scarpa, P. et al. (1994). The role of the right hemisphere in the interpretation of figurative aspects of language. A positron emission tomography activation study. *Brain, 117,* 1241–1253.

Boulenger, V., Hauk, O., & Pulvermüller, F. (2009). Grasping ideas with the motor system: Semantic somatotopy in idiom comprehension. *Cerebral cortex, 19*(8), 1905–1914.

Brownell, H., Lundgren, K., Cayer-Meade, C., Nichols, M., Caddick, K., & Spitzer, J. (2007). Assessing quality of metaphor interpretation by right hemisphere damaged patients. *Brain and Language, 103,* 8.

Brownell, H. H., Potter, H. H., Michelow, D., & Gardner, H. (1984). Sensitivity to lexical denotation and conotation in brain-damaged patients: A double dissociation? *Brain and Language, 22,* 253–265.

Brownell, H. H., Simpson, T. L., Bihrle, A. M., Potter, H. H., & Gardner, H. (1990). Appreciation of metaphoric alternative word meanings by left and right brain-damaged patients. *Neuropsychologia, 28,* 253–265.

Brundage, S. B., & Brookshire, R. H. (1995). A system for scoring proverb interpretations provided by non-brain-damaged adults and aphasic adults. *Clinical Aphasiology, 23,* 165–177.

Bryan, K. L. (1989). *The right hemisphere language battery.* Boston: Far Communications.

Burgess, C., & Chiarello, C. (1996). Neurocognitive mechanisms underlying metaphor comprehension and other figurative language. *Metaphor and symbolic activity, 11,* 67–84.

Cacciari, C., Reati, F., Colombo, M. R., Padovani, R., Rizzo, S., & Papagno, C. (2006). The comprehension of ambiguous idioms in aphasic patients. *Neuropsychologia, 44,* 1305–1314.

Champagne, M., Desautels, M., & Joanette, Y. (2004). Lack of inhibition could contribute to non-literal language impairments in right-hemisphere-damaged individuals. *Brain and Language, 91,* 172–174.

Champagne, M., Stip, E., & Joanette, Y. (2007). Language functions in right-hemisphere damage and schizophrenia: Apparently similar pragmatic deficits may hide profound differences. *Brain, 130*(Pt2), e67.

Chen, E., Widick, P., & Chatterjee, A. (2008). Functional-anatomical organization of predicate metaphor processing. *Brain and Language, 107,* 194–202.

Colston, H. L., & Gibbs, R. W. (2002). Are irony and metaphor understood differently? *Metaphor and Symbol, 17*(1), 57–80.

Eickhoff, S. B., Laird, A. R., Grefkes, C., Wang, L. E., Zilles, K., & Fox, P. T. (2009). Coordinate-based activation likelihood estimation meta-analysis of neuroimaging data: A random-effects approach based on empirical estimates of spatial uncertainty. *Human Brain Mapping, 30*(9), 2907–2926.

Eviatar, Z., & Just, M. A. (2006). Brain correlates of discourse processing: An fMRI investigation of irony and conventional metaphor comprehension. *Neuropsychologia, 44*(12), 2348–2359.

Faust, M., & Weisper, S. (2000). Understanding metaphoric sentences in the two cerebral hemispheres. *Brain and Cognition, 43,* 186–191.

Gagnon, L., Goulet, P., Giroux, F., & Joanette, Y., (2003). Processing of metaphoric and non-metaphoric alternative meanings of words after right- and left-hemispheric lesion. *Brain and Language, 87,* 217–226.

Gibbs, R. W. (1994). *The poetics of mind: Figurative thought, language, and understanding.* New York: Cambridge University Press.

Gibbs, R. W. (2000). Irony in talk among friends. *Metaphor and Symbol, 15*(1), 5–27.

Giora, R. (1997). Understanding figurative and literal language: The graded salience hypothesis. *Cognitive linguistics, 8*, 183–206.

Giora, R., (2007). Is metaphor special? *Brain and Language, 100* (2), 111–114.

Giora, R., Zaidel, E., Soroker, N., Batori, G., & Kasher, A. (2000). Differential effects of right- and left-hemisphere damage on understanding sarcasm and metaphor. *Metaphor and Symbol, 1*(1,2), 63–83.

Gold, R., & Faust, M. (2010). Right hemisphere dysfunction and metaphor comprehension in young adults with Asperger syndrome. *Journal of Autism and Developmental Disorders, 40*(7), 800–811.

Hagoort, P. (2005). On Broca, brain, and binding: a new framework. *Trends in cognitive sciences, 9*(9), 416–423.

Hagoort, P., Hald, L., Bastiaansen, M., & Petersson, K. M. (2004). Integration of word meaning and world knowledge in language comprehension. *Science, 304*, 438–441.

Happé, F. G. (1996). Understanding minds and metaphors: Insights from the study of figurative language in autism. *Metaphor and Symbol, 10*, 275–295.

Hillekamp, U., Knobloch, J., & Buelau, P. (1996). Metaphorische Sprachverarbeitung bei Hirngeschädigten: Anwendung und Analyse eines Metapherntests. *Neurologie and Rehabilitation, 4*, 232–236.

Hillert, D. G., & Buracas, G. T. (2009). The neural substrates of spoken idiom comprehension. *Language and Cognitive Processes, 24* (9), 1370–1391.

Jung-Beeman, M. (2005). Bilateral brain processes for comprehending natural language. *Trends in Cognitive Science, 11*, 512–518.

Klepousniotou, E., & Baum, S. R. (2005a). Unilateral brain damage effects on processing homonymous and polysemous words. *Brain and Language, 93*(3), 308–326.

Klepousniotou, E., & Baum, S. R. (2005b). Processing homonymy and polysemy: Effects of sentential context and time-course following unilateral brain damage. *Brain and Language , 95*(3), 365–382.

Kempler, D., Van Lancker, D., Marchman, V., & Bates, E. (1999). Idiom comprehension in children and adults with unilateral brain damage. *Developmental Neuropsychology, 15*, 327–349.

Kircher, T. T., Leube, D. T., Erb, M., Grodd, W., & Rapp, A. M. (2007). Neural correlates of metaphor processing in schizophrenia. *Neuroimage, 34*(1), 281–289.

Laird, A. R., Eickhoff, S. B., Kurth, F., Fox, P. M., Uecker, A. M., Turner, J. A., et al. (2009). ALE meta-analysis workflows via the brainmap database: Progress towards a probabilistic functional brain atlas. *Frontiers in Neuroinformatics, 3*, 23.

Lakoff, G., Johnson, M. (1980). *Metaphors we live by.* Chicago: University of Chicago Press.

Lauro, L. J., Tettamanti, M., Cappa, S. F., & Papagno, C. (2008). Idiom comprehension: A prefrontal task? *Cerebral Cortex, 18*(1), 162–170.

Lee, S. S., & Dapretto, M. (2006). Metaphorical versus literal word meanings: fMRI evidence against a selective role of the right hemisphere. *NeuroImage, 29*, 536–544.

Lindell, A. K. (2006). In your right mind: Right hemisphere contributions to language processing and production. *Neuropsychology Review, 16*(3), 131–148.

Lundgren, K., Brownell, H., Cayer-Meade, C., & Roy, S. (2006). *Remediation of metaphor comprehension deficit: A pilot study.* Poster presentation at the annual convention of the American Speech-Language Hearing Association, Miami, FL, November 2006.

Lundgren, K., Brownell, H., Roy, S., & Cayer-Meade, C. (2006). A metaphor comprehension intervention for patients with right hemisphere brain damage: A pilot study. Forty-fourth annual meeting of the Academy of Aphasia, Victoria, British Columbia, 15th–17th October, 2006. *Brain and Language, 99*(1–2), 69–70.

Mackenzie, C., Begg, T., Brady, M., & Lee, K. R. (1997). The effects on verbal communication skills of right hemisphere stroke in middle age. *Aphasiology, 11*(10), 929–945.

Markert, K., & Hahn, U. (1997). On the interaction of metonymies and anaphora. In M. E. Pollack (Ed.), *IJCAI-97: proceedings of the fifteenth international joint conference on artificial intelligence* (pp. 1010–1015). San Francisco: Morgan Kaufmann Publishers.

Martin, I., & McDonald, S. (2004). Weak coherence or theory of mind: What causes non-literal language to be misunderstood by high functioning individuals with autism? *Journal of Autism and Developmental Disorders, 34*, 311–328.

Mashal, N., & Faust, M. (2010). The effects of metaphoricity and presentation style on brain activation during text comprehension. *Metaphor and Symbol, 25*(1), 19–33.

Mashal, N., Faust, M., Hendler, T., & Jung-Beeman, M. (2005). The role of the right hemisphere in processing nonsalient metaphorical meanings: Application of principal component analysis to fMRI data. *Neuropsychologia, 43*, 2084–2100.

Mashal, N., Faust, M., Hendler, T., & Jung-Beeman, M. (2007). An fMRI investigation of the neural correlates underlying the processing of novel metaphoric expressions. *Brain and Language, 100*(2), 115–26.

Mashal, N., Faust, M., Hendler, T., & Jung-Beeman, M. (2008). Hemispheric differences in processing the literal interpretation of idioms: Converging evidence from behavioral and fMRI studies. *Cortex , 44*(7), 848–860.

Mashal, N., Faust, M., Hendler, T., & Jung-Beeman, M. (2009). An fMRI study of processing novel metaphoric sentences. *Laterality, 14*(1), 30–54.

Mason, R., Prat, C., & Just, M. (2008). *The components of a theory-of-mind cortical network during narrative comprehension.* Poster presented at the 14th annual meeting of the Organization for Human Brain Mapping, Melbourne, Australia.

Mejía-Constaín, B., Arsenault, M., Monchi, O., Senhadji, N., & Joanette, Y. (2008). *Neural correlates associated with processing metaphoric meaning of words: The impact of age.* Poster presented at the 14th annual meeting of the Organization for Human Brain Mapping, Melbourne, Australia.

Menenti, L., Petersson, K. M., Scheeringa, R., & Hagoort, P. (2009). When elephants fly: Differential sensitivity of right and left inferior frontal gyri to discourse and world knowledge. *Journal of cognitive neuroscience, 21*(12), 2358–2368.

Papagno, C., & Caporali, A. (2007). Testing idiom comprehension in aphasic patients: The effects of task and idiom type. *Brain and Language, 100*(2), 208–220.

Papagno, C., Curti, R., Rizzo, S., & Crippa, F. (2006). Is the right hemisphere involved in idiom comprehension? A neuropsychological study. *Neuropsychology, 20*(5), 598–606.

Papagno, C., Tabossi, P., Colombo, M. R., Zampetti, P. (2004). Idiom comprehension in aphasic patients. *Brain and Language, 89*, 226–234.

Paul, L. K., Van Lancker Sidtis, D., Schieffer, B., Dietrich, R., & Brown, W. S. (2003). Communicative deficits in agenesis of the corpus callosum: Nonliteral language and affective prosody. *Brain and Language, 85*, 313–324.

Pylkkänen, L., Oliveri, B., & Smart, A. J., (2009). Semantics vs. world knowledge in prefrontal cortex. *Language and Cognitive Processes, 24*(9), 1313–1334.

Raine, A. (2006). Schizotypal personality: Neurodevelopmental and psychosocial trajectories. *Annual Review of Clinical Psychology, 2*, 291–326.

Rapp, A. (2009). The role of the right hemisphere for language in schizophrenia. In I. E. Sommer & R. S. Kahn (Eds.), *Language lateralization in psychosis* (pp. 147–156). Cambridge: Cambridge University Press.

Rapp, A. M., Erb, M., Grodd, W., Bartels, M., & Markert, K. (in press). Neural correlates of metonymy resolution.

Rapp, A. M., Leube, D. T., Erb, M., Grodd, W., & Kircher, T. T. (2004). Neural correlates of metaphor processing. *Cognitive Brain Research, 20*(3), 395–402.

Rapp, A. M., Leube, D. T., Erb, M., Grodd, W., & Kircher, T. T. (2007). Laterality in metaphor processing: Lack of evidence from functional magnetic resonance imaging for the right hemisphere theory. *Brain and Language, 100*(2), 142–149.

Rapp, A. M., Mutschler, D. E., & Erb, M. (submitted). Where in the brain is nonliteral language? An ALE-meta-analysis of 21 functional magnetic resonance imaging studies.

Rapp, A. M., Mutschler, D. E., Wild, B., Erb, M., Lengsfeld, I., Saur, R., et al. (2010). Neural correlates of irony comprehension: The role of schizotypal personality traits. *Brain and Language, 113*(1), 1–12.

Rapp, A. M., & Schmierer, P. (2010). Proverbs and nonliteral language in schizophrenia: A systematic methodological review of all studies published 1931–2010. *Schizophrenia Research, 117*(2–3), 422.

Rapp, A. M., & Wild, B. (2011). Nonliteral language in Alzheimer dementia: A review. *Journal of the International Neuropsychological Society, 17*(2), 207–218.

Rinaldi, M. C., Marangolo, P., & Baldassarri, F. (2004). Metaphor comprehension in right brain-damaged patients with visuo-verbal and verbal material: A dissociation (re)considered. *Cortex, 40*, 479–490.

Schmidt, G. L., Kranjec, A., Cardillo, E. R., & Chatterjee, A. (2010). Beyond laterality: A critical assessment of research on the neural basis of metaphor. *Journal of the International Neuropsychological Society, 16*(1), 1–5.

Schmidt, G. L., & Seger, C. A. (2009). Neural correlates of metaphor processing: The roles of figurativeness, familiarity and difficulty. *Brain and cognition, 71*(3), 375–386.

Shibata, M., Abe, J., Terao, A., & Miyamoto, T. (2007). Neural mechanisms involved in the comprehension of metaphoric and literal sentences: An fMRI study. *Brain Research, 1166*, 92–102.

Shibata, M., Toyomura, A., Itoh, H., & Abe, J. (2010). Neural substrates of irony comprehension: A functional MRI study. *Brain Research, 1308*, 114–123.

Somers, M., Sommer, I. E., Boks, M. P., & Kahn, R. S. (2009). Hand-preference and population schizotypy: A meta-analysis. *Schizophrenia Research, 108*(1–3), 25–32.

Sprong, M., Schothorst, P., Vos, E., Hox, J., & van Engeland, H. (2007). Theory of mind in schizophrenia: Meta-analysis. *British Journal of Psychiatry, 191*(1), 5–13.

Stringaris, A. K., Medford, N. C., Giampietro, V., Brammer, M. J., & David, A. S. (2007). Deriving meaning: Distinct neural mechanisms for metaphoric, literal, and non-meaningful sentences. *Brain and Language, 100*(2), 150–162.

Stringaris, A. K., Medford, N. C., Giora, R., Giampietro, V., Brammer, M. J., & David, A. S. (2006). How metaphors influence semantic relatedness judgements: The role of the right frontal cortex. *NeuroImage, 33*, 784–793.

Thoma, P., & Daum, I., (2006). Neurocognitive mechanisms of figurative language processing – Evidence from clinical dysfunctions. *Neuroscience and Biobehavioral Reviews, 30*(8), 1182–1205.

Tompkins, C. A. (1990). Knowledge and strategies for processing lexical metaphor after right or left hemisphere brain damage. *Journal of Speech and hearing research, 33*(2), 307–316.

Tompkins, C. A., Boada, R., & McGarry, K. (1992). The access and processing of familiar idioms by brain damaged and normally aging adults. *Journal of Speech and Hearing Research, 35*, 626–637.

Turkeltaub, P. E., Eden, G. F., Jones, K. M., & Zeffiro, T. A. (2002). Meta-analysis of the functional neuroanatomy of single-word reading: Method and validation. *Neuroimage, 16*, 765–780.

Uchiyama, H., Seki, A., Kageyama, H., Saito, D. N., Koeda, T., Ohno, K., et al. (2006). Neural substrates of sarcasm: A functional magnetic-resonance imaging study. *Brain Research, 1124*(1), 100–110.

Ulatowska, H. K., Bond-Chapman, S., Johnson, J. K. (1995). Processing of proverbs in aphasics and old-elderly. *Clinical Aphasiology, 23*, 179–193.

Ulatowska, H. K., Wertz, R.T., Chapman, S. B., Hill, C. L., Thompson, J. L., Keebler, M. W., et al. (2001). Interpretation of fables and proverbs by African Americans with and without aphasia. *American Journal of Speech-Language Pathology, 10*(1), 40–50.

Van Lancker, D. (1990). The neurology of proverbs. *Behavioral Neurology, 3*, 169–187.

Van Lancker, D. R., & Kempler, D. (1987). Comprehension of familiar phrases by left- but not by right-hemisphere damaged patients. *Brain and Language, 32*, 265–277.

Van Lancker Sidtis, D. (2006). Where in the brain is nonliteral language? *Metaphor and symbol, 21*(4), 213–244.

Wakusawa, K., Sugiura, M., Sassa, Y., Jeong, H., Horie, K., Sato, S., et al. (2007). Comprehension of implicit meanings in social situations involving irony: A functional MRI study. *NeuroImage, 37*(4), 1417–1426.

Wang, A. T., Lee, S. S., Sigman, M., & Dapretto, M. (2006a). Neural basis of irony comprehension in children with autism: The role of prosody and context. *Brain, 129*(4), 932–943.

Wang, A. T., Lee, S. S., Sigman, M., & Dapretto, M. (2006b). Developmental changes in the neural basis of interpreting communicative intent. *Social Cognitive and Affective Neuroscience, 1*(2), 107–121.

Whalen, J. M., Pexman, P. M., & Alastair, J. G. (2009). "Should be fun not!": Incidence and marking of nonliteral language in e-mail. *Journal of Language and Social Psychology, 28*, 263–280.

Wilke, M., & Lidzba, K. (2007). LI-tool: A new toolbox to assess lateralization in functional MR-data. *Journal of Neuroscience Methods, 163*(1), 128–136.

Winner, E., & Gardner, H. (1977). The comprehension of metaphor in brain damaged patients. *Brain, 100*, 717–729.

Yang, F. G., Edens, J., Simpson, C., & Krawczyk, D. C. (2009). Differences in task demands influence the hemispheric lateralization and neural correlates of metaphor. *Brain and Language, 111*(2), 114–124.

Yang, F. P., Fuller, J., Khodaparst, N., & Krawczyk, D. C. (2010). Figurative language processing after traumatic brain injury in adults: A preliminary study. *Neuropsychologia, 48*(7), 1923–1929.

Yu, G., Kim, C., Kim, D. H., & Nam, K. (2006). Semantic activation and cortical areas related to the lexical and idiomatic ambiguity. In I. King et al. (Eds.), *ICONIP 2006, part I* (pp. 290–297). Heidelberg: Springer.

Zaidel, E., Kasher, A., Soroker, N., & Batori, G. (2002). Effects of right and left hemisphere damage on performance of the "right hemisphere communication battery." *Brain and Language, 80*(3), 510–535.

Zempleni, M. Z., (2006). *Functional imaging of the hemispheric contribution to language processing* (Unpublished doctoral dissertation). Rijksuniversiteit Groningen, Netherlands, pp. 84–108.

Zempleni M. Z., Haverkort, M., Renken, R. A., & Stowe, L. (2007). Evidence for bilateral involvement in idiom comprehension: An fMRI study. *Neuroimage, 34*(3), 1280–91.

Zhu, Z., Zhang, J. X., Wang, S., Xiao, Z., Huang, J., & Chen, H. C. (2009). Involvement of left inferior frontal gyrus in sentence-level semantic integration. *NeuroImage, 47*(2), 756–63.

21

Thinking outside the Left Box:
The role of the Right Hemisphere in
Novel Metaphor Comprehension

Miriam Faust

Through the Looking Glass by Lewis Carroll was published in 1871 as a sequel to *Alice's Adventures in Wonderland* (1865) and has remained a popular, intriguing classic. *Through the Looking Glass* features a mirror image world where linguistic rules (in addition to other rules) are frequently violated. In this sense, it is the ultimate example of linguistic creativity. Indeed, the violation of various phonological, syntactic, semantic, and pragmatic rules is a major means by which the author creates the feeling of virtual reality.

This chapter was specifically inspired by Lewis Carroll's use of semantic violations. It will focus on mainly novel metaphoric language that violates semantic rules and use this example to better understand how the rule-based linguistic system of the brain copes with such violations. I will review research suggesting that the violation of semantic rules requires the involvement of the right hemisphere (RH). I will argue that RH contribution to the comprehension of semantic violations, such as novel metaphoric expressions, extends the range of language processing available to the brain and serves as a major tool for verbal creativity. In line with this notion, the creative use of semantic violations in *Through the Looking Glass* may be regarded as some kind of neurolinguistic mirror image to the rule-based language of the dominant, expert left hemisphere (LH), enhancing the feeling of a strange, "behind the mirror" world.

The chapter proceeds as follows. After giving some examples of semantic violations from *Through the Looking Glass*, I review briefly contemporary theorizing and research on metaphor processing by the brain suggesting that at least one component of metaphor comprehension, the ability to tolerate semantic violations, is

The Handbook of the Neuropsychology of Language, First Edition. Edited by Miriam Faust.

associated with the RH. The review focuses mainly on the comprehension of novel metaphors as an example of semantic violations that may support verbal creativity. I will argue that the processing of novel metaphoric expressions requires an ongoing, dynamic interplay between multiple brain areas in both hemispheres and will emphasize the unique contribution of the RH to novel metaphor comprehension. Thus, although it cannot be emphasized too strongly that semantic processing, including the more flexible, creative aspects of semantics, is best viewed as a whole-brain process, previous research indicates that the RH seems to contribute uniquely to specific processes underlying metaphor comprehension. In the final sections I will discuss language as a rule-based system that nevertheless allows for rule violation or semantic "emergence" (Benari, 2005) and suggest that RH unique tolerance to semantic violations is a major resource for the cognitive system (Dascal, 2002), supporting verbal creativity (for a recent meta-analytic review on RH dominance in creative thinking and verbal creativity see Mihov, Denzler, & Förster, 2010).

In *Through the Looking Glass*, Alice, having passed through the looking glass, finds herself among things and people inhabiting the looking glass world, who use the same words that she uses, but who evidently follow some strange, unconventional lexical and semantic rules (e.g., Yaguello, 1981). For example, Humpty Dumpty, one of Carroll's most enduring characters, is remembered principally for his famous definition of the meaning of a word ("When I use a word, it means just what I choose it to mean," p. 81). This definition clearly violates rules of semantic selection and combination. Thus, no wonder that Alice, arriving from the "real" world, has great difficulty in accepting it ("The question is . . . whether you can make words mean so many different things," p. 81).

In addition to this highly flexible and creative use of word meanings by Humpty Dumpty, the characters in the "through the looking glass" world use many other types of creative language. This technique serves to create a world whose logic is different from our own, thereby underlining violations of the semantic structure of words, which is precisely what makes figures of speech possible (Yaguello, 1981). Thus, for example, Carroll uses metaphors, humor, jabberwocky, word games, "portmanteau" expressions (a term coined by Humpty Dumpty, two meanings packed up into one word, p. 83), as well as poetry. The text includes many poetic stanzas and much discussion of poetry. Humpty Dumpty states that he "can explain all the poems that were ever invented – and a good many that haven't been invented just yet" (p. 82), while Alice hopes the knight's song is not too long as "she had heard a good deal of poetry that day" (p. 109). The poems include many novel metaphoric expressions, such as the following from the opening poem: "silver laughter," "moody madness," "nest of gladness," and "shadow of a sigh" (p. 1). In addition, the text includes literal expressions that are used in a novel metaphoric way (e.g., "In fact, the more head downwards I am, the more I keep inventing new things": the knight, p.108) as well as conventional metaphors that are taken literally (e.g., "The dog would lose its temper, wouldn't it? . . . then if the dog went away, its temper would remain!": the red queen, p. 119).

Metaphor Comprehension and the Right Hemisphere

From a neurolinguistic point of view, many of the above-described linguistic phenomena of the mirror image world seem to be highly associated with the unique language of the RH. Although the findings are not entirely consistent, much research indicates that the RH plays a major role in processing metaphors, connotative meanings, humor, lexical ambiguity, and insight problem solving. In general, the RH seems to be involved in those aspects of language process that are based on a highly flexible, open semantic system (e.g., Bowden & Jung-Beeman, 2003; Chiarello, 2003; Faust & Chiarello, 1998; Faust & Mashal, 2007; Fiore & Schooler, 1998; Jung Beeman et al., 2004). RH semantic flexibility and tolerance of semantic violations has been especially emphasized in connection with the processing of metaphoric expressions (e.g., Anaki, Faust, & Kravetz, 1998; Brownell, Simpson, Bihrle, Potter, & Gardner, 1990; Burgess & Chiarello, 2006; Faust & Mashal, 2007; Mashal, Faust, & Hendler, 2005; Schmidt, DeBuse, & Seger, 2007). Thus, metaphor comprehension may involve the retrieval of alternate, distantly related, and even seemingly unrelated meanings in order to integrate unusual or unfamiliar word combinations

Since metaphor comprehension appears to require semantic processing that is subserved by a distinctive neural network, the widespread use of metaphoric expressions is one of the most interesting phenomena of human language (e.g., Lakoff & Johnson, 1980). Perhaps one major reason for their abundance in language is that metaphors ("My job is a jail") permit the efficient expression of ideas that would otherwise be awkward to explain literally (Glucksberg, 2001). Figurative language thus seems especially useful in informing others about one's own attitudes and beliefs in indirect, ambiguous ways (Gibbs, 1994). In addition, metaphoric language plays a central role in reflecting, and perhaps shaping, how people think in a broad range of domains (e.g., Cacciary & Glucksberg, 1994). According to Pinker (2007), using a metaphor requires us to manipulate ideas in a deeper stratum of thought, thus our conceptual system is fundamentally metaphorical. Furthermore, metaphors, both newly invented and conventional, are widely used in poetry, where with a few words, implicit and explicit emotions and associations from one context can powerfully be associated with another, different context. Indeed, Aristotle wrote in his *Poetics* that "the greatest thing by far is to be a master of metaphor."

A metaphor has been traditionally defined as a denotative violation since it conveys information by describing a thing in terms of what it is not (Billow, 1975). Metaphors are often characterized as involving two seemingly unlike things compared, as opposed to literal comparisons involving two things that are clearly alike (Cacciary & Glucksberg, 1994). According to Beck (1987), the understanding of metaphors (such as "This idea is a gem") "forces the mind" to construct a high-order mental linkage of two different, frequently unrelated, category domains, the "topic" or "target" of the metaphor ("idea") and the "vehicle" or "base" of the metaphor ("gem"). This "bridging" effort is required because the idea is not really a gem but rather it shares some properties with a gem (preciousness, uniqueness, but not the color of the gem). Richards (1936) refers to the shared properties between the topic and the vehicle of the metaphor as the "ground" of the metaphor. Thus "understanding a metaphor can be seen as the process by which the metaphor's ground becomes available and salient" (Pynte, Besson, Robichon, & Poli, 1996, p. 294).

Although metaphoric expressions may involve the use of both previously acquired and newly created categories and conceptual linkages (Cacciary & Glucksberg, 1994), the relation between the vehicle and the topic of a metaphor, either conventional or novel, can be characterized as relatively unusual and distant. Metaphoric, as opposed to literal, language comprehension involves some kind of meaning extension through the establishment of correspondence between concepts from disparate knowledge domains (for a review, see Bowdle & Gentner, 2005). Several different models have been postulated to explain the mechanisms that deal with the literal/metaphoric duality (e.g., Glucksberg, 2003; Grice, 1975), focusing mainly on conventional, frequently used, metaphors. Thus, for example, research on the precedence of meaning access (e.g., the claim that figurative and literal meaning is accessed concurrently) is based largely on studies of conventional metaphors (for reviews, see Giora, 2002; Glucksberg, 2001, 2003).

The distinctive nature of the comprehension of unfamiliar or novel metaphors, such as those used in poetry and other creative texts, has been, for the most part, overlooked, in spite of findings suggesting that novel metaphors are processed differently than conventional ones (e.g., Ahrens et al., 2007; Amanzio, Geminiani, Leotta, & Cappa, 2007). Ahrens et al. (2007) conclude, on the basis of their functional magnetic resonance imaging (fMRI) study of the processing of conventional and novel, anomalous metaphoric sentences, that conventional and novel metaphors can no longer be grouped together. Instead, they suggest that in order to make further discoveries on semantic processing, finer-grained distinctions should be used to categorize metaphors into different semantic groups. Similarly, Amanzio et al. (2007), who tested metaphor comprehension in Alzheimer patients and healthy control subjects, concluded that different brain mechanisms are involved in processing conventional and novel metaphors.

The findings of several studies to date, including those from our lab, also suggest that although both conventional and novel metaphors involve some kind of semantic violation, they are different semantic categories involving different semantic and neural processing mechanisms. However, only a few models have proposed distinct operations for novel and conventional metaphors. The career-of-metaphor hypothesis by Bowdle and Gentner (2005) posits different processing of novel and conventional metaphors. According to Gentner's structural-mapping theory (1983), metaphors are comprehended by establishing correspondences between partially isomorphic conceptual structures of the target and base. This comparison process is elicited when comprehending novel metaphors. However, as metaphors get conventionalized they become associated with a metaphoric category and may be processed using categorization as well. Categorization is more rapid and less computationally costly than comparison but requires an existing metaphoric category. When a novel metaphor is encountered, an initial categorization attempt fails due to the lack of a well-defined category. Novel metaphors are thus processed sequentially, and the comparison process begins after determining that the literal meaning cannot be sensibly applied. Furthermore, Gentner and colleagues have suggested that as novel metaphors become increasingly conventional through frequent use, there is an accompanying shift in the mode of processing from comparison to categorization (Gentner & Bowdle, 2001; Gentner & Wolff, 1997).

An additional model that has also implications for the different neural mechanisms involved in conventional and novel metaphor comprehension is the graded salience hypothesis (GSH; Giora, 1997, 2002, 2003). According to this model, the factor determining precedence of meaning access is salience and thus the interpretation of literal and metaphoric expressions is determined by their degree of saliency. The salient meaning, either figurative or literal, is the one always processed first. The figurative meaning in conventional metaphors is commonly more salient than the literal one, thus in most "dead" metaphors the figurative meaning is accessed first. In contrast, when a novel or unfamiliar metaphor is encountered, the salient meaning is the literal one, and the figurative meaning is inferred later by contextual mechanisms. The GSH posits that whereas for conventional metaphors, the salient metaphoric meaning is coded in the mental lexicon, the meaning of novel metaphors must be constructed online. Although the structural-mapping theory does not include neurolinguistic implications, the GSH predicts a selective RH involvement in the comprehension of novel, nonsalient, metaphorical meanings and LH involvement in the comprehension of conventional, salient, metaphorical meanings (Giora, 2002; 2003). This model replaces the LH/literal meaning versus RH/metaphoric meaning dichotomy by a LH/salient meaning versus RH/nonsalient meaning dichotomy.

A third model that may be applied to the hemispheric differences in the comprehension of conventional versus novel metaphors is the fine–coarse semantic coding theory (FCT; Beeman, 1998, Jung-Beeman, 2005; see also Mirous & Beeman, Volume 1, Chapter 16). This model provides an explanation of the role of the RH in metaphor processing. According to this model, the involvement of the RH in the processing of metaphors, and, specifically, in processing novel, unfamiliar metaphoric expressions may not be particular to metaphors, but rather may be one aspect of the unique semantic coding of the RH, characterized by high sensitivity to distant semantic relations. The FCT postulates that immediately after encountering a word, the LH engages in relatively fine semantic coding, strongly focusing on a few closely related word meanings or semantic features, whereas the RH engages in coarse semantic coding, weakly and diffusely activating large semantic fields containing multiple alternative meanings and more distant associates. The larger and less discriminate the semantic field, the more likely it is to overlap with semantic fields activated by other input words, including metaphorically related words.

The metaphorical meaning of a word is usually more semantically distant than its literal meaning. Consequently, the processing of a metaphoric expression may depend on the ability to activate a broader, more flexible set of semantic associations in order to integrate the meanings of the weakly related words into a meaningful linguistic expression. Furthermore, the comprehension of novel metaphoric expressions, such as those taken from poetry, may rely even more on the ability to link several distant associates in order to combine the meanings of seemingly unrelated individual words. The FCT predicts that the RH will benefit more from the unfamiliar semantic relationship between the meanings of single words appearing in a novel metaphoric expression whereas the LH may show an advantage when comprehension depends on the ability to process a highly familiar, either literal or conventional metaphoric, semantic relationship.

This distinction between conventional metaphoric and novel metaphoric expressions with regard to the differential processing by the LH and RH, respectively, is also consistent with the GSH (Giora, 1997, 2002). The integration of the FCT and the GSH could thus imply that a few salient strongly associated meanings, be they literal or metaphoric, are quickly activated in the LH. However, according to the latter integrated account of meaning processing, the RH activates and maintains multiple nonsalient weakly associated meanings, either literal or metaphoric. Both the FCT and the GSH thus predict a LH advantage for processing familiar literal and conventional metaphoric expressions and a RH advantage for processing novel, unfamiliar metaphoric expressions.

Much empirical evidence on metaphor processing by the two cerebral hemispheres is consistent with the GSH and FCT models presented above. The results of semantic priming studies as well as data collected from brain-damaged patients generally suggest that the RH contributes uniquely to the comprehension of metaphoric language. Furthermore, the extent of RH involvement in metaphor comprehension reported in previous studies may be attributed, at least partly, to differences in the linguistic and neural mechanisms involved in processing conventional and novel metaphoric meanings. The findings of several studies support this claim by showing increased RH involvement for novel (e.g., Bottini et al., 1994; Faust & Mashal, 2007; Schmidt et al., 2007) or less familiar (Anaki et al., 1998) metaphoric expressions.

The notion that metaphor, mainly novel metaphor, comprehension involves RH neurolinguistic mechanisms that can cope with semantic violations is what motivated a series of experiments conducted in our lab. This research project was based on the assumption that the processing of literal, conventional metaphoric, and novel metaphoric expressions can be dissociated experimentally and that the processing differences should manifest themselves in the pattern of hemispheric involvement and interaction during comprehension.

To date there have been very few studies that have employed behavioral mehtods, brain imaging, evoked response potentials (ERPs), or transcranial magnetic stimulation (TMS) as a means of exploring RH involvement in conventional versus novel metaphor comprehension. Furthermore, there are almost no data on individual differences in the pattern of hemispheric involvement and interaction during novel metaphor comprehension. Our research project was based on the assumption that novel, but not conventional, metaphors require the online establishment of "mental linkage" between words normally not related, posing an increased load on the semantic system. Since, according to both theoretical accounts (Beeman, 1998; Giora, 1997, 2003; Jung-Beeman, 2005) and previous research (e.g., Anaki et al., 1998; Bottini et al., 1994; Chiarello, 1998, 2003; Faust & Lavidor, 2003; Schmidt et al., 2007), the RH contributes uniquely to the activation and integration of distant, unusual and nonsalient semantic relations, our main hypothesis was that the comprehension of novel metaphoric two-word expressions taken from poetry will show a distinct pattern of neural processing. Specifically, we predicted that compared to the comprehension of both literal and highly conventional metaphoric expressions, the comprehension of novel metaphors will require unique involvement of RH mechanisms.

The Conventional Versus Novel Metaphor Brain Processing Research Project

As described above, metaphoric expressions may vary in familiarity, with novel metaphoric expressions representing the less familiar end of the familiarity continuum. Furthermore, the extent of RH involvement in metaphor processing may depend on the cognitive processes underlying familiar, conventional versus unfamiliar, novel metaphor comprehension. Based on the suggested processing difference between conventional and novel metaphors (Bowdle & Gentner, 2005; Giora, 1997, 2002) as well as on the suggested role of the RH in processing unusual semantic relations (Beeman, 1998; Jung-Beeman, 2005; Giora, 1997, 2002), we conducted a programmatic series of experiments using convergent, complementary experimental methods. In all of the experiments we used the same, simplest form of metaphoric stimuli, i.e., two-word expressions, in order to avoid the confounding effects of sentence-level processes or larger context (see, e.g., Faust, 1998; Faust, Barak, & Chiarello, 2006; Faust, Bar-Lev, & Chiarello, 2003; Peleg & Eviatar, Volume 1, Chapter 4). Furthermore, the novel metaphorical expressions were taken from original Hebrew poetry and thus had high ecological validity and were, at least potentially, meaningful. In all of the experiments, participants were presented with four types of two-word noun–noun or adjective–noun combinations, literal (e.g., "personal confession," "problem resolution," "broken glass"), conventional metaphoric (e.g., "transparent intention," "sweet dream," "lucid mind") and novel metaphoric (e.g., "wilting hope," "ripe dream," "mercy blanket") expressions as well as unrelated word pairs (e.g., "salty rescue," "indirect blanket," "drum outlet"). However, because of Hebrew grammar, the order of words in the translated examples was actually reversed. The different types of word pairs were subjected to extensive pretesting (e.g., meaningfulness, metaphoricity) and carefully controlled for all relevant parameters (e.g., frequency, concreteness, familiarity, syntactic structure; for a detailed description of the linguistic stimuli, see Faust & Mashal, 2007). The experimental task was semantic judgment.

In several behavioral experiments (Faust & Mashal, 2007; Mashal & Faust, 2008; Zeev-Wolf & Faust, 2010), the split visual field paradigm combined with priming was used. In two experiments that were identical in every other respect, we tested the processing of the four types of linguistic expressions by the two cerebral hemispheres across two different time intervals between the two words of the linguistic expressions (stimulus onset asynchronies [SOAs] of 400 ms and 1100 ms). Based on the predictions of the FCT and the GSH as well as on previous research findings on differential patterns of semantic processing by the two cerebral hemispheres, the main hypothesis of both experiments was that the RH will be faster and more accurate than the LH in performing a semantic judgment ("related/unrelated") task for novel metaphoric, but not for either literal or conventional, metaphoric expressions. This left visual field/RH advantage was expected to be more pronounced for the long SOA condition because strategic and post-access prime processing and inhibition were expected mainly to occur within the LH (for reviews, see Chiarello, 2003; Faust & Kahana, 2002)

In the two experiments, participants were presented with the four types of two-word combinations described above and asked to perform a semantic judgment task. The first word of each expression was presented centrally, followed by a focusing signal. The second, target, word was randomly lateralized to the right or left visual field. Participants were instructed to push one of two buttons; "related" if the prime and the target were semantically related and thus constituted a meaningful expression, either literal or metaphoric, or "unrelated" if the two words were not semantically related.

The findings of the two experiments were very similar and generally confirmed the main hypothesis. A RH advantage was found for both accuracy and reaction time (RT), indicating that the novel metaphors were comprehended better and faster when initially presented to the RH. However, as expected, for either literal or conventional metaphors, no RH advantage was found. The putative effect of SOA on the pattern of responding to the different linguistic stimuli was not found. A recent experiment that replicated the behavioral split visual studies used two different SOAs of 150 and 650 ms (Zeev-Wolf & Faust, in preparation). Here too, a left visual field/ RH advantage was expected only for the long SOA condition. The findings confirmed the hypothesis showing a similar pattern of processing for both hemispheres in the short SOA but RH superiority for novel metaphors in the long SOA. The findings are also consistent with the FCT and suggest that distant meanings are initially activated in both hemispheres but maintained only in the RH for further integration.

Although the findings of the three experiments did not show a RH advantage for the other type of unfamiliar expression (i.e., unrelated word pairs), a subsequent split visual study (Mashal & Faust, 2008) was designed to determine whether RH superiority for novel metaphor comprehension reflects genuine sensitivity to distant semantic relations or just a more liberal semantic criterion applied for all unfamiliar expressions, either meaningful or meaningless. We thus used the signal detection paradigm that allows for the separation of sensitivity (d') from response bias (β, response criterion), and computes estimates of each. In each of the two experiments, participants were presented with two types of expressions, half of which were meaningful (either novel or conventional metaphors in the two experiments, respectively) and half, meaningless (unrelated word pairs) and asked to perform a semantic judgment task. The signal detection data analyses provided an estimation (d') of how easy it is to separate "signal" (i.e., either novel metaphors or literal expressions) from "noise" (i.e., unrelated word pairs). The results replicated those of the previous split visual field experiments, showing RH advantage only for the novel metaphors but not for the literal expressions. No hemispheric differences were found for β. Furthermore, the findings showed higher sensitivity (d') for novel metaphors initially presented to the RH as compared to those presented to the LH, indicating a higher ability of the RH to differentiate between novel metaphors and unrelated word pairs. These findings support a unique sensitivity of the RH to distant, unusual semantic relations that is nevertheless highly selective and does not extend to all unfamiliar combinations. The literal pairs, based on familiar, rule-based semantic relationship, showed a significant LH advantage in response criterion.

RH advantage for novel metaphor comprehension was replicated in yet another study (Mashal & Faust, 2009) that was motivated by the above mentioned models postulating different mechanisms for the comprehension of conventional as opposed to novel metaphors (Bowdle & Gentner, 2005; Giora, 1997, 2002, 2003). According to the career-of-metaphor model (e.g., Bowdle & Gentner, 2005), the process of conventionalizing novel metaphors is accompanied by a processing shift from comparison to categorization. Although, as pointed out above, Bowdle and Gentner do not spell out the neurolinguistic implications of their model, this shift could be interpreted neurolinguistically as a shift from LH to RH processing. However, such changes in brain processing as a result of the conventionalization of novel metaphors do not appear to have been tested before.

Using the divided visual field technique, we tested the possibility that the conventionalization of novel metaphors will be accompanied by a shift from RH to LH processing. Participants were presented with novel and conventional metaphoric expressions, literal expressions, and unrelated word pairs and completed the same experiment twice. Following the first experiment, half of the participants were explicitly directed to think about the meanings of the four types of linguistic stimuli. Then the second experiment, which was identical to the first, was carried out by all of the research participants. The results showed hemispheric changes from a RH advantage during initial exposure to similar hemispheric performance as a result of the conventionalization of novel metaphoric expressions only on the part of those participants who had been asked to elaborate the meaning of all of the linguistic stimuli. During the first and second experiments, for all of the research participants, the other types of linguistic expressions did not show a shift in hemispheric advantage.

While the series of the above behavioral experiments supported the notion of RH selective sensitivity to novel, unusual semantic relations, the aim of another study that used the same stimuli was to directly identify the specific RH brain areas involved in novel metaphor comprehension. In this study (Mashal et al., 2005;

Mashal, Faust, Hendler, & Jung-Beeman, 2007), we used a common brain imaging technique, fMRI, to test the claim that the RH has a primary role in processing novel metaphoric expressions. This technique enables localization of brain function by monitoring the hemodynamic changes associated with neural activity. Participants were presented with the four types of two-word expressions used in the above-described experiments and asked to decide whether each expression was meaningful or meaningless. The results showed that when compared with conventional metaphors, there were significant regions of activation for novel metaphors in the right posterior superior temporal gyrus (PSTG), the homologue of Wernicke's area. In addition, significant greater percent signal change for novel metaphors than for both literal expressions and unrelated word pairs was also found in the right PSTG. Stronger activation in the right PSTG for the novel metaphoric expressions than for either literal or conventional metaphoric expressions points to the special role of this brain region in the construction of novel semantic connections.

The fMRI findings were further subjected to principal component analysis (PCA) to analyze brain functioning in terms of networks. The functional connectivity principle points to the interactions and the integration that link the dynamics of specialized regions (Friston, 1998). This principle is based on the assumption that each experimental condition, i.e., each cognitive or linguistic process, may be mediated by a different functional network. Thus, if a specific brain region belongs to the same functional network (i.e., component in terms of PCA) as other regions in one condition but to a different component in another condition, this means that this area interacts differently with other brain areas in each condition and thus might play a different role in processing the various linguistic stimuli.

The PCA analysis identified a special, unique network recruited for the processing of the novel metaphoric expressions, obtained from the second component of the novel metaphor condition. Thus, when processing unfamiliar yet potentially meaningful linguistic expressions, activation in the right homologue of Wernicke's area was highly correlated with activation in frontal areas: Broca's area, left and right insula, and left and right premotor areas.

The causal role played by the right PSTG in the processing of novel metaphoric expressions was further established in two repetitive transcranial magnetic stimulation (rTMS) experiments (Pobric, Mashal, Faust, & Lavidor, 2008). Thus, the causal role of a specific brain region can be estimated by measuring the magnitude of impairment resulting from applying magnetic stimulation to that specific region. In both experiments, participants were presented with English translations of the four types of two-word expressions used in the previously described experiments and asked to perform a semantic judgment task. The findings of the two experiments were very similar and showed that rTMS over the right homologue of Wernicke's area (more precisely over the right posterior superior temporal sulcus, PSTS), that has been previously identified as the critical RH area involved in novel metaphor processing (Mashal et al., 2005, 2007), disrupted processing of novel but not conventional metaphors. However, rTMS over the left inferior frontal gyrus

(IFG) selectively impaired processing of literal word pairs and conventional but not novel metaphors.

In the second experiment, using rTMS over additional brain areas, these findings were replicated (Pobric et al., 2008). Thus, the TMS data analysis revealed that TMS over the right PSTS caused a significant inhibition for novel metaphors, i.e., slowed down the processing of novel metaphoric expressions. However, an additional, unexpected finding was that TMS over the left PSTS caused facilitation in responses to novel metaphors, i.e., enhanced novel metaphor comprehension. Significant interference TMS effects were created for conventional metaphoric and literal expressions when TMS was applied over the left and right IFG, respectively, in comparison to the control condition. This study was the first demonstration of TMS-induced impairment in processing novel metaphoric expressions, and as such confirmed the specialization of the RH in the activation of a broader range of related meanings than the LH, including novel, nonsalient meanings. In addition, the pattern of results strongly indicates that RH involvement in semantic processing is highly selective and limited to novel metaphors, i.e., it does not extend to either conventional metaphors or other unfamiliar nonmetaphoric expressions (unrelated word pairs).

Furthermore, the unexpected finding of the second experiment, showing an opposite pattern of facilitation in processing novel metaphors following TMS over the left PSTS may suggest that interfering with LH activity may facilitate novel metaphor comprehension in the RH. Since previous studies have shown that TMS of one region may disinhibit the homologous regions in the contralateral hemisphere (Seyal, Ro, & Rafal, 1995), such a disinhibition mechanism may have operated in this study. TMS over the left PSTS may have caused the disinhibition of the right PSTS, leading to faster RTs as compared to the control condition. According to this explanation, LH inhibitory semantic processing mechanisms may interfere with RH ability to integrate the individual meanings of two seemingly unrelated concepts into a meaningful metaphoric expression.

To add a temporal dimension to hemispheric asymmetries during metaphor comprehension, we used ERPs. This technique provides measures of brain activity with very high temporal resolution. When coupled with methods for source localization, it can provide an estimation of the neural sources involved (Arzouan, Goldstein, & Faust, 2007a, 2007b; Goldstein, Arzouan, & Faust, 2008). Different processes are reflected as different ERP components, whereas variations in effort or difficulty are manifested as amplitude or latency differences in a specific component. ERP measures can thus assist in pinpointing the processing stages at which metaphorical meaning is achieved. These techniques were applied in several experiments to study the timeline of hemispheric dynamics during the processing of conventional and novel metaphoric two-word expressions

The few studies that have investigated metaphor comprehension using ERPs (e.g., Bonnaud et al., 2002; Coulson & van Petten, 2002; Iakimova et al., 2005; Pynte et al., 1996; for a review, see Arzouan et al., 2007b, and Coulson & Davenport, Volume 1, Chapter 19) focused on a particular ERP component, the N400, which is a negative deflection peaking approximately 400 ms after stimulus presentation. The amplitude of the N400 has been shown to vary systematically with the processing of semantic information and can be thought of as a general index of the ease or difficulty of retrieving stored conceptual knowledge associated with a word (e.g., Kutas & Federmeier, 2000; see also Kutas, Kiang, & Sweeney, Volume 2, Chapter 26). Regarding processing stages later than the retrieval of the semantic information of words, findings in the literature are less consistent. The late positive component (LPC) or P600 usually appears following the N400 and has been thought to reflect sentence-level integration (Kaan et al., 2000) or reanalysis (Friederici, 1995) and memory retrieval processes (Paller & Kutas, 1992; Rugg et al., 1995).

In several ERP experiments (Arzouan et al., 2007a, 2007b), we measured the electrical brain response of participants to the literal, conventional metaphoric, novel metaphoric, and unrelated expressions. The two-word expressions were presented centrally in a random order, one word at a time, each for 200 ms with an interval of 200 ms between words. Participants were instructed to "judge whether the presented two-word expression conveys a meaning (be it literal or metaphoric) or does not convey a meaning as a pair," and press a corresponding key. ERPs to the second word of the expression were derived and entered into a neural-source estimation algorithm (LORETA), and current density at each brain area was compared between expression types.

The findings of the ERP experiments (Arzouan et al., 2007a) showed the N400 amplitude gradient. This gradient started with small N400 for literal relations and increased for conventional metaphors and novel metaphors. Finally, it was largest for unrelated words. Thus, while retrieving the stored conceptual knowledge associated with novel metaphors was more demanding than retrieving knowledge of conventional metaphors or literally related words, meaning was accessed, at least initially, in a similar manner. In addition, the ERP results indicated that the dynamics of hemispheric activity are complex and vary across processing stages and brain areas (Arzouan et al, 2007b; Goldstein et al., 2008). The processing mechanisms used for all types of expressions were similar, as indicated by similar elicited components and parallel fluctuations in brain volume activation. Both hemispheres were active during the comprehension of all expressions as reflected in the absolute current density values and number of active voxels in each hemisphere. However, the relative contribution of each hemisphere at specific processing stages depended on stimulus type. These stages correspond roughly to the N400 and LPC components that reflect semantic and contextual integration. Both the brain volume activity and the current density analyses yielded converging evidence of relative asymmetric processing, increased processing for RH areas relative to LH areas only during novel metaphor comprehension. This asymmetry appears to stem from activity in right temporal and right superior frontal areas. The temporal regions include the right homologue of Wernicke's and surrounding areas. Relative asymmetry toward LH areas was found for all other types of linguistic expressions.

These results are in agreement with those of the imaging studies that have distinguished novel from conventional metaphors. It appears that novel metaphoric expressions activate RH temporal areas more than conventional metaphors or literal expressions. The advantage of ERP data is that it facilitated the identification of the processing stage at which such hemispheric asymmetries occur. The findings for the N400 component also suggest that understanding novel metaphors requires the retrieval of more semantic information about the words in order to bridge the gap between seemingly unrelated words. This claim is supported by the findings of a recent ERP study (Goldstein, Arzouan, & Faust, in preparation) suggesting that the conventionalization of novel metaphoric expressions reduces the semantic integration effort invested by the brain during attempts to comprehend these expressions.

An additional approach to examine changes in hemispheric activity over time is to use statistical nonparametric mapping (SnPM; Nichols & Holmes, 2002). According to this technique, for each condition and on each time point, current density was compared. The findings of our ERP study (Arzouan et al., 2007b) showed that the fluctuations in the number of supra-threshold voxels were mostly parallel in both hemispheres. Nevertheless, asymmetries occurred during various periods. Novel metaphoric expressions elicited more relative RH activity (as reflected by the number of supra-threshold voxels) at two time windows, 350–450 ms and 550–750 ms approximately, with three prominent peaks at about 425, 600 and 710 ms. At those same time windows (and throughout most of the epoch), conventional metaphors showed relative greater LH activity. LT and unrelated expressions elicited more relative LH activity mainly at the first time window. Although this approach estimates the bulk activity of each hemisphere, it does assist in giving a general picture of the dynamics of hemispheric interactions. Thus, the findings suggested that although both hemispheres were active during the comprehension process of all expressions, there are relative LH and RH asymmetries at specific stages as reflected in the absolute current density values and the number of active voxels in each hemisphere.

Initial findings of high activation of RH temporal areas for novel metaphor processing during specific points in time are also found in a pilot study (Zeev-Wolf, Goldstein, & Faust, 2010) using the magnetoencephalography (MEG), an imaging technique used to measure the magnetic fields produced by electrical activity in the brain via extremely sensitive devices (SQUIDs). The MEG technique thus offers both high spatial and high temporal resolution in brain imaging. Findings of this MEG study that used the same paradigm and stimuli as those used in the ERP studies showed a similar grading of the M350, the magnetic counterpart of N400, for the four types of stimuli. Furthermore, during this point in time higher activation was found in RH temporal areas, homologue to Wernicke's area, for novel metaphors, whereas for literal expressions and conventional metaphors we found higher activation in Wernicke's area. Higher activation in RH temporal areas for novel metaphors was also found when these expressions were compared with unrelated word pairs.

Individual Differences in Novel Metaphor
Comprehension in the RH

The unique contribution of RH areas to the processing of novel metaphoric expressions has been repeatedly shown in several studies using convergent experimental methods. However, the findings of two additional studies suggest that there may be marked individual differences in the extent of RH involvement. Furthermore, the findings of these studies suggest that individual differences in the extent of RH involvement in metaphor comprehension are related to verbal creativity and to the ability to tolerate semantic violations.

In a recent divided visual field study (Gold, Faust, & Ben-Artzi, in press), we tested the hypotheses that novel metaphor comprehension is a process of linguistic creativity that seems to rely on RH coarse semantic coding mechanisms (e.g., Faust & Mashal, 2007). This study focused on the relation between linguistic creativity as measured by an offline standard test of verbal creativity and RTs for correct identification of novel metaphors, conventional metaphors, literal, and unrelated word pairs in a group of healthy adults. Linguistic creativity was measured by performance of the Hebrew version of the Mednick Remote Association Test (RAT; Mednick, 1962), based on triads of words each of which is remotely related to a single solution word.

Participants were asked to perform the Hebrew version of the RAT and we tested the relation between linguistic creativity as measured by performance on this test and RTs for correct responses to the four types of expressions. Results indicated that performance on the RAT, as measured by scores on the Hebrew version of this test, was significantly correlated with RTs to novel metaphors only when the metaphors were presented to the left visual field/ RH. In addition, verbal creativity scores were significantly correlated with RT to conventional metaphors in both the LH and the RH. There was no correlation with performance on either the literal or the unrelated word pairs. These results were interpreted as suggesting that the RH contribution to novel metaphor comprehension may be related to the critical involvement of the intact RH in verbal creativity (Bowden & Beeman, 2003). Thus, highly verbally creative persons show higher RH involvement when processing the meanings of the two distantly related words comprising the novel metaphoric expressions. The RAT contains many words that are related to the solution word via conventional metaphoric relations. Therefore, performance on this test and semantic judgment for conventional metaphors were closely related when the semantic task was performed by both hemispheres.

To further study individual differences in the extent of RH involvement in novel metaphor comprehension, we applied the split visual field paradigm to the study of metaphor comprehension in persons with Asperger syndrome (AS; Gold & Faust, 2010). AS is a neurodevelopmental disorder on the autistic spectrum (autistic spectrum disorder – ASD) characterized by social impairments, difficulties in communication, and a set of circumscribed interests and/or a rigid adherence to routines (e.g., Lombardo, Barnes, Wheelwright, & Baron-Cohen, 2007). Although there is no significant delay in language or cognitive development (APA, 1994), persons with AS often exhibit difficulties in comprehending specific linguistic forms, mainly nonliteral language and metaphors (MacKay & Shaw, 2004).

According to Baron-Cohen's model of systemizing versus empathizing in ASD (e.g., Baron-Cohen, 2003), the relative degree of systemizing versus empathizing tendencies can explain behavioral and cognitive characteristics of the general population and of ASD. Since systemizing refers to the inclination to analyze systems and to understand and predict behavior in terms of underlying rules, we assumed that this tendency can be generalized to language processing as well and that different kinds of linguistic stimuli may vary in the degree of systemizing involved in their efficient processing. Thus, the tendency to systemize may interfere with the comprehension of novel metaphoric expressions that involve semantic rule violations.

The study examined the relative contribution of the RH and LH in AS to metaphor comprehension. It was based on previous research suggesting that AS is a specific neuropsychological disorder associated with RH dysfunction and can be understood by analogy to RH damage, developmental disabilities involving RH dysfunction, and nonverbal learning disabilities (e.g., Ellis, Ellis, Fraser, & Deb, 1994). The study's main hypothesis was that RH dysfunction in persons with AS may account for their observed difficulties in metaphor, mainly novel metaphor, comprehension. Specifically, we expected a reduced RH advantage for novel metaphor comprehension in the AS group as compared to a control group of healthy participants.

The findings of this study generally confirmed the hypothesis. Although the control group of healthy participants demonstrated the expected RH advantage for novel metaphor comprehension, AS persons with normal or above normal levels of language ability showed no RH advantage for the comprehension of these stimuli (Gold & Faust, 2010). These findings support the claim that the RH in AS participants may be less efficiently involved in the process of novel metaphor comprehension. Interestingly, the results pointed to a marginally significant tendency towards LH superiority for the comprehension of novel metaphors by the AS participants.

The difficulty that persons with AS experience with the semantic integration required for the processing of novel metaphoric expressions was demonstrated in another study (Gold, Goldstein, & Faust, 2010) that used the ERP method for studying semantic processing of the four types of linguistic stimuli. For persons with AS, N400 amplitudes for novel metaphor comprehension were larger and not different than those for unrelated word pairs. However, for the control group, the N400 amplitudes for novel metaphors were smaller than those for unrelated word pairs.

The findings of the latter studies (Gold et al., in press; Gold & Faust, 2010; Gold et al., 2010) point to a systemizing–nonsystemizing continuum that can serve as a theoretical framework for understanding language processing in the intact brain as well as in various clinical populations. This continuum emphasizes the relative involvement of the two intact cerebral hemispheres depending on degree of systemizing versus nonsystemizing required for processing specific linguistic expressions.

In line with an above-cited study, Gold et al. (in press) showed that the extent of RH involvement in novel metaphor comprehension is highly related to verbal creativity. Accordingly, the idea of a dysfunctional RH in AS can also be extended to account for aspects of language functioning related to linguistic creativity. Thus, the link between difficulties in comprehending novel metaphoric expressions and RH dysfunction may have some wider implications for linguistic creativity in persons with AS. According to this claim, novel metaphoric expressions represent a unique and original combination of two seemingly unrelated concepts (e.g., "ripe dream," "gem eyes"). The ability to semantically relate two concepts, despite the fact that they are not usually linked together and are not coded in the mental lexicon, may require a creative linguistic process in order to establish novel, original semantic relations. This is in contrast to rule-based language processing such as syntax or literal semantic comprehension that may rely on pre-stored information. As mentioned above, creative thinking has previously been related to the RH (Beeman et al., 2004; Faust & Kahana, 2002), and it has been hypothesized that this process may profit from the coarse semantic coding attributed to the RH (Beeman et al., 2004). This notion is consistent with previously reported deficient creative thinking abilities in AS (Craig & Baron-Cohen, 1999). Thus, the difficulties in novel metaphor comprehension experienced by persons with AS may be one aspect of a more general underlying deficit in linguistic creativity related to RH dysfunction. Nevertheless, in accordance with Baron-Cohen's model, the more rule-based aspects of language are usually spared in persons with AS.

Metaphor, Rule Violation, and Emergence: The Contribution of the RH to Semantic Creativity

In this chapter, I offered an interpretation of the differences in semantic processing carried-out by the two cerebral hemispheres. This interpretation was based on a series of studies that used convergent experimental methods and investigated the role of the RH in processing conventional and novel metaphoric two-word expressions. The findings of this series of studies indicate that understanding novel metaphoric two-word expressions taken from poetry involves specific areas of the temporal lobe of the RH that are homologues to Wernicke's area. Furthermore, the ERP and MEG data suggest that RH involvement is manifested during specific points in time associated with semantic retrieval and integration. Such RH involvement was not found for conventional metaphors, literal expressions, or unrelated, meaningless expressions. For these linguistic stimuli, we generally found strong LH involvement. However, the TMS data suggest that LH linguistic mechanisms may interfere with novel metaphor comprehension.

Our research has also demonstrated that there are marked individual differences in the extent of RH involvement in novel metaphor comprehension. Thus, persons who score high on the RAT verbal creativity test, based on unusual word combinations, show higher RH involvement in novel metaphor comprehension. However, persons with AS, who tend to have specific difficulties with linguistic stimuli that are less systemized, i.e., that involve some degree of rule violation, show less RH involvement. Based on the findings of our research, I suggest that hemispheric differences are associated with individual differences in the comprehension of metaphoric word combinations. In turn, this association may be related to the LH rule-based versus the RH emergent, rule-violating semantic processing.

According to this claim, the meaning of a literal or a conventional metaphoric expression can usually be predicted on the basis of a full, systematic and comprehensive description of the semantic relations between the individual words comprising it. Thus, the comprehension of literal expressions is usually based on the processing of semantic relations between interconnected words in the semantic network. Similarly, the comprehension of most conventional, frequently used metaphoric combinations is also based on the retrieval of pre-established, salient semantic relations (e.g., Bowdle & Gentner, 2005; Giora, 2003). The systematic, constraining semantic relation may thus offer a processing advantage for the rule-based semantic system of the LH.

However, when the semantic relations between the two words comprising a linguistic expression are distant and unusual, such as in novel metaphors, the rule-based semantic system of the LH may require a complementary neural system that is able to cope with the potential rule violation created by nonconventional semantic combinations. The comprehension of novel semantic combinations may thus be characterized by "emergence." "Emergence" is used here to refer to a process whose final outcome cannot be fully predicted on the basis of the individual components of the linguistic expression (Benari, 2005). The distant, unusual semantic relations between the two words comprising a novel metaphoric expression may thus require an open and flexible semantic system that is able to tolerate semantic violations and cope with multiple, including less predictable, interpretations. According to the fine–coarse semantic coding hypothesis (Beeman, 1998; Jung-Beeman, 2005), broader semantic fields of the RH may be better able to capture certain types of semantic relations, those that depend on the overlap of distantly related meanings.

Furthermore, such a semantic system may be highly advantageous for cognitive and linguistic processing. Dascal (2002), in his review of language as a cognitive tool, argues that the rule-based linguistic system is constrained and limited in its ability to express the more subtle aspects of communication, i.e., the spirit and the mind and not only the thought. It is for such purposes that the rule-based linguistic system must be complemented by a different system that can compensate for the former system's "mechanical" limitations. Furthermore, Dascal suggests that a particularly significant feature of the linguistic system is that it sometimes achieves its aims by resorting to explicit violations of the system's rules, such as in metaphor, puns, and nonsense poetry. From a cognitive point of view, a rule-based system that uses different kinds of rules and, in addition, permits and even exploits the violation of its own rules is extremely valuable. Such a system does not always treat rule violations as mistakes and thus may support many important cognitive processes that are open-ended, flexible, and creative. Dascal suggests that a successful metaphor created in order to understand a new concept (i.e., a novel metaphor) is an example of a linguistic stimulus that may involve rule violation and nevertheless become a resource for the cognitive system by becoming incorporated into the semantic system.

According to Dascal, the possibility of precision afforded by the rule-based aspects of natural languages should not make us overlook the wide variety of linguistic means for expressing indeterminacy, including indefiniteness, ambiguity, polysemy, unspecificity, imprecision, and vagueness. Although these linguistic aspects of language can be considered a hindrance from the point of view of certain cognitive needs, they are an asset from the point of view of other cognitive needs. The latter may include, for example, the need to consider initial vague intuitions during insight problem solving or to conceptualize ambiguous situations. The findings of previous research showing RH involvement in metaphor processing, insight problem solving and the comprehension of lexical ambiguity (e.g., Anaki et al., 1998; Beeman, 1998; Jung-Beeman, 2005; Faust & Kahana, 2002; Faust & Lavidor, 2003) are consistent with this notion of a neural system that complements the rule-based, precise aspects of language.

In a recent work, Pinker (2007) implicitly also differentiates between two kinds of language. One kind of language serves as a tool with a well-defined and limited functionality. Such language has a finite stock of arbitrary signs and grammatical rules that arrange signs in sentences. On one hand, this kind of language provides a means of sharing an unlimited number of combinations of ideas about who did what to whom, and about what is where. On the other hand, because it digitizes the world, this kind of language is a "lossy" medium, discarding information about the smooth multidimensional texture of experience. A second kind of language provides us with access to metaphoric expression and thus allows us to convey the subtlety and richness of sensations like smells and sounds and to express the ineffable aspects of human experience.

This chapter has attempted to make explicit the distinction between the two kinds of language discussed by Pinker implicitly. It has also provided this distinction with a neurolinguistic framework that associates one kind of language with the LH and the other with the RH. In this sense, the RH affords us with the capability of expressing aspects of experience such as "flashes of holistic insight (like those in mathematical and musical creativity), waves of consuming emotions, and moments of wishful contemplation [that] are simply not the kinds of experience that can be captured by the beads-on-a-string we call sentences" (Pinker, 2007, p. 276–267).

Vagueness, ambiguity, and unpredictability are characteristics of the experiences to which Pinker refers. These characteristics are also all central aspects of creative thinking. Creativity is typically defined as the generation or production of ideas that are both novel and useful (e.g. Amabile, 1996; Dietrich, 2004). Because novel metaphoric combinations do not adhere to semantic rules, the outcome of the process by which they are comprehended is relatively unpredictable. Thus, creativity, by nature, is unpredictable. To cope with such creative aspects of language, a neural system that is tolerant of semantic rule violations is advantageous. Furthermore, according to some previous research (Faust & Kravetz, 1997; Schmidt et al., 2007), novel metaphors may be just one example of a more general ability of the RH to process low constraint, less predictable, linguistic expressions. Novel metaphors taken from poetry are probably just a highly ecologically valid example of low constraining linguistic stimuli.

The coarse semantic coding of the RH (Beeman, 1998), reflecting the activation and maintenance of a wide range of meanings and associations, may support linguistic creativity. Thus, when describing creativity, Amabile, Barsade, Mueller, and Staw (2005) and Simonton (1999) note that the larger the number of relevant elements that are activated during processing the higher is the likelihood that unusual associations or solutions will be generated, and the larger is the pool of novel ideas from which to choose. RH coarse semantic coding may thus contribute to RH dominance in tasks that require verbal creativity. Recent reviews on creative thinking support this claim by emphasizing the retrieval of remote associations during creative problem solving (Helie & Sun, 2010) as well as showing higher RH activation for tasks that involve verbal creativity (Mihov et al., 2010).

Furthermore, RH ability to differentiate between relevant and nonrelevant elements has also been shown in previous research. The findings that RH involvement in the processing of unfamiliar linguistic stimuli is highly selective and does not extend to unrelated, meaningless combinations (e.g., Faust & Mashal, 2007; Mashal & Faust, 2005, 2008) suggest that RH semantic processing is not only novel, but also useful, efficiently differentiating between potentially meaningful expressions taken from poetry and useless, unrelated meanings. Genuine creativity requires some emphasis on constraints in order to meet the usefulness/appropriateness criteria (e.g., Wind & Mahajan, 1997) and thus RH language mechanisms seem to fulfill both basic criteria for creativity, novelty and usefulness.

An important aspect of creativity is that, despite or maybe because of its open-endedness, it does entail much hard work and sustained effort over time (e.g. Amabile, 1996). In this respect, the non rule-based semantic system of the RH requires no less resources than does the rule-based, expert semantic system of the LH. Returning to *Through the Looking Glass*, this hard work is acknowledged by Humpty Dumpty. Following his extremely flexible, unusual use of word meanings and in response to Alice's complaint "that's a great deal to make one word mean," he responds that "when I make a word do a lot of work like that . . . I always pay it extra" (p. 82). This extra pay may refer to the integration of left and right hemisphere semantic processes, which allows us access to the rich resources provided by our linguistic capacity.

Note

The research described in this chapter was partially supported by grant # 2003317 from the US-Israel Binational Science Foundation (BSF) and grant # 724/09 from the Israel Science Foundation (ISF).

References

Ahrens, K., Liu, H. L., Lee, C. Y., Gong, S. P., Fang, S.Y., & Hsu, Y. Y. (2007). Functional MRI of conventional and anomalous metaphors in Mandarin Chinese. *Brain and Language, 100*, 163–171.

Amabile, T. M. (1996). *Creativity in context*. Boulder, GO: Westview Press.

Amabile, T. M., Barsade, S. G., Mueller, J. S., & Staw, B. M. (2005). Affect and creativity at work. *Administrative Science Quarterly, 50*, 367–403.

Amanzio, M., Geminiani, G., Leotta, D., & Cappa, S. (2007). Metaphor comprehension in Alzheimer's disease: Novelty matters. *Brain and Language, 107*, 1–10.

Anaki, D., Faust, M., & Kravetz, S. (1998). Cerebral hemispheric asymmetry in processing lexical metaphors. *Neuropsychologia, 36*, 353–362.

Arzouan, Y., Goldstein, A., & Faust, M. (2007a). Dynamics of hemispheric activity during metaphor comprehension: Electrophysiological measures. *Neuroimage, 38*, 222–231.

Arzouan, Y., Goldstein, A., & Faust, M. (2007b). Brainwaves are stethoscopes: ERP correlates of novel metaphor comprehension. *Brain Research, 1160*, 69–81.

Baron-Cohen, S. (2003). *The essential difference: Men, women and the extreme male brain*. London: Penguin.

Beck, B. (1987). Metaphor, cognition and artificial Intelligence. In R. S. Haskell (Ed.), *Cognition and symbolic structure: The psychology of metaphoric transformation.* (pp. 9–30). Norwood, NJ: Ablex.

Beeman, M. (1993). Semantic processing in the right hemisphere may contribute to drawing inferences from discourse. *Brain and Language, 44*, 80–120.

Beeman, M. (1998). Coarse semantic coding and discourse comprehension. In M. Beeman & C. Chiarello (Eds.), *Right hemisphere language comprehension: Perspectives from cognitive neuroscience* (pp. 255–284). Mahwah, NJ: Erlbaum.

Benari, M. (2005). "Chaos stones," "scum kiss" and "toys grief": Constructing meaning from metaphoric noun–noun combinations. *Criticism and Interpretation: Journal for Interdisciplinary Studies in Literature and Culture, 38*, 7–40. (In Hebrew.)

Billow, R. M. (1975). A cognitive developmental study of metaphor comprehension. *Developmental Psychology, 11*, 415–423.

Bonnaud V., Gil, R., & Ingrand, P. (2002). Metaphorical and non-metaphorical links: A behavioral and ERP study in young and elderly adults. *Clinical Neurophysiology, 32*, 258–268.

Bottini, G., Corcoran, R., Sterzi, R., Paulesu, E. S. P, Scarpa, P., Frackoviak, R. S. J, et al. (1994). The role of the right hemisphere in the interpretation of the figurative aspects of language: A positron emission tomography activation study. *Brain, 117*, 1241–1253.

Bowden, E. M., & Jung-Beeman, M. (2003). Aha! Insight experience correlates with solution activation in the right hemisphere. *Psychonomic Bulletin and Review, 10*, 730–737.

Bowdle, B. F., & Gentner, D. (2005). The career of metaphor. *Psychological Review, 112,* 193–216.

Brownell, H. H., Simpson, T. L., Bihrle, A. M., Potter, H. H., & Gardner, H. (1990). Appreciation of metaphoric alternative word meanings by left and right brain damaged patients. *Neuropsychologia, 28,* 375–383.

Burgess, C., and Chiarello, C. (1996). Neurocognitive mechanisms underlying metaphor comprehension and other figurative language. *Metaphor and Symbolic Activity, 11,* 67–84.

Cacciary, C., & Glucksberg, S. (1994). Understanding figurative language. In M. A. Gernsbacher (Ed.), *Handbook of Psycholinguistics* (pp. 447–477). New York: Academic Press.

Carroll, L. (1871). *Through the looking glass and what Alice found there.* Ware, Hertfordshire, UK: Wordsworth Editions Limited. (1993 edition.)

Chiarello, C. (1998). On codes of meaning and the meaning of codes: Semantic access and retrieval within and between hemispheres. In M. J. Beeman & C. Chiarello (Eds.), *Right hemisphere language comprehension: Perspectives from cognitive neuroscience* (pp. 141–160). Mahwah, NJ: Erlbaum.

Chiarello, C. (2003). Parallel systems for processing language: Hemispheric complemetarity in the normal brain. In: M. T. Banich & M. Mack (Eds.), *Mind, Brain and Language* (pp. 229–247). Mahwah, NJ: Erlbaum.

Coulson, S., & van Petten, C. (2002). Conceptual integration and metaphor: An event-related potential study. *Memory and Cognition, 30,* 958–968.

Craig, J., & Baron-Cohen, S..(1999) Creativity and imagination in autism and Asperger syndrome. *Journal of Autism and Developmental Disorders, 29*(4), 319–326.

Dascal, M. (2002). Language as a cognitive technology. *International Journal of Cognition and Technology, 1*(1), 35–61.

Dietrich, A. (2004). The cognitive neuroscience of creativity. *Psychonomic Bulletin and Review, 11,* 1011–1026.

Dijksterhuis, A., & Meurs, T. (2006). Where creativity resides: The generative power of unconscious thought. *Consciousness and Cognition, 15,* 135–146.

Ellis, H. D., Ellis, D. M., Fraser, W., & Deb, S. (1994). A preliminary study of right hemisphere cognitive deficit and impaired social judgments among young people with Asperger syndrome. *European Child and Adolescent Psychiatry, 3,* 255–266.

Faust, M. (1998). Obtaining evidence of language comprehension from sentence priming. In M. Beeman & C. Chiarello (Eds.), *Right hemisphere language comprehension: Perspectives from cognitive neuroscience* (pp. 161–185). Hillsdale, NJ: Erlbaum.

Faust, M., Barak, O., & Chiarello, C. (2006). The effects of multiple script priming on word recognition by the two cerebral hemispheres: Implications for discourse processing. *Brain and Language, 99,* 247–257.

Faust, M., Bar-Lev, A., & Chiarello, C. (2003). Sentence priming in the two cerebral hemispheres: Influences of lexical relatedness, word order and sentence anomaly. *Neuropsychologia, 41,* 480–492.

Faust, M., & Chiarello, C. (1998). Sentence context and lexical ambiguity resolution by the two hemispheres. *Neuropsychologia, 3,* 827–836.

Faust, M., & Kahana, A. (2002). Priming summation in the cerebral hemispheres: Evidence from semantically convergent and semantically divergent primes. *Neuropsychologia, 40,* 892–901.

Faust, M., & Kravetz, S. (1998). Different levels of sentence constraint and lexical decisions in the two cerebral hemispheres. *Brain and Language, 62,* 149–162.

Faust, M., & Lavidor, M. (2003). Convergent and divergent priming in the two cerebral hemispheres: Lexical decision and semantic judgment. *Cognitive Brain Research, 17,* 585–597.

Faust, M., & Mashal, N. (2007). The role of the right cerebral hemisphere in processing novel metaphoric expressions taken from poetry: A divided visual field study. *Neuropsychologia, 45,* 860–870.

Fiore, S. M., & Schooler, J. W. (1998). Right hemisphere contributions to creative problem solving: Converging evidence for divergent thinking. In M. J. Beeman & C. Chiarello (Eds.), *Right hemisphere language comprehension: Perspectives from cognitive neuro-science* (pp. 349–372). Mahwah, NJ: Erlbaum.

Friederici, A. D. (1995). The time course of syntactic activation during language processing: A model based on neuropsychological and neurophysiological data. *Brain and Language, 50,* 259–281.

Friston, K. J. (1998). Imaging neuroscience: Principals or maps? *Proceedings of the National Academy of Science, USA, 95*(3), 796 –802.

Gentner, D. (1983). Structure mapping: A Theoretical framework for analogy. *Cognitive Science, 7,* 155–170.

Gentner, D., & Bowdle, B. F. (2001). Convention, form and figurative language processing. *Metaphor and Symbol, 16,* 23–247.

Gentner, D., & Wolff, P. (1997). Alignment in the processing of metaphor. *Journal of Memory and Language, 31,* 331–355.

Gibbs, R. W. (1994). Figurative thought and figurative language. In M. A. Gernsbacher (Ed.), *Handbook of psycholinguistics* (pp. 411–446). New York: Academic Press.

Giora, R. (1997). Understanding figurative and literal language: The graded salience hypothesis. *Cognitive Linguistics, 7,* 183–206.

Giora, R. (2002). Literal vs. figurative language: Different or equal? *Journal of Pragmatics, 34,* 487–506.

Giora, R. (2003). *On our mind: Salience, context and figurative language.* New York: Oxford University Press.

Glucksberg, S. (2001). *Understanding figurative language: From metaphors to idioms.* Oxford: Oxford University Press.

Glucksberg, S. (2003). The psycholinguistics of metaphor. *Trends in Cognitive Science, 7,* 92–96.

Gold, R., & Faust, M. (2010). Right hemisphere dysfunction and metaphor comprehension in young adults with Asperger syndrome. *Journal Of Autism And Developmental Disorders, 40,* 800–811.

Gold, R., Faust, M., & Ben-Artzi, E. (in press). Verbal creativity and the role of the right hemisphere in novel metaphor comprehension.

Gold, R., Goldstein, A., & Faust, M. (2010). Semantic integration during metaphor comprehension in Asperger syndrome. *Brain and Language, 113,* 124–134.

Goldstein, A., Arzouan, Y., & Faust, M. (2008). Timing the metaphoric brain: The contribution of ERP and source localization to understanding figurative language. In Z. Breznitz (Ed.), *Brain Research in Language* (pp. 205–224). New York: Springer.

Goldstein, A., Arzouan, Y., & Faust, M. (in preparation). Conventionalizing novel metaphors: Electrophysiological correlates.

Grice, H. P. (1975). Logic and conversation. In P. Cole & J. L. Morgan (Eds.), *Syntax and semantics* (vol. 3, *Speech acts*, pp. 41–58). New York: Academic Press.

Helie, S., & Sun, R. (2010). Incubation, insight and creative problem solving: A unified theory and a connectionist model. *Psychological Review, 117*(3), 994–1024.

Iakimova, G., Passerieux, C., Laurent, J. P., & Hardy-Bayle, M. C. (2005). ERPs of metaphoric, literal, and incongruous semantic processing in schizophrenia. *Psychophysiology, 42,* 380–90.

Jung-Beeman, M. (2005). Bilateral brain processes for comprehending natural language. *Trends in Cognitive Neuroscience, 9*(11), 512–518.

Jung-Beeman, M. J., Bowden, E. M., Haberman, J., Frymiare, J. L., Arambel-Liu, S., Greenblatt, R., et al. (2004). Neural activity when people solve verbal problems with insight. *PLoS Biology, 2,* 500–510.

Kaan, E., Harris, A., Gibson, E., & Holcomb, P. J. (2000). The P600 as an index of syntactic integration difficulty. *Language and Cognitive Processes,15,* 159–201.

Kutas, M., & Federmeier, K. D. (2000). Electrophysiology reveals semantic memory use in language comprehension. *Trends in Cognitive Sciences, 4*(12), 463–470.

Lakoff, G., & Johnson, M. (1980). *Metaphors we live by.* Chicago: University of Chicago Press.

Lombardo, M. V., Barnes, J. L., Wheelwright, S. J., & Baron-Cohen, S. (2007). Self referential cognition and empathy in autism. *PLoS-one, 2*(9), e883.

MacKay, G., & Shaw, A. (2004). A comparative study of figurative language in children with autistic spectrum disorders. *Child Language Teaching and Therapy, 20*(1), 13–32.

Mashal, N., & Faust, M. (2008). Right hemisphere sensitivity to novel metaphoric relations: Application of the signal detection theory. *Brain and Language, 104,* 103–112.

Mashal, N., & Faust, M. (2009). Conventionalization of novel metaphors: A shift in hemispheric asymmetry. *Laterality, 27,* 1–17.

Mashal, N., Faust, M., & Hendler, T. (2005). The role of the right hemisphere in processing nonsalient metaphorical meanings: Application of principal components analysis to fMRI data. *Neuropsychologia, 43*(14), 2084–2100.

Mashal, N., Faust, M., Hendler, T., & Jung-Beeman, M. (2007). An fMRI investigation of the neural correlates underlying the processing of novel metaphoric expressions. *Brain and Language, 100,* 111–122.

Mednick, S. A. (1962). The associative basis of the creative process. *Psychological Review, 69,* 220–232.

Mihov, K. M., Denzler, M., & Förster, J. (2010). Hemispheric specialization and creative thinking: A meta-analytic review of lateralization of creativity. *Brain and Cognition, 72*(3), 442–448.

Nichols, T. E., & Holmes A. P. (2002). Nonparametric permutation tests for functional neuroimaging: A primer with examples. *Human Brain Mapping, 15,* 1–25.

Paller, K. A., & Kutas, M. (1992). Brain potentials during memory retrieval provide neurophysiological support for the distinction between conscious recollection and priming. *Journal of Cognitive Neuroscience, 4,* 375–391.

Pinker, S. (2007). *The stuff of thought.* London: Penguin

Pobric, G., Mashal, N., Faust, M., & Lavidor, M. (2008). The role of the right cerebral hemisphere in processing novel metaphoric expressions: A TMS study. *Journal of Cognitive Neuroscience, 20,* 170–181.

Pynte, J., Besson, M., Robishon, F. H., & Poli, J. (1996). The time course of metaphor comprehension: An event-related potential study. *Brain and Language, 55,* 293–316.

Rapp, A. M., Leube, D. T., Erb, M., Grodd, W., & Kircher, T. T. J. (2004). Neural correlates of metaphor processing. *Cognitive Brain research, 20*, 395–402.

Richards, I. A. (1936). *The philosophy of rhetoric*. London: Oxford University Press.

Rinaldi, M. C., Marangolo, P., & Baldassari, F. (2004). Metaphor comprehension in right brain-damaged patients with visuo-verbal and verbal material: A dissociation (re)considered. *Cortex, 40*, 479–490.

Rugg, M. D., Cox, C. J. C., Doyle, M. C., & Wells, T. (1995). Event-related potentials and the recollection of low and high frequency words. *Neuropsychologia, 33*, 471–484.

Schmidt, G. L., DeBuse, C. J., & Seger, C. A. (2007). Right hemisphere metaphor processing characterizing the lateralization of semantic processes. *Brain and Language, 100*, 127–141.

Seyal, M., Ro, T., & Rafal, R. (1995). Increased sensitivity to ipsilateral cutaneous stimuli following transcranial magnetic stimulation of the parietal lobe. *Annals of Neurology, 38*(2), 264–267.

Simonton, R. (1999). *Origins of genius: Darwinian perspectives on creativity*. New York: Oxford University Press.

Yaguello, M. (1981). *Language through the looking glass: Exploring language and linguistics*. New York: Oxford University Press.

Zeev-Wolf, M., & Faust, M. (in preparation). Hemispheric differences in processing conventional and novel metaphors: A divided visual field study with short and long SOAs.

Zeev-Wolf, M., Goldstein, A., & Faust, M. (2010). Novel metaphor comprehension: Evidence from MEG recordings. Poster presented at the Annual Psychology Scientific Conference, Bar-Ilan University, Israel.

Part V
The Multilingual Brain

22

Word Recognition in the Bilingual Brain

Ton Dijkstra and Walter J. B. van Heuven

Introduction

In the past decades, many behavioral studies have investigated how bilingual readers, listeners, and speakers are able to process and manage two languages more or less at the same time. With respect to word recognition, these behavioral studies have involved both offline and online techniques, using as stimulus materials not just words that exist in only one language, but also "special" words like cognates (translation equivalents with form overlap between the languages involved) and false friends (words that share their form but not their meaning across languages).

The collected body of empirical evidence has given rise to a series of functional models of bilingual word recognition, like the bilingual interactive activation (BIA) and BIA+ models (Dijkstra & van Heuven, 1998, 2002), the inhibitory control (IC) model (Green, 1998), the revised hierarchical model (RHM; Kroll & Stewart, 1994; see also Kroll, Guo, & Misra, Volume 1, Chapter 24), and the language mode framework (Grosjean, 1997). The models agree about some aspects of the nature of the bilingual lexical processing system, but they argue about others. For a full review of these models, see Dijkstra (2005), Thomas & van Heuven (2005), de Groot (Volume 1, Chapter 23), and Kroll et al. (Volume 1, Chapter 24). Both verbal and computer models have been developed to account for empirical effects in terms of basically two dependent variables: reaction time (RT) and accuracy (percent correct).

All models have focused on functional questions of an abstract nature, disregarding how and where the assumed functions are represented in the brain. Thus, it remains to be seen to what extent the available models are compatible with the electrophysiological (event-related brain potential, or ERP) studies and the

The Handbook of the Neuropsychology of Language, First Edition. Edited by Miriam Faust.
© 2012 Blackwell Publishing Ltd. Published 2012 by Blackwell Publishing Ltd.

neuroimaging (functional Magnetic Resonance Imaging, or fMRI) studies that have been reported in recent years.

In this chapter, we investigate to what extent brain-oriented studies on bilingual processing support or reject behaviorally based assumptions about the lexical processing system and the associated executive control (task/decision) system. Neuroimaging studies may shed a new light on psychological theories and models (Henson, 2005), because they bring in new measurement techniques and dependent variables. For instance, behavioral studies have applied tasks like lexical decision, naming, masked priming, and translation recognition; whereas fMRI studies have frequently used covert verb or sentence generation, passive listening, and word repetition. Therefore, a large amount of neuroimaging and electrophysiological data cannot be directly compared to behavioral data, but they are still informative with respect to the assumptions, architecture, and processing characteristics of psycholinguistic models. In fact, *just because* they have not been considered much by psycholinguists, and approach language processing issues from a different angle, they might even be more informative than data obtained by "conventional" techniques (van Heuven & Dijkstra, 2010).

Apart from providing additional and potentially different answers to old questions, neuroimaging studies also help to raise questions of a new nature. Such questions are concerned with the exact mapping of representations and processes proposed in functional models to particular areas and processes in the brain (for a discussion see van Heuven & Dijkstra, 2010). As such, neuroimaging and electrophysiological studies help to provide a physical and biological basis to functional components in psycholinguistic models of (bilingual) language processing.

The present chapter is organized in two parts. In the first part, we discuss to what extent neurostudies are in line with issues that behavioral studies and models agree about. Four issues will be considered here:

1 The bilingual lexicon is integrated across languages.
2 The bilingual lexicon is accessed in a language-independent way.
3 Language exposure affects the activation of words.
4 Bilingual word recognition is governed by an executive control system.

In the second part of the chapter, we consider what neurostudies can tell about issues that behavioral studies and models quarrel about. The following issues, all having to do with context effects on bilingual word processing, will be considered:

5 Sentence context can(not) affect bilingual lexical activation.
6 Global language context can(not) affect bilingual lexical activation.
7 Task demands can(not) affect bilingual lexical activation.

For each issue, we will briefly mention the theoretical position of functional models based on behavioral evidence. This will be followed by a consideration of available neuroscientific evidence on the issue. At the end of each section, we summarize the conclusions arising from neuroscientific evidence.

Neurolinguistic Evidence and Conclusions Shared by Behavioral Studies

The bilingual lexicon is integrated across languages

After several decades of behavioral research, most researchers more or less tacitly agree that the lexicon of bilinguals constitutes one integrated store and that (for languages sharing their script) word recognition involves parallel access to the languages in question (Dijkstra, 2005). Both conclusions appear to hold for orthographic and phonological representations (Dijkstra, 2005), as well as semantic representations (Francis, 1999, 2005).

The assumption of a bilingual lexicon that is integrated across languages lies at the basis of the BIA+, BIA, and IC models for bilingual word recognition. However, there are still models that, implicitly or explicitly, appear to subscribe to the position of separate lexicons in the bilingual. Two examples are the revised hierarchical model, formulated by Kroll and Stewart (1994, p. 150; but compare Talamas, Kroll, & Dufour, 1999) and the SOMBIP model from Li and Farkas (2002), which includes orthographic and semantic maps that separate languages like Chinese and English. In addition, some models assume that lexical access in bilinguals can be more or less language-specific depending on context aspects (as in Grosjean's, 1997, language mode framework). Of course, the overlap in orthographic, phonetic/phonological, and conceptual features between languages sets limits to the degree of language nonselectivity possible (e.g., lexical access to Chinese and English will be language-specific, due to script differences; also see de Groot, 1992; Dong, Gui, & MacWhinney, 2005; van Hell & de Groot, 1998).

The assumption of an integrated lexicon implies that lexical representations belonging to different languages affect each other in the same way as representations within a language. In terms of a spatial metaphor, representations are stored closer together the more similar they are, irrespective of the language to which they belong. The same holds, for instance, for orthographic versus phonological representations within a language; they are stored in separate pools. If the spatial metaphor is true in the brain, a first language and a second language (L1 and L2) should be localized in the same regions. Any deviation from a common storage place suggested by empirical data should be attributable to nonrepresentational differences between L1 and L2, e.g., how they require additional executive control demands in particular task situations.

Many neuroimaging studies have investigated whether or not L1 and L2 processing activate the same regions in the bilingual brain (for a complete review see van Heuven & Dijkstra, 2010). Some studies concluded that brain regions activated by two or more languages were overlapping (e.g., Frenck-Mestre, Anton, Roth, Vaid, &

Viallet, 2005; Hasegawa, Carpenter, & Just, 2002; Hernandez, Dapretto, Mazziotta, & Bookheimer, 2001; Illes et al., 1999), whereas others reported that the languages of the bilinguals activate partially different brain regions (e.g., Chee, Soon, & Lee, 2003; Kim, Relkin, Lee, & Hirsch, 1997; Perani et al., 1996; Tham et al., 2005). For example, Kim et al. (1997) applied a covert sentence-generation task in L1 and L2 with early and late bilinguals and found that the center of activation in the left inferior frontal gyrus (BA 44) was overlapping for early bilinguals, but separate for late bilinguals. In contrast, for both early and late bilinguals, L1 and L2 centers of activation were overlapping in the superior temporal gyrus (BA 22). However, as Abutalebi, Cappa, and Perani (2005) pointed out, the bilingual group in this study was heterogeneous and its language proficiency was not assessed. These aspects limit the interpretability of this study. Furthermore, Marian, Spivey, and Hirsch (2003) have argued that there may be shared L1–L2 brain regions for early stages and separate L1–L2 brain regions at later stages of processing.

Indefrey (2006) concluded on the basis of a meta-analysis of 24 fMRI papers with bilinguals that processing of L1 and L2 takes place in similar brain regions. However, for some bilinguals and in certain tasks reliable differences between L1 and L2 in brain areas were observed. Indefrey argued that factors such as language proficiency, age of L2 acquisition (AoA), and language exposure determine whether brain region differences between L1 and L2 are found.

A possible conclusion is that the neuroscientific evidence supports the assumption of an integrated lexicon, if at the same time differences between and among monolinguals and bilinguals are assumed in terms of processing and cognitive control. We will evaluate this conclusion in the following sections.

The bilingual lexicon is accessed in a language-independent way

Behavioral studies have concluded that the presentation of a letter string to a bilingual initially activates orthographically similar words in both languages. This theoretical view, shared (tacitly sometimes) by all available models, has been referred to as "language-nonspecific access" to the bilingual lexicon. For instance, presenting the English word BLUE to a Dutch–English bilingual will activate not only other English words like CLUE and GLUE, but also Dutch words like BLUT and BLUS. These words, which have the same length as the target word but differ in one letter position, are called (within- and between-language) orthographic neighbors (Coltheart, Davelaar, Jonasson, & Besner, 1977). A behavioral study with Dutch–English bilinguals (van Heuven, Dijkstra, & Grainger, 1998) showed that the number of target and nontarget language neighbors influenced target-word processing in L1 and L2, which can only be explained if word candidates of both languages are activated in parallel.

The number of neighbors (neighborhood density) has also been found to influence the N400 ERP component (negative waveform 300–500 ms after word onset that peaks around 400 ms) in English monolinguals (Holcomb, Grainger, &

O'Rourke, 2002). Words with a large number of neighbors generate a larger N400 effect than words with a small number of neighbors. Midgley, Holcomb, van Heuven, and Grainger (2008) investigated the influence of cross-language neighbors on the N400 in an ERP study with French–English bilinguals. In lists that consisted of only French or English words the number of neighbors (many vs. few) in the other language was manipulated. L2 and L1 words with many cross-language neighbors generated a greater N400 effect than words with few cross-language neighbors. Thus, electrophysiological data provide additional evidence of parallel access to words in different languages.

The nonselective access assumption is further supported by data from Thierry and Wu (2007), who found unconscious translation effects in second language reading. In this study, Chinese–English bilinguals performed a semantic relatedness task with pairs of English words. Some English word pairs (POST – MAILBOX) consisted of English words with repeated Chinese characters when translated from English to Chinese (POST is translated as "you jü" and MAILBOX as "you xiang"), while other English pairs (BATH – SHOWER) translated to Chinese words consisting of completely different Chinese characters (BATH is translated as "xi zao" and SHOWER as "ling yu"). Participants were not aware of the repeated Chinese character manipulation and performed the task in a purely English context. A larger N400 was found for English word pairs with repeated Chinese characters. These results can only be explained by assuming that English words automatically activate their Chinese translations.

Additional neuroimaging evidence in support of language nonselective access comes from studies on interlingual homograph recognition in bilinguals. Interlingual homographs are words that are spelled identically in two languages while their meaning in the two languages is completely different. For example, the English word RAMP is also a correct Dutch word; however, the Dutch meaning of this Dutch–English interlingual homograph is "disaster." Behavioral studies often report slower RTs to such homographs, indicating that the two readings of an interlingual homograph are automatically activated in parallel (e.g., Dijkstra, van Jaarsveld, & ten Brinke, 1998) and interfere at some stage(s) of processing, e.g., during stimulus identification and/or response selection.

Van Heuven, Schriefers, Dijkstra, and Hagoort (2008) investigated the source of interlingual homograph conflicts in two fMRI experiments with Dutch–English bilinguals. They examined the brain responses to Dutch–English interlingual homographs in an English lexical decision task ("Respond yes only if this is an English word") and in a generalized Dutch–English lexical decision task ("Respond yes to any word"). In both tasks, the co-activation of homographs should lead to stimulus competition; however, response competition should only arise in English lexical decision (because only there Dutch words must be responded to with a "no"). Indeed, the imaging data showed that only in the English lexical decision task a response conflict appeared in the pre-supplementary motor area/ dorsal anterior cingulate cortex. In contrast, in both tasks stimulus conflicts appeared in the left prefrontal cortex due to the activation of the two readings of a homograph.

Interestingly, the behavioral results showed significantly slower responses to inter-lingual homographs than to English control words in English lexical decision, but not in generalized lexical decision. The overall results indicate that both readings of the homograph are automatically activated, which leads to conflicts at the stimu-lus level and, depending on the task demands, at the response level as well.

An ERP-study by Kerkhofs, Dijkstra, Chwilla, and de Bruijn (2006; cf. de Bruijn, Dijkstra, Chwilla, & Schriefers, 2001) also supports the nonselective access hypoth-esis of BIA+. In this study, Dutch–English interlingual homographs were preceded by semantically related or unrelated English words (e.g., HEAVEN – ANGEL or BUSH – ANGEL). Furthermore, the word frequency of the English and Dutch reading of the homographs was manipulated. The RTs to interlingual homographs were affected by both English and Dutch frequencies of the interlingual homo-graphs, as in Dijkstra et al. (1998). Remarkably, the N400 amplitude was also influ-enced by the English and Dutch frequencies of the homographs. The N400 for interlingual homographs with a high Dutch frequency was more negative than for interlingual homographs with a low Dutch frequency, while the N400 for interlin-gual homographs with a low English frequency was more negative than for those with a high English frequency. The effect of target language (English) frequency on the N400 to target words has been observed before (Moreno & Kutas, 2005). The reverse effect of Dutch frequency on the N400 of interlingual homographs could be due to the semantic interference by the Dutch reading that hinders the semantic integration reflected by the N400.

In sum, neuroscientific studies appear to support the language nonselective access assumption for bilingual processing. At the same time, ERP- and fMRI-differences have been reported between L1 and L2, and between low- and high-proficiency bilinguals. Such differences, possibly related to relative language exposure, are dis-cussed in the next section.

Language exposure affects the activation of words

When words of a language are used more often in daily life, they become established more strongly in long-term memory. As a consequence, the relative L1–L2 profi-ciency of a bilingual, the age of acquisition at which a word was first encountered, and more general language exposure, are all considered to be important factors determining speed of activation, accuracy of recognition, and impact on the recog-nition of competitor words.

According to the RHM, bilinguals with a weaker L2 have stronger lexical (associa-tive) links from L2 to L1 than from L1 to L2, and stronger links between L1 lexical representations and conceptual representations than between L2 lexical representa-tions and conceptual representations. Based on these assumptions, the RHM pre-dicts that in beginning L2 learners only word translation from L1 to L2 will be conceptually mediated; word translation from L2 to L1 follows the lexical route before tapping into the conceptual level (L2 → L1 → C; e.g., Kroll & Tokowicz,

2005). However, in recent years, several studies have found conceptual mediation effects even in beginning L2 learners (e.g., Altarriba & Mathis, 1997; Comesaña, Perea, Piñeiro, & Fraga, 2009; de Groot & Poot, 1997; Ferré, Sanchez-Casas, & Guasch, 2006; Frenck-Mestre & Prince, 1997).

These findings are in line with BIA+, which assumes that even in beginning L2 learners word candidates from different languages and their meanings are activated in parallel. Asymmetric effects between L1 and L2 are not explained in BIA and BIA+ by strength differences in L1 → L2 and L2 → L1 word form links, but by differences in speed of lexical activation. Due to differences in frequency of usage or L2 proficiency, the activation of L2 words might be slowed relative to L1 words. This assumption has been referred to as the temporal delay assumption (Dijkstra & van Heuven, 2002) and we will come back to it later in this section.

Neuroscientific studies confirm that L1–L2 proficiency affects the activation patterns of L2 relative to L1. Chee, Hon, Lee, and Soon (2001) found that the blood oxygen level dependent (BOLD) signal in an fMRI-study was affected by language proficiency when bilinguals made semantic judgments. The less proficient language of the bilinguals showed a larger BOLD signal change in the left prefrontal and parietal areas as well as additional activation in the right inferior frontal gyrus. More extensive and/or greater levels of brain activation for the less proficient language of bilinguals have been found in other studies as well (e.g., Briellmann et al., 2004; De Bleser et al., 2003; Hasegawa et al., 2002; Hernandez & Meschyan, 2006; Rüschemeyer, Fiebach, Kempe, & Friederici, 2005; Vingerhoets et al., 2003).

The investigation of the role of proficiency for brain regions activated by L1 and L2 in late bilinguals is complicated by the confound of this factor with L2 AoA. A few studies investigated the effects of L2 proficiency and AoA of L2 at the same time. Perani et al. (1998) compared late Italian–English bilinguals with low or high proficiency in English in a positron emission tomography (PET) study (Experiment 1). They also compared early high-proficiency Italian–English bilinguals with early high-proficiency Spanish–Catalan bilinguals (Experiment 2). Language proficiency differences affected the brain regions involved in listening to stories in L1 and L2. For high-proficiency bilinguals, the AoA of L2 did not alter the involved brain areas. Although these data seem to contradict earlier findings by Kim et al. (1997), Perani et al. (1998) pointed out that Kim et al. used a different task and proficiency may have been confounded with AoA. An issue with both studies is that groups of bilinguals with different L1 and L2s were compared (van Heuven & Dijkstra, 2010).

In a later study, Wartenburger et al. (2003) have found that L2 proficiency affected the brain regions involved in semantic decisions by Italian–German bilinguals, while the AoA of L2 influenced mainly the brain regions involved in grammatical judgments. In addition to language proficiency and AoA (further see Hernandez & Li, 2007), the related factor of the amount of daily language exposure or usage (active or passive) also affects the brain regions activated by L2 (Perani & Abutalebi, 2005; Vingerhoets et al., 2003).

As mentioned above, some models (like BIA and BIA+) assume that word candidates of a weaker language may be activated more slowly over time. It may be that on average frequently used words are activated more quickly than infrequently used words, irrespective of the language to which they belong. To the extent that a higher proficiency in a particular language implies a more frequent usage of words in that language, this may imply that L1 words are activated and recognized more quickly than L2 words. (Note that this assumption may not be correct for letter representations, which are shared between languages.) This view seems to imply a temporal delay in the activation of L2 relative to L1 lexical representations. There is some behavioral evidence to support this hypothesis (Dijkstra & van Heuven, 2002).

The delay of L2 relative to L1 has also been observed in terms of temporal patterns of ERP components (e.g., N400) in bilingual word recognition. For example, the N400 effect was delayed for a less proficient L2 (e.g., Ardal, Donald, Meuter, Muldrew, & Luce, 1990; Elston-Güttler & Friederici, 2005; Hahne, 2001; Kutas & Kluender, 1994; Moreno & Kutas, 2005; Weber-Fox & Neville, 1996). In a time-course analysis of brain activity during reading in English and Chinese, Liu and Perfetti (2003) also observed delayed processing of L2. For their Chinese–English bilinguals, processing of the graphic forms was earlier in L1 than L2, and in L1 processing moved quicker to the pronunciation stage and meaning analysis than in L2. In contrast, Kotz (2001) reported no shift in the N400 for L2. However, this study was conducted with early high-proficiency bilinguals.

A temporal delay in the activation of L2 representations in low-proficiency bilinguals might lead to the recruitment of prefrontal brain areas associated with controlled semantic, lexical, and/or phonological retrieval. Within the left prefrontal cortex, different regions have been associated with controlled retrieval of semantic and phonological information (Gold & Buckner, 2002; Poldrack et al., 1999). Stronger activation in these brain regions for low-proficiency bilinguals fits the neuroimaging data on language proficiency discussed above. Importantly, both low- and high-proficiency bilinguals activate representations of both languages in parallel, although there is a relatively delayed activation for the L2 in low-proficiency bilinguals.

In all, the reviewed evidence largely supports the theoretical view of an integrated lexicon that is nonselectively accessed. We note that the observed L1/L2 differences associated with language proficiency, age of L2 acquisition, and language exposure, are not necessarily in contradiction to this assumption. They might reflect differences in processing effort, such as effortful lexical retrieval (De Bleser et al., 2003), increased effort in linking motor codes with visual codes (Hernandez & Meschyan, 2006), increased articulatory demands (Klein, Zatorre, Milner, Meyer, & Evans, 1994), and/or additional executive control demands (e.g., selection difficulties and/or control of interference) in particular tasks (Crinion et al., 2006; Hernandez et al., 2001; Rodriguez-Fornells et al., 2005).

Bilingual word recognition is governed by an executive control system

Researchers in bilingualism have sometimes observed extensive but systematic differences across similar behavioral experiments. They have argued that the activation state of the underlying word identification system may be exploited differently depending on the experimental circumstances, e.g., the requirements of the task at hand (Dijkstra et al., 1998; Green, 1998). The distinction between an executive control system taking care of task demands and a word identification system is shared by several models of bilingual lexical retrieval, e.g., the IC model, BIA+, and BIA. Much less attention is paid to this distinction in some other theoretical frameworks (e.g., those of the RHM and language mode).

The two systems are considered as both functionally and structurally distinct. A spatial metaphor suggests that two different brain areas might be involved. Furthermore, most models assume that there is a hierarchical and temporally structured system in the sense that activation arises in the word identification system before it enters the task/decision system.

To a large extent, neuroanatomical and neurocognitive models of language processing appear to be compatible with these ideas (see Friederici, 2002; Hagoort, 2005; Indefrey & Levelt, 2004; Price, 2000). Studies have identified the prefrontal cortex (PFC) as the brain region involved in the control of cognition and behavior (Miller & Cohen, 2001). The PFC has been associated with language retrieval processes (Gold & Buckner, 2002; Poldrack et al., 1999; Wagner, Paré-Blagoev, Clark, & Poldrack, 2001), selection processes (Thompson-Schill, D'Esposito, Aguirre, & Farah, 1997; Zhang, Feng, Fox, Gao, & Tan, 2004), cognitive control processes such as conflict resolution, monitoring, and subgoaling/integration (Ridderinkhof, Ullsperger, Crone, & Nieuwenhuis, 2004), and working memory (e.g., Baddeley, 2003; Smith & Jonides, 1999). The exact locations of these functions within the prefrontal cortex are still debated. According to Gold and Buckner (2002), the anterior parts of the left inferior prefrontal cortex (LIPC; BA 45/47) and of the posterior LIPC (~BA 44) are involved in the controlled retrieval processes required for many semantic tasks, but are also involved in other nonsemantic tasks as well. They suggest that a posterior region of the left PFC near the precentral gyrus (~ BA 6) is associated with controlled phonology. In contrast, Thompson-Schill et al. (1997) argued that Broca's area in left inferior frontal cortex is involved in the selection of task-relevant information out of competing alternatives. The function of other areas in the prefrontal cortex, such as the dorsolateral prefrontal cortex and the anterior cingulate are also still under discussion (Botvinick, Braver, Barch, Carter, & Cohen, 2001; Ridderinkhof et al., 2004).

Aspects of the task/decision component of the language processing system appear to map onto the PFC, while retrieval processes associated with the PFC (e.g., of Broca's region) might be part of the word identification system. Executive processes play an important role when bilinguals process their less proficient language (Chee et al., 2001; Hernandez & Meschyan, 2006), and/or when bilinguals must resolve conflicts between their languages (Rodriguez-Fornells, De Diego Balaguer, & Münte, 2006; Rodriguez-Fornells, Rotte, Heinze, Nösselt, & Münte, 2002; Rodriguez-Fornells et al., 2005; van Heuven et al., 2008). Within the PFC, these studies observed an increased activity in the dorsolateral and/or middle/inferior PFC and in the anterior cingulate cortex. Language switching requires general executive processing, which activates the dorsolateral prefrontal cortex

(Hernandez et al., 2001). Translation between languages also requires control over language representations in relation with action, and the brain region that has been associated with action control during translation is that of the left basal ganglia (Price, Green, & von Studnitz, 1999). Other studies have found that the left middle prefrontal cortex is important for the control of interference between languages (Rodriguez-Fornells et al., 2005). Furthermore, fMRI studies with bilinguals suggest that subcortical structures such as the putamen and caudate may also be involved in executive control networks. For example, Crinion et al. (2006) concluded that the left caudate plays a role in monitoring and controlling the language in use.

In sum, specific brain regions involved in executive control are the dorsolateral prefrontal cortex, the anterior cingulate, and subcortical structures such as the caudate nucleus. Importantly, the neuroimaging data suggest that the task/decision system consists of multiple components (i.e., monitoring, control) that map onto different regions in the PFC. In fact, the task/decision system in a model such as BIA+ can be considered as part of a large control system, which includes the unification-control components of the memory, unification, and control (MUC) framework (Hagoort, 2005). Furthermore, the brain network model described by Abutalebi and Green (2007) can be considered as a "natural" development of the functional IC model proposed by Green (1998). To conclude, neuroimaging data support the behaviorally based distinction between a task/decision and a word identification system.

Neurolinguistic Evidence and Conclusions Debated by Behavioral Studies

A general issue about which behavioral studies and models disagree is how bilingual word recognition is affected by the context in which it occurs. The term "context" here can refer to many things: situational context, task, or instructions to the participant, but also the list of items, sentence, or discourse, in which the target word occurs. Note that contextual effects on bilingual word recognition operate differently for each of these. For instance, the effects of task demands are essentially nonlinguistic in nature, whereas sentence context effects entail (among others) lexical, syntactic, semantic, and language mechanisms. In the following sections, we consider the effects on bilingual word recognition exerted by (1) sentence context, (2) global language context, and (3) task demands and instructions.

Sentence context can(not) affect bilingual lexical activation

Can the semantic, syntactic, or language aspects of sentence context affect activation in the bilingual word identification system? According to interactive models like BIA, BIA+, the language framework, and (probably) the IC model, that is possible. Only a few behavioral studies with bilinguals have investigated these questions so far (e.g., Duyck, van Assche, Drieghe, & Hartsuiker, 2007; Kroll & Dussias, 2004; Schwartz & Kroll, 2006; van Hell & de Groot, 2008). A tentative conclusion is that sentence context may modulate the degree of language nonselectivity that is observed (e.g., cognate effects might be reduced in highly constraining contexts).

Dijkstra, van Hell, and Brenders (submitted) compared the RTs and brain waves of bilingual participants during the processing of sentences and target words in both L1 and L2. In their study, sentences were presented to the Dutch–English participants word by word. In the RT variant of the experiment, the participants decided if the last presented item was an English word or not (English lexical decision). In the EEG variant, the participants silently read the sentences (and a continuation) word by word. The mean RT for the target word did not differ much when the introductory sentence was English or Dutch. This suggests that the effect of a language switch as such on the RT to a subsequent target word is relatively small.

Nevertheless, a nonidentical cognate like "apple" was processed faster in the sentence context than a comparable control word existing in only one language. This cognate facilitation effect was larger in English sentence context than in Dutch context, and arose also in Dutch lexical decision with translated materials. This finding suggests that the Dutch sentence context exerts a stronger constraint than the English one.

The study also examined how the EEG responded to language switches (also see Moreno, Federmeier, & Kutas, 2002, and Proverbio, Leoni, & Zani, 2004). Again, depending on the sentence context, cognates showed different patterns than control words. After a predictive English sentence context, the English version of the cognate turned out to be easier to integrate than a control word (as reflected in the N400 effect). However, following a Dutch sentence context, the reverse happened: the English cognate was more difficult to integrate. In sum, both the RTs and ERPs in this study indicate that sentence context may modulate effects of word type (cognate status). Result differences for the two dependent variables indicate there is a difference between early identification processes and later decision mechanisms.

There are some puzzling differences between the available studies that suggest that the interaction between lexical and sentence processing components depends on experimental differences, such as presentation method, position of the target in the sentence (middle or end), and nature of the target word (identical cognate or not). Future neuroscientific studies are clearly needed to clarify the origin of semantic effects in bilingual sentence processing.

Global language context can(not) affect bilingual lexical activation

Global language context is interpreted here as the language of the ongoing discourse or even the daily-life language immersion of the bilingual reader or listener. In order to have an effect on bilingual word recognition, a far-reaching top-down effect must be assumed from this global context down on sentence and word processing. Such an effect is explicitly assumed by the language mode framework, but is rejected by the BIA+ framework, which considers bottom-up (signal based) processing factors as much more important.

The effect of global context on the word identification system was investigated by Elston-Güttler, Gunter, and Kotz (2005). In this study, German–English homographs were presented in a sentence context. For example, the sentence "Joan used scissors to remove the" was followed by the sentence final word TAG (a German–English interlingual homograph, which means DAY in English) or a control word (i.e., LABEL). This sentence final word was a prime that was followed by a target word (e.g., DAY). Participants were instructed to make lexical decisions to the target words. Global language context was manipulated in this experiment by showing the bilinguals two different versions of a 20-minute movie before the experiment, one spoken in English (L2) and the other spoken in German (L1). The ERP and behavioral data did not reveal any priming effect in the second half of the experiment. Thus, local sentence context prevented the activation of nontarget readings of the interlingual homograph (see previous section for a further discussion on the effect of local sentence context). In addition, the *global* language context also influenced the priming effect, reflected in a modulation of the N200 and N400 component and in the RTs, but only in the first part of the first block just after the German movie was shown. The results of global language context were explained by changes in task/decision settings of BIA+ and not by an influence of global language context on activity in the word identification system (also see de Bruijn et al., 2001; Lemhöfer, Dijkstra, & Michel, 2004).

Whether bilingual lexical access is influenced by global language context was further investigated by Paulmann, Elston-Güttler, Gunter, and Kotz (2006). A 20-minute film spoken in their native language (German) or in their second language (English) was shown to late bilinguals before the start of the experiment. The experimental task and stimulus materials were identical to those in Elston-Güttler, Gunter, and Kotz (2005), although the prime was not preceded by a sentence context. RTs revealed a significant priming effect for related primes, which in this study was not affected by the language of the film preceding the experiment. The ERP data showed a relatedness effect in the N400 time window. As in the behavioral data, the language of the preceding film did not affect the N400 priming effect. Thus, this experiment also supports the assumption of the BIA+ model that bilingual word recognition is fundamentally nonselective and that global language context does not directly influence the word identification system. It should be noted that according to BIA+ the recognition of repeated words will benefit from a change in their resting level activation, implying that global context effects might arise not exclusively from decision criteria adaptations when words from the context occur in the experiment itself.

Task demands can(not) affect bilingual lexical activation

As described above, the task/decision system has been assumed to operate on the activation of linguistic codes of different types in the word identification system. An unresolved issue is whether it is also possible for the task/decision system to change the activation of language representations in the word identification system. If this would be the case, conflicts between competing representations of both languages could be prevented by suppressing nontarget language representations when that is advantageous.

The BIA+ model assumes that task demands do not change activation in the word identification system. This distinguishes BIA+ from BIA and other models, like IC and RHM. In particular, the IC model assumes that task schemas can inhibit the activation of abstract lexical representations (lemmas). However, an important difference between the BIA+ model and the IC model is that the first is a model of language comprehension and the latter is mostly applied to language production. Language comprehension is fundamentally different from language production in many respects. For example, the directionality of the activation flow between word forms and meaning representations is completely opposite. Via their task/decision system, bilinguals might be able to affect the activation levels of nontarget language words in language production. Thus, as assumed by the IC model and RHM, selection of the correct target language word might be helped by inhibition (however, see La Heij, 2005, and Verhoef, Roelofs, & Chwilla, 2009, for an alternative view, and see Abutalebi & Green, 2007, and Abutalebi & Della Rosa, Volume 1, Chapter 25, for a further discussion of control in language production). Suppression of nontarget language word candidates does not seem as likely in language comprehension, given that the language origin of the input is unknown to the reader or listener. The behavioral data of language comprehension studies, discussed in Dijkstra and van Heuven (2002), so far appear to support BIA+'s assumption that top-down inhibition on lexical activation is absent in reading (Kerkhofs et al. 2006; Martin, Dering, Thomas, & Thierry, 2009; Rodriguez-Fornells et al., 2005; van Heuven et al., 2008).

Neuroimaging data that support the hypothesis that task demands cannot influence the activation of words in the word identification are provided by, for example, van Heuven et al. (2008) and Kerkhofs et al. (2006). In both studies, interlingual homographs were presented to Dutch–English (late) bilinguals in a purely English lexical decision task that did not require any Dutch items to be retrieved. The ERP data of Kerkhofs et al. (2006) showed that the word frequency of interlingual homograph in the target language (English) and the nontarget language (Dutch) influenced the N400 effect. The fMRI data of van Heuven et al. (2008) discussed above showed that conflicts in interlingual homograph processing might take place both at the response level and in the word identification system. Such conflicts would have been circumvented if bilinguals had been able to influence the nontarget language reading of the interlingual homographs. Van Heuven et al.'s (2008) data implied that bilinguals were not able to regulate activation in the word identification system, because conflicts between target and nontarget readings of interlingual homographs still led to brain activation differences between homographs and control words.

However, Rodriguez-Fornells et al. (2002) interpreted their ERP and fMRI data obtained in a go/no-go task in favor of a bilingual model in which bilinguals *can* suppress the activation of nontarget language representations in the word identification system. In their study, Catalan–Spanish bilinguals had to decide whether the first letter of a letter string was a consonant or vowel. Letters strings were Catalan, Spanish, or pseudowords. Importantly, participants were instructed to respond only when Spanish words were presented and to withhold responses to Catalan and pseudowords. The word frequency of both the Spanish and Catalan words was manipulated. Whereas the N400 component in response to Spanish words was modulated by word frequency, the N400 for Catalan words was not. In fact, the ERPs to pseudowords and Catalan words were almost identical, suggesting that Catalan words were not processed up till the semantic level. Using the same task with bilinguals did not reveal any brain activation differences in fMRI between Catalan words and pseudowords. Response differences between Spanish monolingual and Catalan–Spanish bilinguals were found in the left posterior inferior frontal region and the left planum temporale, which the authors associated with phonological processing. The authors proposed that bilinguals performed the go/no-go task by activating only Spanish grapheme–phoneme conversion rules and by inhibiting the direct access route to the lexicon so that Catalan words were not activated.

How can the differences in results of Rodriguez-Fornells et al. (2002) and most behavioral studies be explained? Possibly, their findings are due to the specifics of the go/no-go task that was used and their no-go responses may not have been sensitive enough to pick up nontarget language effects. Furthermore, the bilinguals who participated in this study were early balanced bilinguals. Most bilingual studies have been conducted with late unbalanced bilinguals. Early and late bilinguals might differ fundamentally in their language control abilities and this might explain the absence of nontarget language influence in the early bilinguals. However, the error data of the ERP study showed differences between low and high frequency nontarget Catalan words, which suggests that Catalan words may have been activated after all.

In a recent masked priming study using ERPs, Chauncey, Grainger, and Holcomb (2008) conducted two experiments, differing in prime duration (50 ms vs. 100 ms), in which French–English bilinguals read silently for meaning and responded by key presses to target words that were animal names. ERPs were recorded for critical (nonanimal) words in French and English that did not require any key-press responses but were preceded by unrelated words from the same or the other language. Switch cost was inferred from the difference in magnitude of a predetermined ERP component for a language switch trial versus a language nonswitch trial. Switch costs were already evident at very early intervals of the brainwaves and centered on the N250 component. In other words, Chauncey et al. reported an early automatic modulation of language-specific representations by language membership information. They conclude that these data are probably not affected by executive control or task demands (assumed to occur later in processing), but also argue that there is a top-down influence of language membership directly on lexical processing.

In contrast, ERP data of Martin et al. (2009) provide evidence that task demands have no control over the word identification system. Semantic priming effects in this study were obtained in both the task-relevant and the task-irrelevant language, even though participants were explicitly instructed to disregard the words in the irrelevant language.

In sum, neuroimaging data so far are not at odds with the assumption that a task/decision system cannot influence the activation of nontarget language representations in the language processing system during visual word recognition. This conclusion appears to be more in line with BIA+ than with the IC model, BIA, or RHM (note that this issue is not concerned with the existence of inhibition within the language processing system itself).

Conclusion

In the present chapter, we described a number of assumptions shared or discussed by researchers in bilingual word recognition, and we assessed to what extent the findings of neuroimaging and electrophysiological studies with bilinguals agree with these. Overall, the neuroscientific data support many of the architecture and processing assumptions shared by behavioral models. The distinction between the word identification system and task/decision system is supported by a large number of neuroimaging studies, and with respect to a number of issues that behavioral researchers disagree about, neuroimaging data provide additional evidence based on new dependent variables. Especially when no behavioral (RT or accuracy) differences appear between experimental conditions, differences observed in fMRI and ERP may help to interpret the results in terms of subcomponents that are temporally or spatially distinct (e.g., van Heuven et al., 2008). Neuroimaging and electrophysiological studies of the brain add, in our view, a completely new and revealing dimension to bilingual research (see also Abutalebi, Cappa, & Perani, 2005; van Heuven & Dijkstra, 2010). Most importantly, such studies stress that it is the material organ of the *brain* that represents and processes multiple languages. Given the arrival of dedicated, sophisticated, and precise measurement techniques, the biological and physical sides of bilingualism can no longer be ignored by behavioral scientists.

References

Abutalebi, J., Cappa, S. F., & Perani, D. (2005). What can functional neuroimaging tell us about the bilingual brain? In J. F. Kroll & A. M. B. de Groot (Eds.), *Handbook of bilingualism: Psycholinguistic approaches* (pp. 497–515). Oxford: Oxford University Press.

Abutalebi, J., & Green, D. (2007). Bilingual language production: The neurocognition of language representation and control. *Journal of Neurolinguistics, 20*, 242–275.

Altaribba, J., & Mathis, K. (1997). Conceptual and lexical development in second language acquisition. *Journal of Memory and Language, 36*, 550–568.

Ardal, S., Donald, M. W., Meuter, R., Muldrew, S., & Luce, M. (1990). Brain responses to semantic incongruity in bilinguals. *Brain and Language, 39*, 187–205.

Baddeley, A. (2003). Working memory: Looking back and looking forward. *Nature Reviews Neuroscience, 4*, 829–839.

Botvinick, M. M., Braver, T. S., Barch, D. M., Carter, C. S., & Cohen, J. D. (2001). Conflict monitoring and cognitive control. *Psychological Review, 108*, 624–652.

Briellmann, R. S., Saling, M. M., Connell, A. B., Waites, A. B., Abbott, D. F., & Jackson, G. D. (2004). A high-field functional MRI study of quadri-lingual subjects. *Brian and Language, 89*, 531–542.

Chauncey, K., Grainger, J., & Holcomb, Ph. J. (2008). Code-switching effects in bilingual word recognition: A masked priming study with event-related potentials. *Brain and Language, 105*, 161–174.

Chee, M. W. L., Hon, N., Lee, H. L., & Soon, C. S. (2001). Relative language proficiency modulates BOLD signal change when bilinguals perform semantic judgments. *NeuroImage, 13*, 1155–1163.

Chee, M. W. L., Soon, C. S., & Lee, H. L. (2003). Common and segregated neuronal networks for different languages revealed using functional magnetic resonance adaptation. *Journal of Cognitive Neuroscience, 15*, 85–97.

Coltheart, M., Davelaar, E., Jonasson, J. T., & Besner, D. (1977). Access to the internal lexicon. In S. Dornic (Ed.), *Attention and performance VI* (pp. 535–555). New York: Academic Press.

Comesaña, M., Perea, M., Piñeiro, A., & Fraga, I. (2009). Vocabulary teaching strategies and conceptual representations of words in L2 in children: Evidence with novice learners. *Journal of Experimental Child Psychology, 104*, 22–33.

Crinion, J., Turner, R., Grogan, A., Hanakawa, T., Noppeney, U., Devlin, J. T., et al. (2006). Language control in the bilingual brain. *Science, 312*, 1537–1540.

De Bleser, R., Dupont, P., Postler, J., Bormans, G., Speelman, D., Mortelmans, L., et al. (2003). The organisation of the bilingual lexicon: A PET study. *Journal of Neurolinguistics, 16*, 439–456.

De Bruijn, E. R. A., Dijkstra, T., Chwilla, D. J., & Schriefers, H. J. (2001). Language context effects on interlingual homograph recognition: Evidence from event-related potentials and response times in semantic priming. *Bilingualism: Language and Cognition, 4*, 155–168.

De Groot, A. M. B. (1992). Determinants of word translation. *Journal of Experimental Psychology: Learning, Memory, and Cognition, 18*, 1001–1028.

De Groot, A. M. B., & Poot, R. (1997). Word translation at three levels of proficiency in a second language: The ubiquitous involvement of conceptual memory. *Language Learning, 47*, 215–264.

Dijkstra, T. (2005). Bilingual visual word recognition and lexical access. In J. F. Kroll, & A. M. B. de Groot (Eds.), *Handbook of bilingualism: Psycholinguistic approaches* (pp. 179–201). Oxford: Oxford University Press.

Dijkstra, T., Grainger, J., & van Heuven, W. J. B. (1999). Recognition of cognates and interlingual homographs: The neglected role of phonology. *Journal of Memory and Language, 41*, 496–518.

Dijkstra, T., van Hell, J. G., & Brenders, P. (submitted). Language switches on cognates in bilingual sentence processing: RT and ERP effects.

Dijkstra, T., & van Heuven, W. J. B. (1998). The BIA model and bilingual word recognition. In J. Grainger & A. M. Jacobs (Eds.), *Localist Connectionist Approaches to Human Cognition* (pp. 189–225). Mahwah, NJ: Erlbaum.

Dijkstra, T., & van Heuven, W. J. B. (2002). The architecture of the bilingual word recognition system: From identification to decision. *Bilingualism: Language and Cognition, 5*, 175–197.

Dijkstra, T., van Jaarsveld, H., & ten Brinke, S. (1998). Interlingual homograph recognition: Effects of task demands and language intermixing. *Bilingualism: Language and Cognition, 1*, 51–66.

Dong, Y., Gui, S., & MacWhinney, B. (2005). Shared and separate meanings in the bilingual mental lexicon. *Bilingualism: Language and Cognition, 8*, 221–238.

Duyck, W., van Assche, E., Drieghe, D., & Hartsuiker, R. J. (2007). Visual word recognition by bilinguals in a sentence context: Evidence for nonselective lexical access. *Journal of Experimental Psychology: Learning, Memory, and Cognition, 33*, 663–679.

Elston-Güttler, K. E., & Friederici, A. D. (2005). Native and L2 processing of homonyms in sentential context. *Journal of Memory and Language, 52*, 256–283.

Elston-Güttler, K. E., Gunter, T. C., & Kotz, S. A. (2005). Zooming into L2: Global language context and adjustment affect processing of interlingual homographs in sentences. *Cognitive Brain Research, 25*, 57–70.

Ferré, P., Sánchez-Casas, R., & Guasch, M. (2006). Can a horse be a donkey? Semantic and form interference effects in translation recognition in early and late proficient and nonproficient Spanish–Catalan bilinguals. *Language Learning, 65*, 571–608.

Francis, W. S. (1999). Cognitive integration of language and memory in bilinguals: Semantic representations. *Psychological Bulletin, 125*, 192–222.

Francis, W. S. (2005). Bilingual semantic and conceptual representation. In J. F. Kroll & A. M. B. de Groot (Eds.), *Handbook of bilingualism: Psycholinguistic approaches* (pp. 251–267). Oxford: Oxford University Press.

Frenck-Mestre, C., Anton, J. L., Roth, M., Vaid, J., & Viallet, F. (2005). Articulation in early and late bilinguals' two languages: Evidence from functional magnetic resonance imaging. *NeuroReport, 16*, 761–765.

Frenck-Mestre, C., & Prince, P. (1997). Second language autonomy. *Journal of Memory and Language, 37*, 481–501.

Friederici, A. D. (2002). Towards a neural basis of auditory sentence processing, *TRENDS in Cognitive Sciences, 6*, 78–84.

Gold, B. T., & Buckner, R. L. (2002). Common prefrontal regions coactivate with dissociable posterior regions during controlled semantic and phonological tasks. *Neuron, 35*, 803–812.

Green, D. W. (1998). Mental control of the bilingual lexico-semantic system. *Bilingualism: Language and Cognition, 1*, 67–81.

Grosjean, F. (1997). Processing mixed language: Issues, findings, and models. In A. M. B. de Groot & J. F. Kroll (Eds.), *Tutorials in bilingualism: Psycholinguistic perspectives* (pp. 225–254). Hillsdale, NJ: Erlbaum.

Hagoort, P. (2005). On Broca, brain, and binding: a new framework. *TRENDS in Cognitive Sciences, 9*, 416–423.

Hahne, A. (2001). What's different in second-language processing? Evidence from event-related brain potentials. *Journal of Psycholinguistic Research, 30*, 251–266.

Hasegawa, M., Carpenter, P. A., & Just, M. A. (2002). An fMRI study of bilingual sentence comprehension and workload. *NeuroImage, 15,* 647–660.

Henson, R. (2005). What can functional neuroimaging tell the experimental psychologist? *Quarterly Journal of Experimental Psychology, 58A,* 193–233.

Hernandez, A., & Li, P. (2007). Age of acquisition: Its neural and computational mechanisms. *Psychological Bulletin, 133,* 638–650.

Hernandez, A. E., Dapretto, M., Mazziotta, J., & Bookheimer, S. (2001). Language switching and language representation in Spanish–English bilinguals: an fMRI study. *Neuroimage, 14,* 510–20.

Hernandez, A. E., & Meschyan, G. (2006). Executive function is necessary to enhance lexical processing in a less proficient L2: Evidence from fMRI during picture naming. *Bilingualism: Language and Cognition. 9,* 177–188.

Holcomb, P. J., Grainger, J., & O'Rourke, T. (2002). An electrophysiological study of the effects of orthographic neighborhood size on printed word perception. *Journal of Cognitive Neuroscience, 14,* 938–950.

Illes, J., Francis, W. S., Desmond, J. E., Gabrieli, J. D., Glover, G. H., Poldrack, R., et al. (1999). Convergent cortical representation of semantic processing in bilinguals. *Brain and Language, 70,* 347–63.

Indefrey, P. (2006). A meta-analysis of hemodynamic studies on first and second language processing: Which suggested differences can we trust and what do they mean? *Language Learning, 56,* 279–304.

Indefrey, P., & Levelt, W. J. M. (2004). The spatial and temporal signatures of word production components. *Cognition, 92,* 101–144.

Kerkhofs, R., Dijkstra, T., Chwilla, D. J., & de Bruijn, E. R. (2006). Testing a model for bilingual semantic priming with interlingual homographs: RT and N400 effects. *Brain Research, 1068,* 170–83.

Kim, K. H., Relkin, N. R., Lee, K. M., & Hirsch, J. (1997). Distinct cortical areas associated with native and second languages. *Nature, 388,* 171–4.

Klein, D., Zatorre, R. J., Milner, B., Meyer, E., & Evans, A. C. (1994). Left putaminal activation when speaking a second language: Evidence from PET. *Neuroreport, 5,* 2295–2297.

Kotz, S. A. (2001). Neurolinguistics evidence for bilingual language representation: A comparison of reaction times and event-related brain potentials. *Bilingualism: Language and Cognition, 4,* 143–154.

Kroll, J. F., & Dussias, P. (2004). The comprehension of words and sentences in two languages. In T. Bhatia & W. Ritchie (Eds.), *Handbook of bilingualism* (pp. 169–200). Cambridge, MA: Blackwell.

Kroll, J. F., & Stewart, E. (1994). Category interference in translation and picture naming: Evidence for asymmetric connections between bilinguals memory representations. *Journal of Memory and Language, 33,* 149–174.

Kroll, J. F., & Tokowicz, N. (2005). Models of bilingual representation and processing. In J. F. Kroll & A. M. B. de Groot (Eds.), *Handbook of bilingualism: Psycholinguistic approaches* (pp. 531–553). Oxford: Oxford University Press.

Kutas, M., & Kluender, R. (1994). What is who violating? A reconsideration of linguistic violations in light of event-related brain potentials. In H. J. Heinze, T. F. Münte, & G. R. Mangun (Eds.), *Cognitive electrophysiology* (pp. 261–282). Boston, MA: Birkhauser.

La Heij, W. (2005). Monolingual and bilingual lexical access in speech production: Issues and models. In J. F. Kroll, & A. M. B. de Groot (Eds.), *Handbook of bilingualism: Psycholinguistic approaches* (pp. 289–307). Oxford: Oxford University Press.

Lemhöfer, K. M. L., Dijkstra, T., & Michel, M. (2004). Three languages, one ECHO: Cognate effects in trilingual word recognition. *Language and Cognitive Processes. 19*, 585–612.

Li, P., & Farkas, I. (2002). A self-organizing connectionist model of bilingual processing. In E. Heredia & J. Altarriba (Eds.), *Bilingual sentence processing* (pp. 58–85). North-Holland, Netherlands: Elsevier Science.

Liu, Y., & Perfetti, C. A. (2003). The time course of brain activity in reading English and Chinese: An ERP study of Chinese bilinguals. *Human Brain Mapping, 18*, 167–175.

Marian, V., Spivey, M., & Hirsch, J. (2003). Shared and separate systems in bilingual language processing: Converging evidence from eyetracking and brain imaging. *Brain and Language, 86*, 70–82.

Martin C. D., Dering, B., Thomas, E. M., & Thierry, G. (2009). Brain potentials reveal semantic priming in both the "active" and the "non-attended" language in early bilinguals. *NeuroImage, 47*, 326–333.

Midgley, K. J., & Holcomb, P. J., van Heuven, W. J. B., & Grainger, J. (2008). An electrophysiological investigation of cross-language effects of orthographic neighborhood. *Brain Research, 1248*, 123–135.

Miller, E. K., & Cohen, J. D. (2001). An integrative theory of prefrontal cortex function. *Annual Review Neuroscience, 24*, 167–202.

Moreno, E. M., Federmeier, K. D., & Kutas, M. (2002). Switching languages, switching palabras: An electrophysiological study of code switching. *Brain and Language, 80*, 188–207.

Moreno, E. M., & Kutas, M. (2005). Processing semantic anomalies in two languages: An electrophysiological exploration in both languages of Spanish–English bilinguals. *Cognitive Brain Research, 22*, 205–220.

Paulmann, S., Elston-Güttler, K. E., Gunter, T. C., & Kotz, S. (2006). Is bilingual lexical access influenced by language context? *NeuroReport, 17*, 727–731.

Perani, D., & Abutalebi, J. (2005). The neural basis of first and second language processing. *Current Opinion in Neurobiology, 15*, 202–206.

Perani, D., Dehaene, S., Grassi, F., Cohen, L., Cappa, S. F., Dupoux, E., et al. (1996). Brain processing of native and foreign languages. *NeuroReport, 7*, 2439–2444.

Perani, D., Paulesu, E., Galles, N. S., Dupoux, E., Dehaene, S., Bettinardi, V., et al. (1998). The bilingual brain: Proficiency and age of acquisition of the second language. *Brain, 121*, 1841–52.

Poldrack, R. A., Wagner, A. D., Prull, M. W., Desmon, J. E., Glover, G. H., & Gabrieli, J. D. E. (1999). Functional specialization for semantic and phonological processing in the left inferior prefrontal cortex. *NeuroImage, 10*, 15–35.

Price, C. J. (2000). The anatomy of language: Contributions from functional neuroimaging. *Journal of Anatomy, 197*, 335–359.

Price, C. J., Green, D.W., & von Studnitz, R. (1999). A functional imaging study of translation and language switching. *Brain, 122*, 2221–2235.

Proverbio, A. M., Leoni, G., & Zani, A. (2004). Language switching mechanisms in simultaneous interpreters: An ERP study. *Neuropsychologia, 42*, 1636–1656.

Ridderinkhof, K. R., Ullsperger, M., Crone, E. A., & Nieuwenhuis, S. (2004). The role of the medial frontal cortex in cognitive control. *Science, 306*, 443–447.

Rodriguez-Fornells, A., De Diego Balaguer, R., & Münte, T. F. (2006). Executive control in bilingual language processing. *Language Learning, 56*, 133–190.

Rodriguez-Fornells, A., Rotte, M., Heinze, H. J., Nösselt, T., & Münte, T. F. (2002). Brain potential and functional MRI evidence for how to handle two languages with one brain. *Nature*, *415*(6875), 1026–9.

Rodriguez-Fornells, A., van der Lugt, A., Rotte, M., Britti, B., Heinze, H. J., & Münte, T. F. (2005). Second language interferes with word production in fluent bilinguals: Brain potential and functional imaging evidence. *Journal of Cognitive Neuroscience*, *17*, 422–33.

Rüschemeyer, S.-A., Fiebach, C. J., Kempe, V., & Friederici, A. D. (2005). Processing lexical semantic and syntactic information in first and second language: fMRI evidence from German and Russian. *Human Brain Mapping*, *25*, 266–286.

Schwartz, A. I., & Kroll, J. F. (2006). Bilingual lexical activation in sentence context. *Journal of Memory and Language*, *55*, 197–212.

Smith, E. E., & Jonides, J. (1999). Storage and executive processes in the frontal lobes. *Science*, *283*, 1657–1661.

Talamas, A., Kroll, J. F., & Dufour, R. (1999). Form related errors in second language learning: A preliminary stage in the acquisition of L1 vocabulary. *Bilingualism: Language and Cognition*, *2*, 45–58.

Tham, W. W. P., Rickard Liow, S. J., Rajapakse, J. C., Leong, T. C., Ng, S. E. S., Lim, W. E. H., et al. (2005). Phonological processing in Chinese–English bilinguals biscriptals: An fMRI study. *NeuroImage*, *28*, 579–587.

Thierry, G., & Wu, Y. J. (2007). Brain potentials reveal unconscious translation during foreign-language comprehension. *Proceedings of the National Academy of Sciences USA*, *104*, 12530–12535.

Thomas, M. S. C., & van Heuven, W. J. B. (2005). Computational models of bilingual comprehension. In J. F. Kroll, & A. M. B. de Groot (Eds.), *Handbook of bilingualism: Psycholinguistic approaches* (pp. 202–225). Oxford: Oxford University Press.

Thompson-Schill, S. L., D'Esposito, M., Aguirre, G. K., & Farah, M. J. (1997). Role of the left inferior prefrontal cortex in retrieval of semantic knowledge: A reevaluation. *Proceedings of the National Academy of Sciences USA*, *94*, 14792–14797.

Van Hell, J. G., & de Groot, A. M. B. (1998). Conceptual representations in bilingual memory: Effects of concreteness and cognate status in word association. *Bilingualism: Language and Cognition*, *1*, 193–211.

Van Hell, J. G., & de Groot, A. M. B. (2008). Sentence context modulates visual word recognition and translation in bilinguals. *Acta Psychologica*, *128*, 431–451.

Van Heuven, W. J. B., & Dijkstra, T. (2010). Language comprehension in the bilingual brain: fMRI and ERP support for psycholinguistic models. *Brain Research Reviews*, *64*, 104–122.

Van Heuven, W. J. B., Dijkstra, T., & Grainger, J. (1998). Orthographic neighborhood effects in bilingual word recognition. *Journal of Memory and Language*, *39*, 458–483.

Van Heuven, W. J. B., Schriefers, H., Dijkstra, T., & Hagoort, P. (2008). Language conflict in the bilingual brain. *Cerebral Cortex*, *18*, 2706–2716.

Verhoef, K., Roelofs, A., & Chwilla, D. J. (2009). Role of inhibition in language switching: Evidence from event-related brain potentials in overt picture naming. *Cognition*, *110*, 84–99.

Vingerhoets, G., van Borsel, J., Tesink, C., van den Noort, M., Deblaere, K., Seurinck, R., et al. (2003). Multilingualism: An fMRI study. *NeuroImage*, *20*, 281–2196.

Wagner, A. D., Paré-Blagoev, E. J., Clark, J., & Podrack, R. A. (2001). Recovering meaning: Left prefrontal cortex guides controlled semantic retrieval. *Neuron*, *31*, 329–338.

Wartenburger, I., Heekeren, H. R., Abutalebi, J., Cappa, S. F., Vilringer, & A., Perani, D. (2003). Early setting of grammatical processing in the bilingual brain. *Neuron, 37*, 159–170.

Weber-Fox, C. M., & Neville, H. J. (1996). Maturational constraints on functional specializations for language processing: ERP and behavioral evidence in bilingual speakers. *Journal of Cognitive Neuroscience, 8*, 231–256.

Zhang, J. X., Feng, C.-M., Fox, P. T., Gao, J-.H., & Tan, L. H. (2004). Is left inferior frontal gyrus a general mechanism for selection. *NeuroImage, 23*, 596–603.

23

Vocabulary Learning in Bilingual First-Language Acquisition and Late Second-Language Learning
Annette M. B. de Groot

Even though grammar may be the quintessential component of language, vocabulary is beyond doubt the most indispensable one. This contribution discusses aspects of the acquisition of vocabulary in two very different populations of learners. The first part discusses stages of lexical development in monolingual and bilingual infant first language (L1) learners, focusing on the bilingual case. The stages covered are the development of sublexical knowledge structures and complete word forms, and the association of word form to word meaning. The second part discusses vocabulary acquisition in late second language (L2) learners. Themes that are covered are the stages and methods of acquisition and the effects of various word characteristics on acquisition. Due to the many differences between these two populations of learners that are correlated with the age difference between them, for instance differences in brain size, general cognitive skills, and extant knowledge structures, vocabulary learning differs considerably between them. One specific difference between L1 and L2 vocabulary learning will be highlighted: the fact that L1 vocabulary learning involves the learning of both word form and word meaning, whereas in L2 vocabulary learning the targeted L2 meanings are already largely in place in the form of lexical concepts in the learners' L1.

The Genesis of Vocabulary in Monolingual and Bilingual First Language Acquisition

Monolingual first language acquisition: phonemes and phonotactics

First-language vocabulary learning starts well before the glorious moment a toddler produces its first words around 12 months of age. During the months prior to this

The Handbook of the Neuropsychology of Language, First Edition. Edited by Miriam Faust.
© 2012 Blackwell Publishing Ltd. Published 2012 by Blackwell Publishing Ltd.

first overt sign of a rudimentary lexicon, infants' impressive perceptual skills have led to the build-up of sublexical knowledge structures, phonemes, and phoneme clusters, thus paving the way to this milestone event. Because words are composed of phonemes, the acquisition of a language's phonemes can be regarded a preliminary step in, or even a component part of, vocabulary learning. The acquisition of the phonemes of the ambient language – the native language(s) – starts immediately at birth, proceeding in parallel to a decreasing perceptual sensitivity to innate nonnative phonetic categories and contrasts. During the first 5 or 6 months of life infants can discriminate both native and nonnative minimal phonetic contrasts. In other words, they can perceive small acoustic differences between pairs of speech sounds that represent different phonemes in the ambient language ("native contrasts") as well as acoustically equally small differences between pairs of speech sounds that represent different phonemes in certain nonnative languages but not in the native language ("nonnative contrasts"). After about 6 months of age the ability to perceive nonnative phonetic contrasts starts to decline (Werker & Tees, 1984). At the same time language-specific perception of speech sounds has started to emerge. By the time infants are about 11 months of age, they have largely lost the ability to discriminate nonnative phonetic contrasts, although some of these continue to be perceived (Best & McRoberts, 2003; Best, McRoberts, & Sithole, 1988; Tees & Werker, 1984) and a lost contrast may not be lost forever but be restored through relevant language exposure (Kuhl, Tsao, & Liu, 2003). As stressed by a number of authors (Kuhl, 2004; Kuhl et al., 2003; Sebastián-Gallés & Bosch, 2005), rather than pointing at perceptual loss, this reduced perceptual sensitivity to nonnative speech sounds in fact indexes growth in phonetic development, resulting from perceptual reorganization processes caused by exposure to the ambient language.

The way phonemes combine into phoneme sequences within words is subject to language-specific sequential and positional constraints. For instance, the phoneme strings /str/ and /spr/ occur in English but only at the beginning of a word, not the end, and /ts/ can occur in initial position in German but not in English. Just as vocabulary acquisition involves the learning of the language's phoneme inventory, it requires the development of knowledge regarding these constraints on the sequencing and positioning of phonemes within words. There is some evidence to suggest that this knowledge, known as "phonotactic" knowledge, becomes manifest during the second half of the first year: Jusczyk, Friederici, Wessels, Svenkerud, and Jusczyk (1993) presented English and Dutch word lists to American and Dutch 9-month-old infants, each list containing words of one language only. The majority of the English words violated the phonotactic constraints of Dutch, containing sound sequences that do not occur in Dutch. Conversely, the majority of the Dutch words violated the phonotactic constraints of English. It was found that the American infants listened significantly longer to the English lists than to the Dutch lists, whereas the Dutch infants showed the opposite pattern. These results suggest that the previous 9 months of exposure to the ambient language had sensitized the infants to the phonotactics of their native language. In a further experiment testing

American 6-month-olds the language effect did not materialize. These combined findings suggest that sensitivity to the ambient language's phonotactics has developed between 6 and 9 months.

Two studies by Saffran and her colleagues (Saffran, 2001; Saffran, Aslin, & Newport, 1996) provided relevant information regarding a cognitive mechanism that might underlie this ability of infants to discover the phonotactics of the surrounding language(s). In addition, these studies provided an answer to the question how infants learn to segment continuous speech into sound patterns that correspond to single words. This ability is a further necessary preliminary step in the development of a lexicon. Saffran et al. (1996) first familiarized a group of American 8-month-olds with 2 minutes of fluent synthesized speech. The speech stream consisted of four three-syllabic nonsense "words" (*pabiku, tibudo, golatu, daropi*), repeated in a random order. There were no physical boundaries between the successive words (e.g., *tibudodaropipabikutibudogolatudaropigolatupabiku* . . .) nor did the speech stream contain any prosodic cues to the word boundaries. During a subsequent test phase the infants were presented with repetitions of two of the four "words" presented during training (e.g., *pabiku* and *tibudo*) and with repetitions of two syllable triads that were created by joining the final syllable of one of the words onto the first two syllables of a second word (e.g., *tudaro* and *pigola*, called "part-words" in Saffran, 2001). The crucial difference between these two types of syllable triads was that the sequential (or "transitional") probability between the first, second, and third syllable was always 1.0 within the words whereas it was less (.33) for one of the syllable transitions within the part-words (notice that also the part-words occurred as such in the speech stream; see the example above). If the infants' listening times at test would be different for the words and part-words, this would indicate the infants had extracted from the input the relative frequencies of the transitions between the syllables (high within words; lower within part-words). A difference in listening time for words and part-words was indeed obtained. Accordingly, Saffran and her colleagues concluded that infants possess a statistical learning device that detects sequential probabilities of syllables in speech and that this tool helps them to develop a lexicon by suggesting where the word boundaries are in continuous speech: a syllable sequence of high sequential probability is likely to be a word and one of low sequential probability presumably contains a word boundary somewhere in the middle. This statistical learning device can similarly account for the above finding (Jusczyk et al., 1993) that at 9 months infants can discriminate between the phonotactic patterns of the ambient language and uncommon phonotactic patterns because what distinguishes the two is the sequential probability of the constituent phonemes. Furthermore, just like the sequential probabilities of syllable sequences, the sequential probabilities of phoneme sequences plausibly provide information on word boundaries: a familiar phonotactic pattern is likely to be a sublexical unit of one and the same word, whereas an uncommon phoneme sequence presumably marks a boundary between two words.

In a later study, Saffran (2001) put forward the important argument that only if infants treat the familiar syllabic patterns they have extracted from the speech input as potential words (and not as patterns that are merely familiar to them but are not assigned a special linguistic status), it is legitimate to conclude that this statistical learning device bootstraps vocabulary acquisition. She examined this issue using a modified procedure. Following the same familiarization procedure as used in Saffran et al. (1996), at test the words and part-words were embedded in either an English context (e.g., word: *I like my pabiku*; part-word: *What a nice tudaro*) or in a nonsensical context (word: *Zy fike ny pabiku*; part-word: *Foo day miff tudaro*). A significant listening time difference between words and part-words was obtained when they were embedded in an English context but not when they were embedded in nonsense. Accordingly, the author concluded that "infants are not just detecting the statistical properties of sound sequences. Instead, they are using the statistical properties of sound sequences to acquire linguistic knowledge: possible words in their native language" (Saffran, 2001, p. 165).

The studies by Saffran and her colleagues have thus revealed an important learning mechanism of infants, one that is sensitive to the frequency and internal structure of recurrent patterns in the speech input. The learning process involved, coined "statistical learning" by these authors, does not only start off vocabulary acquisition but is assumed to bootstrap learning in other language domains as well, specifically, the learning of grammar and phonology (see Saffran, 2001, for a review). In its turn, this evidence that statistical learning plays a pivotal role in language learning in general challenges theories of language acquisition that assume it to be largely driven by innate linguistic universals (see Saffran, 2003, for a review).

Bilingual first language acquisition: phonemes and phonotactics

The above description of precursors of vocabulary development was based on studies that examined infants exposed to monolingual input. But of course, many children grow up with two languages either from birth ("simultaneous bilingualism" or "bilingual first language acquisition"), or are exposed to a second language soon after a period of exclusive exposure to the first ("early sequential bilingualism"). This situation gives rise to the question whether and how the above skills and types of knowledge structures develop differently in monolingual-to-be (henceforth: "monolingual") and bilingual-to-be (henceforth: "bilingual") children. There is no reason to believe that the word segmentation procedure described above is operative at different moments in bilingual and monolingual infants, but plausibly language-specific phonological and/or phonotactic knowledge emerges later, or follows a different developmental trajectory, in bilingual infants.

Bilingual infants are exposed to two different speech systems that may contain different numbers of phonemes, different phonetic contrasts, and differences between the prototypical values of shared phonemes. A consequence of these differences between the phonological systems of a bilingual infant's two languages is the occurrence of cross-language distributional overlap of speech sounds that instantiate phonemes belonging to the different languages. For example, the /e/

phoneme in the one language may be realized in speech the same way as the /ɛ/ phoneme in the other language. Maye, Werker, and Gerken (2002) have shown that 6- and 8-month-old monolingual infants exploit distributional information of speech sounds in the language input to develop phoneme categories. Specifically, they found that their infant participants built a single phonetic category when the majority of the speech sounds presented to them clustered around one central value on a particular acoustic dimension (voiced–voiceless) but formed two categories if the presented speech sounds were grouped around two more peripheral values on the phonetic dimension. This finding suggests that bilingual infants, experiencing cross-linguistic distributional overlap of speech sounds, may be hindered in developing the phoneme categories of their two languages, exhibiting a delay as compared with monolingual children and/or perhaps following a different trajectory towards the targeted phonemes.

A second reason for a relatively late emergence of phoneme categories in bilingual infants might be that the language input they receive is divided between their two languages. As a consequence, bilingual infants will be exposed to exemplars of one and the same phoneme less frequently than monolingual infants. Presumably, frequency of exposure to a particular phoneme determines how rapidly it is acquired, thus favoring monolingual infants. For the same reason, the phonotactic development in the two separate languages may be delayed in bilingual infants: a bilingual child will hear a particular phoneme sequence, common in one of his languages, less often than a child exclusively exposed to this language and, plausibly, it will therefore take the bilingual child relatively long to develop the associated knowledge structure.

Among the paucity of studies that examined the developing speech system in bilingual infants there is one that suggests that, despite the complexity of the linguistic input they are exposed to, bilingual infants develop some knowledge of the sublexical elements in their two languages at a very early age: Bosch and Sebastián-Gallés (2001) discovered that Catalan–Spanish 4-month-olds discriminated between Catalan and Spanish speech passages even though Catalan and Spanish belong to the same rhythmical class of languages and an interpretation in terms of perceived rhythm differences cannot therefore account for this result. Although it remains possible that less salient prosodic differences between these two languages enabled them to do so, an equally plausible alternative is that at 4 months bilingual infants have already developed the rudimentary beginnings of the sublexical elements in both their languages.

Still, a further study by these same researchers indicates that at least some phonemes develop later in bilingual infants than in age-matched monolingual controls. Bosch and Sebastián-Gallés (2003a) compared the development of a vowel contrast that exists in Catalan but not in Spanish in Catalan and Spanish monolingual infants and Catalan–Spanish bilingual infants. The vowel contrast under study concerned the vowels /e/ (as in *bait*) and /ɛ/ (as in *bet*). The Spanish phonetic system only contains /e/, which acoustically overlaps with both Catalan /e/ and /ɛ/ and whose prototypical exemplar is intermediate between those of the two Catalan vowels. Two age groups were tested: 4-month-olds and 8-month-olds. Half of the participants in each bilingual and monolingual age group were first familiarized with /e/ exemplars whereas the remainder half were first familiarized with /ɛ/ exemplars. In a subsequent test phase all participants heard exemplars of both the category they had heard during familiarization ("same") and the other category ("different"). The question of interest was which of the infant groups could hear the difference between same and different exemplars, as indicated by different listening times for these two types of stimuli.

In agreement with the common observation that during the first months of life infants are sensitive to both native and nonnative contrasts, all three groups of 4-month-olds, also the Spanish monolingual group, perceived the Catalan contrast. Furthermore, in agreement with the established view that language-specific perception develops in the second semester of life, the Catalan monolingual 8-month-olds still perceived the contrast whereas the Spanish 8-month-olds failed to discriminate between /e/ and /ɛ/ exemplars. Interestingly, despite the fact that the bilingual 8-month-olds had been exposed to the contrast from birth, albeit on average less frequently than their Catalan peers, they failed to perceive it, behaving like the Spanish 8-month-olds. A follow-up experiment testing 12-month-old Catalan–Spanish infants showed that by that age the sensitivity to the Catalan contrast had been restored. The authors concluded that due to the overlapping distributions of exemplars of Spanish /e/ and Catalan /e/ and /ɛ/, the bilingual infants had first developed a single extended phoneme category encompassing all three vowels and therefore failed to discriminate them (cf. Maye et al., 2002; see above). They suggested that this one category is ultimately separated into three (Catalan /e/ and /ɛ/ and Spanish /e/), presumably as a result of extended exposure to both languages. In a second study, the authors replicated part of this bilingual developmental pattern, now testing infants' ability to discriminate between the fricatives /s/ and /z/, which, again, are contrastive in Catalan but not in Spanish (Bosch & Sebastián-Gallés, 2003b): At 4 months infants from monolingual Catalan, monolingual Spanish, and Catalan–Spanish bilingual homes all discriminated between these fricatives when they occurred in word-initial position of monosyllabic stimuli. At 12 months only the Catalan monolingual infants were sensitive to this contrast. No older age groups were tested so that it is impossible to tell when exactly sensitivity to this contrast is restored again in the bilinguals.

The studies by Bosch and Sebastián-Gallés (2003a, 2003b) suggest that cross-language distributional overlap of the speech sounds in bilingual infants' dual language input delays the building of language-specific contrastive phonetic categories. It was already mentioned above that the lower average frequency of exposure to each separate phonetic element might be a further cause of this developmental delay. That exposure frequency indeed plays a role in the development of phonetic categories was suggested by Sundara, Polka, and Molnar (2008). These authors argued that if infants are sensitive to the frequency of occurrence of the phonetic elements in the speech input (which the statistical learning device described above suggests is the case), a high frequency of occurrence might counteract the adverse

effect of cross-language distributional overlap in the development of specific phonetic categories in bilingual infants.

They tested this hypothesis by comparing the ability of monolingual French,
monolingual English, and bilingual French–English 6–8- and 10–12-month-olds,
six groups in all, to discriminate between exemplars of French /d/ (articulated
dentally) and English /d/ (articulated at the alveolar ridge). Exemplars of French
and English /d/ show considerable acoustic overlap and French adults fail to distinguish between them. English adults, however, can hear the difference between them,
possibly because French dental /d/ is perceptually similar to English /ð/. Importantly,
both French /d/ and English /d/ occur very frequently in their respective languages.
As hypothesized by the authors, despite the distributional overlap of French and
English /d/, English–French bilingual infants might therefore remain sensitive to
this contrast. In a habituation procedure similar to the one employed by Bosch
and Sebastián-Gallés (2003a) they found that all three groups of 6–8-month-olds
succeeded in discriminating between French and English /d/. The monolingual
English and French 10–12-month-olds behaved like adult speakers of these languages, the English monolinguals still discriminating French and English /d/ but
the French monolinguals failing to do so. Interestingly, the French–English bilingual
10–12-month-olds also perceived the contrast, exhibiting the same response pattern
as the English monolingual infants this age. These findings warrant the conclusion
that, in addition to the distributional pattern of speech sounds, their occurrence
frequency determines whether or not bilingual infants lag behind their monolingual
peers in developing phonetic categories.

As described earlier, at 9 months monolingual infants recognize the difference
between sound sequences that occur in their native language and those that do not,
thus showing that phonotactic knowledge has emerged (Jusczyk et al., 1993).
Sebastián-Gallés and Bosch (2002) provided a first indication that growing up
bilingual does not inevitably delay phonotactic development. They presented
Catalan monolingual, Spanish monolingual, and Catalan–Spanish bilingual
10-month-olds with lists of nonwords that all had a CVCC structure. Catalan contains consonant clusters in word-final position but Spanish does not. Half of the
presented lists consisted of nonwords with legal Catalan end clusters (e.g., *birt* and
kisk) whereas the nonwords on the other half of the lists contained end clusters that
do not occur in Catalan (e.g., *ketr* and *datl*). Given the absence of consonant clusters
in word-final position in Spanish, all nonwords were illegal in Spanish. The Catalan
monolinguals listened longer to lists of words with legal consonant clusters than to
those with illegal consonant clusters, thus demonstrating sensitivity to the phonotactics of their native language and corroborating the results obtained by Jusczyk et
al. (1993). The Spanish monolinguals listened equally long to both types of word
lists, a finding that agrees with the fact that the words of both lists were illegal in
Spanish, so there was no ground to discriminate between them. The pattern of
results obtained for the bilingual infants depended upon the relative dominance
of their two languages: a subgroup of Catalan-dominant bilinguals (exposed to
Catalan and Spanish 60% and 40% of the time, respectively) exhibited an equally

large difference in listening time to the legal and illegal word lists as their Catalan monolingual peers. In contrast, a much smaller and statistically nonsignificant list-type effect was observed for a subgroup of Spanish-dominant bilinguals (exposed to Catalan and Spanish 40% and 60% of the time, respectively). These results suggest that the development of phonotactic knowledge is not linearly related to the amount of exposure to the phoneme sequences in question because if it were, the Catalan monolinguals should have shown a larger list-type effect than the Catalan-dominant bilinguals. Nevertheless, the statistical null-effect observed for the Spanish-dominant bilinguals indicates that some minimum amount of exposure to the common phoneme sequences of a language is required for phonotactic knowledge to develop and that exposure alone does not suffice for bilingual phonotactic development to keep pace with monolingual phonotactic development. A more general conclusion to draw from the results obtained for the Catalan-dominant bilingual infants is that growing up with two languages does not inevitably delay the development of language-specific phonotactic knowledge.

Word-form recognition and linking word to meaning

The discussion so far has concerned the development of the building blocks of words, the phonemes and common phoneme sequences they consist of. In addition, a statistical learning device was described that presumably plays an important role in this development and that also enables infants to detect the words' sound patterns in fluent speech. A next issue to address is how many months of naturalistic language exposure it takes before infants, exploiting this learning device, actually start recognizing the phonological forms of complete words in connected speech. To become familiar to the infant, a word's sound pattern must probably be encountered a minimum number of times, and reaching this minimally required number of encounters presumably takes longer than the time it takes a language's typical sublexical phoneme sequences to become familiar to the infant. The ground for this claim is that a particular sublexical pattern occurs across a number of different words and is therefore encountered more often than the sound pattern of a complete word. In general, the larger a particular linguistic unit, the less often it is encountered as such in speech. Furthermore, because children growing up with two languages will on average encounter each separate word less often than their monolingual peers, word recognition is plausibly delayed in bilingual children. A further question is at what age infants start to discover the referential nature of words and begin to establish connections between their phonological forms and meanings. If word-form recognition is delayed in bilingual children, then this component process of word knowledge, namely, the linking of word form to word meaning, will also develop later in bilingual infants.

A small number of bilingual studies have addressed the above questions by examining the development of word-form recognition and word-to-meaning linkage in bilingual infants and toddlers between the ages of 9 and 22 months and comparing their performance to age-matched monolingual controls. Vihman, Thierry, Lum, Keren-Portnoy, and Martin (2007) studied word-form recognition in separate groups of 9-, 10-, 11-, and 12-month-old monolingual infants from English-speaking Welsh families and in one group of English–Welsh bilingual 11-month-olds. (In fact, Welsh "monolingual" infants were also tested but their data will be ignored here because there was reason to believe they had been exposed to English as well, to a degree that complicated the interpretation of the data.) For each language, Welsh and English, two sets of words were created, one set (called "unfamiliar") containing words that were presumably all unknown to all of the subjects, the second (called "familiar") containing a number of words (about 35%) likely to be known by the infants. The known–unknown judgments were based on Welsh and English versions of the MacArthur Communicative Development Inventory (CDI; e.g., Fenson et al., 2000), lists of words that the participants' families checked off, indicating which ones they thought their child understood.

The study consisted of two parts, one in which behavioral data were gathered, the second involving the registration of event-related potentials (ERPs). In the behavioral part of the study two loudspeakers were mounted on a wall, on either side of the child, and on every single trial one of them played the words from one of the word-sets for a given language. Across trials, presentation side (right or left) and type of word-set played (familiar or unfamiliar) were randomized. The time the infant looked in the direction of the loudspeaker currently emitting a word-set was registered as the infants' listening time. The bilinguals were tested in both languages, the English monolinguals obviously only on the English materials. In the second part of the study ERPs to the same stimulus materials were collected. The questions of interest were whether the infants' listening time differed for the familiar and unfamiliar word sets and whether familiar and unfamiliar words would give rise to different ERP patterns. Affirmative answers to these questions would suggest that word-form recognition had emerged (in fact confirming the parents' subjective judgments that their child knew at least some of the words).

The 11-month-old English monolinguals, but not the younger ones, listened significantly longer to the familiar English word-set than to the unfamiliar set. The bilingual infants, all 11 months of age, also showed a reliable familiarity effect, in both languages, and the size of this effect was comparable to that observed for the monolinguals. These findings indicate that word-form recognition emerges around 11 months and that it is not noticeably delayed in bilinguals. However, the ERP data suggested a revision of this conclusion, exhibiting a familiarity effect – and, thus, word-form recognition – already at 10 months. This first evidence of word-form recognition at 11 months only in the behavioral data but already one month earlier in the brain data corroborates an observation by previous authors (e.g., Rivera-Gaxiola, Silva-Pereyra, & Kuhl, 2005) that ERPs provide a more sensitive marker of the (emergence of) cognitive skills than behavioral measures do (see McLaughlin, Osterhout, & Kim, 2004, for a similar demonstration in the domain of adult L2 word learning). Because no 10-month-old bilinguals were tested, it is impossible to tell whether they also would have shown the effect as early as at 10 months. Still, on the basis of the available data, it can be concluded that, if word-form recognition is delayed at all in bilingual infants, the delay is a modest one.

In an English–Spanish study Conboy and Mills (2006) also examined bilingual infants' brain responses to known and unknown words, but this study differed crucially from the one by Vihman et al. (2007) in one respect, namely, the age of the participating infants: they were between 19 and 22 months with an average of 20 months. This means that Conboy and Mills' subjects were all presumably long beyond the stage of mere word-form recognition – the developmental stage examined by Vihman and colleagues – and had begun to treat words as meaning-bearing entities with a referential function. This is, for instance, suggested by the fact that 19-month-old monolingual toddlers exhibit an N400-like semantic incongruity effect in the ERP when they listen to words that are either congruent or incongruent with the content of simultaneously presented pictures (Friedrich & Friederici, 2004). That infants this age process the meanings of words is also suggested by the fact that the average monolingual 18-month-old exhibits a sudden growth in productive vocabulary, the so-called "vocabulary spurt," after gingerly having started to produce his first words around 12 months. Nazzi and Bertoncini (2003) hypothesized that this vocabulary spurt reflects a qualitative shift from an "associative" to a "referential" mode of word acquisition and that these two acquisition modes are effectuated by two different lexical acquisition mechanisms. In the first word-acquisition stage an associative mechanism links phonetically underspecified sound patterns to specific objects. In the second stage a referential mechanism pairs phonetically specified sound patterns with categories of objects rather than with specific objects. Nazzi and Bertoncini regard the word-meaning connections resulting from the first stage as "proto-words" and those resulting from the second, the referential stage, as genuine words. The referential acquisition mode allows an increase in cognitive economy and, as a consequence, a reduction in cognitive load: if a particular sound pattern is connected to a whole category of objects, far fewer word–meaning pairings have to be learned than when words are paired with individual objects. The vocabulary spurt observed around 18 months may be the direct effect of this increase in cognitive economy. In addition, the reduced cognitive load would allow the infants to attend to the words' phonological forms more carefully than before, thus gradually replacing the phonetically underspecified word forms by more precisely specified ones. In terms of this model of vocabulary acquisition, and assuming that bilingual infants will not lag substantially behind their monolingual peers, the participants in Conboy and Mills have all presumably reached the associative, and possibly the referential, stage of vocabulary acquisition and the results of that study must be interpreted in that light.

Conboy and Mills (2006) divided their participants in subgroups depending upon their total conceptual vocabulary (TCV) scores, a measure of the total number of concepts, not words, mastered by the child, and examined each child's brain responses to stimuli in both his dominant and the weaker language (as determined by the parents' assessments of how many words their child knew in each language). Their reason for doing so was to determine the effect of differential language experience in the two languages – relatively more and less in the dominant and the weaker language, respectively – on the brain responses to known and unknown words. In their data analysis the investigators focused on three negative components in the ERP signal, between 200–400, 400–600, and 600–900 ms following word onset (and on an early positive component, the P100, to be ignored here). Clear effects of the known–unknown word manipulation were observed, which were qualified by language dominance and TCV and explained in terms of differential meaning processing of these two word types. The high TCV group exhibited an effect of word type in all three time windows and in both the dominant and the weaker language, with the known words eliciting more negative ERP amplitudes than the unknown words in all cases. In the low TCV group these effects occurred only for the dominant language, whereas in the weaker language the known–unknown word effect was only observed in the 600–900 ms time window. Comparing the ERP components' latency and distribution of these bilingual data with those observed in comparable studies testing monolingual infants (e.g., Mills, Coffey-Corina, & Neville, 1997), the authors concluded that in some respects the ERP patterns of both the high and the low TCV bilinguals (all around 20 months of age) resembled those of 13–17-month-old normally developing monolinguals and 20-month-old monolingual late talkers. This suggests that word acquisition is somewhat delayed in bilingual infants. In addition, the different response patterns for the dominant and the weaker language within the low TCV group indicate that the amount of language experience affects brain processes, corroborating similar evidence obtained studies testing adult bilinguals (see e.g., Abutalebi, Cappa, & Perani, 2005; Steinhauer, White, & Drury, 2009).

Three further studies examined the development of word-to-meaning linkage in monolingual (Werker, Cohen, Lloyd, Casasola, & Stager, 1998; Werker, Fennell, Corcoran, & Stager, 2002), and bilingual (Fennell, Byers-Heinlein, & Werker, 2007) toddlers using a behavioral research method. Across these three studies, different age groups were first familiarized with two word–object pairs (Word A – Object A; Word B – Object B), with the (toy) object of each pair shown on a video screen and the (nonsense) word played repeatedly from a speaker just below the screen. The age groups in Werker et al. (1998) concerned infants of 8, 10, 12, and 14 months, whereas the age groups in the remaining two studies concerned toddlers of 14, 17, and 20 months. In Werker et al. (1998) the two words were totally dissimilar (*lif* and *neem*), whereas in the remaining two studies they were similar (*bih* and *dih*). After familiarization – which lasted between about 5 and 10 minutes – the participants were tested on "same" and "switch" trials (e.g., Word A – Object A, vs. Word A – Object B). The researchers argued that if the infants had learned the associative links between the words and the paired objects, the incorrect pairings in the switch trials should surprise them, resulting in longer looking times for the switch trials. In contrast, equally long looking times for both types of trials would suggest they had not learned the word–object links.

The 14-month-olds in Werker et al. (1998; dissimilar words, monolinguals), but not the younger age groups, showed longer looking times for the switch trials than the same trials. Werker et al. (2002; similar words, monolinguals) observed equally long looking times for same and switch trials in the 14-month-olds and different ones in the two groups of 17- and 20-month-olds. Finally, Fennell et al. (2007; similar words, bilinguals) found equally long looking times for same and switch trials in both a group of 14-month-olds and a group of 17-month-olds, whereas a group of 20-month-olds exhibited different looking times for the two types of trials. These results indicate that 14-month-old monolingual toddlers are able to simultaneously attend to the sound pattern of a word and an object associated with this sound, while at the same time establishing a link between the two. Within a short time span of about 5 to 10 minutes they can do so for (at least) two word–object pairings, on condition that the two words have dissimilar phonological forms. According to the authors, this finding challenges the standard view that "prior to the vocabulary spurt, it is a very slow and laborious process for infants to learn to associate new words with objects" (Werker et al., 1998, p. 1301). The authors furthermore argued that earlier evidence suggesting that this skill might already be in place before 14 months (Woodward, Markman, & Fitzsimmons, 1994) probably had to do with the fact that learning and testing took place in a contextually rich, interactive setting instead of under tightly controlled circumstances without any assistance of adults or other contextual support. The equally long looking times of the monolingual 14-month-olds in same and switch trials in Werker et al. (2002) suggest that the mental resources – attentional, perceptual, and memorial – of 14-month-olds do not yet suffice for the component processes to be executed successfully in parallel, if the two words to pair with their respective objects are very similar and thus require very detailed perceptual analysis. Three months later, at 17 months, the monolinguals but not the bilinguals manage to perform the task successfully with a pair of similar words. Finally, at 20 months, bilinguals catch up with their monolingual peers. In conclusion, it appears that attending to the phonetic details of words while at the same time linking these words to objects develops somewhat more slowly in children growing up bilingual. As however noted by Fennell et al. (2007), this may not noticeably delay word learning in children growing up bilingual, because the initial lexicon of infants still contains very few similar-sounding words.

In the above comparison of monolingual and bilingual first-language vocabulary acquisition a number of differences have been identified. The perception of a number of phonetic contrasts (Bosch & Sebastián-Gallés, 2003a, 2003b) and referential word use (Conboy & Mills, 2006; Fennell et al., 2007) was shown to be delayed in bilingual infants and toddlers by a couple of months. But equally noteworthy is the fact that in some cases bilinguals kept pace with their monolingual peers. Sebastián-Gallés and Bosch (2002) found this to be the case for phonotactic development in bilinguals' dominant language and Vihman et al.'s (2007) data indicate it might also hold for word-form recognition. Three of the above studies that *did* point at a delayed development in bilinguals used stimuli that required a very careful perceptual analysis of the presented stimuli (Bosch & Sebastián-Gallés, 2003a, 2003b), presenting pairs of notoriously confusable phonemes or two very similar words (Fennell et al., 2007). These types of stimuli are known to cause lasting discriminative problems in late nonnative speakers of a language (e.g., Broersma, 2006; Weber & Cutler, 2004) and have led to the counterintuitive conclusion that, despite the fact that the nonnative lexicon typically contains fewer lexical elements overall than the native lexicon, more lexical elements compete for selection during nonnative language speech perception than during native language speech perception. That bilingual infants caught up with their monolingual peers after just a few more months of exposure to their two languages testifies to the excellent auditory perceptual skills of infants. The same can be said of the finding that a high frequency of exposure to confusable phonetic items can prevent a delayed development in bilingual infants (Sundara et al., 2008).

All in all, the above experimental studies point at the conclusion that in some ways the development of sublexical and lexical knowledge is slightly delayed in bilingual children as compared with their monolingual age-mates, but that in other respects bilingual children keep pace with their monolingual age-mates. The second part of this conclusion is corroborated by studies that examined lexical development in (Spanish–English) bilingual infants and toddlers (between 8 and 30 months of age) as assessed by means of the MacArthur Communicative Development Inventory rather than experimentally (Pearson & Fernández, 1994; Pearson, Fernández, & Oller, 1993). Perhaps the most noteworthy finding in these (and many other) studies is the wide range of vocabulary sizes exhibited by normally developing children. But of special interest here is the finding that the bilingual children's productive vocabulary in *the two languages together* equaled that of their monolingual age-mates and, moreover, that their receptive vocabulary in *each of their languages* was comparable to that of their monolingual peers. In addition, the Pearson and Fernández study indicated that the vocabulary spurt occurs around the same age in bilingual children as in age-matched monolingual children. Similar findings were obtained in a study that compared vocabulary knowledge in 24- to 27-month-old German–English toddlers and German and English monolingual age-mates (Junker & Stockman, 2002). In conclusion then, all of the above evidence suggests that the relative complexity of the linguistic input to which children growing up to become bilingual are exposed does not appreciably delay their vocabulary development.

Vocabulary Acquisition in Late Second Language Learners

Vocabulary acquisition in late L2 learning differs considerably from vocabulary learning in monolingual and bilingual L1 acquisition, and in a couple of respects late L2 learners clearly have an advantage over L1 learners despite the fact that, perhaps as a consequence of neural commitment of brain tissue to the native language (e.g., Ellis & Lambon Ralph, 2000; Rivera-Gaxiola et al., 2005), they have a lesser aptitude for language learning than young children. Late L2 learners have already figured out how language "works," being aware of the fact that continuous speech is built up from smaller linguistic units with a referential function. In addition, late L2 learners dispose of a larger variety of learning strategies, more cognitive resources, and, perhaps most importantly, a large stock of lexical concepts, namely, the meaning representations of the words they already master in their L1. To the extent that L1 and L2 have lexicalized the same or very similar concepts – in other words, to the extent that L1 words are approximately translatable into single words in the L2 – these L1 meaning representations can serve the L2 as well: an L2 word can be assigned the meaning of its closest word translation in L1. So whereas L1 word learning requires the learning of both form and meaning (in addition to forming a connection between them), at the onset of L2 vocabulary acquisition the targeted L2 meanings are already largely in place. As a consequence, it initially suffices to learn the new forms and to link them onto the meaning representations of the corresponding L1 words. In other words, it initially suffices to merely re-label extant lexical concepts. Because the two terms in a word–translation pair seldom share all aspects of meaning, this parasitic use of the L1 word meanings in L2 word learning inevitably leads to a semantic "accent" in the L2, an overextended and underextended use of words that, for different reasons, also characterizes young L1 users. Through extensive subsequent naturalistic exposure to written and spoken L2, the L1-specific aspects of the inherited L2 meanings can subsequently be chipped off from them and the L2-specific components added onto them. Arguably, this advantage late L2 learners have over L1 learners outweighs a clear disadvantage, namely, the fact that to properly perceive and produce the phonological forms of the L2 words, they will have to relearn lost nonnative contrasts, an undertaking that is often not completely successful (as is, for instance, suggested by a wealth of studies showing age-of-acquisition effects on L2 pronunciation; see also the studies by Broersma, 2006, and Weber and Cutler, 2004, mentioned above).

Methods of second language vocabulary learning

The L1 word meanings already present in memory can most readily be exploited if the forms of the L1 words are present in the L2 learning environment, because through these the extant L1 meanings immediately become available. In naturalistic communication settings this condition will generally not be fulfilled, because the learner does not usually carry a bilingual dictionary around with him, nor is he accompanied by a teacher (perhaps in the form of a bilingual friend) who helps him make the connection with the stored L1 knowledge by providing him with an unknown L2 word's translation in L1 (cf. Sternberg, 1987). In contrast, in the L2 classroom it is a common practice to use methods that directly provide the relevant L1 words.

Two well-known methods of this type are the keyword method and paired-associate learning that both involve an L1 word as a component part of each learning event. Both are so called "direct" methods of L2 vocabulary learning, that is, methods in which the learner's attention is explicitly focused on the individual words to acquire (rather than on the meaning of a text or discourse as a whole, as in so-called "context" methods; see below). L2 word learning by means of the keyword method involves three stages. In the first stage the learner is told an L1 word's name in the L2, for instance, that the French word for *fish* is *poisson* or that the Italian word for *night* is *notte*. In the next step, the learner is provided with (or encouraged to come up with) an L1 word with a similar, or the same, sound as the L2 word (e.g., English *poison* and *naughty*, respectively). This same or similar sound- ing L1 word is the eponymous keyword. In the final stage, he is asked to create, or is provided with, a mental image in which the meanings of keyword and L1/L2 word interact (e.g., he is asked: "Imagine poisoning your pet fish" or "Imagine having a naughty night out"; the examples are from Beaton, Gruneberg, Hyde, Shufflebottom, & Sykes, 2005). When at some later point the learner encounters the new L2 word (*poisson* or *notte*), it will evoke the keyword (*poison* or *naughty*), which, in turn, will arouse the interactive image of the keyword and L1/L2 word from which the L2 word's meaning can subsequently be read off. At that point the native word associ- ated with this meaning (*fish*, *night*) can also be retrieved. It may be obvious from this description that both learning by means of the keyword method and subse- quent retrieval of the learned words are complex processes. Still, the method has been shown to be highly effective, although its efficacy relative to other methods depends on a number of variables, such as the interval between learning and testing, the mode of testing (receptive or productive), and learner characteristics such as the age of the learners and whether or not the learners have substantial prior experi- ence with foreign language learning (see de Groot, 2011, and de Groot & van Hell, 2005, for details).

Of the second of the above-mentioned direct methods of L2 vocabulary acquisi- tion, the paired-associate method, two versions are often used: picture–word asso- ciation and word–word association. In the picture–word version, pairs of stimuli are presented during learning, each pair consisting of the L2 word to acquire and a picture depicting its meaning. In the word–word version the paired terms presented during learning are two words: the L2 word and its translation in L1. The use of the picture–word association method is limited by the fact that it is relatively dif- ficult to draw pictures that unambiguously depict abstract words. As a consequence, studies that have employed the picture–word method have typically confined them- selves to examining the acquisition of concrete L2 words. The use of the keyword method described above is limited for a different reason: it is unsuitable for learning cognates, that is, words that share orthography and/or phonology with their L1 translation (e.g., English *chair* and French *chaise*). The reason is that the L1 cognate form itself (*chair*) will generally be more similar in form to the corresponding L2 word (*chaise*) than any other L1 word that could serve as keyword (*champion*). Therefore, the most straightforward way to learn cognates is to create a direct link between the L1 and L2 cognate forms using the word–word association technique. The use of the word–word association method is not limited to specific subsets of words and can be applied to cognates as well as noncognates and to abstract as well as concrete words.

As mentioned, simply adopting the L1 words' meaning to also serve the L2 leads to overextended and underextended usage of the L2 words, which through extensive subsequent naturalistic exposure to, and use of, the L2 should gradually be refined to come to resemble native-like referential use of the L2 words. In addition to refining the referential meaning of L2 words, subsequent L2 exposure and use should also lead to a native-like "intensional" meaning of each L2 word (that is, a "word web" within the L2 lexicon which connects the L2 word with related L2 words, such as its antonyms, synonyms, and hyponyms; see Henriksen, 1999). Furthermore, subsequent L2 exposure and use should gradually lead towards fluency in using the L2 words. This aspect of L2 word learning is as important as acquiring native-like meaning (and form) representations because, even with the targeted lexical structures fully in place, L2 communication will break down if access to and retrieval of these structures consume more mental resources than the processing system has to spare. Finally, subsequent L2 exposure and use is needed to acquire all the L2 words that were not first learned directly in the curriculum. In fact, many have claimed that by far the majority of L2 words are learned from "context" (that is, from naturalistic L2 exposure and use), even though learning from context is a far less effective method to learn *specific* L2 vocabulary than learning through direct instruction (Sternberg, 1987). The ground for the claim that nevertheless most vocabulary is learned from context is that formal instruction time in the classroom is far too limited to teach more than a basic vocabulary directly.

That learning from context is a relatively ineffective way to acquire specific L2 vocabulary has been repeatedly demonstrated in studies that compared the recall of specific L2 words after a text containing these words had just been read for general comprehension, with recall of these same L2 words after the participants had been engaged in vocabulary-centered activities or had just simply been given the L2 target words' translation in L1 (e.g., Hulstijn, Hollander, & Greidanus, 1996; Laufer, 2003). Merely reading the text led to extremely poor recall scores, while adding the target words' L1 translations in the text's margin significantly improved recall (Hulstijn et al., 1996). Even an explicit instruction to the participants to infer the target words' meaning from context leads to very poor recall, except when the inferred meanings are subsequently verified and memorized (Mondria, 2003). The reason the "context method" is as ineffective as it is presumably is that it does not exploit the fact that the learner already has (approximations of the) meanings of the L2 words to learn in memory (namely, the meanings of their translations in L1). In addition to learning the new L2 words' forms, the learner must therefore also figure out their meanings from context, while all the while these meanings are just sitting there in memory. In Sternberg's (1987) words: "If one has definitions available, then learning from context is not so efficient. Why waste a good definition?" (Sternberg, 1987, p. 95).

Word-type effects in L1–L2 word-association learning

As mentioned, the word–word association method (and also the keyword method) *does* provide definitions of the L2 words to acquire in the form of their L1 translations and is therefore an effective method to acquire specific L2 vocabulary. It enables the learner to focus on form learning. Interestingly, the ease with which L2 words (in the narrow sense of new labels for old lexical concepts) are learned by means of this method depends on a number of characteristics of both the new labels to learn (the L2 words' forms) and the L1 words and concepts that are already in place. One common finding is that L2 words are easier to learn if the corresponding L1 words have concrete referents than when they have abstract referents (e.g., de Groot, 2006; van Hell & Candia Mahn, 1997). A second is that L2 words are easier to learn when they have a phonotactic structure typical of L1 words than when they have a phonotactic structure atypical of the learner's L1 (e.g., Ellis & Beaton, 1993; de Groot, 2006). A third is that L2 words with a cognate translation in the L1 are easier to learn than those with a noncognate L1 translation. A final finding is that it is easier to learn L2 words if the corresponding L1 words occur frequently in L1 use than when the latter are infrequent, but this effect is less robust than the other three (de Groot, 2006; de Groot & Keijzer, 2000; Lotto & de Groot, 1998).

Of these four word-type effects, those of cognate status and phonotactical typicality are intuitively the most obvious, because both concern aspects of the new forms to learn: the orthographic and/or phonological form similarity between the L2 words and the corresponding L1 translations (cognate status) and whether or not the new forms have a sound structure that is familiar to the learner. That also L1 word concreteness and word frequency exert an effect on L2 labeling is more surprising, because typically the L2 word forms paired with concrete and frequent L1 words during learning do not systematically differ from those paired with abstract and infrequent L1 words, respectively. This suggests that the representations of the L1 words with which the new L2 forms are paired during learning must somehow cause the effects of L1 concreteness and frequency.

The effect of phonotactical typicality probably partly results from the fact that the learning of L2 words requires the rehearsal of their phonological forms in working memory (e.g., Gathercole & Thorn, 1998). This rehearsal process is hindered if the phonological forms of the new vocabulary are atypical. A further reason is that phonological structures in long-term memory similar to the phonological forms of the L2 words to learn are known to be recruited during learning and to facilitate the learning process (e.g., Service & Craik, 1993). For phonotactically typical L2 words, but not for phonotactically atypical ones, such supporting structures exist in long-term memory. For the same reason cognate translations of L1 words may be easier to learn than noncognate translations. After all, by definition, a cognate L2 word closely resembles at least one other structure in long-term memory, namely, the form of its L1 translation. A further source of the cognate effect is likely facilitated retrieval due to the fact that upon the presentation of a written or spoken word, the memory representations of words with a similar form, be they similar words in the same language or actual cognates or "pseudocognates" in another language (e.g., Hall, 2002), are automatically activated. (A pair of pseudocognates – also called "false cognates" or "accidental cognates" – consists of two words belonging to different languages that share form but not meaning across these languages. Notice that the keyword method discussed above exploits this same process of automatic triggering of similar memory representations: what was called a "keyword" there is a "pseudocognate" in the present terminology.) In other words, if, following training, one element of a cognate translation pair is presented as the recall cue, this stimulus automatically reminds of the other element in the pair.

Regarding the concreteness effect on L2 vocabulary acquisition, de Groot and Keijzer (2000) hypothesized that it might result from different amounts of information stored for concrete and abstract L1 words in memory, on the assumption that the more information stored for the L1 words the easier it is to link their new names, the L2 words, onto them. Two versions of this view were considered, one in terms of Paivio's (1986) "dual coding" theory, which holds that concrete words but not abstract words are represented in memory by means of both an image representation and a verbal representation whereas for abstract words only a verbal representation exists. The second view does not distinguish between verbal and image representations in memory but assumes that all stored knowledge is built from "amodal" information units. In addition, it assumes that the (meaning) representations of concrete words consist of a larger number of these information units than those of abstract words, possibly because only the former have referents that can be experienced by one or more senses: they can be observed and felt, sometimes heard and tasted. These perceptual experiences will lead to the storage of meaning elements that the representations of abstract words lack (see, e.g., de Groot & Keijzer, 2000; de Groot & van Hell, 2005, for more details and supporting evidence). In various publications (e.g., Lotto & de Groot, 1998) it was suggested that the (smaller and less robust) effect of L1 word frequency can also be explained in terms of differential information density of memory representations, those representing frequently used words containing more information units than those representing less frequently used words.

Conclusion

In a way, this review started where a previous review of vocabulary-acquisition studies (de Groot & van Hell, 2005) ended. That earlier review exclusively concerned late L2 vocabulary learning and ended with the statement that the learning processes involved in late L2 vocabulary acquisition and early bilingual vocabulary acquisition "differ crucially because, in early bilingual vocabulary acquisition . . . the acquisition of word form and word meaning proceed in parallel, whereas in late FL [foreign language] vocabulary learning, a meaning for the new word to be learned is already in place" (de Groot & van Hell, 2005, p. 25). It then continued stating that future reviews of studies on foreign language (FL = L2 in the present terminology) vocabulary learning might shift the focus to this neglected issue. This is exactly what was done above. This exercise has hopefully convinced the reader that vocabulary acquisition in monolingual and bilingual L1 acquisition and late L2 vocabulary learning involve very different processes that exploit different skills and knowledge structures. The difference stressed in this review was the presence of approximate meanings of the vocabulary to acquire in late L2 learners' memory but not in L1 learners' memory. In our earlier review we mentioned a second neglected issue, namely, the role of typological distance between L1 and L2 in late L2 vocabulary learning, noting that "the larger the distance between L1 and the FL to be learned . . . the more alien the meanings of the FL words will be to the learner" (p. 25). This implies that in cases of distant L1–L2 language pairs, L2 vocabulary acquisition methods that exploit the L1 meaning representations in the learning process are less effective and it might make sense to shift the balance in the initial stages of learning towards a stronger role for contextual learning. With such a shift to contextual learning, late L2 vocabulary learning would more closely resemble L1 vocabulary learning than when it can maximally exploit extant L1 lexical concepts.

References

Abutalebi, J., Cappa, S. F., & Perani, D. (2005). What can functional neuroimaging tell us about the bilingual brain? In J. F. Kroll & A. M. B. de Groot (Eds.), *Handbook of bilingualism: Psycholinguistic approaches* (pp. 497–515). New York: Oxford University Press.

Beaton, A. A., Gruneberg, M. M., Hyde, C., Shufflebottom, A., & Sykes, R. N. (2005). Facilitation of receptive and productive vocabulary learning using the keyword method: The role of image quality. *Memory, 13*, 458–471.

Best, C. T., & McRoberts, G. W. (2003). Infant perception of non-native consonant contrasts that adults assimilate in different ways. *Language and Speech, 46*, 183–216.

Best, C. T., McRoberts, G. W., & Sithole, N. M. (1988). Examination of perceptual reorganization for nonnative speech contrasts: Zulu click discrimination by English-speaking adults and infants. *Journal of Experimental Psychology: Human Perception and Performance, 14*, 345–360.

Bosch, L., & Sebastián-Gallés, N. (2001). Evidence of early language discrimination abilities in infants from bilingual environments. *Infancy, 2*, 29–49.

Bosch, L., & Sebastián-Gallés, N. (2003a). Simultaneous bilingualism and the perception of a language-specific vowel contrast in the first year of life. *Language and Speech, 46*, 217–243.

Bosch, L., & Sebastián-Gallés, N. (2003b). Language experience and the perception of a voicing contrast in fricatives: Infant and adult data. In M. J. Solé, D. Recasens, & J. Romero (Eds.), *Proceedings of the 15th International Congress of Phonetic Sciences* (pp. 1987–1990). Barcelona: Causal Productions.

Broersma, M. (2006). *Accident-execute: Increased activation in nonnative listening.* Paper presented at Interspeech 2006-ICSLP, ninth international conference on spoken language processing, Pittsburgh PA.

Conboy, B. T., & Mills, D. L. (2006). Two languages, one developing brain: Event-related potentials to words in bilingual toddlers. *Developmental Science, 9*, F1–F12.

De Groot, A. M. B. (2006). Effects of stimulus characteristics and background music on foreign language vocabulary learning and forgetting. *Language Learning, 56*, 463–506.

De Groot, A. M. B. (2011). *Language and cognition in bilinguals and multilinguals: An introduction.* New York: Psychology Press.

De Groot, A. M. B., & Keijzer, R. (2000). What is hard to learn is easy to forget: The roles of word concreteness, cognate status, and word frequency in foreign-language vocabulary learning and forgetting. *Language Learning, 50*, 1–56.

De Groot, A. M. B., & van Hell, J. G. (2005). The learning of foreign language vocabulary. In J. F. Kroll & A. M. B. de Groot (Eds.), *Handbook of bilingualism: Psycholinguistic approaches* (pp. 9–29). New York: Oxford University Press.

Ellis, A. W., & Lambon Ralph, M. A. (2000). Age of acquisition effects in adult lexical processing reflect loss of plasticity in maturing systems: Insights from connectionist networks. *Journal of Experimental Psychology: Learning, Memory, and Cognition, 26*, 1103–1123.

Ellis, N. C., & Beaton, A. (1993). Psycholinguistic determinants of foreign language vocabulary learning. *Language Learning, 43*, 559–617.

Fennell, C. T., Byers-Heinlein, K., & Werker, J. F. (2007). Using speech sounds to guide word learning: The case of bilingual infants. *Child Development, 78*, 1510–1525.

Fenson, L., Pethick, S., Renda, C., Cox, J. L., Dale, P. S., & Reznick, J. S. (2000). Short-form versions of the MacArthur Communicative Development Inventories. *Applied Psycholinguistics, 21*, 95–116.

Friedrich, M., & Friederici, A. D. (2004). N400-like semantic incongruity effect in 19-months-olds: Processing known words in picture contexts. *Journal of Cognitive Neuroscience, 16*, 1465–1477.

Gathercole, S. E., & Thorn, A. S. C. (1998). Phonological short-term memory and foreign-language learning. In A. F. Healy & L. E. Bourne (Eds.), *Foreign-language learning: Psycholinguistic studies on training and retention* (pp. 141–185). Mahwah, NJ: Erlbaum.

Hall, C. J. (2002). The automatic cognate form assumption: Evidence for the parasitic model of vocabulary development. *International Review of Applied Linguistics in Language Teaching (IRAL), 40*, 69–87.

Henriksen, B. (1999). Three dimensions of vocabulary development. *Studies in Second Language Acquisition, 21*, 303–317.

Hulstijn, J. H., Hollander, M., & Greidanus, T. (1996). Incidental vocabulary learning by advanced foreign language students: The influence of marginal glosses, dictionary use, and reoccurrence of unknown words. *The Modern Language Journal, 80*, 327–339.

Junker, D. A., & Stockman, I. J. (2002). Expressive vocabulary of German–English bilingual toddlers. *American Journal of Speech-Language Pathology, 11*, 381–394.

Jusczyk, P. W., Friederici, A. D., Wessels, J. M. I., Svenkerud, V. Y., & Jusczyk, A. M. (1993). Infants' sensitivity to the sound patterns of native language words. *Journal of Memory and Language, 32*, 402–420.

Kuhl, P. K. (2004). Early language acquisition: Cracking the speech code. *Nature Reviews/Neuroscience, 218*, 831–843.

Kuhl, P. K., Tsao, F.-M., & Liu, H.-M. (2003). Foreign-language experience in infancy: Effects of short-term exposure and social interaction on phonetic learning. *Proceedings of the National Academy of Sciences, 100*, 9096–9101.

Laufer, B. (2003). Vocabulary acquisition in a second language: Do learners really acquire most vocabulary by reading? Some empirical evidence. *Canadian Modern Language Review, 59*, 567–588.

Lotto, L., & de Groot, A. M. B. (1998). Effects of learning method and word type on acquiring vocabulary in an unfamiliar language. *Language Learning, 48*, 31–69.

Maye, J., Werker, J. F., & Gerken, L. (2002). Infant sensitivity to distributional information can affect phonetic discrimination. *Cognition, 82*, B100–B111.

McLaughlin, J., Osterhout, L., & Kim, A. (2004). Neural correlates of second-language word learning: Minimal instruction produces rapid change. *Nature Neuroscience, 7*, 703–704.

Mills, D. L., Coffey-Corina, S., & Neville, H. J. (1997). Language comprehension and cerebral specialization from 13 to 20 months. *Developmental Neuropsychology, 13*, 397–445.

Mondria, J. A. (2003). The effects of inferring, verifying, and memorizing on the retention of L2 word meanings. *Studies in Second Language Acquisition, 25*, 473–499.

Nazzi, T., & Bertoncini, J. (2003). Before and after the vocabulary spurt: Two modes of word acquisition? *Developmental Science, 6*, 136–142.

Paivio, A. (1986). *Mental representations: A dual-coding approach.* New York: Oxford University Press.

Pearson, B. Z., & Fernández, S. C. (1994). Patterns of interaction in the lexical growth in two languages of bilingual infants and toddlers. *Language Learning, 44*, 617–653.

Pearson, B. Z., Fernández, S. C., & Oller, D. K. (1993). Lexical development in bilingual infants and toddlers: Comparison to monolingual norms. *Language Learning, 43*, 93–120.

Rivera-Gaxiola, M., Silva-Pereyra, J., & Kuhl, P. K. (2005). Brain potentials to native and non-native speech contrasts in 7- and 11-month old American infants. *Developmental Science, 8*, 162–172.

Saffran, J. R. (2001). Words in a sea of sounds: The output of infant statistical learning. *Cognition, 81*, 149–169.

Saffran, J. R. (2003). Statistical language learning: Mechanisms and constraints. *Current Directions in Psychological Science, 12*, 110–114.

Saffran, J. R., Aslin, R. N., & Newport, E. L. (1996). Statistical learning by 8-months-old infants. *Science, 274*, 1926–1928.

Sebastián-Gallés, N., & Bosch, L. (2002). Building phonotactic knowledge in bilinguals: Role of early exposure. *Journal of Experimental Psychology: Human Perception and Performance, 28*, 974–989.

Sebastián-Gallés, N., & Bosch, L. (2005). Phonology and bilingualism. In J. F. Kroll & A. M. B. de Groot (Eds.), *Handbook of bilingualism: Psycholinguistic approaches* (pp. 68–87). New York: Oxford University Press.

Service, E., & Craik, F. I. M. (1993). Differences between young and older adults in learning a foreign vocabulary. *Journal of Memory and Language, 32*, 608–623.

Steinhauer, K., White, E. J., & Drury, J. E. (2009). Temporal dynamics of late second language acquisition: Evidence from event-related brain potentials. *Second Language Research, 25*, 13–41.

Sternberg, R. J. (1987). Most vocabulary is learned from context. In M. G. McKeown & M. E. Curtis (Eds.), *The nature of vocabulary acquisition* (pp. 89–105). Hillsdale, NJ: Erlbaum.

Sundara, M., Polka, L., & Molnar, M. (2008). Development of coronal stop perception: Bilingual infants keep pace with their monolingual peers. *Cognition, 108*, 232–242.

Tees, R. C., & Werker, J. F. (1984). Perceptual flexibility: Maintenance or recovery of the ability to discriminate non-native speech sounds. *Canadian Journal of Psychology, 38*, 579–590.

Van Hell, J. G., & Candia Mahn, A. (1997). Keyword mnemonics versus rote rehearsal: Learning concrete and abstract foreign words by experienced and inexperienced learners. *Language Learning, 47*, 507–546.

Vihman, M. M., Thierry, G., Lum, J., Keren-Portnoy, T., & Martin, P. (2007). Onset of word form recognition in English, Welsh, and English–Welsh bilingual infants. *Applied Psycholinguistics, 28,* 475–493.

Weber, A., & Cutler, A. (2004). Lexical competition in non-native spoken-word recognition. *Journal of Memory and Language, 50,* 1–25.

Werker, J. F., Cohen, L. B., Lloyd, V. L., Casasola, M., & Stager, C. L. (1998). Acquisition of word–object associations by 14-month-old infants. *Developmental Psychology, 34,* 1289–1309.

Werker, J. F., Fennell, C. T., Corcoran, K. M., & Stager, C. L. (2002). Infants' ability to learn phonetically similar words: Effects of age and vocabulary size. *Infancy, 3,* 1–30.

Werker, J. F., & Tees, R. C. (1984). Cross-language speech perception: Evidence for perceptual reorganization during the first year of life. *Infant Behavior and Development, 7,* 49–63.

Woodward, A. L., Markman, E. M., & Fitzsimmons, C. M. (1994). Rapid word learning in 13- and 18-month-olds. *Developmental Psychology, 30,* 553–566.

24

What ERPs Tell Us About Bilingual Language Processing

Judith F. Kroll, Taomei Guo, and Maya Misra

Although more people in the world are bilingual than monolingual, it is only recently that language researchers have considered the implications of bilingualism for language processing more generally (e.g., Kroll & de Groot, 2005). The upsurge of event-related potential (ERP) and functional magnetic resonance imaging (fMRI) research on language processes has provided a new opportunity to evaluate the consequence of having two languages in the same mind and brain. Contrary to the view that bilinguals are a special population of language users, we take an approach that assumes that bilinguals are in fact universal language users whose performance will more generally inform theories of the constraints and plasticity of language processes and of their interactions with domain-general cognitive processes. Because other contributions to this volume focus extensively on issues of bilingual word recognition (see Dijkstra & van Heuven, Volume 1, Chapter 22), we instead consider another set of research questions on bilingualism that have recently begun to exploit the power associated with comparisons of behavioral and electrophysiological methods. One examines the processes engaged during speech planning when a bilingual must select only one of the two available languages to produce. The second investigates the extent to which the processing of the second language (L2) engages the first language (L1) during the earliest stages of L2 acquisition and once individuals become relatively proficient in the L2. Each of these contexts reflects the persistent activity of the language not in use. We consider the empirical evidence from behavioral and ERP studies that demonstrate the presence of cross-language activity. We then consider the implications of these results for claims about the neural basis for a bilingual advantage in executive function tasks that require the resolution of competition more generally.

The Handbook of the Neuropsychology of Language, First Edition. Edited by Miriam Faust.
© 2012 Blackwell Publishing Ltd. Published 2012 by Blackwell Publishing Ltd.

Overview

A theme in the current research on bilingualism is that both languages are active even under conditions in which it should be logically possible to restrict processing to one language alone. The parallel activity of the bilingual's two languages has been well documented in the domains of visual and spoken word recognition (e.g., Dijkstra, 2005; Marian & Spivey, 2003). The observation in behavioral research is that the activation of lexical alternatives in both languages increases the functional competition that must be resolved to identify a target word. Recent fMRI studies have also begun to identify the neural basis of the hypothesized cross-language competition and its resolution (e.g., van Heuven, Schriefers, Dijkstra, & Hagoort, 2008; Dijkstra & van Heuven, Volume 1, Chapter 22). The bottom-up nature of processing in word recognition makes it not particularly surprising to find activation of candidates in both of the bilingual's two languages. More surprising is the fact that these effects have been observed even when words are presented in sentence context, providing cues that in theory should make it possible to identify the language of the target word with higher certainty (e.g., Duyck, van Assche, Drieghe, & Hartsuiker 2007; Libben & Titone, 2009). Only when the sentence context is highly constrained semantically (e.g., Schwartz & Kroll, 2006; van Hell & de Groot, 2008) or when highly proficient bilinguals are able to "zoom in" to the target language, does evidence of the cross-language activity diminish (e.g., Elston-Güttler, Gunter, & Kotz, 2005).

The persistent activity of the language not in use is also observed in two other contexts in which we might not expect to see it. In planning speech, the events that initiate the production sequence are necessarily based on conceptually mediated processing, such as the intention to express a thought, to name a picture, or to translate a word from one language to the other. Because the act of production is under the speaker's control, it is therefore surprising to see that like word recognition, there is activity of both of the bilingual's languages even when speaking is required in one language alone (e.g., Costa, 2005; Kroll, Bobb, & Wodniecka, 2006). However, the nature of the activated candidates differs in word production and word recognition because speaking is engaged through meaning and only later are word forms available. The question of what is active, how far into speech planning that activity extends, and on what basis language selection eventually allows bilinguals to control spoken utterances has been investigated in the past using behavioral methods and more recently using both ERPs and fMRI methods (for a review of fMRI studies in bilinguals, see Abutalebi & Della Rosa, Volume 1, Chapter 25). Because speech planning is a temporally sequenced task, the use of ERPs is particularly well suited to investigate these issues.

The second counterintuitive example of activity in both of the bilingual's two languages concerns the evidence for the role of the L1 translation equivalent in recognizing and processing words in the L2. Research on bilingual word recognition (e.g., Dijkstra, 2005; Jared & Kroll, 2001; Schwartz, Kroll, & Diaz, 2007), demonstrates that relatively proficient bilinguals activate within-language lexical form relatives, related in orthography and/or phonology to target words. However, unless words in the two languages are cognates, translations that share aspects of their lexical form, activation of the translation equivalent is not usually found, unless the individual is an L2 learner at a relatively early stage of acquiring the L2 (e.g., Kroll & Stewart, 1994). A number of recent studies, however, have shown that even highly proficient bilinguals access the L1 translation equivalent under some circumstances (e.g., Thierry & Wu, 2007). A critical issue then is to understand how those circumstances might be identified, whether they depend on the form of bilingualism or the time course of processing. Like the issues concerning speech planning, ERPs, as a temporally sensitive tool, provide a useful approach for investigating this issue.

In the remainder of this chapter we consider each of these topics, focusing on the way that the recent ERP data might be used to adjudicate between alternative theoretical claims. We then discuss the implications of parallel activation of the two languages for claims concerning the cognitive advantages that have been associated with bilingualism (e.g., Bialystok, 2005). Here again, the comparison of behavioral and neurocognitive data on the cognitive consequences of bilingualism provides a useful analytic tool for identifying mechanisms responsible for the observed cognitive consequences (see van Hell & Tokowicz, 2009, for a related review of ERP studies of syntactic processing in L2).

Bilingual Speech Planning

When monolingual speakers plan to produce even a single word utterance, a series of processes must be engaged to map the intended thought to words and their associated phonology (e.g., Levelt, 1989). The past literature has debated the way in which the component processes of speech planning are sequenced and the degree to which the production system itself is open to interactions across levels of planning (e.g., Dell, 1986; Levelt, Roelofs, & Meyer, 1999; Rapp & Goldrick, 2000; see also Goldrick, Volume 1, Chapter 7). For bilinguals, there is an additional requirement to specify the language of spoken utterances. If bilinguals were able to commit to one language only at an early stage of planning, their performance should resemble that of monolingual speakers. However, all evidence to date suggests that under many, if not most, circumstances, it is difficult for bilinguals to prevent the activity of the language not in use. At issue is how far into planning the activation of the nontarget language extends and what mechanism eventually allows the selection of the intended language and intended utterance to be engaged. It is beyond the scope of the present chapter to do more than briefly review the evidence and debate on this issue, but there are a number of recent detailed discussions on this topic (e.g., Costa, 2005; Finkbeiner, Gollan, & Caramazza, 2006; Kroll et al., 2006). In what follows, we review the main findings of research on bilingual spoken word production, highlighting in particular the way in which

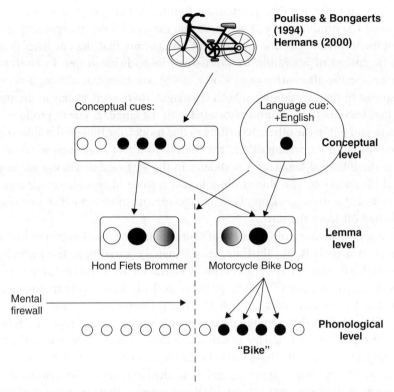

Figure 24.1 A model of bilingual spoken word production (adapted from Hermans, 2000, and Poulisse & Bongaerts, 1994). The "mental firewall" refers to the idea in language specific models that information may be activated in the language not in use but that candidates that result from that activation are not themselves considered for selection (e.g., Costa, 2005).

recent ERP evidence illuminates questions about the locus of cross-language activations and its resolution.

Models of bilingual word production

An illustrative model of bilingual speech planning for a Dutch–English bilingual is shown in Figure 24.1. The model is intended to represent each of the major alternative views about the planning process. According to the competition-for-selection or language nonspecific view (e.g., Green, 1998; Kroll, Bobb, Misra, & Guo, 2008), the flow of information from the event that initiates planning (in this example a picture of a bicycle) activates information at multiple levels of representation in a cascading process. Thus, the conceptual representation of the bicycle will activate abstract lexical representations in both languages (e.g, Dutch and English), and they in turn will activate their respective phonological forms. Although there may be an active language cue that directs attention to intended language in which the utterance should be produced (e.g., English, so that the word "bike" is eventually spoken), the competition-for-selection model does not assume that the cue itself is able to limit the spread of activation to alternatives in both languages. In contrast, the language specific alternative (e.g., Costa, 2005) assumes that although activation may spread to representations in both languages, there is effectively a "mental firewall" that encodes the intention associated with the language cue to produce in one language and not in the other. According to this model, the bilingual is able to ignore the activation on the wrong side of the firewall to direct attention only to alternatives in the intended language. Candidates in the language not in use are not considered for selection. The almost ubiquitous presence of cross-language activation itself rules out a strong version of a language-specific model in which one language is switched off from the start.

Behavioral evidence from a variety of sources has been taken as critical in evaluating these two models. To illustrate, cross-language variants of the picture–word Stroop task ask whether visual or auditory distractor words in one language interfere with the production of a picture's name in the bilingual's other language (e.g., Costa, Miozzo, & Caramazza, 1999; Hermans, Bongaerts, De Bot, & Schreuder, 1998). The result in these bilingual experiments is that Stroop-type interference is observed regardless of language match when the distractor is semantically related to the target to be named. There is also facilitation when the distractor is phonologically related to the target, again regardless of the language of the distractor. While there is some disagreement in this work about whether there is an effect of phonology via the translation, the basic result in these experiments would appear to support the competition-for-selection model since information from the two languages appears largely interchangeable. However, there is also a counterintuitive result when the distractor is itself the name of the picture in the language to be ignored. Although the competition-for-selection model might predict that this condition would produce the most interference of all since it is precisely the word in the wrong language that the speaker is attempting to avoid, the data show that it produces facilitation (see Hermans, 2004, for arguments concerning the translation facilitation result and why it does not itself adjudicate between these alternative interpretations).

Other methods that have been used to examine bilingual production have also produced a mix of results, although most of them provide very clear support for the idea that alternatives in both of the speaker's languages are available prior to speaking even one language alone (see Costa, 2005, and Kroll et al., 2006, 2008, for detailed reviews of these studies). There is robust cognate facilitation in simple picture naming (e.g., Costa, Caramazza, & Sebastián-Gallés, 2000) and the magnitude of cognate facilitation is not reduced in bilinguals who speak different-script languages where cognate status is only based on phonological similarity across translations (Hoshino & Kroll, 2008). Because words are not themselves present in the simple picture naming task, the cognate facilitation effect has been interpreted to mean that activation flows all the way to the phonology of both language alternatives in the scenario depicted in Figure 24.1. When the cross-language phonology converges, facilitation is observed.

In behavioral studies, there is also an effect of language mixture and language switching that suggests that when bilinguals speak the L2, there is necessarily activation of the L1 that must eventually be inhibited to enable L2 production (e.g., Kroll, Dijkstra, Janssen, & Schriefers, 2000; Meuter & Allport, 1999; and see Linck, Kroll, & Sunderman, 2009, for other evidence of inhibition of the L1 in L2 production). A comparison of blocked and mixed picture naming shows that L1 suffers a processing cost in the mixed language context, whereas L2 is relatively unaffected, suggesting that L1 was active regardless of the requirement to keep it active (e.g., Kroll et al., 2000). In the language switching task, the time to name pictures or numbers in the L1 is slower following L2 than when L2 follows L1. That is, there is an asymmetry in the magnitude of switch costs. A great deal has been made of this asymmetry, whether these effects reflect inhibitory processes or not, and whether they are differential as a function of the proficiency level of the bilingual (e.g., Costa & Santestban, 2004; Finkbeiner, Almeida, Janssen, & Caramazza, 2006). Costa and Santesteban found an asymmetry in switch costs for nonproficient L2 speakers but symmetry for proficient bilinguals. However, even when there was symmetry in the switch costs, the L1 was slower than the L2, suggesting a pattern of inhibitory processing (e.g., Kroll et al., 2008). What seems clear in recent work is that the switch cost asymmetry does not provide the entire story on selection processes as it may disappear when bilinguals switch between two languages spontaneously (e.g., Gollan & Ferreira, 2009).

ERP studies on lexical selection in bilingual language processing

More recently, ERPs have been used to examine the earliest stages of speech planning and to investigate the basis of language selection. In the past, there were few ERP studies of spoken production because of concerns about movement artifact. A combination of technical and design innovations have now made it possible to investigate the time course of planning during actual or tacit naming (e.g., Schmitt, Rodriguez-Fornells, Kutas, & Münte, 2001; van Turennout, Hagoort, & Brown, 1997). Compared to other imaging methods, ERPs have high temporal resolution and permit a sensitive analysis of ongoing cognitive processes on the basis of the mean amplitude, peak, and/or peak latency of distinct ERP components. Behavioral measures alone may reflect only the aggregate result of this process, but ERPs have the promise to illuminate the time course of the earliest stages engaged when bilinguals begin to plan the words they intend to speak. A comparison of the behavioral and ERP measures may provide a particularly effective means to track processes that unfold rapidly over time.

ERP studies of lexical selection in bilingual language processing have focused on the question of whether bilinguals need to inhibit the activation of the nontarget language by considering the role of a specific ERP component, the N2 (sometimes also referred to as the N200). The N2 is a negative ERP component with a fronto-central distribution over the scalp which reaches its peak at approximately 300 ms after stimulus onset. Some researchers believe it reflects the individual's inhibition of a response (e.g., Falkenstein, Hoormann, & Hohnsbein, 1999), while others think that it may reflect the individual's perception of response conflict (Nieuwenhuis, Yeung, van den Wildenberg, & Ridderinkhof , 2003). Although there is still controversy about the interpretation of the N2, there is an agreement that it may be used as an index of a general control process (Nieuwenhuis, Yeung, & Cohen, 2004).

According to the inhibitory control model (Green, 1998), bilinguals select words in the intended language by inhibiting the activation of the unintended language, and the degree of inhibition will be enhanced if the activation of the unintended language is strong. Therefore, language switching conditions should lead to a more negative N2 component. To date, three ERP studies on bilingual language selection have used the switching paradigm to investigate this issue and these studies have produced a mixed pattern of results. Jackson, Swainson, Cunnington, and Jackson (2001) initially reported that language switch conditions elicited a stronger N2 component than no-switch conditions. They called this the N2 effect of language switching and claimed to provide physiological evidence for the bilingual inhibitory control model. However, subsequent ERP studies examining similar conditions have not fully replicated their results.

In the Jackson et al. (2001) study, bilingual participants were asked to name one of the digits (1 to 9) in either L1 or L2 according to its background color. In order to avoid naming artifacts in the EEG data and expectations about upcoming stimuli, the digits were presented on the screen for either 250 ms or 1000 ms, and participants were instructed to name the digits after they disappeared from the screen. Reaction times were collected at the short presentation time, while ERPs for the switching effects were analyzed for the long presentation time. Behaviorally, the study replicated the findings of the previous language switching studies (e.g., Meuter & Allport, 1999). Critically, in the ERP data, Jackson et al. found that the L2 switching condition elicited a more pronounced N2 than the L2 nonswitching condition, while there was no significant N2 effect for L1. They concluded that these data demonstrated the existence of inhibition of L1 in L2 production, but also pointed out that the asymmetric switch cost in the ERP data is different from the behavioral switch cost, in which a greater switching cost is observed for the L1 than for the L2.

Christoffels, Firk, and Schiller (2007) performed an ERP study with German–Dutch bilinguals to further investigate the effects of language switching and language mixing in spoken production. Unlike the digit naming task used by Jackson et al. (2001), Christoffels et al. (2007) used a picture naming task and a sample of bilinguals who actively used their native language in everyday life. Furthermore, this study did not use delayed naming as Jackson et al. (2001) did, but instead simply asked participants to name pictures as quickly and accurately as possible, a procedure more similar to the previously published behavioral studies of language switching. In two blocked language naming conditions, bilinguals named pictures in either L1 or L2 only. In the mixed naming conditions, they named pictures in either L1 or L2 depending on the background color of pictures which cued one of the two languages. Significant N2 effects were found for L1 but not for L2. However, it should be noted that the direction of the N2 effect was opposite to that in the Jackson et al. (2001) study. That is, a larger N2 was elicited in L1 nonswitching condition than in L1 switching condition, although Christoffels et al. (2007) also interpreted their results as providing evidence for bilingual inhibition. Furthermore, a significant language context effect was revealed by comparing the blocked naming condition and nonswitch trials from the mixed naming condition for each language. Both languages revealed a greater negativity for nonswitch trials in the mixed naming conditions relative to the blocked naming conditions. Christoffels et al. (2007) concluded that a more global level of bilingual inhibition indicated by the language list context effect should be distinguished from the local level inhibition indicated by the trial-to-trial language switching effect.

In a more recent ERP study, Verhoef, Roelofs, and Chwilla (2009) asked relatively proficient but unbalanced Dutch–English bilinguals to name pictures in the appropriate language, according to a visually presented cue (the Dutch flag or the British flag), as quickly and accurately as possible. Like Christoffels et al. (2007), they did not use the delayed naming task, but unlike the previous studies they included two different delays between the language cue and the stimulus (i.e., stimulus cue intervals, SCIs), one at 750 ms and the other at 1500 ms. No significant N2 effect was found in language switch conditions relative to the nonswitch conditions, but there was a significant effect of the SCI on the N2 effect. Specifically, except for the L1 nonswitch condition, the other three conditions elicited a more negative N2 component at the long SCI than at the short SCI. As such, these results failed to support the predictions of the bilingual inhibitory control model and Verhoef et al. argued instead for the L1-repeat-benefit hypothesis, according to which bilinguals do not necessarily inhibit the activation of the nontarget language during speech production.

To summarize, the first two of the recent ERP studies using the language switching paradigm found a significant N2 effect for switch trials and provided ERP evidence for the bilingual inhibitory control model. The Verhoef et al. (2009) study showed that the response preparation time had a significant effect on the N2 component, leading them to posit an interpretation of the results that does not require active inhibition of candidates in the language not to be spoken. A possible reason for the apparent discrepancies across studies is that these studies differed in the presentation procedures that were used. Specifically, Jackson et al. (2001) and Christoffels et al. (2007) presented a naming cue and a stimulus digit or picture simultaneously. In this case, bilinguals cannot begin to select the correct language and the correct word until they see the cue and the stimulus. As both languages are activated to a high level, the selection process is difficult, making inhibition necessary. However, the Verhoef et al. (2009) study presented a visual naming cue 750 or 1500 ms before the onset of the picture to be named, potentially making it easier for bilinguals to prepare for a picture's name in advance and thus less competitive to select an appropriate language. From this point of view, the results of these studies may not be in conflict with each other. Under conditions that enhance competition,

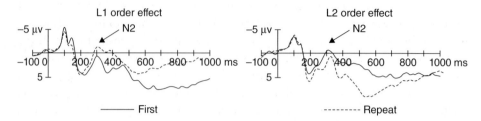

Figure 24.2   Grand average ERP waveforms at electrode site Cz for blocked picture naming in L1 and L2 as a function of the order of the language blocks. Data are adapted from Misra et al. (under review).

greater inhibitory control may be required prior to language selection. Increased preparation time may reduce the effective stress on the system and lessen the requirement for inhibition.

If this account is correct, then conditions that effectively bias speech planning to one of the bilingual's two languages should also reduce the observed inhibition. In a recent ERP study in our lab (Misra, Guo, Bobb, & Kroll, under review), we compared picture naming in blocked conditions when Chinese–English bilinguals named a set of pictures in L1 followed by a block of pictures in L2 or the reverse, naming in L2 before L1. The results, a portion of which are shown in Figure 24.2, revealed a clear inhibitory effect for the L1 when naming in L1 followed naming in L2. Naming in the L1 after naming the same pictures in L2 produced more negative waveforms than initially naming the pictures in L1. What is surprising is that this block order effect occurred even though the pictures were only repeated after many intervening trials, suggesting, like the results of the Christoffels et al. (2007) study, that there is a global effect of inhibition of the L1. This inhibitory effect is similar to a switch cost, but its distribution is much wider, indicating that different neural mechanisms may be involved in global and local inhibition. The opposite pattern was observed for L2, where waveforms for the second block were more positive than the first. Because pictures were repeated across blocks in the design of this study, the effect in L2 is likely to reflect repetition priming, with benefits following naming of the same pictures in L1. Of course the same repetition priming of pictures should be present for picture naming in the L1, suggesting that the apparent inhibition of L1 seen in Figure 24.2 is, if anything, an underestimate of the true magnitude of inhibition. It is interesting to note that in other paradigms we have also found evidence for global inhibition, for example under conditions in which L2 learners are immersed in a study-abroad context in which there are reduced opportunities to use the L1 (see Linck et al., 2009). Likewise, recent fMRI studies show that language selection during bilingual speech appears to impose specific processing associated with areas of the brain associated with inhibitory control (e.g., Abutalebi & Green, 2007).

Research on the neural basis of speech planning in bilinguals is at an early stage of development but the initial results of the first studies examining these issues suggest that the emerging ERP evidence is beginning to converge with the results of behavioral studies that show that both languages are active during speech planning and that it may be necessary to suppress the more active language to enable planning to proceed for the weaker of the bilingual's two languages.

Activation of the L1 Translation Equivalent

Research on L2 acquisition suggests that during early stages of learning, adult learners rely heavily on the transfer of information from the L1 at all levels of linguistic knowledge, from the lexicon and phonology to the grammar (e.g., MacWhinney, 2005; but see Dussias, 2003, and Nosarti, Mechelli, Green, & Price, 2010, for examples of cross-language influences from L2 to L1). One line of research has examined the way that transfer occurs at the lexical level to enable the development of the foundational vocabulary knowledge that will ultimately contribute to proficient L2 language use. These studies have been conducted with actual adult L2 learners and also in laboratory simulations in the context of vocabulary training studies (e.g., see de Groot & van Hell, 2005, for a review).

The revised hierarchical model (Kroll & Stewart, 1994) was initially proposed to account for findings that suggested that early in L2 learning there is reliance on the L1 translation equivalent to access the meaning of the L2 word (e.g., Kroll, Michael, Tokowicz, & Dufour, 2002; Kroll & Stewart, 1994; Talamas, Kroll, & Dufour, 1999). According to the model, adult learners exploit the existing mappings between words and concepts in their L1 to enable new L2 words to be added to the lexical network. Once they have established mappings between words and concepts in L2, the links that first mediated access via the L1 were hypothesized to no longer be necessary. This account of the role of the L1 translation equivalent in accessing the meaning of L2 words was actively debated after the revised hierarchical model was published in 1994. A series of studies using different paradigms claimed that there was little evidence for lexical mediation and that instead, even learners at early stages of L2 acquisition were capable of directly understanding the meanings of L2 words (e.g., Altarriba & Mathis, 1997; de Groot & Poot, 1997; Duyck & Brysbaert, 2004). Other studies provided support for the developmental progression suggested by the revised hierarchical model, with initial reliance on the translation equivalent giving way to direct semantic processing for the L2 (e.g., Sunderman & Kroll, 2006; Talamas et al., 1999; and see Kroll, van Hell, Tokowicz, & Green, 2010, for a review and analysis of the discrepant findings).

ERP evidence on acquisition

An ERP study by Thierry and Wu (2007) renewed interest in the debate about the role of translation equivalents during L2 processing. ERP studies of L2 processing have sometimes revealed implicit processes that cannot be observed in the behavioral record. For example, McLaughlin, Osterhout, and Kim (2004) demonstrated that foreign language learners in a classroom setting who had only had a few months of exposure to the L2, began to reveal sensitivity to the L2 in the ERP record (indexed by a N400 response) at the same time that their behavioral performance remained at chance (see Tokowicz & MacWhinney, 2005, for related evidence on the processing of the L2 grammar; and Osterhout et al., 2008, for a more extensive review of this approach). Thierry and Wu hoped to capitalize on the potential for ERPs to reveal aspects of processing not revealed in behavior and asked relatively proficient Chinese–English bilinguals to perform a semantic relatedness judgment in English, their L2. The bilinguals were living in the UK and had extensive immersion experience in English. Unbeknownst to the participants, the Chinese translations of the English words sometimes contained shared characters. The presence of shared Chinese characters was independent of whether the English words were semantically related or not. If proficient Chinese–English bilinguals can access the meaning of words in English without mediation via the Chinese translation, then performance on an English-only task should not be influenced by the form of the L1 translation and in other respects should resemble the performance of monolingual speakers in English. Thierry and Wu found that the amplitude of the N400 response was reduced for conditions in which the translations of the English words shared a character in Chinese. The result suggests that even relatively proficient bilinguals access the L1 translation when processing words in the L2. A control group of monolingual speakers of English showed none of these effects, suggesting that they were a genuine reflection of bilingualism and not a special property of the experimental materials.

The Thierry and Wu (2007) ERP data are potentially problematic for all sides of the acquisition debate. From the perspective of the revised hierarchical model, only learners at early stages should be sensitive to the L1 translation equivalent. The Chinese–English bilinguals in the Thierry and Wu study were easily at a level of proficiency that should have enabled L2 to function independently. From the perspective of those who argue that the meaning of L2 words is available directly (e.g., Brysbaert & Duyck, 2010), these findings provide an exception and further suggest that behavioral measures of response time and accuracy may not be adequately sensitive to adjudicate this issue. Behaviorally, the Chinese–English bilinguals in the Thierry and Wu study did not respond differentially to the presence of repeated Chinese characters. In that respect, their results were similar to behavioral findings with other proficient L2 speakers (e.g., Sunderman & Kroll, 2006; Talamas et al., 1999).

One interpretation of these results is that different-script bilinguals, like the Chinese–English bilinguals in the Thierry and Wu (2007) study, follow a different developmental course of L2 learning than same-script bilinguals. Most of the previous behavioral studies have examined the performance of same-script bilinguals, like the English–Spanish bilinguals in Sunderman and Kroll's (2006) study. Studies of bilingual word recognition that have examined the performance of same-script bilinguals (e.g., Dutch–English, Spanish–English, or German–English bilinguals) have shown that cross-language ambiguity gives rise to the parallel activation of similar lexical forms in both languages (e.g., Dijkstra, 2005). When languages share orthography, there is greater opportunity for cross-language ambiguity than under circumstances in which only the phonology can be similar. It may be the case that when the activation of visually related forms in the other language are blocked, as in the case of different-script bilingualism, the translation is more likely to be activated directly. Another recent behavioral study (Morford, Wilkinson, Villwock, Piñar, & Kroll, 2011) provides some support for this hypothesis. Morford et al. replicated the Thierry and Wu study but using deaf bilinguals whose two languages, American Sign Language (ASL) and written English, do not share the same modality. Again, the bilingual participants judged the semantic relatedness of two English words. In the Morford et al. study, some of the related and unrelated pairs had ASL translations that were similar in form. Both relatively proficient and less proficient ASL–English bilinguals were sensitive to the presence of the similarity in the form of the translation, suggesting that the L1 translation is activated even when it is not logically required by the task, even when the bilinguals are highly proficient in the L2, and even when the two languages do not share the same modality.

The time course of activating the translation equivalent

To investigate the basis of the apparent discrepancies across studies concerning the role of the L1 translation, Guo, Misra, Tam, and Kroll (under review) used an ERP paradigm with Chinese–English bilinguals, like the Thierry and Wu (2007) study, but with the translation recognition task used in the earlier behavioral studies that has demonstrated a developmental shift from reliance on the translation to relative independence with increasing L2 skill. The conditions in the Guo et al. study were similar to those used by Talamas et al. (1999) and Sunderman and Kroll (2006). Two words, one in each language, were presented, with the L2 word followed by the L1 word. On half of the trials, the L1 was the correct translation of the L2 words. On the remaining trials, it was an incorrect translation. The task was simply to judge whether the second word was the correct translation of the first word. Critically, the incorrect translations included trials in which there was an L1 word that resembled the form of the correct L1 translation (translation neighbors) and trials in which the L1 word was related in meaning (semantic distractors) to the correct translation. Other incorrect translation trials were matched controls that were completely unrelated to the target word. If different-script bilinguals are more likely than same-script bilinguals to access the translation equivalent of the L2 word, then the relatively proficient Chinese–English bilinguals in the Guo et al. study were predicted to produce interference when the incorrect translation was similar in form to the correct translation. This predicted pattern differs from the behavioral data

reported by Sunderman and Kroll for relatively proficient English–Spanish bilinguals who showed no effect of distractors similar in form to the translation equivalent, although less proficient L2 learners were sensitive to the translation distractors.
Guo et al. also hypothesized that, like the Thierry and Wu study, the ERP record
might reveal sensitivity to the translation equivalent that was not apparent in the
behavioral record.

Guo et al. (under review) found that relatively proficient Chinese–English bilinguals produced significant interference in the behavioral data for distractors that
were translation neighbors, as well as for semantically related distractors. Response
times to reject incorrect translations in each of the critical conditions were longer
than response times to reject unrelated controls. The magnitude of interference was
similar for the two types of distractors. Like Thierry and Wu (2007) and Morford
et al. (in press), these data show that even highly proficient bilinguals who are
immersed in the L2 environment appear to access the translation equivalent when
they process words in the L2. Furthermore, like Thierry and Wu's results, Guo et al.
found ERP results that supported these differences. Also, the ERPs revealed differences in the processing underlying the two behavioral interference effects. Figure
24.3 shows the grand averages for the ERP data for the Cz electrode site. The data
in the top panel are for the semantically related and unrelated word pairs. The data
in the bottom panel are for the translation neighbors and unrelated controls.
Crucially, unlike the behavioral data, which showed a similar pattern of interference
for both types of distractors, the ERP data suggest that there is a distinct time course
of processing associated with the two distractor conditions.

Guo et al. (under review) speculated that the nature of the ERP design itself, and
in particular the use of a relatively long stimulus onset asynchrony (SOA) of 750 ms

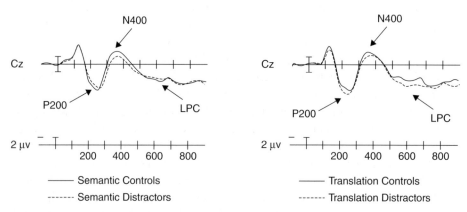

Figure 24.3 Grand average ERP waveforms at electrode site Cz for translation recognition
performance for L1 words following L2 words related in meaning (semantic distractors) to
the translation equivalent or unrelated to the L1 word (top panel), and for L1 words following L2 words related in form to the translation equivalent (translation neighbors) or unrelated to the L1 words (bottom panel). Data are adapted from Guo et al. (under review).

between the two words might have contributed to the results. On this account, it is possible that relatively proficient bilinguals access the L1 translation when the conditions of processing encourage or require it, but that under ordinary time pressures, their skill in the L2 allows them to access meaning directly. To test this hypothesis, they performed a behavioral study in which the SOA was reduced to 300 ms. Under these conditions there were robust effects for the semantic distractors, but little effect of the translation neighbors. Taken together, the combined ERP and behavioral data suggest that proficient bilinguals do indeed access the translation equivalent, but only after they have already accessed the meaning of the L2 word. Without the differential time course data in the ERP record, it would have been otherwise difficult to understand that what seemed like discrepant results are actually two different aspects of the same process. For learners, it may be necessary to mediate access to meaning for L2 via the L1. For proficient bilinguals, the translation may become active as other semantic alternatives emerge and when the time course is sufficient to reveal its presence. These different effects of the translation equivalent stand in contrast to the robust effect of lexical neighbors themselves that are observed for both L2 learners and skilled bilinguals (e.g., Dijkstra, 2005; Sunderman & Kroll, 2006; van Heuven et al., 2008). These are two different manifestations of the activity of the language not in use, one that has clear developmental implications and the other that appears to be ubiquitous across the course of development.

Access to semantics

There is another side to this debate that has also been informed by ERP research with bilinguals. Although there is a great deal of support for the claim that the semantics are largely shared across the bilingual's two languages (e.g., Francis, 2005) and fMRI evidence suggesting that the same neural tissue supports both the L1 and L2 (e.g., Abutalebi, Cappa, & Perani, 2005), there is still disagreement about whether all bilinguals, regardless of their learning histories and proficiency, are able to fully access the semantics for the L2 (e.g., Kotz & Elston-Güttler, 2004; Silverberg & Samuel, 2004). Kotz and Elston-Güttler examined the N400 priming effect that is typically observed in ERP studies investigating semantic priming. The question in their study was whether highly proficient but late bilinguals would reveal the N400 priming effect and, if so, whether it would be modulated by the nature of the semantic relation. They found that late bilinguals produced the N400 effect but only for words that were related by virtue of a high degree of association. For words with a categorical relation, the high proficiency late bilinguals appeared to be insensitive to priming within the ERP record. Less proficient bilinguals produced neither type of priming. It will remain to be seen how this issue is eventually resolved, because data from a range of sources lead to rather different conclusions about whether skill alone is the factor that determines whether or not bilinguals have complete access to the semantics in the L2.

The Cognitive Consequences of Bilingualism

In the studies reviewed above, we presented evidence that provides compelling support for the claim that both languages are always active when bilinguals process one language alone. What is the consequence of the continual need to juggle the competition across the two languages? Recent studies on the cognitive consequence of bilingualism suggest that the expertise acquired by learning to effectively select the language to be used imparts a number of distinct advantages to cognition itself that extend beyond language processing. We consider some of that evidence here and, in particular, the studies that suggest that bilingual language experience has consequences that are manifest in brain function as well as behavior.

In an extensive series of studies with young bilingual children, Bialystok and colleagues have shown that bilingual children outperform their monolingual counterparts on tasks that require irrelevant information to be ignored and conflict among competing alternatives to be resolved (see Bialystok, 1999, 2005, for reviews of this work). These cognitive advantages are observed for a wide range of bilingual children, suggesting that they are not simply a reflection of group differences between bilinguals and monolinguals.

More recently, similar findings have been obtained in adults and elderly bilinguals by using cognitive tasks such as the Simon task that index performance in the domain of executive control. In one version of the Simon task, participants are instructed to judge the color (e.g., pressing a left button for red or pressing a right button for blue) of a square while ignoring its location (e.g., left or right) on the computer screen. The squares with the congruent color and location are termed "congruent trials," while those with incongruent color and location are termed "incongruent trials." For the latter trials, participants need to inhibit an inappropriate response (e.g., press a left button) in order to make a correct response (e.g., press a right button to a blue box presented on the left). The response-time difference between the incongruent trials and congruent trials is termed as the Simon effect, and is a good measure of an individual's ability to block interference. If bilinguals indeed have a potential advantage in cognitive control compared with monolinguals, then they should produce a smaller Simon effect. This is precisely what was observed in a study by Bialystok, Craik, Klein, and Viswanathan (2004). The striking result is that bilingualism appears to provide special protection against the rate of cognitive aging. Although the magnitude of the Simon effect increases overall as individuals age, and that is true for both bilinguals and monolinguals, the rate of decline is slower for bilinguals than for age-matched monolinguals.

Other recent studies have attempted to identify the particular components of executive function that are affected by bilingualism (e.g., Bialystok, Craik, & Ryan, 2006). Although the consequences of bilingualism are sometimes more dramatic in very young bilingual children and in elderly bilinguals, for whom cognitive resources may be stressed and more likely to reveal these effects, the recent literature makes clear that the bilingual advantage in executive function can also be observed in young adult bilinguals who are at the top of their cognitive form (e.g., Costa, Hernandez, & Sebastián-Gallés, 2008).

A number of recent studies have begun to investigate the neural basis of the observed cognitive benefits. For example, Bialystok et al. (2005) investigated this issue using magnetoencephalography (MEG). In this study, Cantonese–English bilinguals, French–English bilinguals, and English monolinguals performed the Simon task while their MEG signals were recorded. A significant Simon effect was found in all three groups of participants. However, the neural mechanism for the Simon effect observed in bilinguals and monolinguals was different. In bilinguals, faster responses were correlated with increased activation of the superior and middle temporal cingulate and the superior and inferior frontal areas. In monolinguals, only the middle frontal regions were found to be related to the faster responses (and see Mechelli et al., 2004, for structural imaging evidence on the difference between bilingual and monolingual brains).

Although the evidence for a bilingual advantage in executive control is fascinating, these data are correlational and their causal basis is largely unknown. If bilinguals gain expertise by virtue of the constant requirement to reduce competition across the two languages, then we might expect to see a general advantage for bilinguals with a range of different types of language experience. A recent study by Emmorey, Luk, Pyers, and Bialystok (2008) tested the specific hypothesis that the bilingual advantage in executive control arises in response to resolving competition during spoken production. That is, the very act of language selection on which we focused earlier in this chapter, is proposed to be the locus of the cognitive consequences to executive control. Because bilinguals can only speak one language at a time, a choice must be made each time a word is spoken. To test this hypothesis, Emmorey et al. compared the performance of unimodal bilinguals who speak each of their two languages with bimodal bilinguals who speak one language and sign the other. The bimodal bilinguals in this study were children of deaf adults (CODAs), who grew up as early bilinguals in ASL and English. Previous research on bimodal bilinguals has shown that very similar cross-language interactions are observed between sign and speech as between two spoken languages (e.g., Emmorey, Borinstein, Thompson, & Gollan, 2008). However, bimodal bilingualism differs from unimodal bilingualism in the respect that it is possible to code blend, i.e., to produce signs and speech in parallel. Thus a choice is not required for selection for bimodal bilinguals in the same way that it is for unimodal bilinguals. If the bilingual advantage is due to the specific requirement to choose one alternative from competing speech candidates, then only unimodal bilinguals should be advantaged. If the effect is attributable to a more abstract level of competition, then both types of bilinguals should show the advantage. All bilingual participants performed a flanker task and their performance was compared to monolingual controls. The results showed that only the unimodal (speech–speech) bilinguals were advantaged relative to the monolinguals. The bimodal (speech–sign) bilinguals were no different than the monolinguals. The pattern of results is consistent with the hypothesis that it is competition along the speech channel that is critical in producing more domain-general benefits to cognition.

Although the results of the Emmorey, Luk, et al. (2008) study are of great interest, recent findings on bilingual infants challenge the conclusion that it is speech alone that produces the bilingual advantage to attentional control. Kovács and Mehler (2009) reported findings that show that even 7-month bilingual infants have an advantage in executive function ability compared to age-matched monolingual controls. Bilingual infants raised in a bilingual household demonstrated that they could exploit cues to anticipate the side of a computer screen on which they would see a puppet. Because 7-month-old infants do not speak, the results suggest that bilingual advantages to cognitive control cannot be due only to language selection during speech production. Understanding the way in which the language processes we described earlier in this chapter map to these cognitive changes is a topic of great promise for future research.

Conclusion

In this chapter we have reviewed a set of findings on bilingual language processing that suggest that bilinguals actively juggle the competition across their two languages to enable spoken production and to acquire proficient skill in the L2. The mental juggling that they appear to do has consequences for language performance, as indexed in behavioral studies and also in the time course of processing as indexed by the ERP record. The behavioral and electrophysiological data that we have presented suggests that the comparison across methods provides an important source of evidence to constrain theories of bilingual language processing. Because much of this research is still in its infancy, there remain many questions that are as yet unanswered. We anticipate this next phase of neurocognitive studies will be critical not only in resolving ongoing debates about bilingual performance and L2 learning, but also for demonstrating that research on bilingualism provides a unique tool for informing theories of language and cognition more generally.

Note

The writing of this article was supported by NIH Grant R01-HD053146 to Judith F. Kroll, Taomei Guo, and Maya Misra and NSF Grant BCS-0955090 to Judith F. Kroll. Correspondence can be directed to Judith F. Kroll, 641 Moore Building, Department of Psychology, Pennsylvania State University, University Park, PA 16802 USA. E-mail: jfk7@psu.edu.

References

Abutalebi, J., Cappa, S. F., & Perani, D. (2005). What can functional neuroimaging tell us about the bilingual brain? In J. F. Kroll & A. M. B. de Groot (Eds.), *Handbook of bilingualism: Psycholinguistic approaches* (pp. 497–515). New York: Oxford University Press.

Abutalebi, J., & Green, D. W. (2007). Bilingual language production: The neurocognition of language representation and control. *Journal of Neurolinguistics, 20*, 242–275.

Altarriba, J., & Mathis, K. M. (1997). Conceptual and lexical development in second language acquisition. *Journal of Memory and Language, 36*, 550–568.

Bialystok, E. (1999). Cognitive complexity and attentional control in the bilingual mind. *Child Development, 70*, 636–644.

Bialystok, E. (2005). Consequences of bilingualism for cognitive development. In J. F. Kroll & A. M. B. de Groot (Eds.), *Handbook of bilingualism: Psycholinguistic approaches* (pp. 417–432). New York: Oxford University Press.

Bialystok, E., Craik, F. I. M., Grady, C., Chau, W., Ishii, R., Gunji, A., et al. (2005). Effect of bilingualism on cognitive control in the Simon task: Evidence from MEG. *NeuroImage, 24*, 40–49.

Bialystok, E., Craik, F. I. M., Klein, R., & Viswanathan, M. (2004). Bilingualism, aging, and cognitive control: Evidence from the Simon task. *Psychology and Aging, 19*, 290–303.

Bialystok, E., Craik, F. I. M., & Ryan, J. (2006). Executive control in a modified antisaccade task: Effects of aging and bilingualism. *Journal of Experimental Psychology: Learning, Memory, and Cognition, 32*, 1341–1354.

Brysbaert, M., & Duyck, W. (2010). Is it time to leave behind the revised hierarchical model of bilingual language processing after 15 years of service? *Bilingualism: Language and Cognition, 13*, 359–371.

Carlson, S. M., & Meltzoff, A. N. (2008). Bilingual experience and executive functioning in young children. *Developmental Science, 11*, 282–298.

Christoffels, I. K., Firk, C., & Schiller, N. O. (2007). Bilingual language control: An event-related brain potential study. *Brain research, 1147*, 192–208.

Costa, A. (2005). Lexical access in bilingual production. In J. F. Kroll & A. M. B. de Groot (Eds.), *Handbook of bilingualism: Psycholinguistic approaches* (pp. 308–325). New York: Oxford University Press.

Costa, A., Caramazza, A., & Sebastián-Gallés, N. (2000). The cognate facilitation effect: Implications for the model of lexical access. *Journal of Experimental Psychology: Learning, Memory, and Cognition, 26*, 1283–1296.

Costa, A., Hernandez, M., & Sebastián-Gallés, N. (2008). Bilingualism aids conflict resolution: Evidence from the ANT task. *Cognition, 106*, 59–86.

Costa, A., Miozzo, M., & Caramazza, A. (1999). Lexical selection in bilinguals: Do words in the bilingual's two lexicons compete for selection? *Journal of Memory and Language, 41*, 365–397.

Costa, A., & Santesteban, M. (2004). Lexical access in bilingual speech production: Evidence from language switching in highly proficient bilinguals and L2 learners. *Journal of Memory and Language, 50*, 491–511.

De Groot, A. M. B., & Poot, R. (1997). Word translation at three levels of proficiency in a second language: The ubiquitous involvement of conceptual memory. *Language Learning, 47*, 215–264.

De Groot, A. M. B., & van Hell, J. G. (2005). The learning of foreign language vocabulary. In J. F. Kroll & A. M. B. de Groot (Eds.), *Handbook of bilingualism: Psycholinguistic approaches* (pp. 9–29). Oxford: Oxford University Press.

Dell, G. S. (1986). A spreading activation theory of retrieval in sentence production. *Psychological Review, 93*, 283–321.

Dijkstra, T. (2005). Bilingual word recognition and lexical access. In J. F. Kroll & A. M. B. de Groot (Eds.), *Handbook of bilingualism: Psycholinguistic approaches* (pp. 179–201). New York: Oxford University Press.

Dussias, P. E. (2003). Syntactic ambiguity resolution in L2 learners: Some effects of bilinguality on LI and L2 processing strategies. *Studies in Second Language Acquisition, 25*, 529–557.

Duyck, W., & Brysbaert, M. (2004). Forward and backward number translation requires conceptual mediation in both balanced and unbalanced bilinguals. *Journal of Experimental Psychology: Human Perception and Performance, 30*, 889–906.

Duyck, W., van Assche, E., Drieghe, D., & Hartsuiker, R. J. (2007). Visual word recognition by bilinguals in a sentence context: Evidence for nonselective access. *Journal of Experimental Psychology: Learning, Memory, and Cognition, 33*, 663–679.

Elston-Güttler, K. E., Gunter, T. C., & Kotz, S. A. (2005). Zooming into L2: Global language context and adjustment affect processing of interlingual homographs in sentences. *Cognitive Brain Research, 25*, 57–70.

Emmorey, K. , Borinstein, H. B., Thompson, R., & Gollan, T. H. (2008). Bimodal bilingualism. *Bilingualism: Language and Cognition, 11*, 43–61.

Emmorey, K., Luk, G., Pyers, J. E., & Bialystok, E. (2008). The source of enhanced cognitive control in bilinguals. *Psychological Science, 19*, 1201–1206.

Falkenstein, M., Hoormann, J., & Hohnsbein. J. (1999). ERP components in go/no-go tasks and their relation to inhibition. *Acta Psychologica, 101*, 267–291.

Finkbeiner, M., Almeida, J., Janssen, N., & Caramazza, A. (2006). Lexical selection in bilingual speech production does not involve language suppression. *Journal of Experimental Psychology: Learning, Memory, and Cognition, 32*, 1075–1089.

Finkbeiner, M., Gollan, T., & Caramazza, A. (2006). Lexical access in bilingual speakers: What's the (hard) problem? *Bilingualism: Language and Cognition , 9*, 153–166.

Francis, W. S. (2005). Bilingual semantic and conceptual representation. In J. F. Kroll & A. M. B. de Groot (Eds.), *Handbook of bilingualism: Psycholinguistic approaches* (pp. 251–267). New York: Oxford University Press.

Gollan, T. H., & Ferreria, V. S. (2009). Should I stay or should I switch? A cost-benefit analysis of voluntary language switching in young and aging bilinguals. *Journal of Experimental Psychology: Learning, Memory, and Cognition, 35*, 640–665.

Green, D. (1998). Mental control of the bilingual lexico-semantic system. *Bilingualism: Language and Cognition 1*, 67–81.

Guo, T., Misra, M., Tam, J. W., & Kroll, J. F. (under review). *On the time course of accessing meaning in a second language: An electrophysiological investigation of translation recognition.*

Hermans, D. (2000). *Word production in a foreign language* (Unpublished doctoral dissertation). University of Nijmegen, Nijmegen, The Netherlands.

Hermans, D. (2004). Between-language identity effects in picture–word interference tasks: A challenge for language-nonspecific or language-specific models of lexical access? *International Journal of Bilingualism, 8*, 115–125.

Hermans, D., Bongaerts, T., De Bot, K., & Schreuder, R. (1998). Producing words in a foreign language: Can speakers prevent interference from their first language? *Bilingualism: Language and Cognition, 1*, 213–229.

Hoshino, N., & Kroll, J. F. (2008). Cognate effects in picture naming: Does cross-language activation survive a change of script? *Cognition, 106*, 501–511.

Jackson, G. M., Swainson, R., Cunnington, R., & Jackson, S. R. (2001). ERP correlates of executive control during repeated language switching. *Bilingualism: Language and Cognition, 4*, 169–178.

Jared, D., & Kroll, J. F. (2001). Do bilinguals activate phonological representations in one or both of their languages when naming words? *Journal of Memory and Language, 44*, 2–31.

Kotz, S. A., & Elston-Güttler, K. (2004). The role of proficiency on processing categorical and associative information in the L2 as revealed by reaction times and event-related brain potentials. *Journal of Neurolinguistics, 17*, 215–235.

Kovács, A. M., & Mehler, J. (2009). Cognitive gains in 7-month-old bilingual infants. *Proceedings of the National Academy of Sciences, 106*, 6556–6560.

Kroll, J. F., Bobb, S. C., Misra, M. M., & Guo, T. (2008). Language selection in bilingual speech: Evidence for inhibitory processes. *Acta Psychologica, 128*, 416–430.

Kroll, J. F., Bobb, S., & Wodniecka, Z. (2006). Language selectivity is the exception, not the rule: Arguments against a fixed locus of language selection in bilingual speech. *Bilingualism: Language and Cognition, 9*, 119–135.

Kroll, J. F., & de Groot, A. M. B., Eds. (2005). *Handbook of bilingualism: Psycholinguistic approaches*. New York: Oxford University Press.

Kroll, J. F., Dijkstra, A., Janssen, N., & Schriefers, H. (2000). *Selecting the language in which to speak: Experiments on lexical access in bilingual production.* Paper presented at the 41st annual meeting of the Psychonomic Society, New Orleans, LA.

Kroll, J. F., Michael, E., Tokowicz, N., & Dufour, R. (2002). The development of lexical fluency in a second language. *Second Language Research, 18*, 137–171.

Kroll, J. F., & Stewart, E. (1994). Category interference in translation and picture naming: Evidence for asymmetric connections between bilingual memory representations. *Journal of Memory and Language, 33*, 149–174.

Kroll, J. F., van Hell, J. G., Tokowicz, N., & Green, D. W. (2010). The revised hierarchical model: A critical review and assessment. *Bilingualism: Language and Cognition, 13*, 373–381.

Levelt, W. J. M. (1989). *Speaking: From intention to articulation*. Cambridge, MA: MIT Press.

Levelt, W. J. M., Roelofs, A., & Meyer, A. S. (1999). A theory of lexical access in speech production. *Behavioral and Brain Sciences, 22*, 1–75.

Libben, M. R., & Titone, D. A. (2009). Bilingual lexical access in context: Evidence from eye movements during reading. *Journal of Experimental Psychology: Learning, Memory, and Cognition, 35*, 381–390.

Linck, J. A., Kroll, J. F., & Sunderman, G. (2009). Losing access to the native language while immersed in a second language: Evidence for the role of inhibition in second language learning. *Psychological Science, 20*, 1507–1515.

MacWhinney, B. (2005). A unified model of language acquisition. In J. F. Kroll & A. M. B. de Groot (Eds.). *Handbook of bilingualism: Psycholinguistic approaches* (pp. 49–67). New York: Oxford University Press.

Marian, V., & Spivey, M. J. (2003). Competing activation in bilingual language processing: Within- and between-language competition. *Bilingualism: Language and Cognition, 6*, 97–115.

McLaughlin, J., Osterhout, L., & Kim, A. (2004). Neural correlates of second-language word learning: Minimal instruction produces rapid change. *Nature Neuroscience, 7*, 703–704.

Mechelli, A., Crinion, J. T., Noppeney, U., O'Doherty, J., Ashburner, J., Frackowiak, R. S. K., et al. (2004). Structural plasticity in the bilingual brain: Proficiency in a second language and age at acquisition affect grey-matter density. *Nature, 431,* 757.

Meuter, R. F. I., & Allport, A. (1999). Bilingual language switching in naming: Asymmetrical costs of language selection. *Journal of Memory and Language, 40,* 25–40.

Misra, M., Guo, T., Bobb, S. C., & Kroll, J. F. (under review). *ERP evidence for inhibition in bilingual word production.*

Morford, J. P., Wilkinson, E., Villwock, A., Piñar, P., & Kroll, J. F. (2011). When deaf signers read English: Do written words activate their sign translations? *Cognition, 118,* 286–292.

Nieuwenhuis, S., Yeung, N., & Cohen, J. D. (2004). Stimuli modality, perceptual overlap, and the go/no-go N2. *Psychophysiology, 41,* 157–160.

Nieuwenhuis, S., Yeung, N., van den Wildenberg, W., & Ridderinkhof, K. R. (2003). Electrophysiological correlates of anterior cingulate function in a go/no-go task: Effects of response conflict and trial type frequency. *Cognitive, Affective, Behavioral Neuroscience, 3,* 17–26.

Nosarti, C., Mechelli, A., Green, D. W., & Price, C. J. (2010). The impact of second language learning on semantic and nonsemantic first language reading. *Cerebral Cortex, 20,* 315–327.

Osterhout, L., Poliakov, A., Inoue, K., McLaughlin, J., Valentine, G., Pitkanen, I., et al. (2008). Second language learning and changes in the brain. *Journal of Neurolinguistics, 21,* 509–521.

Poulisse, N., & Bongaerts, T. (1994). First language use in second language production. *Applied Linguistics, 15,* 36–57.

Rapp, B., & Goldrick, M. (2000). Discreteness and interactivity in spoken word production. *Psychological Review, 107,* 460–499.

Schmitt, B. M., Rodriguez-Fornells, A., Kutas, M., & Münte, T. F. (2001). Electrophysiological estimates of semantic and syntactic information access during tacit picture naming and listening to words. *Neuroscience Research, 41,* 293–298.

Schwartz, A. I., & Kroll, J. F. (2006). Bilingual lexical activation in sentence context. *Journal of Memory and Language, 55,* 197–212.

Schwartz, A. I., Kroll, J. F., & Diaz, M. (2007). Reading words in Spanish and English: Mapping orthography to phonology in two languages. *Language and Cognitive Processes, 22,* 106–129.

Silverberg, S., & Samuel, A. G. (2004). The effects of age of acquisition and fluency on processing second language words: Translation or direct conceptual access? *Journal of Memory and Language, 51,* 381–398.

Sunderman, G., & Kroll, J. F. (2006). First language activation during second language lexical processing: An investigation of lexical form, meaning, and grammatical class. *Studies in Second Language Acquisition, 28,* 387–422.

Talamas, A., Kroll, J. F., & Dufour, R. (1999). Form related errors in second language learning: A preliminary stage in the acquisition of L2 vocabulary. *Bilingualism: Language and Cognition, 2,* 45–58.

Thierry, G., & Wu, Y. J. (2007). Brain potentials reveal unconscious translation during foreign language comprehension. *Proceeding of National Academy of Sciences, 104,* 12530–12535.

Tokowicz, N., & MacWhinney, B. (2005). Implicit and explicit measures of sensitivity to violations in second language grammar. *Studies in Second Language Acquisition, 27,* 173–204.

Van Hell, J. G., & de Groot, A. M. B. (2008). Sentence context affects lexical decision and word translation. *Acta Psychologica, 128,* 431–451.

Van Hell, J. G., & Tokowicz, N. (2009). Event-related potentials and second language learning: Syntactic processing in late L2 learners at different L2 proficiency levels. *Second Language Research, 25,* 1–32.

Van Heuven, W. J. B., Schriefers, H., Dijkstra, T., & Hagoort, P. (2008). Language conflict in the bilingual brain. *Cerebral Cortex, 18,* 2706–2716.

Van Turennout, M., Hagoort, P., & Brown, C. M. (1997). Electrophysiological evidence on the time course of semantic and phonological processes in speech production. *Journal of Experimental Psychology: Learning, Memory, and Cognition, 23,* 787–806.

Verhoef, K., Roelofs, A., & Chwilla, D. J. (2009). Role of inhibition in language switching: Evidence from event-related brain potentials in overt picture naming. *Cognition, 110,* 84–99.

25

How the Brain Acquires, Processes, and Controls a Second Language

Jubin Abutalebi and Pasquale Anthony Della Rosa

Introduction

The cerebral basis of bilingualism has drawn the interest of researchers for more than a century. The origins of this research field may be traced back to early accounts of selective language loss and recovery in bilingual aphasia (Pitres, 1896; for an extensive discussion of bilingual aphasia, see Marini, Urgesi, & Fabbro, Volume 2, Chapter 36) which gave rise to vivid discussions concerning potential different brain locations for multiple languages. In the past two decades, with the advent of newly developed functional neuroimaging techniques, we have been able to trace an identikit of the neural correlates of bilingualism. Prior to the advent of functional neuroimaging, many researchers postulated that bilinguals may have languages represented in different brain areas or even in different hemispheres (Albert & Obler, 1978). This picture was essentially based on the fact that it is not rare to observe a bilingual aphasic who recovers only with one language, while the other is lost. The latter observation gave rise to the hypothesis that the brain area for one language was damaged and that for the other was not. However, functional magnetic resonance imaging (fMRI) studies have so far contradicted this assumption (for review, see Abutalebi, 2008; Indefrey, 2006; Perani & Abutalebi, 2005).

The main focus of the present work is to provide an overview of the most relevant results that have so far been achieved. In particular, our main aim is to focus not on the question whether two languages are differentially represented in the brain but rather on how the brain processes two languages, i.e., the neurodynamics of bilingualisms. This will be done in a schematic manner for each of the major components of language processing, i.e., grammatical processing, phonological processing, and lexico-semantic processing. A particular emphasis will be put on the neural

The Handbook of the Neuropsychology of Language, First Edition. Edited by Miriam Faust.
© 2012 Blackwell Publishing Ltd. Published 2012 by Blackwell Publishing Ltd.

mechanisms that allow us to "acquire" a second language (L2) with respect to an already existing L1 system. Due to a lack of sufficient research papers focusing on prosody and pragmatics in bilingual language processing, these latter aspects are not covered in our review. Likewise, we will mainly focus on hemodynamic studies such as fMRI and positron emission tomography (PET) investigations and not on electrophysiological studies such as event-related potential (ERP) because of the limited space available. The reader interested in a comprehensive treatment of ERP studies focusing on bilingualism may refer to a recent review by Kotz (2009; see also Kroll, Guo, & Misra, Volume 1, Chapter 24).

The Neural Representation of L2

In order to successfully acquire an L2 different types of grammatical (i.e., morpho-logical, syntactic) as well as phonological and lexico-semantic knowledge need to be stored and well established in our mind. Whereas in the acquisition of a first language during childhood the shaping and organization of the mental representa-tions of such knowledge lead to a fairly effortless tuning of all cognitive processes subtending language, the same hardly ever occurs for L2 when it is acquired later in life where language processing abilities rarely "perform" at L1 levels.

Notably, an important question to unravel is whether L2 acquisition obeys the "critical" time period which is paralleled in neural terms with maturational changes in the brain (McDonald, 2000). Although it has been clearly demonstrated that successful L1 acquisition can occur only during a certain age span, the same rules are not so fixed for L2 acquisition. L1 and L2 acquisition show clear dissimilarities with respect to learning processes and successful mastering of all language compe-tences, which have brought researchers to hypothesize a "fundamental difference" between L1 and L2 acquisition (Meisel, 1991). An influential position, namely the critical period hypothesis (CPH; Birdsong, 2006; Hernandez & Pi, 2007; Johnson & Newport, 1989; Lenneberg, 1967; Penfield & Roberts, 1959) claims that there is a critical period in acquiring full competence (grammar, phonology, and lexico-semantic representations) in two (or more) languages and we will discuss its impli-cations with respect to all the most prominent psycholinguistic models and neuroimaging findings in the past years.

Acquisition and processing of L2 grammar

The CPH postulates the existence of a critical period for acquisition of segmental phonology, inflectional morphology, and syntax. All changes happening to the human language faculty induced by neural maturation are supposed to constitute the grounding of the substantial differences arising throughout the acquisition and attainment of grammatical competences between L1 and L2 learners (Birdsong, 2006; Chomsky, 1975; Hernandez & Pi, 2007; Johnson & Newport, 1989; Lenneberg,

1967). The rationale for this assumption is that an L1 is generally acquired implicitly whereas an L2 is acquired explicitly in the sense that its grammar may be taught. The declarative/procedural model (Ullman, 2001) provides a rationale for the supposition of differential representation by claiming that in normal monolinguals, words are represented in a declarative (i.e., explicit) memory system whereas grammatical rules are represented in a cognitive system that mediates the use of procedures (i.e., implicit memory that is processed without conscious awareness). When an L2 is acquired after the critical period, it cannot rely on the implicit resources that are used for L1 grammatical processes, and thus grammatical processing in L2 is carried out by explicit resources (Ullman, 2001; 2004). Since implicit and explicit knowledge are mediated by distinct neural systems (i.e., Broca's area and the basal ganglia for the first type and left temporal areas for the second), late L2 acquisition bilinguals would use different and more posterior brain areas (left temporal areas) with respect to L1 (Broca's area and the basal ganglia) whenever they compute L2 grammar (Ullman, 2001). In contrast to Ullman's view, Green (2003) argues instead that the acquisition of L2 arises in the context of an already specified, or partially specified, language system (i.e., L1). According to the convergence theory (Green, 2003), if Broca's area has learned to compute grammatical processing for L1 during the initial stages of language acquisition, it will perform the same kind of computation also for an L2. Differences may arise in the initial stages of L2 acquisition, where a need of additional brain areas for processing the newly acquired L2 is required, but once L2 reaches a comparable degree of proficiency, its neural representation will converge towards L1 (Broca's area and basal ganglia in the case of grammar processing).

However, to what extent is there functional neuroimaging evidence of these different claims? A strong source of evidence in favor of the convergence theory comes from studies of artificial grammar learning. In a landmark study, Opitz and Friederici (2004) investigated with fMRI the acquisition of language-like rules of an artificial language. Increased proficiency for the artificial language was associated with increased recruitment of Broca's area. In a further study, Friederici, Bahlman, Helm, Schubotz, and Anwander (2006) confirmed those findings. These results support the notion that the acquisition of an L2 (albeit an artificial one) is achieved through an existing network mediating syntax in L1. In more naturalistic settings (i.e., studies investigating bilinguals) the available evidence clearly points out that both low- and high-proficiency bilinguals engage for L2 the same neural structures responsible for L1 grammatical processing. For example, studies investigating single word processing in L2 such as verb conjugation (Sakai, Miura, Narafu, & Muraishi, 2004) and past-tense word processing (Tatsuno & Sakai, 2005) showed increased activity around the areas mediating L1 syntax (i.e., Broca's area). Furthermore, Sakai et al. (2004) showed that the acquisition of grammatical competences in late bilingual twins is achieved through the same neural structures for processing L1 grammar. Twins were used as subjects in order to investigate whether shared genetic factors influence their language abilities and neural substrates for Japanese (L1) and English (L2). For 2 months, the students participated in intensive training in English verbs (either regular or irregular verbs) as part of their standard classroom education. The authors reported that "in spite of notable differences between L1 and L2 in the students' linguistic knowledge and in their performance" in conjugating verbs, Broca's area was responsible for conjugating verbs in L2 (Sakai et al., 2004, p. 1233). These findings suggest an identical cortical substrate underlying L2 grammar acquisition for both languages. Along similar lines, two further fMRI studies in adults reported comparable evidence for shared brain structures underlying native language and the acquisition of L2 grammar (Musso et al., 2003; Tettamanti et al., 2002). A further relevant study is the fMRI investigation by Golestani et al. (2006) that required moderately fluent late bilinguals in French and English either to read, covertly, words in L1 or in L2 or to produce sentences from these words, again covertly, in either L1 or in L2. No systematic difference was found in the left prefrontal region activated in L1 as compared to L2 and no shifts in the extent of activation with increased syntactical proficiency (measured outside the scanner). But interestingly, the distances between peak activation (i.e., strength of activity) in each language decreased with an increase in L2 proficiency. The authors suggested that such convergence between L1 and L2 might reflect the use of neural regions more tuned to syntax. A further relevant finding of the Golestani et al. study (2006) was that increased proficiency in L2 was correlated to increased involvement of the basal ganglia. Golestani et al. (2006) claim that the involvement of the basal ganglia may be for rule-based processing. However, again, such a finding is not consistent with the direct application of the declarative/procedural model to the bilingual case because the model proposes that the basal ganglia are not involved in syntactic encoding in L2.

To sum up, the available evidence shows that independently of language proficiency (low or high degree of L2 proficiency), late L2 acquisition bilinguals engage the same neural structures as in L1 for grammar processing in L2 (e.g., Rueschemeyer, Zysset, & Friederici, 2006; Suh et al., 2007). Within these brain structures there may be differences concerning the extension and/or the peak activation of brain activity in the sense that a late learned L2 may recruit additional neural resources around the areas mediating L1 syntax (Golestani et al., 2006; Jeong et al., 2007; Rueschemeyer, Fiebach, Kempe, & Friederici, 2005; Sakai et al., 2004; Tatsuno & Sakai, 2005; Wartenburger et al., 2003).

In detail, the aim of the Wartenburger et al. (2003) study was to test the claim that syntactic processing is more influenced by the critical period than by any other linguistic function. This study is remarkable insofar as it manipulated both proficiency and the age of acquisition of languages while looking at changes in brain activation in response to grammatically correct sentences and sentences with violations of semantic rules (selection restriction) and syntactic rules (number, gender, or case agreement). When comparing L2 processing between the two highly proficient groups, more bilateral activation in inferior frontal gyrus (IFG) emerged for late bilinguals during syntactic judgments with respect to early ones, while no difference arose for semantic judgments. The authors suggested that compared to other linguistic competences, the acquisition of an L2 grammar may be strongly constrained by the age factor, at least at the neural level (since the authors found no difference at the behavioral level for the two groups of highly proficient bilinguals).

However, a recent study (Hernandez, Hofmann, & Kotz, 2007) using naturally occurring regular and irregular morphology to verify the critical period framework for syntactic processing in highly proficient early and late bilinguals highlighted only an increase in activity in BA 44/45 for processing irregular (vs. regular) items. Furthermore, activity in the prefrontal cortex was significantly higher in the late bilingual group compared to the early one suggesting that additional syntactic processing is requested when a late bilingual is confronted with naturally occurring irregular items in an L2. Similar results were also reported by Luke, Liu, Wai, Wan, and Tan (2002) with subjects that learned L2 at the relative end-state of the critical period.

What may we conclude from these studies investigating grammatical processing in bilinguals and what are the repercussions for the neural basis of L2 grammatical competence acquisition? First of all, these studies show us that the same set of brain areas responsible for L1 grammar acquisition and processing is also involved for acquiring and processing an L2, independently of age of L2 acquisition and proficiency. Second, there may be differences regarding the extent of brain activity in the sense that an L2 that is processed with a lower degree of proficiency would entail additional areas located around Broca's area (but not in posterior brain areas as suggested by Ullman, 2001). Third, the differences in the extent of brain activity seem to vanish once the proficiency is comparable to that of L1, hence the neural representation of L2 converges to that of L1 as suggested by Green (2003). However, it remains to be determined why exactly there is more activity for an L2 (especially when spoken with a low or not native-like proficiency) in Broca's area and surrounding areas. Following Indefrey (2006), bilinguals might compensate for lower efficiency by driving this region more strongly. It is noteworthy that a recent functional connectivity analysis (i.e., a statistical approach to measure the strength of connections between brain areas) reported that the strength of connections of brain areas related to syntax production is stronger during L2 than L1 sentence production (Dodel et al., 2005). An alternative interpretation is based upon the principles of "the efficiency of neural organization," i.e., the amount of neurons necessary to perform a given task. In the latter case, performance can be negatively correlated with either the extent or the peak of activation. Studies reporting negative longitudinal changes (i.e., a decrease of brain activity) such as when a more extended L2 network converges to that of the L1 following a learning period (Sakai et al., 2004; Tatsuno & Sakai, 2005) may support the notion of the efficiency of neural organization.

Acquisition and processing of L2 phonology

Languages differ in many properties, including their phoneme inventories. Correctly perceiving and producing the sounds of a second language is a very difficult task, as evidenced both by widespread anecdotal evidence and by a number of formal studies (for a review, see Strange, 1995). Problems of this kind are observed even in those who have been exposed to a second language for considerable periods of time and who have therefore had plenty of opportunities to learn its sounds (Pallier, Bosch, & Sebastián-Gallés, 1997; Sebastián-Gallés & Soto-Faraco, 1999). Adults find it difficult to discriminate acoustically similar phonetic contrasts that are not used in their native language whereas young infants discriminate phonetic contrasts even if they are not used in the language they are learning. Therefore, similar to grammar processing (see above), critical or sensitive periods were advocated also for phonological processing (Singleton, 2005). However, the ease with which foreign sounds are perceived and produced may vary; the degree of difficulty may depend on the phonetic similarity between L1 and L2 sounds.

From a neuroanatomical perspective, in monolinguals phonetic perception and production appears to involve specialized networks in the left hemisphere; the chief among these areas are the Wernicke's area in the left temporal lobe, the supramarginal and angular gyrus in the parietal lobe, and also Broca's area in the frontal lobe, as shown by functional neuroimaging in both adults (Zatorre, Evans, Meyer, & Gjedde, 1992; for reviews, see Démonet et al., 2005, and Indefrey & Levelt, 2004) and young infants (e.g., Dehaene-Lambertz & Baillet, 1998; Dehaene-Lamberts, Dehaene, & Hertz-Pannier, 2002). Recent neuroimaging studies also provide evidence for a shared neural network for production and perception of phonemes (e.g., Heim & Friederici, 2003). The temporal dynamics in this network during perception shows a primacy for Wernicke's over Broca's area, while the reversed pattern occurs for producing phonemes. Heim and Friederici (2003) interpreted this finding with respect to the functionality of the different regions within the shared network, with Wernicke's area being the sound form store and Broca's area a processor necessary to extract relevant phonological information from that store.

As mentioned above, similarly to grammar processing, we may again wonder whether L2 phonological representations are acquired, stored, and processed in a different manner at the brain level.

A series of studies specifically investigating phonological processing is now available in the literature. For instance, Callan, Jones, Callan, and Yamada (2004) investigated the neural processes underlying the perception of phonemes using fMRI. The same phonemes (i.e., English syllables starting with a /r/, /l/, or a vowel) were used for native English speakers and English-L2 speakers (i.e., low-proficient Japanese–English bilinguals). Greater activity for second- over native-language speakers during perceptual identification of /r/ and /l/ relative to vowels was found in Broca's area, Wernicke's area, and parietal areas (including the supramarginal gyrus), while more extended activity for native-language speakers was found in the anterior parts of the temporal lobe. For English-L2 speakers, Callan et al.(2004) suggested that the more extended involvement of neural structures for nonnative phoneme identification may be related to the use of internal models of speech articulation and articulatory-orosensory representations that are used to overcome the difficulty in L2 phoneme identification.

A further finding of the Callan et al. study (2004) was greater activity in the right frontal regions in native Japanese compared to native English speakers for /r/ and /l/ relative to vowel perceptual identification. These findings are consistent with the findings of previous fMRI studies (Callan et al., 2003; Pillai et al., 2003; Wang, Sereno, Jongman, & Hirsch, 2003) that, apart from a greater involvement of the left frontal areas, also reported greater recruitment of the right frontal regions for L2 phonetic processing. Specifically, in the study of Callan et al. (2003) native Japanese speakers underwent one month of perceptual identification training in order to learn the /r–l/ phonetic contrast in English as compared to a relatively easy /b–g/ contrast. Brain activity was present to a much greater extent in Broca's area, and other frontal lobe areas for the difficult /r–l/ contrast than for the easy /b–g/ contrast even before training. Enhancement in brain activity after training, relative to before training, occurred bilaterally in several brain regions including Wernicke's area, the supramarginal and angular gyrus, Broca's area, and other frontal lobe areas. Notably, the authors also reported the engagement of the basal ganglia, the anterior cingulate cortex (ACC), and the dorsolateral prefrontal cortex (i.e., two areas in the frontal lobe that are related to cognitive control processes), which might be related to selection and control processes (see below for the neural basis of control processes). Interestingly, the change in brain activity with learning the /r–l/ contrast did not resemble that of the easily discriminated /b–g/ contrast, suggesting that different and/or additional neural processes may be used for processing difficult phonetic contrasts even as performance improves.

Learning nonnative phonetic contrasts was also investigated by Golestani and Zatorre (2004) who used fMRI to study 10 native English monolinguals while they performed an identification task before and after training with a Hindi dental– retroflex nonnative phonetic contrast. Successful learning of the nonnative phonetic contrast resulted in the recruitment of the same areas involved during the processing of native contrasts, including the left frontal and temporal lobe areas. Additionally, Golestani and Zatorre (2004) showed that successful learning is accompanied by more efficient neural processing in the Broca's area and the caudate nucleus which, as suggested by the authors, may be related to the allocation of potential control resources for processing the newly learned foreign language speech sounds. In line with this assumption, it was shown that low-proficient bilinguals engage Broca's area to a greater extent for L2 during a phonological task (i.e., nonword processing; Marian et al., 2007).

Moreover, Golestani and Zatorre (2004) also found a positive correlation between a behavioral learning measure and activity in the parietal lobes (i.e., left and right angular gyri): there was less deactivation of these regions for better learners than for poorer learners. The strong positive correlation between learning and activation in the left angular gyrus supports the idea that activity in this region is modulated by learning, such that poorer learners deactivate this region more than faster learners do. This observation does fit well with a series of voxel-based morphometry (VBM) studies conducted by Golestani and colleagues (Golestani, Molko, Dehaene, Le Bihan, Pallier, 2007; Golestani & Pallier, 2007; Golestani, Paus, &

Zatorre, 2002) who have shown structural brain differences within the parietal lobes for fast phonetic learners as compared to slow phonetic learners. In general, fast phonetic learners (i.e., subjects who successfully learn to distinguish or produce phonetic contrasts not present in their native language) have increased white matter density in the right parietal lobe, but even more so in the left parietal lobe. While the VBM studies of Golestani and colleagues investigated the white matter density of brain volumes, a different VBM study showed grey matter density differences in the left parietal lobe between different groups of bilinguals (Mechelli et al., 2004). Early bilinguals had increased grey matter density within this area. Notably, late bilinguals may also have comparable grey matter density in this brain area, but only when L2 proficiency is high. These striking results of the above-mentioned VBM studies fit with data from the classical aphasiological literature, suggesting that the left inferior parietal lobule is the site of the so-called "language talent" area in bilinguals (Poetzl, 1930).

In summary, although the functional neuroimaging literature on phonological processing in bilinguals is rather limited (as compared to the multitude of studies investigating grammatical and lexico-semantic processing), some tentative conclusions may be drawn. Similarly to grammatical processing, the available evidence shows that an L2 is essentially acquired and processed through the same neural structures mediating L1 phonology. As to the extension of brain activity, the studies reviewed above indicate overall that an L2 is in need of greater recruitment of neural resources. One reason for this observation might be that all these studies used late and low-proficient bilinguals (i.e., Callan et al., 2003; Callan et al., 2004; Pillai et al., 2003; Wang et al., 2003), or monolingual subjects who for the purpose of the experiment had to learn a phonetic contrast in a foreign language (Golestani & Zatorre, 2004). In the latter case, it is possible that the greater brain activity may reflect the accommodation of a new set of sounds by the existing native speech system rather than acquisition of a nonnative phonetic contrast in a second-language context. In the former case (i.e., L2 speakers), it is plausible that processing sounds in the less proficient language is subserved by less well-tuned neural representations and/or may require greater cognitive effort, and it therefore requires greater neuronal activity than processing sounds in L1.

The lexical semantic domain

Concerning the acquisition of lexical semantic knowledge, no predictions emerge in accordance with the CPH, whereas a recent theory of neurolinguistic development (Locke, 1997, pp. 265–326) assumes "an optimum biological moment for the appropriate organization and use of the mental lexicon." According to this theory, if the availability of appropriate stimulation is lacking during the phase of lexical material storage (5–20 months), children will probably show difficulties when asked to perform analytical operations and recognize recurrent structural patterns (20–37 months).

In the context of the multilingual brain, many studies have addressed the question of whether the neuroanatomical organization of the bilingual mental lexicon may also be affected by neural maturation.

One class of models delineates two different levels of representation within the architecture of the bilingual's memory that are "hierarchically" related (Potter, Von Eckardt, & Feldman, 1984; Snodgrass, 1984). For example, the revised hierarchical (RH) model (Kroll & Stewart, 1994; see also Kroll, Guo, & Misra, Volume 1, Chapter 24) claims that separate lexical memory systems contain words for each of the two languages, whereas concepts are stored in an abstract memory system common to both languages. At the early stage of L2 development, L2–L1 mediation mainly occurs between translations at the lexical level; with further L2 development (i.e., highly proficient late bilinguals), L2 lexical codes are more tightly bound to their specific conceptual representations.

Another class of "interactive" models postulates instead three levels of representations (i.e., the bilingual interactive activation model; Dijkstra & van Heuven, 2002; see also Dijkstra & van Heuven, Volume 1, Chapter 22; and the interactive model proposed by Silverberg and Samuel, 2004). The lexical level contains words and "above" them, at the conceptual level (lemma level), their meanings are represented, whereas "below" them we find their orthographic and phonological features (letters and phonemes) at the lexeme level.

The hierarchical and the interactive models put forward different hypotheses concerning the relationship between the period of acquisition of L2 and the shaping and nature of the semantic conceptual representations for L1 and L2 words, although both bilingual interactive activation plus (BIA+) and RH models postulate that L1 and L2 share common conceptual representations, irrespective of the age at which L2 was acquired. In contrast, Silverberg and Samuel (2004) claim that only in early bilinguals common semantic representations will cluster at the conceptual level. However, higher levels of proficiency in L2 produce lexical semantic mental representations that more closely resemble those constructed in L1 and, according to Green's "convergence hypothesis" (2003), many of the qualitative differences between native and L2 speakers may disappear as proficiency increases.

It is therefore interesting to see whether functional neuroimaging evidence supports the psycholinguistic notions of a shared system for an L2 and L1 when the proficiency of the former increases. Irrespective of the experimental paradigm employed (such as picture naming, verbal fluency, word completion, and word repetition), functional neuroimaging studies consistently reported common activations in similar left frontal and temporoparietal brain areas, when the degree of L2 proficiency was comparable to L1 (Chee, Tan, & Thiel, 1999; Ding et al., 2003; Hernandez, Martinez, & Kohnert 2000; Hernandez, Dapretto, Mazziotta, & Bookheimer, 2001; Klein, Zatorre, Milner, Meyer, & Evans, 1994; Klein, Milner, Zatorre, Meyer, & Evans, 1995; Klein, Milner, Zatorre, Zhao, & Nikelski, 1999; Klein, Watkins, Zatorre, & Milner, 2006; Perani et al., 2003; Pu et al., 2001). Notably, the same set of areas are commonly engaged when monolinguals perform the same task. The activations found for L2 were similar to, if not identical with, those underlying

L1 lexical retrieval in the same individuals, underlining the fact that a bilingual can utilize the same neural structures to perform identical tasks for both languages. Moreover, this happened irrespective of differences in orthography, phonology, or syntax among languages (Chee et al., 1999). On the other hand, bilinguals with low proficiency in L2 engaged additional brain activity, mostly in prefrontal areas (Briellmann et al., 2004; Chee, Hon, Ling Lee, & Soon, 2001; De Bleser et al., 2003; Marian et al., 2007; Pillai et al., 2003; Vingerhoets et al., 2003; Yetkin, Yetkin, Haughton, & Cox, 1996). It is also worth mentioning that these findings were confirmed by employing paradigms such as lexical decision and semantic judgment tasks in bilinguals (for example, lexical decision: Illes et al., 1999; Pillai et al., 2003; semantic judgment: Chee et al., 2001; Wartenburger et al., 2003; Rueschemeyer et al., 2005; Rueschemeyer et al., 2006). Indeed, low proficient bilinguals activated more extensively the prefrontal cortex.

Apart from the degree of language proficiency, the amount of relative exposure towards a given language may also have an impact upon the cerebral organization of languages (Abutalebi, Tettamanti, & Perani, 2009). Two of our own fMRI investigations have reported that exposure rather then proficiency may determine specific activity patterns in the bilingual brain (Perani et al., 2003; Abutalebi et al., 2007). In one study (Perani et al., 2003), two groups of early highly proficient bilinguals living in Barcelona (either Spanish-born or Catalan-born individuals) were scanned with fRMI while performing a word fluency task. Strikingly, Spaniards living in Barcelona (Catalonia) and hence mostly exposed to Catalan (i.e., their L2), activated less the left prefrontal cortex for L2 than Catalans, who were less exposed to Spanish (their L2).

In line with our conclusions on grammatical and phonological processing, we may also draw parallels to the lexical-semantic domain. Again, L2 is essentially processed through the same neural networks underlying L1 processing. L2-related differences are found for low-proficiency and/or less exposed bilinguals in terms of greater engagement of the left prefrontal cortex or the selective engagement of prefrontal areas located outside the classical language areas (more anterior to language areas). As to our initial question whether L1 and L2 rely upon a shared system, we may conclude that this also holds for the lexico-semantic domain since there is no brain evidence that two different systems are responsible for two different languages. A remarkable study in this regard is the study by De Bleser et al. (2003) who reported that brain activity for producing L1 words and L2 cognates exactly overlap, while L2 noncognates were in need of additional brain activity around the same brain areas mediating L1 word production (i.e., left prefrontal cortex).

In general, how may we interpret the overall finding of greater engagement of the left prefrontal cortex when processing a second language, which is not mastered in a native-like fashion, not only in lexical tasks but also, as shown above, during grammatical and phonological tasks? Elsewhere, we have argued that the activity within the prefrontal cortex may reflect executive control over access to short- or long-term memory representations such as grammatical, phonological, or lexical representations to assist L2 processing (Abutalebi, 2008). The main idea is that a low-proficient L2 will be processed through neural pathways related to "controlled processing" (i.e., with the active engagement of brain areas related to cognitive control). These brain areas (of which the prefrontal cortex is a main component) are responsible for a conscious control of our actions and in the case of bilingualism they would allow us, for instance, to block potential interferences from the dominant language while speaking the weaker language. On the other hand, a "strong" L2 system (i.e., a high-proficient L2) is processed in a more native-like fashion and, hence, in a more automatic manner without the engagement of brain areas related to cognitive control. In the next sections, we will show that cognitive control is a chief component of bilingualism per se, especially during the process of L2 acquisition. For a proper understanding, we have first to characterize the so-called prefrontal effect (Abutalebi & Green, 2007; Abutalebi, 2008).

Effects of Successful Language Acquisition and the Prefrontal Response

As reported above, differential activity found for a low-proficient L2 is located (1) in the same L1-related language areas which are, however, more extensively activated (either in the extent or the peak of brain activity), and/or (2) in brain areas located more anterior to the classical language areas such as in BA 9, BA 46, and BA 47 (i.e., brain areas located in the prefrontal cortex) that are related to cognitive control (Miller & Cohen, 2001). We have also reported that once a native-like proficiency is achieved, these prefrontal activations disappear, strongly supporting the neural convergence hypothesis (Green, 2003; Perani & Abutalebi, 2005). The convergence of neural representation of an L2 with that of an L1 does not make it impossible that in certain cases the reverse will apply. For instance, when individuals learn to read in L2 first, the substrate for reading L1 will converge with that of L2 (Abutalebi, Keim, et al., 2007).

Now, establishing evidence of neural convergence requires that we consider the effects of proficiency on L2 processing. A suitable example is lexical retrieval. A beginning L2 learner will necessarily struggle to produce the correct name for a picture or to name a word, and such difficulty may have a number of reasons. The neural connections between the concept, lemma, and word form may be still weak and, in general, lexical retrieval may take more time for a low-proficient L2 (Kroll & Stewart, 1994; Snodgrass, 1993). Such differences in relative strength of one language system over the other may offer one source for expected differences in prefrontal activation for L2 and L1. A second potential reason for difficulty may be interference from a dominant concept name. The L2 learner must block unwanted "prepotent" L1 lexical items during L2 word production. As aforementioned, the "prefrontal effect" may reflect between-language competition involving the controlled, rather than the automatic processing of L2. Certainly, once a speaker achieves higher levels of proficiency in L2, overt intrusions (Poulisse & Bongaerts, 1994) become less frequent. A decrease in interference is to be expected to the extent that the system underlying the use of L2 is differentiated from that of L1 (Hernandez, Li, & McWhinney, 2005). A further strong reason may be that with higher L2 proficiency, the actual process of generating a lexical item will be more practiced and so will demand less cognitive effort. We may expect then that with increasing proficiency, the L2 learner may be less in need of controlled processing in normal language. Thus, between-language competition can be resolved more automatically.

At the brain level, less dependency on control mechanisms is translated to decreases in prefrontal activity. A strong message that we wish to deliver here to the reader is that it would be false to infer that L1 and L2 are differentially represented at the neural level on the basis of neuroimaging data. Consider the following very simple question: Why should the L2 learner have her L2 more extensively represented at the brain level (in terms of more brain areas, i.e., the prefrontal effect)? Consider that a low-proficient L2 speaker such as our learner may know only, for example, no more than 1500 words as compared to the 15000 or so words in her native language. Following any principle of neural efficiency, it would be a paradox that these 1500 words are represented in larger brain areas. As a consequence, the prefrontal effect cannot be a question of language-specific neuroanatomical representations (L2 and L1 lexical items are differentially represented), but necessarily an issue of differences in processing demands! The neural effort to process a weak system such as the L2 of a learner is higher than to process a strong system, such as the L2 of a high-proficiency L2 speaker.

As outlined above, it is important to distinguish between controlled and automatic retrieval. Once sufficient L2 proficiency is achieved, retrieval, correct selection, and maintenance of lexical items will become more tuned and more automatic because subjects are familiar with the task and, therefore, the prefrontal response would not be necessary anymore because L2 is processed in a more automatic manner.

In the following section, we will illustrate that controlled processing (we will refer to it as "language control" in bilinguals) is not achieved solely through the intervention of the prefrontal cortex but, like many other cognitive functions, through a dedicated network of brain areas. Interestingly, this network of brain areas is also responsible for language functions specific to bilingualism such as language switching and translation. Since language control constitutes a particular and specific aspect of bilingualism, we will provide a psycholinguistic background of the phenomenon which is then followed by the neural evidence of how language control is achieved.

Controlling Two Languages

Why "casa" and not "house"? How do bilinguals control two languages

How is it that bilinguals keep information from one language from constantly interfering with processing of the other language? The potential for interference is, at least in theory, massive, particularly in view of the overlap in neural tissue, as outlined above. The cognitive machinery subtending all linguistic abilities is extremely complex: To say the word "peace" seems very simple to achieve, but it involves the coordination and integration of pragmatic, semantic, syntactic, phonological, and articulatory processes and representations (e.g., Caramazza, 1997; Dell, 1986; Levelt, 1989). The attentional/control mechanisms responsible for coordinating all these processes are already maximally entailed when speaking one language and are taxed even more in cases of bilingualism. A bilingual speaker should not simply be considered the sum of two monolingual speakers (Grosjean, 1982, 1998, 2000). Compared to monolingual individuals, bilingual speakers must manage competing phonological, syntactic and prosodic systems, as well as distinct mappings of orthography to phonology (Abutalebi & Green, 2007). For example, a bilingual person has to ensure that the intended message is conveyed in the proper language for the communicative context. In Figure 25.1, we illustrate an English–Italian bilingual deciding whether to call a house "house" in English or "casa" in Italian while speaking to a bilingual friend. This apparently simple decision looks similar in theory to decisions that monolinguals also experience when they decide how to name the object on which you lay down in your living room and watch TV:

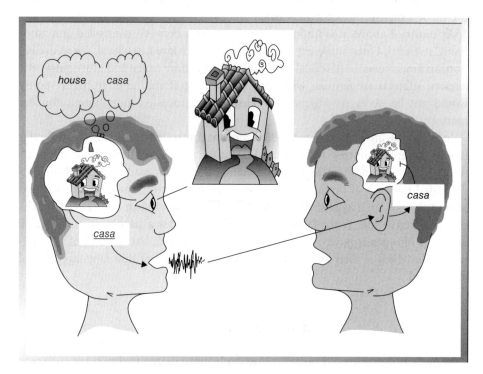

Figure 25.1   An English–Italian bilingual in a conversation while deciding whether to call a house "house" in English or "casa" in Italian as an example of language competition during language production. This process is accomplished by means of language control (see text).

a sofa or a couch? For monolingual speakers, this dilemma between synonyms rarely occurs. For bilingual speakers, most words in one language have a corresponding translation equivalent in the other language and anarchy would reign at our lexical level in the absence of a mechanism to control the two languages allowing us to speak (e.g., Kroll, Bobb, & Wodniecka, 2006). An important issue in this context is how this control mechanism guarantees output in the desired language.

It has been proposed that bilingual control is attained by triggering a differential level of activation in the two lexicons and this may be accomplished by increasing the level of activation of the target language (Grosjean, 1998, 2000; La Heij, 2005; Poulisse & Bongaerts, 1994), or by reactively suppressing the lexical nodes in the nontarget language (Green, 1986, 1998).

For the so-called inhibitory models, selection of a word in a defined language is accomplished through an inhibitory mechanism that suppresses the activation of the lexical representations of the nontarget language (e.g., Green, 1986, 1998; Meuter & Allport, 1999). Once a lexical node has been activated "below" the conceptual system, suppression takes place in a "reactive" manner and the amount of inhibition is proportional to the level of activation of a particular word form (i.e., the stronger the activation of an item, the stronger is the inhibition required to hamper its production). Thus, in the context of L1, when a word is produced, not much inhibition is necessary to suppress L2 lexical items, as the baseline level of activation of L2 lexical items is lower than the L1 counterparts. In turn, when speaking in L2, L1 items must be strongly suppressed through a higher degree of inhibition in order to allow L2 lexical items to break through. Green (1998) advanced a very interesting account of bilingual speech processing and language control within the inhibitory control (IC) model. Briefly, this model proposes that the steps necessary to carry out a task are stored in schemas and to speak a defined language may be considered equivalent to performing a task. Schema selection is competitive, and is determined on the basis of the level of activation of a specific schema. Activation levels can be modulated in a bottom-up fashion by external inputs and in a top-down manner by attentional and motivational components.

In this sense, given the previously reported evidence revealing that L1 and L2 have overlapping or partly overlapping neuroanatomical bases, bilingual individuals must necessarily possess effective neural mechanisms to control and regulate the activation of their two language systems (Abutalebi and Green, 2007, 2008; Green, 1986, 1998; Wang et al., 2007, 2008, 2009). This issue will be the focus of the next section.

How the brain deals with language control in bilinguals

Using various language paradigms, functional neuroimaging studies carried out in bilingual subjects have started characterizing the neural basis of language control processes. We will consider paradigms such as language switching, language translation, and language selection because these paradigms have in common an important cognitive load: a current task must be inhibited (i.e., speaking in language A) in favor of the new task (speaking in language B) in the case of switching and translating, and withholding a potential prepotent response (i.e., from a nontarget dominant language) when selecting items of a weaker language in the case of language selection. Thus, these tasks are thought to heavily rely upon cognitive control mechanisms.

The first study carried out was a PET study on bilinguals performing translation and switching tasks based on visually presented words (Price, Green, & von Studnitz, 1999). The authors reported that switching between languages increased activation in Broca's area and the left supramarginal gyrus (i.e., a brain area located in the parietal lobule). Conversely, word translation increased activation in the ACC and basal ganglia structures. The involvement of the basal ganglia along with activity in the left prefrontal cortex was also reported by the fMRI study of Lehtonen et al. (2005) during sentence translation in a group of Finnish–Norwegian bilinguals. Language switching in picture naming (compared to nonswitching trials) increased fMRI responses in the left prefrontal cortex (Hernandez et al., 2000; Hernandez et al., 2001; Wang et al., 2007). Notably, when switching is performed into the less-proficient language, the prefrontal activity is paralleled by activity in the ACC (Wang et al., 2007).

Two further studies showed that, when controlling interference from the nontarget language during naming (Rodriguez-Fornells et al., 2005) and during reading (Rodriguez-Fornells, Rotte, Heinze, Noesselt, & Muente, 2002) in the target language, there is specific brain activity in the left prefrontal cortex. Similar findings were found by employing an adaptation paradigm (Chee, 2006). In adaptation paradigms, similar stimuli such as items belonging to the same language are contrasted to stimuli belonging to two different languages. For instance, Chee et al. (2003) studied word repetition within and across languages and, notably, only the "across language" condition led to more extended left prefrontal activity (see also Klein et al., 2006, for similar findings). In a further adaptation paradigm, Crinion et al. (2006) reported that left caudate activity was sensitive to the "across language" but not to a "within language" condition.

In line with these findings, Abutalebi et al. (2008) have shown that the specific activity of the left caudate is confined in bilinguals to the situational context. Only naming in L1 in a bilingual context (i.e., where L2 stimuli may have occurred to create a fully bilingual setting) increased activation in the left caudate and ACC. Strikingly, this pattern of activity was absent when the same bilingual subjects were placed in a purely monolingual L1 naming context (i.e., by using the same L1 stimuli that occurred also in the bilingual context). As to the validity of these findings and their practical and theoretical application to bilingualism, we underline that the above-mentioned studies investigated only language production, and, moreover, with the exception of the study of Lehtonen et al. (2005), production was investigated only at the single-word level. It is therefore remarkable that in a recent study focusing on the auditory perception of language switches during comprehension of narratives (Abutalebi et al., 2007) a neural network consisting of the ACC and the left caudate was reported when subjects perceived a switch into the weaker language (i.e., the less exposed language). In general, language comprehension is thought to be a more passive and automatic task than language production (Abutalebi, Cappa, & Perani, 2001). Ultimately, the finding of a cognitive control network during comprehension strongly highlights the fact that the bilingual brain is equipped with a dedicated cognitive mechanism responsible for the correct selection of the intended language. We also emphasize that there is now ample clinical evidence of the language control mechanism in bilinguals. Clinical studies have consistently reported that lesions to a left prefrontal-basal ganglia circuit not only cause involuntarily switching between languages, but may also cause interferences from the nontarget language during naming tasks (e.g., Abutalebi, Della Rosa, Tettamanti, Green, & Cappa, 2009; Abutalebi, Miozzo, & Cappa, 2000; Marien, Abutalebi, Engelborghs, & De Deyn, 2005).

In summary, the emerging picture shows that language control in bilinguals is achieved through a set of brain areas, i.e., the caudate nucleus, the prefrontal cortex, the ACC and eventually the supramarginal gyrus (see figure 25.2). These brain regions are classically related to executive control in humans (Abutalebi & Green, 2007; Braver & Barch, 2006). However, as to our fundamental question if language control is a main component of bilingual language processing and, if so, at which level it occurs, the data reviewed here do not favor those psycholinguistic models that do not postulate inhibition and control mechanism during language selection (Costa & Caramazza, 1999; Roelofs, 2003). If a dedicated cognitive control network in the brain is necessary to achieve language selection correctly, then it is desirable that cognitive models take into consideration this neurobiological evidence. Furthermore, the available neural evidence on language control in bilinguals shows that multiple neural levels of control (prefrontal – ACC – basal ganglia and parietal) are involved, and so cognitive accounts that focus on a single level of control (e.g., competition between lemmas or competition between goals) may be insufficient to

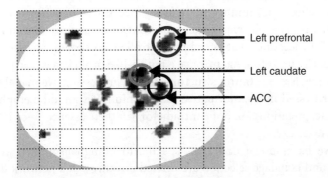

Figure 25.2 The figure highlights brain areas engaged during language switching between L1 and L2 in nine German–Italian bilinguals (unpublished data from our lab). Language switching mainly activates the left caudate, the ACC, and the prefrontal cortex; these areas are also involved in nonlinguistic tasks requiring executive control.

explain properly lexical retrieval in bilinguals (see, for discussion, Abutalebi & Green, 2007). As to the effects of proficiency upon the cognitive control mechanism, there are good indications that cognitive control networks are specifically engaged when it comes to the task of processing a low-proficient L2. For instance, the studies that disentangled the single switching trials in order to observe whether it is more difficult to switch into L1 or into L2 have so far reported that prefrontal along with ACC and caudate activity is even more necessary when switching into the less proficient L2 (Abutalebi et al., 2008; Wang et al., 2007).

Conclusion

In this chapter, we have reviewed and analyzed to what extend functional neuroimaging may show us how the brain acquires, processes, and controls an L2. First of all, concerning language acquisition, the available neurobiological evidence clearly underlines that those brain areas responsible for L1 are also involved in the acquisition of an eventual L2. Moreover, the above-reviewed works support a dynamic view concerning language acquisition. "Dynamic" because, as aforementioned, there may be proficiency-related changes in the brain, i.e., once an L2 learner has gained sufficient proficiency, she will engage exactly the same brain areas as she would for her native language. We underline that this evidence was also reported for grammar and phonology acquisition in late L2 learners, contrary to what one may expect because of the notion of critical periods. As we have seen, at the initial stages of L2 acquisition there are neural differences particularly prominent in the left prefrontal cortex. Indeed, two kinds of neural differences between L1 and L2 were observed: on the one hand, increased L2-related brain activity in and around the areas mediating L1 such as Broca's area, and on the other, the specific engagement of additional brain areas such as areas related to cognitive control (i.e., left prefrontal cortex, ACC, basal ganglia). As proposed by Indefrey (2006), L2 speakers could compensate for lower efficiency by driving these regions more strongly and the greater activity observed for L2 may reflect the number of neurons necessary to perform a given task. Alternatively, the specific engagement of control structures may underline the nature of L2 processing, that is, more controlled processing as compared to L1 (Abutalebi & Green, 2007). Again, once a native-like proficiency is achieved, our L2 learner may rely less on control structures for L2 processing; we may then suppose that L2 is processed in a more "native-like" fashion. It should be emphasized that these two interpretations are not contradictory in their essence since it is plausible that they may co-exist.

Finally, we have shown that tasks specific to bilingualism such as switching, translation, and language selection are carried out through a network dedicated to executive control (to which we refer as the "language control" network in bilinguals). Again, the role of language proficiency seems to be prominent since low-proficient bilinguals activate the language control network more strongly. As we have suggested in a recent paper (Abutalebi et al., 2007), the observation of the engagement of this control network may be a neural signature of a "non-native like L2 processing." One interesting point that still needs to be addressed is whether the selective engagement of executive control areas in bilinguals (as compared to monolinguals) when speaking in one of their languages may lead to neural advantages for nonlinguistic "domain-general" executive functions. Initial behavioral data seem to confirm this assumption since bilinguals seem to be faster and more accurate in attentional tasks (Costa, Hernandez, & Sebastián-Gallés, 2008; Craig & Bialystok, 2006). Future neuroimaging studies will reveal whether bilingualism per se may induce beneficial neurofunctional and structural changes in the human brain.

References

Abutalebi, J. (2008). Neural processing of second language representation and control. *Acta Psychologica, 128*, 466–478.

Abutalebi, J., Annoni, J. M., Seghier, M., Zimine, I., Lee-Jahnke, H., Lazeyras, F. et al. (2008). Language control and lexical competition in bilinguals: An event-related fMRI study. *Cerebral Cortex, 18*, 1496–505.

Abutalebi, J., Brambati, S. M., Annoni, J. M., Moro, A., Cappa, S. F., & Perani, D. (2007). The neural cost of the auditory perception of language switches: An event-related fMRI study in bilinguals. *Journal of Neuroscience, 27*, 13762–13769.

Abutalebi, J., Cappa, S. F., & Perani, D. (2001). The bilingual brain as revealed by functional neuroimaging. *Bilingualism: Language and cognition, 4*, 179–190.

Abutalebi, J., Della Rosa, P. A., Tettamanti, M., Green, D. W., & Cappa, S. F. (2009). Bilingual aphasia and language control: A follow-up fMRI and intrinsic connectivity study. *Brain and Language, 109*, 141–156.

Abutalebi, J., & Green, D. (2007). Bilingual language production: The neurocognition of language representation and control. *Journal of Neurolinguistics, 20*, 242–275.

Abutalebi, J., & Green, D. (2008). Control mechanisms in bilingual language production: Neural evidence from language switching studies. *Language and Cognitive Processes, 23*, 557–582.

Abutalebi, J., Keim, R., Brambati, S. M., Tettamanti, M., Cappa S. F., De Bleser, R., et al. (2007). Late acquisition of literacy in a native language. *Human Brain Mapping, 28*, 19–33.

Albert, M. L., & Obler, L. K. (1978). *The bilingual brain: Neuropsychological and neurolinguistic aspects of bilingualism*. London: Academic Press.

Birdsong, D. (2006). Age and second language acquisition and processing: A selective overview. *Language Learning, 56*, 9–49.

Briellmann, R. S., Saling, M. M., Connell, A. B., Waites, A. B., Abbott, D. F., & Jackson, G. D. (2004). A high-field functional MRI study of quadrilingual subjects. *Brain and Language, 89*, 531–542.

Callan, D. E., Jones, J. A., Callan, A. K., & Yamada, R. A. (2004). Phonetic perceptual identification by native- and second-language speakers differentially activates brain regions involved with acoustic phonetic processing and those involved with articulatory–auditory/orosensory internal models. *NeuroImage, 22*, 1182–1194.

Callan, D. E., Tajima, K., Callan, A. M., Kubo, R., Masaki, S., Akahane-Yamada, R. (2003). Learning-induced neural plasticity associated with improved identification performance after training of a difficult second language phonetic contrast. *NeuroImage, 19,* 113–124.

Caramazza, A. (1997). How many levels of processing are there in lexical access? *Cognitive Neuropsychology, 14,* 177–208.

Chee, M. W. L. (2006). Dissociating language and word meaning in the bilingual brain. *Trends in Cognitive Sciences, 10,* 527–529.

Chee, M. W. L., Hon, N., Ling Lee, H., & Soon, C. S. (2001). Relative language proficiency modulates BOLD signal change when bilinguals perform semantic judgments. *NeuroImage, 13,* 1155–1163.

Chee, M. W. L., Soon, C. S., & Lee, H. L. (2003). Common and segregated neuronal networks for different languages revealed using functional magnetic resonance adaptation. *Journal of Cognitive Neuroscience, 15,* 85–97.

Chee, M. W. L., Soon, C. S., Lee, H. L., & Pallier, C. (2004). Left insula activation: A marker for language attainment in bilinguals. *Proceedings of the National Academy of Sciences of the United States of America,101,* 15265–15270.

Chee, M. W. L., Tan, E. W. L., & Thiel, T. (1999). Mandarin and English single word processing studied with functional magnetic resonance imaging. *Journal of Neuroscience, 19,* 3050–3056.

Chomsky, N. (1975). *Reflections on language,* New York: Pantheon.

Costa, A., & Caramazza, A. (1999). Is lexical selection in bilinguals language-specific? Further evidence from Spanish–English bilinguals and English–Spanish bilinguals. *Bilingualism: Language and Cognition, 2,* 231–244.

Costa, A., Hernandez, M., & Sebastián-Gallés, N. (2008). Bilingualism aids conflict resolution: Evidence from the ANT task. *Cognition, 106,* 59–86.

Craik, F. I. M., & Bialystok, E. (2006). Cognition through the lifespan: Mechanisms of change. *Trends in Cognitive Sciences, 10,* 131–138.

Crinion, J., Turner, R., Grogan, A., Hanakawa, T., Noppeney, U., Devlin, J. T., et al. (2006). Language control in the bilingual brain. *Science, 312,* 1537–1540.

De Bleser, R., Dupont, P., Postler, J., Bormans, G., Speelman, D., Mortelmans, L., et al. (2003). The organisation of the bilingual lexicon: A PET study. *Journal of Neurolinguistics, 16,* 439–456.

Dell, G. S. (1986). A spreading-activation theory of retrieval in sentence production. *Psychological Review, 93,* 283–321.

Démonet, J. F., Thierry, G., & Cardebat, D. (2005). Renewal of the neurophysiology of language: Functional neuroimaging. *Physiological Review, 85,* 49–95.

Dijkstra, A., & van Heuven, W. J. B. (2002). The architecture of the bilingual word recognition system: From identification to decision. *Bilingualism: Language and Cognition, 5,* 175–197.

Ding, G. S., Perry, C., Peng, D. L., Ma, L., Li, D. J., Xu, S. Y., et al. (2003). Neural mechanisms underlying semantic and orthographic processing in Chinese–English bilinguals. *NeuroReport, 14,* 1557–1562.

Dodel, S., Golestani, N., Pallier, C., ElKouby, V., Le Bihan, D., & Poline, J. B. (2005). Condition-dependent functional connectivity: Syntax networks in bilinguals. *Philosophical Transactions of the Royal Society Biological Sciences, 360,* 921–935.

Friederici, A. D., Bahlmann, J., Helm, S., Schubotz, R. I., & Anwander, A. (2006). The brain differentiates human and non-human grammars: Functional localization and structural connectivity. *Proceedings of the National Academy of Sciences of the United States of America, 103,* 2458–2463.

Golestani, N., Alario, F. X., Meriaux, S., Le Bihan, D., Dehaene, S., & Pallier, C. (2006). Syntax production in bilinguals. *Neuropsychologia*, *44*, 1029–1040.

Golestani, N., Molko, N., Dehaene, S., LeBihan, D., & Pallier, C. (2007). Brain structure predicts the learning of foreign speech sounds. *Cerebral Cortex*, *17*, 575–582.

Golestani, N., & Pallier, C. (2007). Anatomical correlates of foreign speech sound production. *Cerebral Cortex*, *17*, 929–934.

Golestani, N., Paus, T., & Zatorre, R. J. (2002). Anatomical correlates of learning novel speech sounds. *Neuron*, *35*, 997–1010.

Golestani, N., & Zatorre, R. J. (2004). Learning new sounds of speech: Reallocation of neural substrates. *NeuroImage*, *21*, 494–506.

Green, D. W. (1986). Control, activation and resource. *Brain and Language*, *27*, 210–223.

Green, D. W. (1998) Mental control of the bilingual lexico-semantic system. *Bilingualism: Language and Cognition*, *1*, 67–81.

Green, D. W. (2003). The neural basis of the lexicon and the grammar in L2 acquisition. In R. van Hout, A. Hulk, F. Kuiken & R. Towell (Eds.), *The interface between syntax and the lexicon in second language acquisition* (pp. 197–218). Amsterdam: John Benjamins.

Grosjean, F. (1982). *Life with two languages: An introduction to bilingualism*. Cambridge, MA: Harvard University Press.

Grosjean, F. (1998). Studying bilinguals: Methodological and conceptual issues. *Bilingualism: Language and Cognition*, *1*, 131–149.

Grosjean, F. (2000). The bilingual's language modes. In J. Nicol (Ed.), *One mind, two languages: Bilingual language processing*. Oxford: Blackwell.

Heim, S. T., & Friederici, A. D. (2003). Phonological processing in language production: time course of brain activity. *NeuroReport*, *14*, 2031–2033.

Hernandez, A. E., Dapretto, M., Mazziotta, J., & Bookheimer, S. (2001). Language switching and language representation in Spanish–English Bilinguals: An fMRI study. *Neuroimage*, *14*, 510–520.

Hernandez, A. E., Hofmann, J., & Kotz, S. A. (2007). Age of acquisition modulates neural activity for both regular and irregular syntactic functions. *NeuroImage*, *36*, 912–923.

Hernandez, A. E., & Li, P. (2007). Age of acquisition: Its neural and computational mechanisms. *Psychological Bulletin*, *133*, 638–50.

Hernandez, A. E., Martinez, A., & Kohnert, K. (2000). In search of the language switch: An fMRI study of picture naming in Spanish–English bilinguals. *Brain and Language*, *73*, 421–431.

Illes, J., Francis, W. S., Desmond, J. E., Gabrieli, J. D. E., Glover, G. H., Poldrack, R., et al. (1999). Convergent cortical representation of semantic processing in bilinguals. *Brain and Language*, *70*, 347–363.

Indefrey, P. (2006). A Meta-analysis of hemodynamic studies on first and second language processing: Which suggested differences can we trust and what do they mean? *Language Learning*, *56*, 279–304.

Indefrey, P., & Levelt, W. J. M. (2004). The spatial and temporal signatures of word production components. *Cognition*, *92*, 101–144.

Johnson, J. S., & Newport, E. L. (1989). Critical period effects in second language learning: The influence of maturational state on the acquisition of English as a second language. *Cognitive Psychology*, *21*, 60–99.

Klein, D., Milner, B., Zatorre, R., Meyer, E., & Evans, A. (1995). The neural substrates underlying word generation: A bilingual functional-imaging study. *Proceedings of the National Academy of Sciences of the United States of America*, *92*, 2899–2903.

Klein, D., Milner, B., Zatorre, R. J., Zhao, V., & Nikelski, J. (1999). Cerebral organization in bilinguals: A PET study of Chinese–English verb generation. *NeuroReport, 10*, 2841–2846.

Klein, D., Watkins, K. E., Zatorre, R. J., & Milner, B. (2006). Word and non-word repetition in bilingual subjects: A PET study. *Human Brain Mapping, 27*, 153–161.

Klein, D., Zatorre, J. R., Chen, J. K., Milner, B., Crane, J., Belin, P., et al. (2006). Bilingual brain organization: A functional magnetic resonance adaptation study. *NeuroImage, 31*, 366–375.

Klein, D., Zatorre, R., Milner, B., Meyer, E., & Evans, A. (1994). Left putaminal activation when speaking a second language: Evidence from PET. *Neuroreport, 5*, 2295–2297.

Kotz, S. A. (2009). A critical review of ERP and fMRI evidence on L2 syntactic processing. *Brain and Language, 109*, 68–74.

Kroll. J. F., Bobb, S., & Wodniecka, Z. (2006). Language selectivity is the exception, not the rule: Arguments against a fixed locus of language selection in bilingual speech. *Bilingualism: Language and Cognition, 9*, 119–135.

Kroll, J. F., & Stewart, E. (1994). Category interference in translation and picture naming: Evidence for asymmetric connections between bilingual memory. *Journal of Memory and Language, 33*, 149–174.

La Heij, W. (2005). Selection processes in monolingual and bilingual lexical access. In J. F. Kroll and A. M. B. de Groot (Eds.), *Handbook of bilingualism: Psycholinguistic approaches* (pp. 289–307). New York: Oxford.

Lehtonen, M., Laine, M., Niemi, J., Thomson T., Vorobyev, V. A., & Hughdal, K. (2005). Brain correlates of sentence translation in Finnish–Norwegian bilinguals. *NeuroReport, 16*, 607–610.

Lenneberg, E. H. (1967). *Biological foundations of language*. New York: Wiley.

Levelt, W. J. M. (1989). *Speaking: From intention to articulation*. Cambridge, MA: MIT Press.

Locke, J. L. (1997). A theory of neurolinguistic development. *Brain and Cognition, 58*, 265–326.

Marian, V., Shildkrot, Y., Blumenfeld, H. K., Kaushanskaya, M., Faroqi-Shah, Y., & Hirsch, J. (2007). Cortical activation during word processing in late bilinguals: Similarities and differences as revealed by functional magnetic resonance imaging. *Journal of Clinical and Experimental Neuropsychology, 29*, 247–265.

Mariën, P., Abutalebi, J., Engelborghs, S., & De Deyn, P. P. (2005). Acquired subcortical bilingual aphasia in an early bilingual child: Pathophysiology of pathological language switching and language mixing. *Neurocase, 11*, 385–398.

McDonald, J. (2000). Grammaticality judgments in a second language: Influences of age of acquisition and native language. *Applied Psycholinguistics, 21*, 395–423.

Mechelli, A., Crinion, J. T., Noppeney, U., O'Doherty, J., Ashburner, J., Frackowiack, R. S., et al. (2004). Structural plasticity in the bilingual brain. *Nature Brief Communications, 431*, 757.

Meisel, J. M. (1991). Principles of universal grammar and strategies of language use: On some similarities and differences between first and second language acquisition. In L. Eubank (Ed.), *Point counterpoint: Universal grammar in the second language* (pp. 231–276). Amsterdam, Philadelphia: John Benjamins.

Meuter, R. F. I., & Allport, D. A. (1999). Bilingual language switching in naming: Asymmetrical costs of language selection. *Journal of Memory and Language, 40*, 25–40.

Miller, E. K., & Cohen, J. (2001) An integrative theory of prefrontal cortex function. *Annual Review of Neuroscience, 24*, 167–202.

Musso, M., Moro, A., Glauche, V., Rijntjes, M., Reichenbach, J., Buechel, C., et al. (2003). Broca's area and the language instinct. *Nature Neuroscience, 6,* 774–81.

Opitz, B., & Friederici, A. D. (2004). Interactions of the hippocampal system and the prefrontal cortex in learning language-like rules. *NeuroImage, 19,* 1730–1737.

Penfield, W., & Roberts, L. (1959) *Speech and brain-mechanisms.* New York: Atheneum.

Perani, D., & Abutalebi, J. (2005). Neural basis of first and second language processing. *Current Opinion of Neurobiology, 15,* 202–206.

Perani, D., Abutalebi, J., Paulesu, E., Brambati, S., Scifo, P., Cappa, S. F., et al. (2003). The role of age of acquisition and language usage in early, high-proficient bilinguals: A fMRI study during verbal fluency. *Human Brain Mapping, 19,* 170–182.

Pillai, J., Araque, J., Allison, J., Sethuraman, S., Loring, D., Thiruvaiyaru, D., et al. (2003). Functional MRI study of semantic and phonological language processing in bilingual subjects: Preliminary findings. *NeuroImage, 19,* 565–576.

Pitres, A. (1895). Etude sur l'aphasie chez les polyglottes. *Revue de médecine, 15,* 873–899.

Poetzl, O. (1930). Aphasie und Mehrsprachigkeit. *Zeitschrift fuer die gesamte Neurologie und Psychiatrie, 124,* 145–162.

Potter, M. C., Von Eckardt, B., & Feldman, L. B. (1984). Lexical and conceptual representations in beginning and more proficient bilinguals. *Journal of Verbal Learning and Verbal Behavior, 23,* 23–38.

Poulisse, N. & Bongaerts, T. (1994). First language use in second language production. *Applied Linguistics, 15,* 36–57.

Price, C. J., Green, D., & von Studnitz, R. A. (1999). Functional imaging study of translation and language switching. *Brain, 122,* 2221–2236.

Pu, Y., Liu, H. L., Spinks, J. A., Mahankali, S., Xiong, J., Feng, C. M., et al. (2001). Cerebral hemodynamic response in Chinese (first) and English (second) language processing revealed by event-related functional MRI. *Magnetic Resonance Imaging, 19,* 643–647.

Rodriguez-Fornells, A., Rotte, M., Heinze, H. J., Noesselt, T., & Muente, T. F. (2002). Brain potential and functional MRI evidence for how to handle two languages with one brain. *Nature, 415,* 1026–1029.

Roelofs, A. (2003). Goal-referenced selection of verbal action: Modelling attentional control in the Stroop task. *Psychological Review, 110,* 88–125.

Rueschemeyer, S. A., Fiebach, C. J., Kempe, V. & Friederici, A. D. (2005). Processing lexical semantic and syntactic information in first and second language: fMRI evidence from German and Russian. *Human Brain Mapping, 25,* 266–286.

Rueschemeyer, S. A., Zysset, S., & Friederici, A. D. (2006). Native and non-native reading of sentences: An fMRI experiment. *NeuroImage, 31,* 354–365.

Sakai, K. L., Miura, K., Narafu, N., & Muraishi, Y. (2004). Correlated functional changes of the prefrontal cortex in twins induced by classroom education of second language. *Cerebral Cortex, 14,* 1233–1239.

Sebastián-Gallés, N., & Soto-Faraco, S. (1999). On-line processing of native and non-native phonemic contrasts in early bilinguals. *Cognition, 72,* 111–123.

Silverberg, S. & Samuel, A. G. (2004) The effect of age of second language acquisition on the representation and processing of second language words. *Journal of Memory and Language, 51,* 381–398.

Singleton, D. (2005). The critical period hypothesis: A coat of many colours. *International Review of Applied Linguistics in Language Teaching, 43,* 269–285.

Snodgrass J. G. (1984). Concepts and their surface representations. *Journal of Verbal Learning and Verbal Behavior, 23,* 3–22.

Snodgrass, J. G. (1993). Translating versus picture naming. In R. Schreuder & B. Weltens (Eds.), *The bilingual lexicon* (pp. 83–114). Amsterdam: John Benjamins.

Suh, S., Yoon, H. W., Lee, S., Chung, J. Y., Cho, Z. H., & Park, H. W. (2007). Effects of syntactic complexity in L1 and L2: An fMRI study of Korean–English bilinguals. *Brain Research, 1136,* 178–189.

Tatsuno, Y., & Sakai, K. L. (2005). Language related activations in the left prefrontal regions are differentially modulated by age, proficiency and task demands. *Journal of Neuroscience, 16,* 1637–1644.

Tettamanti, M., Alkadhi, H., Moro, A., Perani, D., Kollias, S., & Weniger, D. (2002). Neural correlates for the acquisition of natural language syntax . *NeuroImage, 17,* 700–709.

Ullman, M. T. (2001). A neurocognitive perspective on language: The declarative/procedural model. *Nature Reviews Neuroscience, 2,* 717–726.

Ullman, M. T. (2004). Contributions of memory circuits to language: The declarative/procedural model. *Cognition, 92,* 231–270.

Vingerhoets, G., van Borsel, J., Tesink, C., van den Noort, M., Deblaere, K., Seurinck, R., et al. (2003). Multilingualism: An fMRI study. *NeuroImage, 20,* 2181–2196.

Wang, Y., Kuhl, P. K., Chen, C., & Dong, Q. (2009). Sustained and transient language control in the bilingual brain. *NeuroImage, 47,* 414–422.

Wang, Y., Sereno, J. A., Jongman, A., & Hirsch, J. (2003). fMRI evidence for cortical modification during learning of mandarin lexical tone. *Journal of Cognitive Neuroscience, 15,* 1019–1027.

Wang, Y., Xue, G., Chen, C., Xue, F., & Dong, Q. (2007). Neural bases of asymmetric language switching in second-language learners: An ER-fMRI study. *NeuroImage, 35,* 862–870.

Wartenburger, I., Heekeren, H. R., Abutalebi, J., Cappa, S. F., Villringer, A., & Perani, D. (2003). Early setting of grammatical processing in the bilingual brain. *Neuron, 37,* 159–170.

Yetkin, O., Yetkin, F. Z., Haughton, V. M., & Cox, R. W. (1996). Use of functional MR to map language in multilingual volunteers. *American Journal of Neuroradiology, 17,* 473–477.

Acknowledgments

Figures 1.1, 1.2, 1.3	Created by Christine Chiarello, Suzanne E. Welcome, and Christiana M. Leonard
Tables 1.1, 1.2	Created by Christine Chiarello, Suzanne E. Welcome, and Christiana M. Leonard
Figures 2.1, 2.2a, 2.2b, 2.2c, 2.3, 2.4, 2.5, 2.6, 2.7	Created by Henri Cohen
Table 2.1	Created by Henri Cohen
Figures 3.1, 3.2	Created by Michal Lavidor
Table 3.1	Created by Michal Lavidor
Figure 4.1	Reprinted from O. Peleg & Z. Eviatar (2009). Semantic asymmetries are modulated by phonological asymmetries: Evidence from the disambiguation of heterophonic versus homophonic homographs. *Brain and Cognition, 70*, 154–162. Used with permission of Elsevier.
Figures 4.2, 4.3	Created by Orna Peleg and Zohar Eviatar
Table 4.1	Reprinted from O. Peleg & Z. Eviatar (2009). Semantic asymmetries are modulated by phonological asymmetries: Evidence from the disambiguation of heterophonic versus homophonic homographs. *Brain and Cognition, 70*, 154–162. Used with permission of Elsevier.
Figures 5.1, 5.2, 5.3, 5.4	Created by Debra L. Long, Clinton L. Johns, Eunike Jonathan, and Kathleen Baynes
Table 5.1	Created by Debra L. Long, Clinton L. Johns, Eunike Jonathan, and Kathleen Baynes from elements presented in D. L. Long

The Handbook of the Neuropsychology of Language, First Edition. Edited by Miriam Faust.
© 2012 Blackwell Publishing Ltd. Published 2012 by Blackwell Publishing Ltd.

	& K. Baynes (2002). Discourse representation in the two cerebral hemispheres. *Journal of Cognitive Neuroscience, 14,* 228–242.
Table 5.2	Created by Debra L. Long, Clinton L. Johns, Eunike Jonathan, and Kathleen Baynes from elements presented in D. L. Long, K. Baynes, & C. S. Prat (2005). The propositional structure of discourse in the two cerebral hemispheres. *Brain and Language, 95,* 383–394.
Figure 6.1	Adapted from T. T. Rogers, M. A. Lambon Ralph, P. A. Garrard, S. Bozeat, J. L. McClelland, J. R. Hodges, et al. (2004). Structure and deterioration of semantic memory: A neuropsychological and computational investigation. *Psychological Review, 111,* 205–235.
Figures 6.2, 6.3	Created by Christine E. Watson
Figure 6.4	Adapted from D. C. Plaut (2002). Graded modality-specific specialization in semantics: A computational account of optic aphasia. *Cognitive Neuropsychology, 19,* 603–639.
Figures 6.5a, 6.5b	Adapted from A. M. Woollams, M. A. Lambon Ralph, D. C. Plaut, & K. Patterson (2007). SD-squared: On the association between semantic dementia and surface dyslexia. *Psychological Review, 114,* 316–339.
Figure 7.1	Created by Matthew Goldrick
Tables 7.1, 7.2, 7.3	Created by Matthew Goldrick
Figures 8.1a 8.1b, 8.2	Created by Prahlad Gupta
Figure 9.1	Created by William W. Graves, Jeffrey R. Binder, Mark S. Seidenberg, and Rutvik H. Desai
Figures 10.1, 10.2, 10.3	Created by Chia-lin Lee and Kara D. Federmeier
Figures 11.1, 11.2, 11.3	Created by Peter Indefrey
Figures 13.1, 13.2	From D. Chwilla & H. Kolk (2005). Accessing world knowledge: Evidence from N400 and reaction time priming. *Cognitive Brain Research, 25,* 589–606. Copyright 2005, with permission from Elsevier Science.
Figure 13.3	From D. Chwilla, H. Kolk, & C. Vissers (2007). Immediate integration of novel meanings: N400 support for an embodied view of language comprehension. *Brain Research, 1183,* 109–123. Copyright 2007, with permission from Elsevier Science.
Table 15.1	Created by Kristina A. Kellett, Jennifer L. Stevenson, and Morton Ann Gernsbacher
Figures 17.1, 17.2, 17.3, 17.4, 17.5	Created by Diana Van Lancker Sidtis

Figures 20.1a, 20.1b From A. M. Rapp, D. E. Mutschler, & M. Erb (submitted). Where in the brain is nonliteral language? An ALE-meta-analysis of 21 functional magnetic resonance imaging studies.

Tables 20.1, 20.2 Created by Alexander Michael Rapp

Figures 24.1, 24.2, 24.3 Created by Judith F. Kroll, Taomei Guo, and Maya Misra

Figures 25.1, 25.2 Created by Jubin Abutalebi and Pasquale Anthony Della Rosa